Frontiers of Virology 2

Y. Becker · G. Darai (Eds.)
E.-S. Huang (Guest Editor)

Molecular Aspects of Human Cytomegalovirus Diseases

With 98 Figures and 51 Tables

Springer-Verlag
Berlin Heidelberg New York
London Paris Tokyo
Hong Kong Barcelona
Budapest

Editors:

Professor Yechiel Becker
Department of Molecular Virology
Faculty of Medicine
Hebrew University of Jerusalem
POB 1172
Jerusalem 910010, Israel

Professor Gholamreza Darai
Institut für Medizinische Virologie
Universität Heidelberg
Im Neuenheimer Feld 324
W-6900 Heidelberg, Germany

Guest Editor:

Eng-Shang Huang, Ph. D.
Lineberger Comprehensive Cancer Research Center
The University of North Carolina
CB # 7259, Rm. 117, Lineberger Building
Chapel Hill, NC 27599-7295, USA

ISBN 3-540-55948-5 Springer-Verlag Berlin Heidelberg New York
ISBN 0-387-55948-5 Springer-Verlag New York Berlin Heidelberg

Library of Congress Cataloging-in-Publication Data. Molecular aspects of human cytomegalovirus diseases / Y. Becker, G. Darai (eds.); E.-S. Huang (guest ed.) p. cm. – (Frontiers of virology; 2) Includes bibliographical references and index. ISBN 3-540-55948-5 (alk. paper). – ISBN 0-387-55948-5 (alk. paper) 1. Cytomegalovirus infections – Molecular aspects. I. Becker, Yechiel. II. Darai, Gholamreza. III. Huang, E.-S. (Eng-Shang) IV. Series. [DNLM: 1. Cytomegalic Inclusion Disease – pathology. 2. Cytomegaloviruses – pathogenicity. WC 500 M7175] QR201.C94M65 1992 616'.0194 – dc20 92-49467

Printed in Germany

Typesetting: Triltsch, Würzburg
27/3145-5 4 3 2 1 0 – Printed on acid-free paper

Frontiers of Virology: Aims and Plans

Virology at the end of the twentieth century is still a frontier of the biological sciences with new viruses emerging as disease-causing agents of man, animal, and plant. Ever since 1796 when Edward Jenner named the causative agent of smallpox "virus" (toxin), knowledge on virus diseases has slowly accumulated. The vast influenza epidemic (the "Spanish flu") at the end of World War I revealed that virologists lacked the scientific tools to identify the epidemic and protect against it. During the middle of the twentieth century, the methods for the diagnosis of viruses and for research were markedly improved. New technologies were developed to identify the structure and organization of viruses, ranging from bacterial to plant viruses and from human to animal viruses. In the past 50 years, virology has developed as a part of immunology and molecular biology, providing these biological sciences with tools and at the same time utilizing their biochemical, molecular, and immunological advancements to further knowledge on the mechanisms by which viruses cause a variety of diseases. Thus, virology remains in the forefront of science.

With this idea that virology is constantly developing, the present series, *Frontiers of Virology*, was conceived. We intend to select topics on which knowledge from a number of biological fields of research, including conceptual and technical breakthroughs, can merge in the field of virology and move it further ahead. We plan to put the emphasis on discoveries which will help to curb virus diseases. We hope that *Frontiers of Virology* will be of interest not only to virologists, molecular biologists, and immunologists, but also to physicians with expertise in infectious diseases.

We wish to express our thanks to Dr. Jürgen Wieczoreck, Springer-Verlag, for his general support and encouragement to develop the series *Frontiers of Virology*.

Y. Becker, Jerusalem
G. Darai, Heidelberg

Preface

Human cytomegalovirus (HCMV) is a ubiquitous herpesvirus that rarely causes symptomatic disease in the immunocompetent host. Yet this virus has been at the frontier of virology since it was found to be involved in symptomatic diseases in immunocompromised individuals. Such clinical manifestations range from developmental abnormalities, mental retardation, deafness, mononucleosis, chorioretinitis, and fatal diseases like interstitial pneumonitis and disseminated HCMV infections.

HCMV is prevalent in the human population around the world, and sexual transmission of the virus is common. The AIDS epidemic has led to an increased interest in the role of HCMV in AIDS patients, since it was found to be the primary or secondary cause of death in 25% of immunocompromised HIV-1-infected patients. The role of HCMV genes in activation of HIV-1 promoters is discussed in this book.

Since organ transplant patients are immunodeficient, HCMV has also become a menace to the organ transplant patient. The suppression of the T helper cells by cyclosporin A in seropositive transplant patients led to the emergence of HCMV from its latent state, and thence interstitial pneumonia with a high mortality rate in a large number of patients. The newly introduced immunosuppressive drug FK506 for organ transplantation promises to be highly effective in suppressing the immune response, and maybe without the reactivating HCMV.

The state of knowledge of HCMV as a human pathogen is lucidly summarized in the chapters of this book, bringing the reader fully up to date with the current knowledge concerning HCMV and all the known clinical and medical aspects of disease caused by, and associated with, HCMV. In addition, an insight into the function of HCMV genes in disease mechanisms is presented. The molecular aspects of HCMV genes and proteins are also presented in chapters devoted to these subjects.

The book is divided into four parts. Part I deals with human cytomegalovirus and human diseases, Part II describes human cytomegalovirus infections in the immunocompromised host, Part III covers the diagnosis, treatment, and prevention of human cytomegalovirus diseases, and Part IV presents data on molecular aspects of human cytomegalovirus. Each section of the book comprises chapters written by experts, providing basic medical and molecular knowledge in addition to a more specific understanding of HCMV infections.

The editors of the book wish to thank all those who have contributed chapters for their willingness to share their knowledge and allowing this comprehensive synthesis of current knowledge of HCMV as a problem of great current medical importance. We would also like to thank Dr. Wieczorek for his support and for making the publication of this book possible. The editorial assistance of Waltraud Janssen is much appreciated.

Spring 1993

Y. Becker, Jerusalem
G. Darai, Heidelberg
E.-S. Huang, Chapel Hill

Contents

List of Authors

Adam, E., Division of Molecular Virology, Baylor College of Medicine, Texas Medical Center, One Baylor Plaza, Houston, TX 77030, USA

Albrecht, T., Department of Microbiology, University of Texas Medical Branch, Galveston, TX 77550, USA

Becker, Y., Department of Molecular Virology, Faculty of Medicine, The Hebrew University of Jerusalem, POB 1172, Jerusalem 910010, Israel

Boldogh, I., Department of Microbiology, University of Texas Medical Branch, Galveston, TX 77550, USA
permanent address: Department of Microbiology, Medical University of Debrecen, 4012 Debrecen, Hungary

Chang, M. H., Department of Pediatrics, College of Medicine, National Taiwan University, Taipei, Taiwan, Republic of China

Choudhury, S., Department of Microbiology, Georgetown University Medical Center, 3900 Reservoir Rd. N.W., Washington, DC 20007, USA

DeBakey, M. E., Department of Surgery, Baylor College of Medicine, Texas Medical Center, One Baylor Plaza, Houston, TX 77030, USA

Drew, W. L., Department of Pathology, Laboratory Medicine, and Medicine, Mount Zion Hospital and Medical Center of the University of California, 1600 Divisadero Street, San Francisco, CA 94120, USA

Dudding, L., Departments of Obstetrics and Gynecology, Microbiology and Immunology, and Comprehensive Cancer Center, The University of North Carolina at Chapel Hill, Chapel Hill, NC 27599-7295, USA

Ferreiro, J. A., Department of Pathology and Brain Research Institute, UCLA Medical Center, CHS Room 18-170, Los Angeles, CA 90024-1732, USA

Fiala, M., Department of Neurology, University of California Medical Center, Los Angeles, CA 90024-1732, USA

Fons, M. P., Department of Microbiology, University of Texas Medical Branch, Galveston, TX 77550, USA

Ghazal, P., Department of Immunology, The Scripps Research Institute, La Jolla, CA 92037, USA

Gibson, W., Virology Laboratories, Johns Hopkins School of Medicine, 725 North Wolfe Street, Baltimore, MD 21205, USA

Graves, M. C., Department of Medicine, University of California (Irvine), School of Medicine, Orange, CA 92668, USA

Grody, W. W., Departments of Pathology, Molecular Pathology, and Medical Genetics, University of California Medical Center, Los Angeles, CA 90024-1732, USA

Hamilton, J. D., Department of Medicine, Duke University Medical Center and Department of Veterans Affairs Medical Center, 508 Fulton Street, Durham, NC 27705, USA

Haskill, S., Department of Obstetrics and Gynecology, and Comprehensive Cancer Center, The University of North Carolina at Chapel Hill, Chapel Hill, NC 27599-7295, USA

Higenbottam, T. W., Heart-Lung Transplant Research Unit, Papworth Hospital, Cambridge CB3 8RE, UK

Ho, M., Department of Infectious Diseases and Microbiology, Graduate School of Public Health, and Departments of Medicine and Pathology, School of Medicine, University of Pittsburgh, Pittsburgh, PA 15261, USA

van der Horst, C. M., Division of Infectious Disease, University of North Carolina, Campus Box # 7030, Chapel Hill, NC 27599-7030, USA

Huang, E.-S., Lineberger Comprehensive Cancer Research Center, The University of North Carolina at Chapel Hill, School of Medicine, C # 7295, Rm. 117, Lineberger Building, Chapel Hill, NC 27599-7295, USA

Jahn, G., Institute for Clinical and Molecular Virology, University of Erlangen-Nürnberg, 8520 Erlangen, Germany

Kowalik, T. F., Lineberger Comprehensive Cancer Research Center, The University of North Carolina at Chapel Hill, School of Medicine, C # 7295, Rm. 117, Lineberger Building, Chapel Hill, NC 27599-7295, USA

Lee, C. Y., Department of Pediatrics, College of Medicine, National Taiwan University, Taipei, Taiwan, Republic of China

Marshall, G. S., Department of Pediatrics, University of Louisville School of Medicine, Louisville, KY 40292, USA

Melnick, J. L., Division of Molecular Virology, Baylor College of Medicine, Texas Medical Center, One Baylor Plaza, Houston, TX 77030, USA

Navarro, D., University of Valencia, School of Medicine, Valencia, Spain

Nelson, J. A., Departments of Pathology and Immunology, Division of Virology, The Scripps Research Institute, Clinic, La Jolla, CA 92037, USA

Pereira, L., Department of Stomatology, Division of Oral Biology, University of California San Francisco, HSW-604, San Francisco, CA 94143, USA

Plotkin, S. A., Pasteur-Merieux Serums et Vaccins, Marnes-la-Coquette, France and Connaught Laboratories, Swiftwater, PA, USA and Willowdale, Ontario, Canada

Rosenthal, L. J., Department of Microbiology, Georgetown University Medical Center, 3900 Reservoir Rd. N.W., Washington, DC 20007, USA

Scott, J. P., Heart-Lung Transplant Research Unit, Papworth Hospital, Cambridge CB3 8RE, UK

Serody, J. S., Division of Infectious Disease, University of North Carolina, Campus Box # 7030, Chapel Hill, NC 27599-7030, USA

Smyth, R. L., Heart-Lung Transplant Research Unit, Papworth Hospital, Cambridge CB3 8RE, UK
Present address: Oncology Unit, Ward C3, Royal Liverpool Children's Hospital, Alder Hey, Liverpool L12 2AP, UK

Stenberg, R. M., Department of Microbiology and Immunology, Eastern Virginia Medical School, 7700 West Olney Road, Norfolk, VA 23501-1696, USA

Valyi-Nagy, T., Department of Microbiology, University of Texas Medical Branch, Galveston, TX 77550, USA
permanent address: The Wistar Institute, 36th and Spruce Streets, Philadelphia, PA, USA

Vinters, H. V., Department of Neuropathology, University of California Medical Center, Los Angeles, CA 90024-1732, USA

Wallwork, J., Heart-Lung Transplant Research Unit, Papworth Hospital, Cambridge CB3 8RE, UK

Wiley, C. A., Department of Pathology, University of California San Diego, La Jolla, CA 92093, USA

Winston, D. J., Division of Hematology/Oncology, University of California Medical Center, 10833 Le Conte Avenue, Los Angeles, CA 90024-1678, USA

Section I Human Cytomegalovirus and Human Diseases

Chapter 1 The Pathogenicity of Human Cytomegalovirus: An Overview

Eng-Shang Huang and Timothy F. Kowalik

Summary

Defining causality between an agent– be it a virus, bacteria, or chemical – and a disease is the principal aim of biomedical research. Achievement of this lofty goal is hampered when the suspected agent is commonly found in the environment or in populations. Such is the case with human cytomegalovirus (HCMV). Its ubiquity diminishes the impact of its omnipresentation in many pathologies. Despite this lack of a direct cause-effect pattern between HCMV and most of the diseases it is associated with, the application of molecular biology technology has permitted us to begin to define basic underlying mechanisms by which this virus can influence, as well as cause, disease. Much of this chapter is an initial attempt at discerning important molecular biological features of HCMV which have the potential to play significant roles in the pathogenicity and oncogenicity of this virus. In so doing, patterns emerge between HCMV molecular biology and the types of pathological phenomena this virus is associated with directly or as a coetiological agent. Common themes include induction of transcriptional activators and the cell cycle, production of specific cytokines by HCMV infection, and hampering host immunities. The latter part of this chapter reviews many of the diseases and clinical features of HCMV infections. Both sections cross-reference subsequent chapters in this volume where more detailed analyses of these particular issues are provided.

Introduction

Cytomegaloviruses (CMV) are a group of double-stranded DNA viruses within the herpes family which share great structural and biological similarities [215]. In both in vivo infection and infection of tissue cultures, this group of viruses displays strong species specificity and induces the distinctive cytopathic

Lineberger Comprehensive Cancer Center, Departments of Medicine, Microbiology and Immunology and Curriculum of Genetics, University of North Carolina at Chapel Hill, School of Medicine, CB # 7295, Rm. 117, Lineberger Building, Chapel Hill, NC 27599-7295, USA effect of cell enlargement (cytomegaly) with typical Cowdry's type A intranuclear and cytoplasmic inclusions [34]. Cytomegaloviruses have been found widely in humans, mice, monkeys, guinea pigs, horses, chimpanzees, etc. Although there is a great deal of structural and biological similarity among these viruses, there is nevertheless a lack of genetic relatedness among human, mouse, and simian CMV as determined by nucleic acid hybridizations at high stringency hybridization conditions [94]. CMV grows in the host of homologous origin with the exception of simian CMV, which will grow in human fibroblasts and can probably cause disease in human; this is based on the finding of an unusual CMV strain (Colburn) isolated from brain tissue of a boy suffering from encephalopathy. The Colburn strain resembles simian CMV [93a].

The biochemical and biological natures of human cytomegalovirus (HCMV) are extremely complex, as is its pathogenesis. On one hand, this virus is a ubiquitous herpes group virus that rarely causes symptomatic disease in immunocompetent human beings. On the other hand, it has been found to associate with a great variety of clinical manifestations, ranging from developmental abnormalities, mental retardation, deafness, mononucleosis, chorioretinitis to fatal diseases such as interstitial pneumonitis and disseminated HCMV infection in immunocompromised individuals. Active CMV infections have been found in numerous cancer patients and patients with AIDS. This omnipresentation makes it difficult for investigators to prove a causal role for HCMV in specific diseases. As with the other herpesviruses, HCMV is able to establish a lifelong latent infection after primary infection. Reactivation of HCMV is frequently encountered during pregnancy, after perfusion, organ transplantation, and at other stages when the immune system is compromised. Data obtained from molecular biological studies of HCMV indicate the oncogenic potential of this virus is comparable to that of other herpesviruses.

As mentioned above, a major concern of studies implicating this ubiquitous and usually latent virus with a particular pathological disorder is causality. In in vivo infections and infections of tissue culture cells, HCMV displays strong species specificity. It will not induce diseases in any species other than humans. Ethical considerations obviously prevent the direct experimentation with pathological agents in humans and, therefore, definitive proof of other species-derived, CMV-causing diseases in humans is lacking. Even though it is difficult to demonstrate a direct cause and effect between HCMV and a particular disease, recent advances in molecular biology research provide us sufficient data to suggest basic mechanisms by which HCMV could induce many of the diseases associated with this virus. In addition, the appearance of HCMV with a particular disorder usually results in a worsened clinical prognosis and warrants consideration of potential viral mechanisms for such an effect. Therefore, in this communication we shall briefly describe the classic infectious disease aspects of HCMV infections and devote our effort to explore the molecular pathological aspects of HCMV-induced pathogenesis.

Considerations Toward Elucidating the Mechanisms of HCMV Pathogenesis

Several important epidemiological, biochemical, and biological factors should be taken into consideration for a better understanding of the mechanisms of HCMV pathogenesis.

Epidemiological Aspects of HCMV Infection

1. HCMV infection seems to be nearly universal in the human population. The frequency and age incidence of infection varies with socioeconomic level and to some extent depends on geographic location. Based on seroepidemiological studies, more than 60% of the general population have CMV complement-fixating antibodies after age 35; some areas in Africa and the Far East reach 100% seropositivity by enzyme-linked immunosorbent assay (ELISA) [87].

2. HCMV was found in the urine of 3.5% of healthy pregnant women in the United States [86], in the cervix of 13%–15% of healthy pregnant women in Taiwan [5] and Africa (our unpublished data), and in the cervix of 10%–20% of asymptomatic pregnant Japanese women [149].

3. Infectious HCMV was found in the semen of 30% of asymptomatic homosexual men in the San Francisco area [43, 138] and the research triangle area of North Carolina [93]. By tissue culture isolation, we were able to detect HCMV in the semen of 15% of asymptomatic newlywed males in Zimbabwe (E.S. Huang, unpublished data). HCMV particles can be demonstrated inside the sperm head as well as in the extracellular fluid [93, 116, 151].

4. The congenital HCMV infection rate, as indicated by viruria during the first 48 h of life, in the United States was found to be as high as 1.2% [198]. Excretion of virus was demonstrated in over 60% of infants between 5 and 9 months of age in a study conducted at Sendai National Hospital, Sendai, Japan [149]. The prevalence rate of viruria in children ranges from 3% to 27%, while the incidence rate for the first year of life varies from 15% to 18% [121].

5. Intrauterine HCMV infection has been estimated to be responsible for damage to CNS in 800 to 2000 children born in England and Wales each year [201].

6. HCMV-induced viral interstitial pneumonia has been observed in 35%–90% of organ transplant recipients. The mortality rate for patients suffering from interstitial pneumonitis is high in seronegative transplant recipients and in patients without anti-CMV chemotherapy [7, 84, 87, 133, 155, 165].

7. Active HCMV infection has been demonstrated in more than 95% of homosexual men with AIDS [41, 42, 44].

Biological Aspects of HCMV Infection

1. The 230 kilobase pair HCMV genome has a coding capacity of more than 200 proteins. Many of these proteins are subsequently subjected to posttranscriptional modifications by proteolytic cleavage, phosphorylation, glycosylation, etc. [27]. The host-immune responses to these proteins may play a very important role in the pathogenesis of HCMV infection [161, 203] (Pereira et al., in Chap. 21, this volume).

2. HCMV has a strong major immediate-early (IE) promoter-enhancer with a complicated array of *cis*-regulating elements. Expression of the major HCMV IE proteins is under the control of virus-associated and cellular proteins. Host-cell factors affect viral gene expression and determine the permissiveness of HCMV infection (see Stenberg, Chap. 17, and Ghazal and Nelson, Chap. 18, this volume).

3. HCMV has active major IE gene products which can not only regulate the expression of viral genes but also can transactivate numerous heterologous viral and cellular promoters. Many promoters regulating the expression of enzymes involved in cellular proliferation are transactivated upon HCMV infection [12, 45, 51, 91].

4. HCMV has virion-associated proteins with protein kinase activities [22, 36, 38, 128, 135] which might be able to activate or inactivate important signal transduction factors or oncogenes upon infection via protein phosphorylation.

5. The open reading frame (ORF) of a putative HCMV glycoprotein (0.07–0.11 map units) has 20% homology with the major histocompatibility complex (MHC) class Iα chain. β-2 Microglobulin may bind to this α-chain-like viral glycoprotein and facilitate viral attachment and penetration during HCMV infection [11]. Immunotolerance of HCMV infection may also be due to this sequence homology.

6. HCMV IE region 2 shares sequence homology and immunologic cross-reactivity to HLA-DR β chain of class II MHC [62]. This sequence homology and immunological cross-reactivity might contribute to graft rejection after transplantation. In addition, three HCMV ORF – UL33, US27 and US28 – encode three G protein-coupled receptor family proteins, which implies that a complicated interaction exists between HCMV and its host. This may provide a potential pathway for virus transformation of its host [28].

7. HCMV possesses DNA sequences that are able to transform mammalian cells in vitro (see by Rosenthal and Ghoudhury, Chap. 20, this volume).

8. HCMV does not encode a virus-specific thymidine kinase [51].

HCMV-Host Interaction

1. HCMV can be reactivated in organ transplant patients despite preexisting high titers of antibodies against HCMV. Virus can also be transmitted from pregnant women to fetuses despite high titers of maternal antibodies.

2. HCMV induces Ig Fc receptor synthesis and virus-infected cells can bind β_2-microglobulin [130].

3. HCMV induces cytokine synthesis in virus-infected monocytes and macrophages [45]. Infection also results in host-cell macromolecular synthesis.

4. HCMV can replicate in developing sperm and persists in semen and cervical tissue.

5. HCMV infects a wide range of human organs and tissues.

Cytomegalic Inclusion Disease and HCMV

In the early 1900s, HCMV-infected inclusion body-bearing cells were originally considered as a consequence of protozoan infection [122] or a cellular response to syphillitic infection [158] because of the presence of intranuclear as well as cytoplasmic inclusion bodies. The presence of protozoan-like cells in lung, kidney, liver, and parotid glands tissue of a leutic fetus was described early in 1904 by Jesionek and Kiolemeoglou [103], and a similar observation was made later in the same year by Ribbert [164]. Ribbert even mentioned that he first saw such large "protozoan-like" cells in the kidney sections of a stillborn infant in 1881 [87, 164]. This protozoan theory was continued until the discovery of a transmissible virus associated with inclusion-bearing cells in the submaxillary glands of guinea pigs by Cole and Kuttner [32]. The concept of viral involvement in this kind of pathological change was further supported by the demonstration and description of intranuclear inclusions induced by virus infections by Cowdry [34].

Apparent cytomegalic inclusion disease (CID) was reported by Farber and Wolbach [53] by examining a series of 183 postmortem submaxillary glands from infants who died of various causes. Among these, 14% had intranuclear and cytoplasmic inclusions in their glands. In 1950, the term "generalized cytomegalic inclusion disease" was proposed by Wyatt et al. [222] in their study of congenital lethal cytomegalic infections. Because the inclusion-bearing cells were invariably present in the collection tubules of kidneys, Wyatt et al. [222] had suggested to use the appearance of these cells in urine as indicators to monitor diseased infants [87]. In 1952, Fetterman of the Children's Hospital in Pittsburgh made a cytological examination of the urine of a 3-day-old premature infant with juandice, purpura, hepatosplenomegaly, and intracerebral calcification and found enormous cytomegalic cells with large intranuclear inclusions. This infant died the next day, and typical cytomegalic inclusions were found in the brain, lung, liver, thyroid, kidney, etc., indicating generalized CID. This was the first case of CID diagnosed during life [54, 87].

In 1954, Margaret Smith succeeded in isolating and propagating murine CMV in mouse embryonic tissue culture [188]. Following this pioneering work, she was able to isolate HCMV from the salivary glands and kidneys of infants who died of CID [189]. Independently, Weller and his coworkers in Boston isolated the Davis strain of HCMV from a liver biopsy of a 3-month-old infant suspected of toxoplasmosis, and the Kerr and Esp strains from the urine of two living infants suffering from CID [213]. Rowe and his coworkers in Bethesda at the same period inadvertently isolated AD-169 strain HCMV instead of adenovirus from human adenoidal tissue of an older child [174]. Since then HCMV has been recognized as a ubiquitous agent associated not only with CID in neonates, but also with heterophile-negative mononucleosis syndrome in immunologically competent normal adults [109, 110], hepatitis, gastrointestinal ulceration, retinitis, and even encephalopathy in immunocompromised patients. The histological events leading to the discovery of HCMV and the pathobiological impact of HCMV infection have been given in detail by Monto Ho in his second edition of "Human Cytomegalovirus: Biology and Infection" [87].

Molecular Pathology of HCMV Infection

It is crucial for us to understand virus and host-cell interactions at the molecular level before we can make a final conclusion of the viral etiology of a particular disease. With the exception of fibroblasts, understanding the consequences of HCMV infection in different cell types is not well developed. In addition, study of the effects of such infections on the surrounding microenvironment as well as on the human body as a whole are virtually nonexistent at this moment.

Several factors may determine the success of initiating and establishing HCMV infections: (a) cellular receptors for HCMV attachment on the host surface, (b) virus-specific glycoproteins gB and gH for attachment and entry, (c) the availability in cells of various nuclear factors, such as NF-κB, SP-1, AP-1, etc., that are needed for HCMV IE gene promoter activity, and (d) the existence of cellular repressor molecules that limit the expression of HCMV IE genes.

Viral Receptors and Viral Entry

The enveloped viruses display ligand proteins on their membrane surface that bind selectively to specific receptors on the cell. Following viral ligand-receptor interactions, the virus is then internalized and the intracellular infection process begins. This ligand-receptor interaction is the initial event in an infection and is one of the important factors determining the susceptibility of a cell type to a virus infection. Application of soluble peptides carrying the receptor-binding epitope for the viral ligand or the use of antibody against this epitope will inhibit virus infectivity. Therefore, the presence of receptors for HCMV on the cell surface and the application of antibodies against the viral ligand could affect HCMV pathogenesis. Using ^{35}S-labeled HCMV particles, Taylor et al. [207] found that HCMV binds to many cell types, but interacts especially well

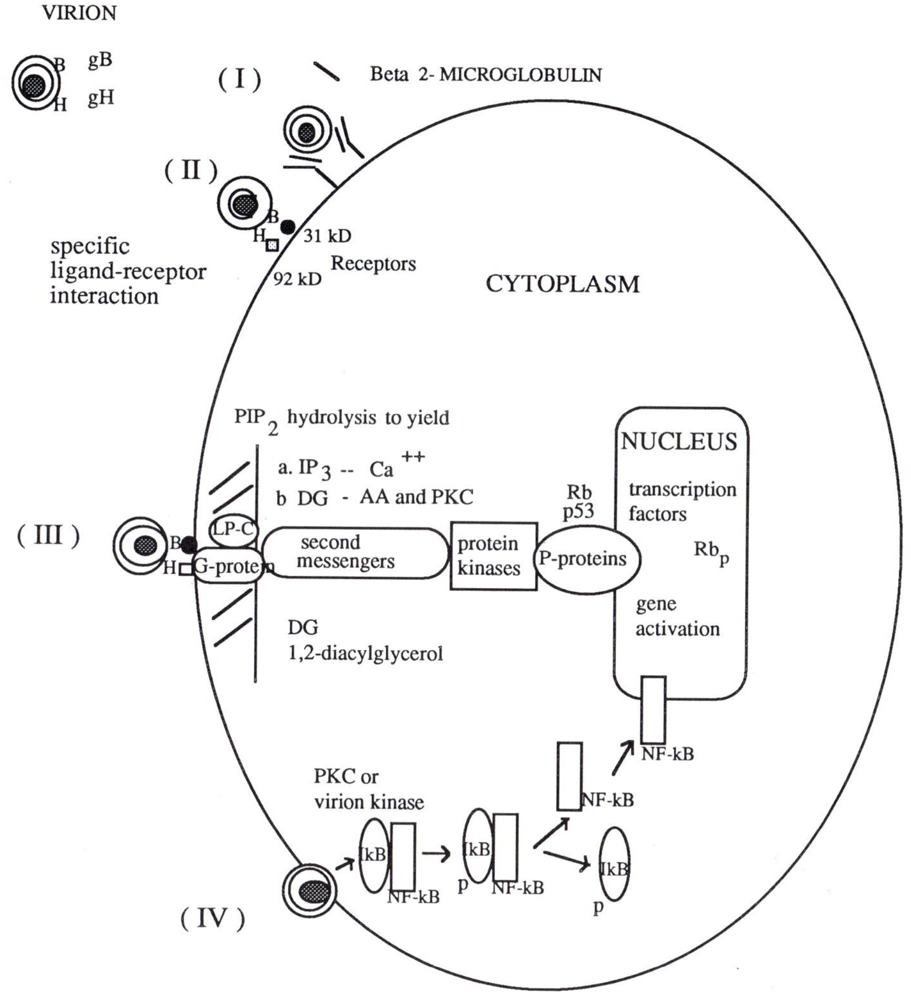

Fig. 1. Human cytomegalovirus specific ligand–receptor interactions and proposed models for the activation of cellular genes by HCMV prior to the expression of HCMV immediate early genes. *I*, HCMV glycoproteins gH (*H*) and gB (*B*) are responsible for HCMV ligand–cellular receptor interactions. gH is an 86-kD glycoprotein which interacts with a 92-kD receptor on the cell curface at the time of attachment. gB (55–130 kD) glycoprotein, binds predominantly to a 31-kD cellular protein at the stage after virus attachment, but before viral gene expression; *II*, proteins from HCMV bind β_2 -M. β_2-M is the light chain of the class I HLA that normally associates with class I heavy (α) chain to form the MHC antigens on the cell surface. Therefore, HCMV and β_2-M complex could potentially enter into the host cell via its interaction with class I heavy chain antigen; *III*, HCMV activates cellular gene expression via G-protein(s) and second messengers. This model is adapted from Albrecht et al. [2]. See also Chap. 19, this volume; *IV*, HCMV transactivates cellular genes via IϰB and the NF-ϰB pathway. Phosphorylation of IϰB causes IϰB to separate from NF-ϰB and allows NF-ϰB to translocate into the nucleus. *PKC*, protein kinase C; *p*, phosphorylated; *RB*, retinoblastoma; *AA*, arachidonic acid; IP_3, inositol 1,4,5-triphosphate; *LP*, phospholipase-C

with human foreskin fibroblasts. Quantitative analysis indicated that the maximal binding of HCMV to human fibroblasts reached approximately 2500–3000 particles per cell [33].

HCMV Glycoprotein gH and gB. To date, two groups of HCMV glycoproteins, gB and gH, have been reported to be responsible for HCMV ligand-cellular receptor interactions [161] (for details see Pereira et al., in Chap. 21, this volume). HCMV gH, with a molecular mass of around 86 kD, apparently interacts with a specific cellular receptor(s) [105], while the gB homologue, with a molecular mass of 55–130 kD, is required for viral infectivity at a stage after virus attachment but before the expression of HCMV-specific genes [24]. Various binding studies revealed that HCMV gH interacts with a 92-kD cellular receptor, while the HCMV-gB homologue binds predominantly to a 31-kD protein with minor bands at 180, 96, and 90 kD (see Fig. 1) [2]. The distribution of the HCMV gH receptor on various cell lines correlates with the appearance of HCMV IE and late antigens when cells are infected with HCMV. The HCMV gH glycoprotein does not bind to the gB receptors on the cell surface [162].

β_2-Microglobulin. Grundy et al. [77, 78] demonstrated that proteins from HCMV binds to β_2-microglobulin (β_2-M). β_2-M is a small nonglycosylated globular peptide (molecular weight 12 000) which noncovalently associates with the glycosylated heavy (α) chain of class I antigen to form MHC antigens on the outer side of the plasma membrane. β_2-M does not form part of the antigenic site of the HLA molecule, but it is essential for the processing and expression of the class I MHC molecules. If β_2-M is absent, the expression of class I antigenic determinants is retarded [98]. β_2-M also occurs as a free soluble molecule in serum and urine. Because HCMV binds to β_2-M and β_2-M associates with the heavy chain class I antigen, Grundy et al. [78] hypothesized that the virus may use β_2-M binding as a mechanism of infection. Subsequently, Beck and Barrell [11] presented evidence from DNA sequence analysis that HCMV encodes a glycoprotein molecule (HCMV-H301, UL18) which shares sequence homology to the MHC class I HLA antigen. This protein was then proposed to be responsible for the observed β_2-M association with HCMV. Furthermore, the binding to and cellular deprivation of β_2-M by HCMV may interfere with the processing and expression of class I MHC, which in turn would effect the class I-dependent immune response. In fact, Browne et al. [23] showed that HCMV-infected cells have drastically reduced expression of HLA on the cell surface even though they have normal levels of class I HLA mRNA.

Cellular Factors and CMV IE Promoter

HCMV is capable of binding to human umbilical vein endothelial (HUVE) cells to the same degree as it binds to fibroblasts [33]. But the progression of

HCMV infection and expression of HCMV genes in HUVE cells are retarded as compared to that in human foreskin fibroblasts. Treatment of HUVE with sodium butyrate at the time of infection accelerates the progression of viral infection and gene expression, indicating that additional factors play a role(s) in the progression of HCMV infection. Likewise, the expression and replication of HCMV is restricted in peripheral blood mononuclear cells (PBMNS) of normal immunocompetent individuals. Both mitogenic and antigenic stimulation of PBMNS can enhance and increase HCMV gene expression. Therefore, the state of cell differentiation or activation by chemical or biological agents could be critical determinants that dictate viral gene expression and replication (for detail, see Ghazal and Nelson, Chap. 18, this volume).

Upon absorption, uncoating, and entry of viral DNA into the nucleus, expression of the HCMV genome is sequentially regulated. According to the kinetics of gene expression, the genes encoded by HCMV can be categorized into three kinetic classes: immediate-early (IE), early (E), and late (L) genes (for details, see Gibson, Chap. 16, and Stenberg, Chap. 17, this volume). IE genes of HCMV encode a group of regulatory proteins with strong transactivating activities. IE expression is not only needed to activate subsequent E gene expression, but the IE gene products also transactivate the promoters of numerous important cellular genes associated with macromolecule synthesis. HCMV E genes encode enzymes and factors involved in viral DNA replication and downstream structural protein synthesis.

The expression of HCMV major IE genes is under the control of the major IE promoter (MIEP). Initial activation of the MIEP is heavily dependent on host-cell factors and possibly a virion-associated tegument protein analogous to the tif protein in HSV (our unpublished data). HCMV MIEP is an extremely strong and complicated promoter. Its enhancer region (see Fig. 2) contains at least four classes of specific repeat units that have many nuclear factor binding motifs [19, 179]. These motifs include consensus binding sequences for NF-κB binding proteins (-GGGACTTTCC- within 18 bp repeats), AP-1 (-TGACTCA- in an AP18 type repeat), CREB/ATF(-TGACGTCA- in 19 bp repeats), SP-1 (GC boxes in 17, 18, and 19 bp repeats) and a glucocorticoid responsive element. A serum response element is located between -530 to -539 from IE1 mRNA capping site and a retinoic acid responsive element around -242 to -305. The presence of these consensus sequences within HCMV major IE enhancer domain, between -65 to -539, allows this virus to respond to wide varieties of nuclear transcription factors, serum factors, and hormones and to exert high levels of IE gene expression in a wide variety of cells [125].

In addition to the enhancer elements mentioned above, NF-1 and other cellular factor binding regions were found between -540 to -800 from the capping site [85, 101]. The NF-1 binding sites within this region were found to coincide with regions shown to be hypersensitive to DNase I in the active promoter-enhancer, but not sensitive when the promoter was silent [143]. It was, therefore, speculated that NF-1 might play an important role in cell type-specific IE gene expression [101, 125]. An additional DNase I hypersensitive area was also found in the region further upstream, between position

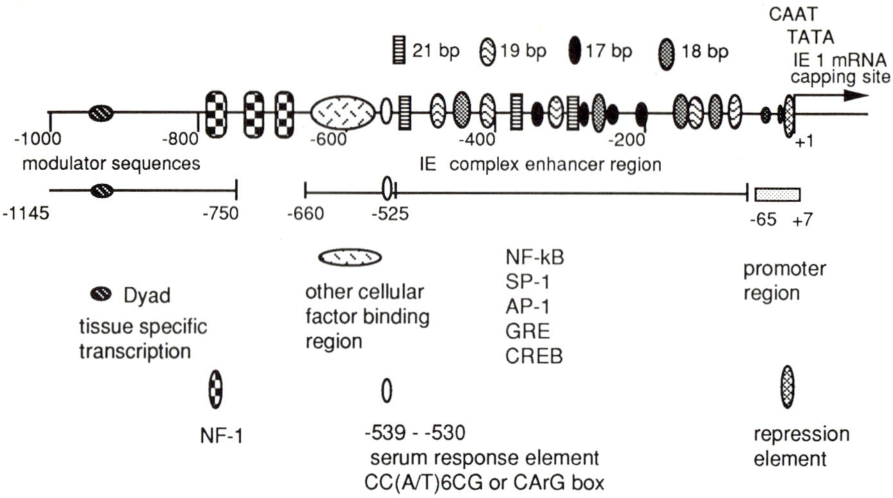

Fig. 2. Schematic diagram and relative location of various consensus sequences and *cis*-regulating elements on the human cytomegalovirus major immediate-early promoter. The base sequence numbers are relative to the IE1 mRNA capping site (+1). (Adapted from Ghazal and Nelson, Chap. 18, this volume, [138 a])

−750 to −1145, and suggested that this area could be a target for cellular transregulatory factors [145]. By in vitro transient expression assays, Nelson and his colleagues demonstrated that this DNase I hypersensitive element was able to modulate gene expression in nonpermissive cells in a negative manner. On the other hand, this element was observed to positively influence downstream gene expression in permissive cells [145]. Furthermore, by means of deletion mutagenesis and DNA gel retardation, Shelbourn et al. [183] identified a 19-bp symmetrical palindromic dyad sequence within this modulator region which played an important role in transcriptional repression of downstream gene expression in undifferentiated teratocarcinoma cells. The factor(s) bound to this palindromic dyad sequence was removed or replaced when cells differentiated. All of these facts clearly suggest that the upstream domain between −540 and −1145 of the enhancer region of HCMV MIEP appears to modulate IE gene expression in a cell type-specific and differentiation-dependent manner [125] (Ghazal and Nelson, Chap. 18, this volume). Repression of virus growth by cellular factors and subsequent release by appropriate stimuli is an important concept when trying to understand HCMV biology.

The control of IE gene expression by cellular nuclear proteins and the coordinate regulation of interactions between IE gene products and downstream viral- or cellular-target promoters are important determinants affecting the outcome of HCMV infections (Stenberg, Chap. 17; Ghazal and Nelson, Chap. 18, this volume). Interactions of the major IE promoter with cellular-specific regulatory proteins would dictate the levels of HCMV IE gene expression and consequently affect the outcome of an HCMV infection. The expression of HCMV MEIP differs under permissive and nonpermissive conditions. This difference is independent of viral proteins and appears to be largely dependent on the availability of various nuclear proteins associated with transcription in virus-infected cells.

HCMV Major IE Genes: The Central Theme in HCMV Pathogenesis

The nature of HCMV IE genes and their products is described in detail by Gibson in Chap. 16 and Stenberg in Chap. 17 of this volume. Three regions of HCMV IE genes which express at the IE stage of infection have been mapped on the HCMV genome [203]. One region, mapped between 0.73 and 0.751 mapping units of HCMV genome, gives rise to the most abundant IE gene products, IE1 and IE2. IE gene 1 encodes a 72-kD protein which regulates the expression of another IE protein, IE2, and induces NF-ϰB to activate promoters with NF-ϰB enhancer motifs (GGGACTTTCC) [138 a]. The IE2 gene encodes several different sizes of proteins (84 kD, 55 kD, 28 kD, etc.) by differential splicing of the same premessenger RNA. These IE2 products, independently or in conjunction with IE1, can broadly activate the expression of viral early genes and cellular genes. In contrast, one of the IE2 gene products can repress IE1 gene expression via a *cis* sequence (CGTTTAGTGAACCGT) at the start site, −14 to +1, of the IE1-IE2 transcription cluster.

In a related consideration, HCMV IE genes require and induce proteins which bind to and activate the enhancer domains of many promoters and thereby stimulate the expression of exogenous genes. Some of these activators play central roles in defining the differentiated state of blood cells. Most important of these is probably NF-ϰB. The DNA binding and resulting transcriptional activation of NF-ϰB was originally described as central to the activation of the promoter regulating the expression of the ϰB polypeptide chain of immunoglobulins and was thought to be restricted to maturing B cells [182]. NF-ϰB has since been shown to be important in regulating the expression of genes encoding interleukins, MHC class I and II genes, Fc receptor, cell adhesion molecules as well as genes encoding acute phase proteins [8, 67, 118]. In addition, the regulated expression of genes for at least two viruses, HCMV and HIV, are integrally tied to NF-ϰB activity.

HCMV infection of fibroblasts rapidly induces nuclear NF-ϰB binding activity by at least two mechanisms. The immediate response is due to release of cytosolic stores of NF-ϰB [112 a]. This occurs by inactivating the cytosolic inhibitor of NFϰB, IϰB, possibly by viral component(s) or a virion-associated protein kinase (see Fig. 1). These cytosolic stores of NF-ϰB act as second messengers transposing signals received at the cell surface to the nucleus and activating appropriate responses. The uncoupling of this system could make infected cells unresponsive to extracellular signals which normally utilize this system. Signals transduced through protein kinase C and A are speculated to regulate subsets of the NF-ϰB system [9, 66, 88, 106, 184]. The sustained activation of NF-ϰB by HCMV is most likely due to transcriptional activation of the genes encoding the two characterized NF-κB proteins, p50 and p65 [112a]. Activation of NF-κB is at least partly due to the HCMV MIE proteins. Based on these facts and considerations, we postulate that HCMV can enhance or induce NF-κB-mediated gene expression by two mechanisms: first, via phosphorylation of IκB at the initial stages of virus-cell interactions and second, via the transactivation of target promoters by IE proteins after HCMV IE gene expression.

In addition to the induction of NF-κB binding proteins, infection of human HEL fibroblast by HCMV also induces SP-1 and AP-1 binding proteins (E. S. Huang et al., in preparation). HCMV major IE gene products can also activate the promoter of the cellular housekeeping dihydrofolate reductase (DHFR) gene via E2F consensus sequences [209a]. HCMV IE gene products can activate the IL-1β promoter which in turn causes high levels of IL-1β protein synthesis [45]. Other cytokines, such as macrophage colony stimulation factor (CSF-1) and tumor necrosis factor-α (TNF-α), and key enzymes involved in cell proliferation, such as DNA polymerase [91], thymidine kinase [51], RNA polymerase [206], and topoisomerase II [12] can be induced upon HCMV infection. HCMV IE gene proteins are speculated to be either directly or indirectly (via NF-κB, SP-1, E2F, etc.) involved in transactivating the promoters of these genes.

HCMV IE gene products not only can specifically transactivate promoters of homologous genes but also can transactivate the selected promoters of genes from other viruses, such as HSV TK, HIV LTR, HPV 18 NCR and SV40 late genes [37] (our unpublished data). In addition, in collaboration with Dr. L. B. Ting of Yang Ming Medical College, we have also found that HCMV IE genes can transactivate the HBV C and S promoters in hepatocytes and the more differentiated hepatoma cell lines. This phenomenon implies the possibility of a coetiological role for HCMV in certain diseases induced by other viruses.

HCMV and AIDS – Synergy with HIV

A rather contemporary association of HCMV with a disease is with acquired immunodeficiency syndrome (AIDS). In fact, HCMV was originally suspected as the causative agent in patients suffering from this malady. This was based on several facts: (1) the extremely high rates of HCMV infection in homosexual men with AIDS, almost 100% had evidence of active HCMV infection, (2) serological data and the detection of HCMV antigen and nucleic acid in Kaposi's sarcoma tissue [41, 68, 69], (3) HCMV was a primary or secondary cause of death in 25% of AIDS patients [126], and (4) the observed suppression of cell-mediated immunity in primary HCMV infections [61, 168, 172]. With the identification of human immunodeficiency virus (HIV) as the etiological agent of AIDS, interest in HCMV decreased. Still, disseminated HCMV, HCMV-induced interstitial pneumonia, and HCMV retinitis complications in AIDS patients indicate a poor prognosis and high mortality. HCMV has remained as a well-documented cause of morbidity and mortality among AIDS patients with HIV infection. Furthermore, it is clear that factors other than HIV play important roles in the progression of HIV infection toward AIDS. The interest in HCMV as one of these cofactors has, therefore, reemerged [61]. As the AIDS phenomenon has grown to incorporate blood bank recipients and the heterosexual as well as homosexual populations, some trends have become apparent. Those most likely to develop HCMV-associated complications tend to have multiple sex partners and poor hygiene, emphasizing HCMV as a sexually transmitted agent and having the greatest relevance here (see Drew, Chap. 5, this volume).

The exact mechanisms by which HCMV or HIV reactivate from latency and the role(s) each plays in influencing this reactivation remains unclear. However, several studies provide evidence of how this may occur. Whether HCMV activates HIV or vice versa is unclear and may be a moot point for studies show that either virus can transactivate gene expression of the other virus in vitro. The in vivo correlations to these studies are probably infections involving T cells and monocyte/macrophages in the circulation and glial cells in the central nervous system. Actively replicating HCMV and HIV within the same cell in vivo has been demonstrated in glial cells in the brain and in cytomegalic inclusion cells in the lung [56, 144]. Whether or not these are the sources of viral activation will be difficult, if not impossible, to prove.

The synergistic and cofactoral roles of HCMV in AIDS can be assessed by the following in vitro and in vivo observations:

1. HCMV Infection Stimulates the Expression of Monocyte- and Macrophage-associated Mediator Genes. In HCMV-infected monocytes and macrophages the expression of IL-1β, TNF-α, MAD-9 and CSF-1 are greatly extended and enhanced [45]; MAD-9 is the same as human monocyte-derived neutrophil chemotatic factor (MDNCF, [225]), neutrophil-activating factor (NAF, [156]), and neutrophil-activating protein (NAP-1, [117]) that has been shown to be a chemotactic factor for neutrophils and lymphocytes. These cytokines in turn are able to induce the expression of HIV-1 in chronically infected promonocytic cells and human T lymphocytes releasing HIV from latency [58, 97, 123, 150, 173]. Therefore, it is suggested that HCMV infections can influence the outcome of HIV infections at a distance.

2. Transactivation of HIV Promoter by HCMV IE Products. Recent molecular studies may shed light onto the mechanisms by which HCMV and HIV-1 act in synergy within the same cell. The results all revolve around regulation and stimulation of the second messenger and promoter transactivator, NF-κB. Davis et al. [37] and others [159] observed that HCMV infection strongly transactivated the promoter region (LTR) of HIV. Nabel and Baltimore [141] observed NF-κB binding sites in the LTR and found that these regions could bind NF-κB and stimulate transcription. Subsequently, several groups discovered that the majority of HCMV-induced transactivation of the HIV LTR was due to presence of these NF-ϰB sites. However, a recent study has brought this into question, suggesting that only the minimal promoter or TATA box was sufficient for this activation. Further comparative studies are needed to clarify this discrepancy. As the HCMV major IE promoter activation is regulated by NF-ϰB sites in at least fibroblasts, it thus appears that both viruses have a vested interest in stimulating NF-ϰB activity.

In the past few years, data has emerged suggesting a possible means by which these viruses may act in synergy to stimulate NF-ϰB activity. The mechanisms by which HCMV stimulates NF-ϰB activity are described above. HIV has been shown to use a unique means to initiate the activation of NF-ϰB [97, 169]. One of the components of NF-ϰB is p50. This protein is actually encoded within a large RNA transcript encoding a protein of p105 kD. The p50 protein represents the N-terminal half of p105 and is proteolytically processed in the cell [52]. Riviere et al. [169] have demonstrated in vitro that the HIV protease, usually thought of in terms of processing the HIV polyproteins, can cut p105 at or near the normal processing site. The result is a p50-like protein with properties identical to purified p50. They also provide evidence for this activity in HIV-infected cells. This action in dually infected cells would most likely increase the processing rate of p50, whose gene is rapidly overexpressed during HCMV infections [112a], and may subvert innate regulatory mechanisms by which the cell controls the levels of p50 protein and NF-ϰB activity. Clearly, the activation mechanisms of NF-ϰB by HCMV and HIV compliment each other.

3. HCMV Infection Can Enhance the Expression of Surface Bound HLA-DR Antigens and Fc IgG Receptors, All of Which are Involved in HIV-1 Binding to or Entry into Target Cells [131, 202]. The receptor for HIV-1 on T and B lymphocytes, monocytes, and macrophages is the CD4 antigen. Infection of these cells by HIV-1 is blocked by monoclonal antibodies to CD4 [35] and by recombinant soluble CD4 [39, 57]. Expression of transfected CD4 on the cell surface of HeLa and other human cells renders them susceptible to HIV infection [127]. In addition, HIV antigen-antibody complexes can also infect monocytes, macrophages, and fibroblasts by means of receptors for the Fc portion of immunoglobulins (FcR) or complement receptors [89, 170, 205]. In vivo, HCMV shows little tissue tropism, as it is found in most human tissues and organs. Infection by HCMV can induce the expression of IgG Fc receptors, which in turn could permit HIV to infect a wide range of cell types [131]. Once HIV or HIV-antibody complexes enter HCMV-infected cells via CD4 or by means of the induced Fc receptor, HIV gene expression and replication could then be enhanced by transactivation of the HIV LTR via the HCMV IE gene products [37].

In the more severe cases of AIDS, both HIV and HCMV are actively replicated and disseminated. Again, HCMV potentially plays a role in enhancing the overall replication of HIV. The synergism or two-way enhancement between HIV and HCMV was reported by Skolnik et al. [187] in a culture system. In this study, HIV superinfection of T cells abortively infected with

HCMV could lead to productive infection of HCMV. Frenkel et al. [61] reported that the prevalence of active HCMV infection in HIV-positive individuals was significantly higher in symptomatic than asymptomatic children. In addition, there was a significant association between HCMV infection and mortality among symptomatic children. Webster et al. [211] also reported that HCMV infection correlated with an accelerated disease progression in HIV-infected hemophiliacs.

HCMV and Human Cancers

Due to the ubiquity of this virus, it is extremely difficult, almost impossible, to provide epidemiological evidence with biostatistical significance for the causal association of HCMV with any human malignancy. It has been previously demonstrated that HCMV or its genome can be readily detected in various human cancers [93]. But its omnipresentation argues against a direct etiological role and is mostly considered as an opportunistic infection. Nevertheless, this virus possesses many of the biological and biochemical characteristics associated with that of many other oncogenic DNA viruses and herpesviruses (see Rosenthal and Choudhury, Chap. 20, this volume) and therefore further consideration of a role for HCMV in cancer is warranted.

Activation of fos, jun and myc Cellular Protooncogene Expression

HCMV has been shown to be able to activate important cellular protooncogenes (*fos*, *jun* and *myc*) right at the time of viral attachment, prior to HCMV IE gene expression [13] (see Albrecht et al., Chap. 19, this volume). Albrecht's group has provided experimental evidence that the HCMV envelope, in addition to facilitating viral entry, selectively transduces signalling systems and subsequently *fos*, *jun*, and *myc* gene expression. The activation process starts with the ligands on the viral envelope binding to membrane receptors. The binding of this ligand(s) to a cellular receptor complex linked to phospholipase-C (via a G protein) can lead to the hydrolysis of phosphatidyl inositol diphosphate (PIP_2) and subsequently activate two secondary messenger systems [2] as shown in Fig. 1. One of these, inositol 1,4,5-triphosphate (IP_3), is formed by the hydrolysis of phosphatidyl inositol diphosphate (PIP_2) and induces the release of Ca^{2+} from the endoplasmic reticulum and calciosomes. The second product of PIP_2 hydrolysis, 1,2-diacylglycerol (DG), can activate protein kinase C and increase arachidonic acid (AA) metabolism.

Activation of Cellular Machinery Involved in Cell Proliferation

HCMV infection of the cell activates the cellular replication machinery or, more accurately, derepresses cellular enzymes associated with cell proliferation. Under normal lytic infections, this machinery is used primarily for viral DNA and viral progeny synthesis. But under nonpermissive environments HCMV infection or reactivation of latent virus could result in cellular DNA synthesis and uncontrolled cell growth. More specifically, productive HCMV infection induces a "G1/S"-like state resulting in the formation of DNA-protein complexes which have recently been identified as important for activating cell cycle progression through G1 and S phase. The proteins involved are cyclins whose periodicity suggest, and some recent studies demonstrate, that they play important roles in regulating the cell cycle.

Complementation experiments in yeast have shown that many cyclins are involved in key commitment stages of the cell cycle. These steps include initiating G1 and progressing past what has been called the restriction point (early G1) in higher eukaryotes (which is somewhat analogous to START in the yeast system), the transition through G1/S, establishing S phase, and commitment to mitosis in G2/M. Many of these cyclins form higher ordered structures which create protein kinase activities specific for nuclear targets such as histone H1 proteins [157]. Some of these complexes involve the cell cycle regulated (by phosphorylation) retinoblastoma (Rb) gene product (p105Rb). This protein as well as p53, another component of cell cycle regulation, have been described as "antioncogenes" and "tumor suppressors" for their ability to reverse aspects of cell transformation when overexpressed in cell cultures; mutations in Rb were originally identified as the cause of familial retinoblastoma and p53 is commonly mutated in colon cancers.

Recent studies have demonstrated that at least two cell cycle-regulated protein complexes bind DNA through the transcription factor E2F [10, 29, 40, 140, 185]. This factor was originally described as a cellular factor necessary for activation of the adenovirus E2 gene. In adenovirus infections, the virally encoded oncoprotein E1A releases cellular stores of E2F enabling another adenovirus product, E4, to bind two E2F molecules and specify its interaction to the E2 promoter, thereby activating expression of the E2 protein [146]. In uninfected cells, the E2F protein is associated with at least two different complexes. These protein-DNA interactions occur in the G1 and S phases of the cell cycle. One contains E2F and p105Rb, where p105Rb is in the "inactive" underphosphorylated form. It is suspected that this complex is transcriptionally inactive and may play a role in suppressing genes regulated by E2F. The other complex contains E2F in association with p107 (a protein closely related to p105Rb), cyclin A, and $p33^{cdk2}$. Cyclin A is present in G1 through S phases and has recently been shown necessary for completion of these stages. In addition, its degradation has been shown to be necessary for mitosis to proceed to completion. And $p33^{cdk2}$ is a tyrosine protein kinase, which in interactions with cyclins, is given substrate specificity.

The role of the DNA-bound E2F/p107/cyclin A/$p33^{cdk2}$ complex is unclear; however the combination of a transcription factor and proteins intimately associated with cell cycle progression suggest an important function for this grouping. In fact, a recent study of HCMV-infected cells suggest this complex may be necessary for transcriptional activation of genes regulated by E2F

[209 a]. When HCMV infects primary fibroblasts, a complex similar, if not identical, to the DNA-binding E2F/p107/cyclin A/$p33^{cdk2}$ complex is strongly induced. The presence of this complex correlates with the transcriptional activation of the DHFR promoter which is regulated by E2F and whose expression is intimately tied to DNA replication and G1/S. Concomitantly, p105Rb is hyperphosphorylated, a form which does not associate with E2F (T. F. Kowalik and E. S. Huang, unpublished observations). In addition, many of the other genes whose expression precedes DNA replication (DNA polymerases, RNA polymerase, thymidine kinase, topoisomerase II, ornithine decarboxylase, etc.) are also induced upon infection with HCMV [12, 51, 91, 206]. Furthermore, ornithine decarboxylase, an enzyme associated with cell transformation, synthesis is also enhanced upon HCMV infection [96]. The promoters of several of these genes have recently been found to contain E2F *cis* element.

Why HCMV would then induce such a complex now becomes clear. The virus is stimulating a G1/S-like phase to activate the cellular machinery which is needed to replicate its own genome. The other incentive to activate transcription through E2F is to stimulate several virally encoded early genes which appear to be regulated by E2F. These include the 2.2-kb and 2.7 kb E transcripts described by Spector's laboratory [111, 190, 204, 220] and pp65 and pp71, whose E2F sites were identified as octamer sequences by Stenberg (see Chap. 17, this volume). This latter situation is interesting in that the HCMV major IE gene products are sufficient to transcriptionally activate E2F containing promoters and pp65/71 have recently been shown to stimulate the major IE promoter [36 a, 121 a] (J. F. Baskar et al., in preparation). The result is the potential creation of a positive feedback loop; expression of the IE genes activates expression of pp65 and pp71, which in turn enhance the activity of the major IE promoter.

The effect that HCMV infection would have on p53 is not clear. As stated earlier, p53 has been shown to be associated with several cancers and is believed to play a role in downregulating cell growth by suppressing expression of many genes while activating others. The mechanism(s) by which p53 causes these responses is not clear. The apparent necessity to sequester p53 by viruses, especially transforming viruses, has been observed with SV40 and papillomaviruses. Both viruses produce a protein, large T and E6, respectively, which specifically binds to p53. A protein with such a function has not yet been demonstrated for HCMV. In fact, the level of p53 expression and phosphorylation during HCMV infection appears to remain constant (T. F. Kowalik and E. S. Huang, unpublished observation). However, we have observed that overexpression of p53 results in suppressed expression of the major IE promoter (E. S. Huang et al., unpublished observation), suggesting that HCMV may need to inactivate p53 activity for optimal IE gene expression.

Activation of Enzymes Associated with Cellular Macromolecular Synthesis and Cell Proliferation

Instead of shutting down host-cell macromolecule synthesis, as does herpes simplex virus, HCMV is able to stimulate the synthesis of numerous enzymes relating to cellular DNA synthesis. Enzymes studied include thymidine kinase, DNA polymerase, topoisomerase, RNA polymerase, and ornithine decarboxylase, etc., as described above. The ability to stimulate the synthesis of these enzymes provides the biochemical criteria for the oncogenic potential of this virus. Furthermore, Gonczol and Plotkin [72] demonstrated that HCMV infection induced the secretion of extracellular macromolecules with biochemical and biological characteristics resembling that of growth factors. Susan Michelson's laboratory also found that HCMV infection of fibroblasts induced a type II heparin-binding growth factor which stimulated human endothelial cell proliferation [4]. These results imply the possible role of HCMV in oncogenesis as well as angiogenesis.

Ornithine decarboxylase is an enzyme involved in the first rate-limiting reaction in the biosynthesis of protamine which is then frequently linked to cellular DNA synthesis. Increase of this enzyme activity was found to be associated with and to precede DNA synthesis. The level of this enzyme in normal stationary phase cells is relatively low, but increases substantially upon infection of cells with tumor viruses [96]. In HCMV-infected fibroblasts, a great degree of stimulation of this enzyme activity was found by 12-h postinfection. Another important enzyme affected by HCMV infection is plasminogen activator. This is an enzyme which is able to convert plasminogen into plasmin, and the plasmin, in turn, is able to hydrolyze fibrin. This enzyme appears to be closely related to malignant transformation. Transformation of cells by DNA and RNA tumor viruses frequently leads to enhanced synthesis of plasminogen activator. The stimulation of plasminogen activator in HCMV-infected cells does not require virus DNA synthesis. Therefore, it is suggested that the stimulation of this enzyme activity in an early gene function of HCMV [223].

HCMV Transforming DNA Sequences

The concept of oncogenicity of HCMV has been further supported by the ability of this virus to morphologically transform various mammalian cells in vitro. Albrecht and Rapp [3] first demonstrated, and Boldogh et al. [16] later confirmed, that UV-irradiated HCMV is able to transform hamster embryonic fibroblasts. The transformed cell lines were tumorigenic in golden Syrian hamsters. The resultant tumors were poorly differentiated fibrosarcomas and HCMV antigens were found in the cytoplasm and on the cell surface. Nelson et al. [142] transfected NIH3T3 cells with cloned AD169 strain HCMV DNA fragments to identify the transforming region(s) of HCMV. From mapping and transfection experiments they have found that the transforming region was in the 2.9-kb XbaI/HindIII-NE fragment (or the XbaI-N fragment). By exonuclease III and S1 sequential digestion of the 2.9 kb XbaI/HindIII-NE transforming subfragment, they were able to define the transforming region to the size of 172 bp. This implies that morphological transformation of NIH3T3 cells can be achieved by small pieces of viral DNA without any obvious ORF. The DNA sequence of this small piece of transforming sequence revealed a stem like hairpin structure resembling that of bacteria insertion elements.

In Syrian hamster embryo (SHE) cell system, Clanton et al. [30] were able to morphologically transform SHE cells with cloned Towne strain XbaI E fragment. This Towne XbaI E fragment was found to be homologous to the BglII transforming fragments N and C of herpes simplex virus-2 (HSV-2), but lacking homology to the 2.9-kb subfragment (mtr I) mentioned above (see Rosenthal and Choudhury, Chap. 20, this volume). Rosenthal's group has further subfragmented the Towne XbaI E fragment with BamHI and found that the subclones containing Xba/BamHI fragments EM and EJ were each active in transforming NIH3T3 and Rat-2 cells, but synergy in transformation was observed when both fragments were used together. These two transforming fragments were subsequently termed mrtII and mtrIII, respectively. The details of the stem-loop structures, transforming activity and possible ORFs are described in Chap. 20 of Rosenthal and Choudhury (this volume).

On the other hand, spontaneous release of HCMV from established cell lines derived from human tissues has been reported [63, 216, 217]. A virus strain called Major was spontaneously released from a prostate cell line from a child. This cell line grew in vitro to a passage level well above the expected life span. This virus was, therefore, used to study transforming ability by low multiplicity of infection (0.001 PFU/cell). After a crisis period, foci of morphologically transformed cells appeared and transformed cell lines were established. Viral specific antigens could be detected by immunofluorescence and immunocytotoxicity tests [63]. Viral DNA had been found in one of the transformed cell lines at 0.3 genome equivalents per cell at early passage (p48), but become undetectable after prolonged cultivation in vitro [92]. In human fibroblasts, we were able to obtain several HCMV transformed cell lines by both DNA transfection using XbaI or HindIII fragmented HCMV DNA or by low multiplicity of infection of HEL or WI38 cells with infectious virus (0.001 PFU per cell). HCMV-specific antigen and viral specific mRNA could be detected in transformed foci by immunofluorescent tests and by in situ DNA-RNA cytohybridization. A total of three continuous cell lines were established from cultures transfected with Xba I HCMV DNA fragment, and eight from HCMV low multiplicity infected HEL and WI38 cells. These transformed cell lines were able to grow in soft agar and produce tumors in athymic nude mice. HCMV DNA sequences corresponding to mtr I could be detected in all 11 transformed cell lines by the polymerase chain reaction, but not by routine Southern blot hybridization using radioactive DNA probes derived from HindIII E or XbaI E fragment of HCMV Ad169 or Towne strain, respectively.

HCMV in Human Cancer Tissues

As stated previously a major setback in the epidemiological analyses of the association of HCMV with human cancers is viral ubiquity and the high prevalence of HCMV antibodies in asymptomatic control populations. To date, HCMV has been found at high frequencies in carcinomatous tissues from Kaposi's sarcoma [15, 41, 69], prostatic adenocarcinoma [14, 178], adenocarcinoma of the colon [83, 95], and cervical cancers [92, 132]. Seroimmunology, virus isolation, and nucleic acid hybridization were the technologies mostly employed for studying these associations. Again, whether HCMV is a passenger virus or plays an etiological or coetiological role will require extensive investigation (for details see Rosenthal and Choudhury, Chap. 20, this volume).

Kaposi's Sarcoma. Kaposi's sarcoma (KS) is a multifocal idiopathic pigmented hemorrhagic sarcoma with an extremely obscure nature. The classic KS is a rare disease in Europe and America, but high in Blacks in some equatorial countries of Africa. It is one of the most common solid tumors in Kenya, where it constitutes close to 2.5% of all malignant tumors [114]. The prevalence rate is also higher among Italian or Jewish descendants as compared to other races in Europe and America [176]. Through an extensive seroepidemiological study and molecular hybridization detection scheme, Giraldo and his colleagues showed a significant association between HCMV infection and classic KS in European and American KS patients [68, 69]. More recently, an increased incidence of KS has been found in patients with AIDS [177]. The clinical features of AIDS-KS are considerably different from that of the classic form, occurring in younger patients, generally widespread and often involving the skin, mucous membranes of the gastrointestinal tract, lymph nodes, and other organs. HCMV antigens and DNA have also been demonstrated in KS biopsy specimens from homosexual men with AIDS [41, 191].

It has been recently demonstrated in culture systems that IL-6, tat transactivating protein of HIV, and oncostatin M are important growth factors for AIDS-KS-derived cells [136, 137]. A variety of other cytokines, including IL-1β, TNF-α, TGF-β and IL-4, have been shown to modulate IL-6 activity and to have effects on the proliferation of cultured AIDS-KS cells. As HCMV infections of monocytes and differentiated macrophages greatly enhances the synthesis of IL-1β, TNF-α and CSF-1, we believe that HCMV could at least play a cofactor role in the pathogenesis and proliferation of AIDS-KS.

Oncostatin M, a cytokine produced by activated lymphoid cells, is one of the most potent mitogens for KS cells in culture. It has the ability to transform the morphological phenotype of cells to spindle cells and to facilitate the proliferation of AIDS-KS derived cells in semisolid agar. Oncostatin M RNA and immunoreactive protein could be found in AIDS-KS-derived cell isolates. It has been, therefore, suggested that oncostatin M may play an important role in the pathogenesis of AIDS-KS [136]. It may well be of importance for us to study the effects of HCMV on oncostatin M expression in both permissive and nonpermissive HCMV-infected cells.

Cervical and Liver Cancers. Cervical tissue is a leading candidate for development of cancer in women. This is especially the case in societies with less access to proper hygiene and preventative screening. Cervical carcinoma is a classic example of multiple progression from hyperplastic growth through neoplastic transformation and metastasis. Epidemiological studies have shown a strong correlation between cervical carcinoma and human papillomaviruses (HPV). In the vast majority of cervical carcinomas, as well as precancerous lesions of human uterine cervix, HPV DNA sequences (such as HPV types 6, 11, 16 and 18) are frequently found [47, 70]. However, the same HPV types are also found in normal cervical epithelial cells in other individuals and no HPV has been observed in some cervical carcinomas. It is therefore thought that HPV may be necessary for most cases of cervical carcinoma but is not sufficient for this state alone. A second "hit" or insult is apparently required for the fully transformed state. Laboratory studies have substantiated this hypothesis observing that the activated c-*ras* protooncogene together with HPV can efficiently transform cells. A role for herpesviruses as this second hit has also been hypothesized.

At least two herpesviruses, HCMV and HSV-2, have been shown to be sexually transmitted and frequently found in the cervix. HSV-2 is associated with anogenital lesions, as are some HPV types. HCMV is the leading cause of virally associated birth defects and has been observed frequently in cervix, semen, and sperm. Both viruses have biological activities befitting of a coactivator. HCMV has been shown to be commonly associated with cervical carcinoma, although its prevalence is less than that of HPV (see Rosenthal and Choudhury, Chap. 20, this volume; [92, 132]). Preliminary studies have shown a synergistic ability of HPV and HCMV to transform mouse fibroblasts [112]. Similar observations were also demonstrated by Goldstein et al. [71] in the enhanced transformation of mouse cells by bovine papillomavirus following HCMV infection. In addition, infection of primary foreskin keratinocytes with HCMV results in transactivation of the HPV promoter regulating the expression of its oncogenic E6 and E7 proteins (T. F. Kowalik et al., in preparation). Obviously, a clear demonstration of causality or coetiology of HCMV in cervical cancer is very difficult and only circumstantial arguments, backed by laboratory experimentation, can be made.

A similar scenario with HCMV having a coetiological role with hepatitis B virus (HBV) is plausible. HCMV has a perpensity for infecting the liver. In neonates, HCMV has been implicated as the leading cause of hepatitis (see Chang and Lee, Chap. 3). No similar cause and effect case can be made for adult hepatitis where several hepatitis viruses have been shown to cause this disease. The long-term harboring of HBV has been associated with an increased likelihood of contracting liver cancer. The dual association of HCMV and HBV in liver disease suggests that coetiology should be considered. In the laboratory, it has been shown that HCMV infection can stimulate the expression of the promoter-enhancer sequences of the HBV core and surface antigens, respectively (E.-S. Haung and L.-B. Ting, unpublished data). Epidemiological and continued molecular studies are needed to further develop this hypothesis.

Prostate Adenocarcinoma and Benign Hypertrophy of the Prostate. Adenocarcinoma and benign hypertrophy of the prostate are two of the most common illnesses of the American male. The etiologies of these diseases are still unknown. Some preliminary observations imply that HSV and HCMV might play some role in the induction of prostatic malignancy. Lymphocytes from patients with prostatic adenocarcinoma were cytotoxic to HCMV-infected and HCMV-transformed cells that bore viral membrane antigens [178]. The peripheral lymphocytes from 84% of patients with prostatic carcinoma were able to kill HCMV-transformed cells. In addition, sera from prostatic cancer patients were able to block the specific cytotoxicity generated by their lymphocytes [178]. These cellular immunologic data strongly suggest an association of HCMV infection with adenocarcinoma of the prostate, and the long-term persistence of the oncogenic Major strain HCMV in a cell line derived from prostatic tissue makes this speculation even more attractive [160]. Furthermore, Boldogh et al. [14] analyzed surgically removed human prostate samples, including normal, benign hypertrophic, and adenocarcinomatous specimens, for the presence of HCMV and HSV by nucleic acid hybridization and immunofluorescent tests. Experimental results showed 33% of benign hypertrophy and 40% of adenocarcinoma, and only 15.4% of normal prostates carried HCMV DNA or antigens.

HCMV and Atherosclerosis

Atherosclerosis has many of the hallmarks anticipated in an HCMV infection. This disease is characterized by atherosclerotic plaques consisting of complex accumulations produced by arterial smooth muscle cells, deposition of lipids, and associated fibrosis. The arterial smooth muscle cells have been stimulated to proliferate at the plaque site, possibly due to injury of the endothelial lining of the artery resulting in the exposure of smooth muscle cells to hormones, low density lipid and other growth-promoting factors (see Melnick et al., Chap. 4, this volume). In addition, the many enlarged cells associated with this lipid deposition are macrophage derivatives. Targeting of the monocyte/macrophage lineage and fibroblasts by HCMV in vivo and in vitro and the ability of this virus to cause the overexpression of many genes upon the appropriate stimulus (e.g., hormones, lipoproteins, and growth factors associated with serum and platelets) in these and other cells has been implicated as manifestations of HCMV infections (see Albrecht et al., Chap. 18 and Melnick et al., Chap. 4, this volume). In addition, HCMV viremia is frequently encountered, and virus-infected cells are often detected in lesions taken from patients with atherosclerosis. High levels of antibodies to HCMV were found to associate with clinically manifested atherosclerotic disease. Furthermore, the biological properties of HCMV are consistent with the pathological involvement of this virus at several levels of the atherogenic process (for details see Melnick et al., Chap. 4, this volume). Therefore, we should not overlook the role of HCMV in this pathological event by viewing its ubiquity.

Disease States and Clinical Features Associated with HCMV Infection

In general, HCMV is a herpesvirus with low pathogenicity. The outcome of HCMV infection is frequently determined by the status and competency of host immunity and, in the case of intrauterine fetal HCMV infection, the developmental stage at the time of infection.

Congenital HCMV Infection

Approximately 1%–2% of infants are infected in utero and another 6%–60% become infected during the first 6 months of life as the result of birth canal or breast milk transmissions [87, 163]. Primary infection has varied from 0.7%–4% (with an average of 2%–2.5%) per gestation among susceptible seronegative women [6, 195]. Risk of congenital HCMV infection following primary infection of the mother during the pregnancy is around 54%. The chance of such a baby being symptomatically infected is around 41% [87].

Immune mothers may also give birth to congenitally infected infants by viral reactivation and transplacental infection, but the result is usually asymptomatic [196]. However, there are exceptions. Ahlfors et al. [1] reported a case of a neonate suffering from HCMV induced hepatosplenomegaly and petechiae at birth and later was found to be bilaterally deaf. In this case, HCMV was isolated from urine 1 week after birth, and the mother was found to have been seropositive 2 years prior to pregnancy. Congenital HCMV infection also can occur in consecutive pregnancies. Embil et al. [49] reported a case of two consecutive children born of an 18-year-old Caucasian. The first child had disseminated CMV infection and died within 30 days after birth. The second child was born within a year and had viruria at birth for 8.5 months and viremia at 5 months of age but was otherwise asymptomatic. Stagno et al. [197] also reported two siblings born 3 years apart with congenital HCMV infections. The first child had viruria at birth, severe growth retardation, hepatosplenomegaly, and severe psychomotor retardation at later ages. The second child had viruria at birth but was normal in other aspects. In most cases, congenital HCMV transmission from immune mothers is usually asymptomatic or less severe in their clinical manifestation (see [87] for details).

The clinical features of symptomatic congenital infections have been extensively described in previous reviews [80, 87, 212, 221]. Harry T. Wright described the clinical features of CID of infancy as a symptomatic complex which included (1) jaundice; (2) petechiae; (3) chorioretinitis; (4) microcephaly; (5) central nervous system disease (such as seizures, spastic diplegia, deafness and microphthalmia); (6) HCMV pneumonia; (7) hepatosplenomegaly; (8) psychomotor retardation; (9) mental retardation; (10) diarrhea; (11) thrombocytopenia; (12) cerebral calcifications; (13) chronic gastroenteritis; and (14) prematurity [221]. In addition, patients with severe and prolonged illness due to

HCMV have growth retardation, appearing in approximately 35% of CID infants. In a longitudinal study of 20 patients with CID, McCracken and associates [129] observed several patients that had abnormal findings related to the heart and liver. Over one third of the infants had structural abnormalities in the organs derived from the first embryonic arch; these included high arched palate, soft and hard cleft palates, micrognathia, facial weakness, and deafness. These clinical manifestations are more likely to result from primary infections occurring during the first trimester of gestation.

In addition to the complex syndrome of CID described above, Hanshaw [81] also pointed out additional abnormalities resulting from HCMV teratogenic effects. These include unusual ocular abnormalities (such as microphthalmia, cataracts, blindness, and malformation of the interior eye chamber), cardiovascular anomalies (such as atrial septal defect, anomalous venous return), gastrointestinal anomalies (esophageal atresis and malformed pylorus), genitourinary anomalies (such as hypospadias), pulmonary anomalies (such as thymic hypoplasia), and musculoskeletal anomalies (such as clubfeet and spastic diplegia). On the long-term follow-up of 20 infants with congenital cytomegalic inclusion diseases, Wright [221] further described the expanded syndromes appearing at later stages of life. These include eye defects, hearing loss, abnormal EEG, congenital heart disease, unusual dermatoglyphics, retarded bone age, hypoplastic lumbar spine, unusual urine chromatography, and inguinal hernia. Prolonged follow-up studies of surviving infants with congenital HCMV infection should lead to the recognition of more expanded syndromes due to HCMV infection.

A number of late sequelae of congenital infections have been described, including persistent HCMV shedding, low IQ, sensorineural hearing loss, and other various auditory defects (for details see review in [87]). In studying the microbial causes of mental retardation, Stern et al. [200] found that HCMV was the most important agent among three common suspects (HCMV, rubella and toxoplasma) in causing metal deficiency. HCMV accounted for about 10% of microcephalic types of mental retardation. Rubella and toxoplasmosis together were responsible for 2%–3% of cases of mental retardation.

Perinatal HCMV Infection

Perinatal HCMV transmission often results from infected uterine cervix, birth canal, milk and colostrum, and other maternal reservoirs. Substantial proportions of infants (8%–60%) become infected during the first 6 months of life; most of them are asymptomatic. On the other hand, perinatal infection can be symptomatic or even end in death if HCMV is transmitted to the immature neonate via transfusions [87]. Kumar et al. [113] reported on 21 perinatally infected infants. Seven were symptomatic and developed pneumonitis, lymphadenopathy, hepatosplenomegaly, and rash, but seemed to develop normally. In contrast, Whitely et al. [214] only observed one out of 96 perinatally acquired HCMV infections which developed into HCMV pneumonitis with lower respiratory obstruction. In general, immature infants are more susceptible to perinatal HCMV infections. These infections may result in symptomatic presentations such as pneumonitis, neuromuscular disability [20], bronchopulmonary dysplasia [180], and delay in speech [75].

HCMV Infection in Immunocompetent Individuals

In immunocompetent individuals, HCMV infection usually is asymptomatic, or, at the most, produces a self-limited mononucleosis syndrome. With distinctions from Epstein-Barr virus(EBV)-induced mononucleosis, HCMV mononucleosis is serologically identified to be heterophile-negative and occurs in an older age group; it is uncommon in children. Primary infection is presumably generalized. Transmission of infections can be through body fluids (including saliva, semen, urine, and blood) via oral or orogenital contact or by blood transfusion. Viral latency can be established after primary infection. Recurrent infections occur frequently during pregnancy and in immunosuppressed states. HCMV antibodies of IgM, IgG, and IgA classes can be detected in immunocompetent people during primary and recurrent infections and vary in the antibody titers and time course of appearance. Unlike the humoral immune response, cell-mediated immunity is depressed in symptomatic primary infections. The blood cells from acute HCMV mononucleosis patients have been observed to be hyperresponsive to certain nonspecific mitogens and interferon production diminished [167].

The outcome of HCMV infection in immunocompetent patients is heavily dependent on HCMV-specific protective immunities, both at the humoral and cellular levels. In congenital infection, preexisting maternal immunity prevents severe HCMV-induced disease [195]. The same is observed in organ transplant patients where the preexisting immunity to HCMV limits diseases and syndromes associated with HCMV infection (see Ho, Chap. 10, this volume; [87]). In natural HCMV infections, immunocompetent humans respond to virus-encoded envelope proteins (gp65 or GC1, gp86 or gH, gp65 or gB), capsid proteins (p155, p37, and p12), tegument proteins (pp200, pp149, pp71, and pp65), and nonstructural proteins (pp49 DNA binding protein, pp72 major IE1, and pp84 major IE2). Among them, only antibodies against viral envelope glycoprotein have functional neutralization activity [21]. In view of the fact that passive immunization with HCMV antibodies reduced both the incidence of infection and clinical manifestation of HCMV-related interstitial pneumonia in bone marrow and organ transplant patients, it is therefore believable that protective antibodies to HCMV do exist [21]. Humoral antibodies are important in antibody dependent cell lysis and in inhibition of virus absorption, fusion, assembly, and cell-to-cell spread.

A number of structural and nonstructural HCMV proteins, particularly glycoproteins, have been demonstrated to provoke helper T (T_h) and cytotoxic/suppressor T-cell (T_c) responses. It has been shown that MHC class I-restricted cytotoxic T lymphocytes displaying CD8 play an important role in host defense to HCMV infection. Cytotoxic T_c cells recognizing the major IE proteins of HCMV were important for recovery from acute HCMV infection and for preventing reactivation of latent virus [17, 64]. Also, Lindsley et al. [121 b] demonstrated MHC class II (DR)-restricted cytotoxicity against HCMV in the T-lymphocyte subset with the CD4 marker (helper/inducer cells). Therefore, both T_h and T_c lymphocytes are involved in MHC-restricted cytotoxicity.

There are two more kinds of cytotoxic cell killing which do not require histocompatibility between effectors and target cells. One is the antibody-dependent, cell-mediated cytotoxicity (ADCC) which requires a killer cell (K cell) that possesses Fc receptors on the cell surface [107]. Another kind of cytotoxic response is mediated by the natural killer (NK) cell, a non-B, non-T, large granular lymphocyte that carries Fc receptor for IgG on its surface. Antibody is not needed for its killing effect. The role of these two classes of cytotoxic lymphocytes in controlling HCMV infection is not known at this time and needs to be investigated.

Carney et al. [26] observed that during acute HCMV mononucleosis, the ratio of T_h and T-suppressor subsets altered (less than 1, inbetween 0.1 and 0.5) without marked change in the total number of T cells; there was an increase in CD8 cytotoxic/suppressor cells and a slight decrease or normal level of CD4 helper cells. This ratio change is quite different from that occurring in patients with HIV-induced AIDS, in whom an absolute decrease in CD4 helper cells is observed. This abnormality in lymphocyte subsets in HCMV mononucleosis persisted as long as 10 months, while EBV-induced mononucleosis only lasted for a few months [168]. Furthermore, CD8 cells from patients with CMV mononucleosis were hyposensitive to mitogenic stimulation by concanavalin A [25].

In infants and children with congenital or perinatal HCMV infection, the abnormalities in cell-mediated immunity appear different from that observed in adults with HCMV mononucleosis. In chronically or persistently infected infants or children, their lymphocytes failed to elicit the blastogenic response and failed to induce interferon production when challenged with HCMV antigen in vitro [65, 153, 154, 199]. This defect is more profound and persists longer, for years, than that in adult patients with mononucleosis [154]. The inability of antigen recognition in this case appears to be HCMV specific, because the blastogenic responses to other mitogens appear normal [153].

Levin et al. [120] and Rinaldo et al. [167] observed diminished interferon production in cells from patients with HCMV mononucleosis in response to HCMV antigenic and mitogenic stimulation. During the convalescent stage, interferon production returned to near normal levels. On the other hand, in in vitro experiments, Dudding et al. [45] were able to demonstrate the stimulation of cytokine messsages upon the infection of peripheral monocytes with HCMV.

In the mouse model, Becker and his colleagues have shown that dendritic Langerhans cells and Thy.1+ effector cells play very important roles in immune response following HSV-1 infection in the skin [192, 193]. Langerhans cells are derived from the bone marrow and express the cortical thymocyte antigen CD1 and MHC class II antigens in humans. These cells are epidermal, antigen-presenting cells that function by taking up antigens in the skin, migrating to the lymph nodes where they are designated interdigitating cells, and then triggering the immune response [194]. Unfortunately, not much research has been done regarding the role of these dendritic cells in the suprabasal epidermis, in epithelium, and in alveoli during HCMV infection. It is important for us to determine the mechanism of antigenic presentation which is essential for provoking both humoral and cellular immunities during HCMV infection (see Y. Becker, Chap. 22, this volume).

As mentioned above, HCMV may have the ability to induce cross-reactive immune responses to normal cellular antigens or induce viral immunotolerance components due to shared sequence or antigenic homology of HCMV proteins with cellular components. These molecular homologies include IE2 of HCMV with human HLA-DR β chain of class II MHC [11], and the HCMV UL18 putative glycoprotein with MHC class I α chain [62]. Furthermore, the binding of β_2-M to HCMV may effect the expression of class I MHC molecules, which may in turn hamper the host-cell immunity.

The clinical manifestations of HCMV infection in immunocompetent older children and adults are usually mild and patients appear reasonably well. However, not only primary HCMV infection, but also reactivation/reinfection by HCMV can result in mononucleosis in these individuals [90]. Classical manifestations of HCMV mononucleosis include malaise, headache, myalgia, protracted fever, abnormalities in liver functions, hepatosplenomegaly, and atypical lymphocytosis. Other clinical complications such as interstitial pneumonitis, subclinical myocarditis, pericarditis, CNS involvement (Guillain-Barré syndrome and other neuritis), acute and chronic encephalitis, aseptic meningitis, thrombocytopenic purpura, hemolytic anemia, gastroenteritis, hepatitis, retinitis and epidermolysis occasionally occur in severe cases of HCMV mononucleosis [6, 87].

HCMV and Guillain-Barré Syndrome. Klemola et al. [110] first reported a case of Guillain-Barré syndrome with HCMV mononucleosis. In this report, a 27-year-old man had a fever for 4 days with motor and sensory deficits starting distally and progressing proximally from the extremities. Three weeks later he had symmetrical paresis of Vth and VIIth nerve, marked paresis of the upper and lower extremities, and sensory loss reaching the chest. Recovery began 1 month after onset and was complete in 6 months. Increase in CMV CF-antibody titer was detected and HCMV was isolated from urine specimens. Later on, Leonard and Tobin [119] reported nine cases from England and Schmitz and Enders [181] reported 19 cases from Germany, supporting the association of HCMV with Guillain-Barré syndrome. Most of the cases began with signs of upper respiratory infections, fever, headache, and progressive peripheral neuropathy. Involvement of the respiratory muscles was also common.

HCMV and Charcot-Marie-Tooth Disease. Charcot-Marie-Tooth disease is a familial, demyelinating, peripheral neuropathy which exhibits decreased nerve conduction velocities with contractures of feet and hands [48]. Williams et al. [217] identified an HCMV strain, CMT-6, spontaneously released from a cell line derived from intact human skin of a Charcot-Marie-Tooth disease patient. Subsequently, by DNA-DNA reassociation kinetics analysis they were able to detect the HCMV genome in three of four skin fibroblast cell lines derived from Charcot-Marie-Tooth disease patients at 0.2–2 genome equivalents per cell level [216]. The significance of this finding is not clear; further studies have to be undertaken to make any conclusions.

HCMV and Postperfusion Syndrome. Postperfusion syndrome can result from primary infection or virus reactivation in children as well as in adults following the administration of large volumes of blood or blood products [31, 60, 115] (see Hamilton, Chap. 9, this volume). A typical form of postperfusion syndrome occurs between 3 and 6 weeks after administration of blood. In the normal individual, adult or child, it is usually indistinguishable from spontaneous mononucleosis. With a mild disease, the course of postperfusion syndrome is self-limited with a duration of approximately 3 weeks [221]. Previous studies indicated that fever occurred between 21 and 34 days after surgery. Splenomegaly, atypical lymphocytosis, lymphadenopathy, and occasional rash were considered part of the syndrome (see review [87]). Splenomegaly appears more often in patients with postperfusion syndrome than in patients with spontaneous HCMV mononucleosis. It persists for weeks to months after infection with relative lymphocytosis in the absence of leukocytosis. Symptomatic disease is particularly obvious following blood transfusions in premature or immunocompromised neonates [224].

HCMV and Diabetes Mellitus. The association of HCMV with diabetes mellitus has been suggested, but is still inconclusive [87, 152, 210]. The pancreas, including the islets of Langerhans, is a target of HCMV in congenital infections [102]. In one study, approximately 44% of the children who died of disseminated HCMV infection had characteristic HCMV inclusion bodies in islet cells [102]. Pak et al. [152] studied the lymphocytes of 59 cases of type 1 diabetic patients and found that HCMV genomes were detected in 22% of the diabetic patients but only in 2.6% of the controls. Patients with HCMV in their lymphocytes had a higher frequency of islet cell antibody (62%) and cytotoxic β-cell surface antibody (69%) than patients without HCMV in lymphocytes. In this case, the association of HCMV with type 1 diabetes mellitus has biostatistic significance, $p < 0.05$. Numazaki et al. [148] successfully infected cultures of fetal islets of Langerhans with HCMV. HCMV CPE was found 4 days after infection. Infectious progeny was recovered and viral late antigen was detected. However, β-cells were not infected and insulin production was not affected by HCMV infection. Further studies of this nature are needed for this important implication [87].

HCMV Hepatitis. HCMV is one of the important etiological agents of neonatal hepatitis. Either congenital or perinatal infection of HCMV can cause neonatal hepatitis (see Chang and Lee, Chap. 3, this volume). Hanshaw et al. [82] demonstrated that close to 39% of children with hepatomegaly or chronic liver diseases had evidence of HCMV infection. McCracken et al. [129] also found that 18 of 20 infants with hepatitis had congenital infection. Abnormal liver function was observed six times more often in the virus-positive group than in the controls. In one study carried out in Taiwan, 78% of the 46 infants with neonatal hepatitis showed positive for HCMV by PCR, while 54% of these 46 infants with hepatitis had evidence of CMV infection with either urine culture or positive serology (Chang and Lee, Chap. 3, this volume). All of these results strongly suggest that liver diseases can be caused by HCMV. Although abnormal liver functions are frequently observed in HCMV mononucleosis of the adult population, severe hepatitis with profound abnormalities of liver function are encountered on rare occasions within immunocompetent individuals. One important molecular biological aspect of HCMV infection in the liver is the possible interaction between HCMV and HBV. As mentioned above, our preliminary data indicates that HCMV IE gene products can transactivate the expression of HBV core as well as surface antigen promoters in hepatocytes and more differentiated hepatocarcinoma cell lines (E.S. Huang and L.P. Ting, unpublished data). Therefore, the coetiological role of HCMV in hepatocarcinoma also requires attention.

HCMV and Hematological Disorders. The ability of HCMV to infect many blood cell types both latently and productively warrants consideration of the results of these interactions. Likely primary targets for typical blood-borne HCMV infection in vivo are monocytes, macrophages, the endothelial cells lining blood vessels, and even megakaryocytes – each of which has been shown susceptible to HCMV infection in vitro. Infection of these cells usually results in persistent infections producing altered expression of genes encoding cytokines [45]. It is unclear at this moment whether the infection of megakaryocytes by HCMV will result in thrombocytopenia. Hemolytic anemia and thrombocytopenia are frequent in and often result in severe manifestations in congenital HCMV infections [55, 226], but may also occur in adults as a complication of HCMV mononucleosis.

HCMV and Other Clinical Manifestations. Gastrointestinal disease is the most prominent manifestation of HCMV infection in a population of heart and heart-lung transplant patients with an incident of 9.9%, occurring most frequently in HCMV-seronegative recipients of organs from HCMV-seropositive donors [104]. Clinical manifestations include gastritis, gastric ulceration, duodenitis, esophagitis, pyloric perforation, and colonic hemorrhage. Gastrointestinal tract and dermatological involvements were relatively rare complications in the past, but become increasingly more important in patients with AIDS (see review [87]; Vinters and Ferreiro, Chap. 2, this volume). HCMV-induced pneumonitis and retinitis are frequently observed in organ transplant patients, but are not such dominant complications as in patients with AIDS (see "Clinical Manifestations in Immunocompromised Individuals"). Miscellaneous reports of association of HCMV with acute ulcerative colitis, conjunctivitis, and vasculitis have been documented in the past. Details can be obtained from the review by Ho [87].

Clinical Manifestations in Immunocompromised Individuals

Populations at greatest risk of HCMV infection and HCMV-induced diseases are those undergoing organ transplants and those with malignancies receiving immunosuppressive chemotherapy, and particularly patients with AIDS [6]. In immunocompromised hosts more severe and profound syndromes are observed when infected with HCMV, either as primary or recurrent infections. Similarly, morbidity and mortality are also increased with HCMV infection in patients of this group. Due to the severe and complex immune deficiency in AIDS patients, HCMV often causes disseminated infections frequently involving multiple organ systems in these subjects. The most common sites of pathological involvement include adrenals (75%), lung (58%), gastrointestinal tract (30%), CNS (20%), and oculus (10%) [108].

The severity, frequency and clinical manifestation of HCMV infections in transplant recipients, cancer patients, and other immunosuppressed groups are quite variable [6]. In most of the cases, mononucleosis syndrome with fever is the common sign observed. After mononucleosis syndrome, pneumonia is the most frequent manifestation of HCMV infection in immunosuppressed patients. It is more prevalent and severe in bone marrow transplant patients, with mortality rates close to 40% [133]. Gastroenteritis and chorioretinitis are two manifestations most frequently described in association with HCMV in patients with AIDS [100] (Fiala et al., Chap. 8, this volume). Furthermore, HCMV also plays a very important role in neurologic abnormalities of patients with AIDS (see Wiley and Nelson, Chap. 7 and Fiala et al., Chap. 8, this volume).

HCMV Pneumonitis. Next to the kidneys, the lung is the most common site in which HCMV induces significant pathological changes both focal or disseminated. Giant HCMV inclusion cells are seen in the alveolar and bronchial epithelium. Related pathological findings vary from interstitial pneumonitis to diffuse alveolar damage in HCMV-induced pulmonary damage (see Vinters and Ferreiro, Chap. 2, this volume). HCMV-induced interstitial pneumonitis is frequently seen in patients with AIDS and in recipients of allogeneic organ or bone marrow transplants [73, 74, 175, 186, 218, 219]. The incidence of HCMV pneumonitis or the incidence of idiopathic pneumonitis are lower in recipients of syngeneic or autologous organ transplants than that of allogeneic transplants [76, 218, 219]. Furthermore, the pathogenesis of HCMV infection in the lungs of recipients of allogeneic transplants is more severe than, and differs remarkably from that of, syngeneic or autologous transplant recipients. It has been suggested that some effects induced by transplanted allogeneic cells attribute to this obvious variation in the outcome of the manifestation of

HCMV infected lungs rather than differences in the immunosuppression status of patients [76].

HCMV-induced interstitial pneumonia frequently develops between 30 and 80 days after allogeneic bone marrow transplantation, at the time that immunologic events occur [59]. Although HCMV is detected in bronchial alveoli, it is often present at relatively low quantities with a level disproportional to the degree of pulmonary infiltrations. It is suggested that vigorous virus replication does not occur in HCMV pneumonia and that host components might contribute to the disease itself [59]. Forman [59] suggested several risk factors for HCMV interstitial pneumonitis, including allogeneic bone marrow transplantation, acute graft-vs.-host disease, prior HCMV exposure of donor and recipient, and occurrence of active HCMV infection in lung and blood.

Grundy et al. [79] have used the murine CMV (MCMV) model to study the effect of graft-vs.-host on the induction of CMV pneumonitis. They found that MCMV increased the severity of the graft-vs.-host reaction and the development of interstitial pneumonitis in the MCMV model and that this was not related to viral replication, but rather to some component of the immune response involved in the graft-vs.-host reaction. Analysis of cells in the lungs of mice with interstitial pneumonitis showed an influx of Thy 1.2-positive cells of donor origin. The depletion of Thy 1.2-positive cells from the donor inoculum prevented the development of interstitial pneumonitis. It was, therefore, suggested that the immune response triggered by MCMV and mediated by donor lymphocytes against recipient cells in the lung was involved in the pathogenesis of CMV pneumonitis [76, 79].

HCMV Retinitis. CMV-induced chorioretinitis rarely occurs in normal individuals, but is increased substantially in immunocompromised patients, particularly in patients with AIDS. Approximately 30%–50% of AIDS patients have ocular lesions with diagnostic and prognostic significance [208]. In a study at Johns Hopkins University with a series of 157 patients with AIDS, 46 (29%) developed HCMV retinitis. Patients with ganciclovir treatment survived significantly longer than those who did no recieve this drug [99]. Clinically, when retinitis appears in AIDS patients, a poor prognosis and often a rapidly fatal outcome are expected.

HCMV retinitis may be unilateral or bilateral, unifocal or multifocal with syndromes characterized by blurred vision, decreased vision, and scotomata. In progressive retinitis, the retina frequently shows a widespread, necrotic, often hemorrhagic area. On fundoscopic examination white granular necrotic patches can be superimposed on intraretinal hemorrhages. HCMV inclusions can be found in the retina and retinal pigment epithelium. HCMV chorioretinitis can be recurrent months to years after the initial lesions heal [6]. Details related to HCMV retinitis are provided by Fiala et al. in Chap. 8 (this volume).

HCMV and Neurological Abnormalities in Patients with AIDS. HCMV infection of the CNS is very common in patients with AIDS. Approximately 20%

of autopsied cases of AIDS had evidence of HCMV involvement [139, 209]. Both central and peripheral neurological symptoms can be found. HCMV-induced encephalopathy in AIDS includes subacute encephalitis, microgial nodules, focal parenchymal necrosis, necrotizing ventriculitis, and CMV infarction [215 a] (Wiley and Nelson, Chap. 7 and Fiala et al., Chap. 8, this volume). HCMV inclusion bodies can be found in astrocytes, neurons, and capillary endothelial cells. Furthermore, HCMV has been implicated in the etiology of peripheral nerve inflammation. Cytomegalic cells and HCMV antigens were seen at the site of focal nerve root or peripheral nerves in patients with peripheral neuritis. Schwann cells are also among HCMV targets (for details see Chaps. 7 and 8, this volume).

Conclusion

Because of the ubiquitous and mysterious nature of HCMV, most of the medical problems associated with HCMV have not been adequately studied. It is believable that many more diseases or clinical manifestations, in addition to what we understand today, are associated with HCMV infection. In general, this virus does not create a significant problem in an immunocompetent host, but severe syndromes can result from either primary or recurrent infection in immunocompromised individuals or in developing fetuses. The pathogenicity of HCMV and the outcome of the virus infection frequently are determined and affected by many factors in the host (or host cells) as well as viral origins. HCMV has an extremely strong MIEP and a set of very active IE gene products. The MIEP possesses consensus sequences for a great variety of nuclear factors. Therefore, the existence of positive and negative nuclear regulatory factors within infected cells, the stage of cell differentiation, the specific humoral and cellular immunities, the availability of viral receptors on the cell surface, and the host cell environment (including the microenvironment surrounding the virus and host cell, which greatly influences the tissue-specific gene expression) are all important factors toward determining the fate of HCMV infection, such as permissiveness, latency, and reactivation. One major public health concern is that HCMV exists commonly in human semen (and in sperm) and the cervix. It can, therefore, infect fetuses, interfere with embryonic development, and cause developmental abnormalities. HCMV infection has also been attributed to numerous cases of mental retardation worldwide. Furthermore, the oncogenic potential of HCMV is strongly suggested by its ability to induce host-cell macromolecule synthesis, particular enzymes associated with cell proliferation, and its ability to transform mammalian cells in vitro. Induction of latency and subsequent reactivation of HCMV is comparable to that of other oncogenic herpesviruses. HCMV is also the most common opportunistic viral agent in patients with AIDS. It has all of the essential characteristics necessary to be considered as a coetiological agent in the progression of HIV infection towards the development of AIDS. Thus, the problems of HCMV infection observed today in organ transplant recipients and immunocompromised patients are much like the visible portion of icebergs. We shall have more poignant discussion related to the pathogenesis of HCMV in the future when sufficient attention and study of this virus has been made.

References

1. Ahlfors K, Harris S, Ivarsson S, Svanberg L (1981) Secondary maternal cytomegalovirus infection causing symptomatic congenital infection. N Engl J Med 305:284
2. Albrecht T, Fons MP, Boldogh I, AbuBakar S, Deng CZ, Millinoff D (1991) Metabolic and cellular effects of human cytomegalovirus infection. Transplant Proc 23 [Suppl 3]:48–55
3. Albrecht T, Rapp F (1973) Malignant transformation of hamster embryo fibroblasts following exposure to ultraviolet-irradiate human cytomegalovirus. Virology 55:53–61
4. Alcami J, Barzu T, Michelson S (1991) Induction of an endothelial cell growth factor by human cytomegalovirus infection of fibroblasts. J Gen Virol 72:2765–2770
5. Alexander ER (1967) Maternal and neonatal infection with cytomegalovirus in Taiwan. Pediatr Res 1:210
6. Alford CA Jr, Britt WJ (1990) Cytomegalovirus. In: Fields B et al. (eds) Virology, 2nd edn. New York
7. Andersen HK, Spenser ES (1969) Cytomegalovirus infection among renal allograft recipients. Acta Med Scand 186:7–19
8. Baeuerle PA (1991) The inducible transcription activator NF-κB: regulation by distinct protein subunit. Biochim Biophys Acta 1072:63–80
9. Baeuerle PA, Baltimore D (1988) IκB: a specific inhibitor of the NF-κB transcription factor. Science 242:540–546
10. Bandara LR, Adamaczewski JP, Hunt T, LaThangue NB (1991) Cyclin A and the retinoblastoma gene product complex with cellular transcription factor. Nature 352:249–251
11. Beck S, Barrell BG (1988) Human cytomegalovirus encodes a glycoprotein homologous to MHC class I antigens. Nature 331:269–272
12. Benson JD, Huang ES (1990) Human cytomegalovirus induces expression of cellular topoisomerase II. J Virol 64:9–15
13. Boldogh I, AbuBakar S, Albrecht T (1990) Activation of proto-oncogenes: an immediate early event in human cytomegalovirus infection. Science 247:561–564
14. Boldogh I, Baskar JF, Mar EC, Huang ES (1983) Human cytomegalovirus and herpes simplex type 2 virus in normal and adenocarcinomatous prostate glands. J Natl Cancer Inst 70:819–825
15. Boldogh I, Beth E, Huang ES, Kyalwazi KS, Giraldo G (1981) Kaposi's sarcoma: IV. Detection of CMV DNA, CMV RNA and CMNA in tumor biopsies. Int J Cancer 28:469–474
16. Boldogh I, Gonczol E, Vaczi L (1978) Transformation of hamster embryonic fibroblast cell by UV-irradiated human cytomegalovirus. Acta Microbiol Hung 25:269–275
17. Borysiewicz LK, Graham S, Hickling JK, Mason PD, Sissons JG (1988) Human cytomegalovirus specific cytotoxic T cells: their precursor frequency and stage specificity. Eur J Immunol 18:269–275
18. Borysiewicz LK, Hickling JK, Graham S, Sinclair J, Cranage MP, Smith GL, Sissons JG (1988) Human cytomegalovirus-specific cytotoxic T cells. Relative frequency of stage-specific CTL recognizing the 72-kD immediate early protein and glycoprotein B expressed by recombinant vaccinia viruses. J Exp Med 168:919–931

19. Boshart M, Weber F, Jahn G, Dorsch-Hasler K, Fleckenstein B, Schaffner W (1985) A very strong enhancer is located upstream of an immediate early gene of human cytomegalovirus. Cell 41:521–530
20. Brasfield DM, Stagno S, Whitley RJ, Cloud G, Cassell G, Tiller RE (1987) Infant pneumonitis associated with cytomegalovirus, chlamydia, pneumocystis, and ureaplasma: follow-up. Pediatrics 79:76–83
21. Britt WJ (1991) Recent advanced in the identification of significant human cytomegalovirus-encoded proteins. Transplant Proc 23 [Suppl 3]:64–68
22. Britt WJ, Auger D (1986) Human cytomegalovirus virion-associated protein with kinase activity. J Virol 59:185–188
23. Browne H, Smith G, Beck S, Minson T (1990) A complex between MHC class I homologue encoded by human cytomegalovirus and beta 2-microglobulin. Nature 347:770–772
24. Cai W, Gu B, Person S (1988) Role of glycoprotein B of herpes simplex virus type 1 in viral entry and cell fusion. J Virol 62:2596–2604
25. Careny WP, Lacoviello V, Hirsch MS (1983) Functional properties of T lymphocytes and their subsets in cytomegalovirus mononucleosis. J Immunol 130:390–393
26. Carney WP, Rubin RH, Hoffman RA, Hansen WP, Healey K, Hirsch MS (1981) Analysis of T lymphocyte subsets in cytomegalovirus mononucleosis. J Immunol 126:2114–2116
27. Chee MS, Bankier AT, Beck S, Bohni R, Brown CM, Cerny R, Horsnell T, Hutchison CA III, Kouzarides T, Martignetti JA, Preddie E, Satchwell SC, Tomlinson P, Weston KM, Barrell BG (1990) Analysis of the protein-coding content of the sequence of human cytomegalovirus strain AD169. Curr Top Microbiol Immunol 154:125–169
28. Chee MS, Satchwell SC, Preddie E, Weston KM, Barrell BG (1990) Human cytomegalovirus encodes three G protein-coupled receptor homologues. Nature 344:774–777
29. Chellappan SP, Hiebert S, Mudryj M, Horowitz JM, Nevins JR (1991) The E2F transcription factor is a cellular target for the RB protein. Cell 65:1053–1061
30. Clanton DJ, Jariwalla RJ, Kress C, Rosenthal LJ (1983) Neoplastic transformation by a cloned human cytomegalovirus DNA fragment uniquely homologous to one of the transforming regions of herpes simplex virus type 2. Proc Natl Acad Sci USA 80:3826–3830
31. Contreras TJ, Lang DJ, Pivacek LE, Valeri CR (1979) Occurrence of HBsAg, anti-HBs, and anti-CMV following the transfusion of blood products. Transfusion 19:129–136
32. Cole R, Kuttner AG (1926) A filterable virus present in the submaxillary glands of guinea pigs. J Exp Med 44:855–873
33. Cooper NR, Nowlin D, Taylor HP, Compton T (1991) Cellular receptor for human cytomegalovirus. Transplant Proc 23 [Suppl 3]:56–59
34. Cowdry EV (1934) The problem of intranuclear inclusion in virus disease. Arch Pathol 18:525–542
35. Dalgleish AG, Beverley PC, Clapham PR, Crawford DH, Greaves MF, Weiss RA (1984) The CD4 (T4) antigen is an essential component of the receptor for the AIDS retrovirus. Nature 312:763–767
36. Davis MG, Huang ES (1985) Nucleotide sequence of a human cytomegalovirus DNA fragment encoding a 67-kilodalton phosphorylated viral protein. J Virol 56:7–11
36a. Davis MG, Huang ES (1987) Dissection of the regulatory functions of the immediate early region of human cytomegalovirus. Abstract, p 4. Twelfth International Herpes Workshop, Philadelphia, PA. July 30 – August 4, 1987
37. Davis MG, Kenney SC, Kamine J, Pagano JS, Huang ES (1987) Immediate-early gene region of human cytomegalovirus transactivates the promoter of human immunodeficiency virus. Proc Natl Acad Sci USA 84:8642–8646
38. Davis MG, Mar EC, Wu YM, Huang ES (1984) Mapping and expression of a human cytomegalovirus major viral protein. J Virol 52:129–135
39. Deen KC, Mcdougal JS, Inacker R, Folena-Wasserman G, Arthos J, Rosenberg J, Madden PJ, Axel R, Sweet RW (1988) A soluble form of CD (T4) protein inhibits AIDS virus infection. Nature 331:82–84

40. Devoto SH, Mudryj M, Pines J, Hunter T, Nevins JR (1992) A cyclin A-protein kinase complex possesses sequence-specific DNA binding activity: $p33^{cdk2}$ is a component of the E2F-cyclin A complex. Cell 68:167–176
41. Drew WL, Conant MA, Miner RC, Huang ES, Ziegler JL, Groundwater JR, Gullett JH, Volberding P, Abrams DI, Mintz L (1982) Cytomegalovirus and Kaposi's sarcoma in young homosexual men. Lancet 2:125–127
42. Drew WL, Huang ES (1988) Etiology: role of cytomegalovirus. In: Ziegler JL, Dorfman RF (eds) Kaposi's sarcoma. Dekker, New York, pp 113–128
43. Drew WL, Mintz L, Miner RC, Sands M, Ketterer B (1981) Prevalence of cytomegalovirus in homosexual men. J Infect Dis 143:188–192
44. Drew WL, Mocarski ES, Sweet E, Miner RC (1984) Multiple infections with CMV in AIDS patients: documentation by southern blot hybridization. J Infect Dis 150:952–953
45. Dudding L, Haskill S, Clark BD, Auron PE, Sporn S, Huang ES (1989) Cytomegalovirus infection stimulates expression of monocyte-associated mediator genes. J Immunol 143:3343–3352
46. Duh EJ, Maury WJ, Folks TM, Fauci AS, Rabson AB (1989) Tumor necrosis factor alpha activates human immunodeficiency virus-type 1 through induction of nuclear factor binding to the NF-kappa B sites in the long terminal repeat. Proc Natl Acad Sci USA 86:5964–5978
47. Durst M, Gissmann L, Ikenberg H, zur Hausen H (1983) A papilloma DNA from a cervical carcinoma and its prevalence in cancer biopsy samples from different geographic regions. Proc Natl Acad Sci USA 80:3812–3815
48. Dyck PJ, Lambert EH (1968) Lower motor and primary sensory neuron diseases with peroneal muscular atropy (part I and II). Arch Neurol 18:603–625
49. Embil JA, Ozere RL, Haldane EV (1970) Congenital cytomegalovirus infection in two siblings from consecutive pregnancies. J Pediatr 77:417–421
50. Ensoli B, Barillari G, Salahuddin SZ, Gallo RC, Wong-Staal F (1990) Tat protein of HIV-1 stimulates growth of cells derived from Kaposi's sarcoma lesions of AIDS patients. Nature 345:84–86
51. Estes JE, Huang ES (1977) Stimulation of cellular thymidine kinases by human cytomegalovirus. J Virol 24:13–21
52. Fan CM, Maniatis T (1991) Generation of p50 subunit of NF-κB by processing of p105 through an ATP-dependent pathway. Nature 354:395–398
53. Farber S, Wolbach SG (1932) Intranuclear and cytoplasmic inclusions ("protozoan-like bodies") in the salivary glands and other organs of infants. Am J Pathol 8:123–135
54. Fetterman GH (1952) A new laboratory aid in the clinical diagnosis of inclusion disease of infancy. Am J Clin Pathol 22:424–425
55. Fiala M, Kattlove H, Lemkin T (1973) Cytomegalovirus mononucleosis with severe thrombocytopenia. Ann Intern Med 79:450–451
56. Finkle C, Tapper MA, Knox KK, Carrigan DR (1991) Coinfection of cells with the human immunodeficiency virus and cytomegalovirus in lung tissues of patients with AIDS. J Acquir Immune Defic Syndr 4:735–737
57. Fisher RA, Bertonis JM, Meier W, Johnson VA, Costopoulos DS, Liu T, Tizard R, Walker BD, Hirsch MS, Schooley RT et al. (1988) HIV infection is blocked in vitro by recombinant soluble CD4. Nature 331:76–78
58. Folks TM, Justement J, Kinter A, Dinarello CA, Fauci AS (1987) Cytokine-induced expression of HIV-1 in a chronically infected promonocyte cell line. Science 238:800–802
59. Forman SJ (1991) Bone marrow transplantation. Transplant Proc 23 [Suppl 3]:110–114
60. Foster KM (1966) Post-transfusion mononucleosis. Aust Ann Med 15:305–310
61. Frenkel LD, Gaur S, Tsolia M, Scudder R, Howell R, Kesarwala H (1990) Cytomegalovirus infection in children with AIDS. Rev Infect Dis 12 [Suppl 7]:S820–826
62. Fujinami RS, Nelson JA, Walker L, Oldstone MBA (1988) Sequence homology and immunologic cross-reactivity of human cytomegalovirus with HLA-DR B chain: a means for graft rejection and immunosuppression. J Virol 62:100–105

63. Geder L, Lausch R, O'Neill F, Rapp F (1976) Oncogenic transformation of human embryo lung cells by cytomegalovirus. Science 192:1134–1137
64. Gehrz RC, Liu YNC, Eckhardt J, Klaus A (1991) Relevance of immune responses to pathogenesis of cytomegalovirus associated diseases. Transplant Proc 23 [Suppl 3]:55–84
65. Gehrz RC, Marker SC, Knoor SO, Kalis JM; Balfour HH Jr (1977) Specific cell-mediated immune defect in active cytomegalovirus infection of young children and their mothers. Lancet 2:844–847
66. Ghosh S, Baltimore D (1990) Activation in vitro of NF-$\varkappa$B by phosphorylation of its inhibitor IkB. Nature 344:678–682
67. Gilmore T (1990) NF-$\varkappa$B, KBF1, dorsal and rel-related matters. Cell 62:841–843
68. Giraldo G, Beth E, Henle W, Henle G, Mike V, Safai B, Huraux JM, McHardy J, de-The G (1980) Antibody patterns to herpesvirus in Kaposi's sarcoma: II. Serological association of American Kaposi's sarcoma with cytomegalovirus. Int J Cancer 22:126–131
69. Giraldo G, Beth E, Huang ES (1980) Kaposi's sarcoma and its relationship to cytomegalovirus (CMV): III. CMV DNA and CMV early antigens in Kaposi's sarcoma. Int J Cancer 26:23–29
70. Gissmann L, Wolnick L, Ikenberg H, Koldenovsky U, Schurch HG, zur Hausen H (1983) Human papilloma type 6 and 11. DNA sequence in genital and laryngeal papilloma and in some cervical cancers. Proc Natl Acad Sci USA 80:560–563
71. Goldstein SC, Byrne JC, Rabson AS (1987) Human cytomegalovirus (HCMV) enhance bovine papilloma virus (BPV) transformation in vitro. J Med Virol 23:157–164
72. Gonczol E, Plotkin SA (1984) Cells infected with human cytomegalovirus release a factor(s) that stimulates cell DNA synthesis. J Gen Virol 65:1833–1837
73. Gorensek MJ, Stewart RW, Keys TF, McHenry MC, Babiak T, Goormastic M (1988) Symptomatic cytomegalovirus infection as a significant risk factor for major infections after cardiac transplantation. J Infect Dis 158:884–887
74. Gorensek MJ, Stewart RW, Keys TF, McHenry MC, Goormastic M (1988) A multivariate analysis of the risk of cytomegalovirus infection in heart transplantation recipients. J Infect Dis 157:515–522
75. Granstrom ML, Leinikki P, Santavuori P, Pettay O (1977) Perinatal cytomegalovirus infection in man. Arch Dis Child 52:354–359
76. Grundy JE (1990) Virologic and pathologic aspects of cytomegalovirus infection. Rev Infect Dis 12 [Suppl 7]:S711–S719
77. Grundy JE, McKeating JA, Sandersom AR, Griffiths PA (1988) Cytomegalovirus and β-2 microglobulin in urine specimens. Transplantation 45:1075–1079
78. Grundy JE, McKeating JA, Ward P, Sanderson A, Griffiths PA (1987) β2-Microglobulin enhances the infectivity of cytomegalovirus and when bound to the virus enables class I HLA molecules to be used as a virus receptor. J Gen Virol 68:793–803
79. Grundy JE, Shanley JD, Shearer GM (1985) Augmentation of graft vs host reaction by cytomegalovirus infection resulting in interstitial pneumonitis. Transplantation 39:548–553
80. Hanshaw JB (1968) Cytomegaloviruses. In: Gard S, Hallauer C, Meyer KF (eds) Cytomegaloviruses, Rinderpest Virus, Lumpyskin Disease Virus. (Virology Monograph, Vol. 3). Springer New York, pp 1–23
81. Hanshaw JB (1970) Developmental abnormalities associated with congenital cytomegalovirus infection. Adv Teratol 4:64–93
82. Hanshaw JB, Betts RF, Simon G, Boynton RC (1965) Acquired cytomegalovirus infection: association with hepatomegaly and abnormal liver-function tests. N Engl J Med 272:602–609
83. Hashiro GM, Horikami S, Loh PC (1979) Cytomegalovirus isolations form cell cultures of human adenocarcinomas of colon. Intervirology 12:84–88
84. Hedley-Whyte ET, Craighead JE (1965) Generalized cytomegalic inclusion disease after renal homotransplantation – report of a case with isolation of virus. N Engl J Med 272:473–475

85. Henninghausen L, Fleckenstein B (1986) Nuclear factor interacts with five DNA elements of the human cytomegalovirus major immediate early gene. EMBO J 5:1367–1371
86. Hilderbrandt RJ, Sever JL, Margileth AM, Callagan DA (1967) Cytomegalovirus in the normal pregnant women. Am J Obstet Gynecol 98:1125–1128
87. Ho M (1991) Cytomegalovirus: biology and infection, 2nd edn. Plenum, New York
88. Hohmann HP, Remy R, Aigner L, Brockhaus M, van Loon APGM (1992) Protein kinases negatively affect nuclear factor-λB activation by tumor necrosis factor-α at two different stages in promyelocytic HL60 cells. J Biol Chem 267:2065–2072
89. Homsy L, Meyer M, Tateno M, Clarkson S, Levy JA (1988) The Fc and not CD4 receptor mediates antibody enhancement of HIV infection in human cells. Science 244:1357–1360
90. Horwitz CA, Henle W, Henle G (1979) Diagnostic aspects of the cytomegalovirus mononucleosis syndrome in previously healthy persons. Postgrad Med 66:153–158
91. Huang ES (1975) Human cytomegalovirus: III. Virus-induced DNA polymerase. J Virol 16:298–310
92. Huang ES, Boldogh I, Mar EC (1983) Human cytomegaloviruses: evidence for possible association with human cancer. In: Philips LA (ed) Viruses associated with human cancer. Dekker, New York, pp 161–193
93. Huang ES, Davis MG, Baskar JF, Huong SM (1986) Molecular epidemiology and oncogenicity of human cytomegalovirus. In: Harris CC (ed) Biochemical and molecular epidemiology of cancer. Liss, New York, pp 313–322 (UCLA symposium on molecular and cellular biology, new series, vol 40)
93a. Huang ES, Kilpatrick B, Lakeman A, Alford CA (1978) Genetic analysis of a cytomegalovirus-like agent isolated from human brain. J Virol 26:718–723
94. Huang ES, Pagano JS (1974) Human cytomegalovirus. II. Lack of relatedness to herpes simplex I and II, Epstein-Barr virus and non-human cytomegalovirus. J Virol 13:642–645
95. Huang ES, Roche JK (1978) Cytomegalovirus DNA and adenocarcinoma of the colon: evidence for latent viral infection. Lancet 1:957–960
96. Isom HJ (1979) Stimulation of ornithine decarboxylase by human cytomegalovirus. J Gen Virol 42:265–278
97. Israel N, Hazan U, Alcami J, Munier A, Arenzana-Seisdedos F, Bachelerie F, Israel A (1989) Tumor necrosis factor stimulates transcription of HIV-1 in human T lymphocytes, independently and synergistically with mitogen. J Immunol 143:3956–3960
98. Ivan R, Brostoff J, Male D (1989) Chap. 4, p 8 Immunology, 2nd edn. Gower, London
99. Jabs DA, Engler C, Bartlett JG (1989) Cytomegalovirus retinitis and acquired immunodeficiency syndrome. Arch Ophthalmol 107:75–80
100. Jacobson MA, Mills J (1988) Serious cytomegalovirus disease in the acquired immunodeficiency syndrome (AIDS). Clinical findings, diagnosis, and treatment. Ann Intern Med 108:585–594
101. Jeang KT, Rawlins DR, Rosenfeld PJ, Shero JH, Kelley TJ, Hayward GS (1987) Multiple tandemly repeated binding sites for cellular nuclear factor 1 that surround the major immediate-early promoters of simian and human cytomegalovirus. J Virol 61:1559–1570
102. Jenson AB, Rosenberg HS, Notkins AL (1980) Pancreatic islet cell damage in children with fatal viral infection. Lancet 2:354–358
103. Jesionek A, Kiolemenoglou B (1904) Ueber einen Befund von protozoen-artigen Gebilden in den Organen eines hereditar-luetischen Foetus. Muench Med Wochenschr 15:1905–1907
104. Kaplan CS, Petersen EA, Icenogle TB, Copeland JG, Villar HV, Sampliner R, Minnich L, Ray CG (1989) Gastrointestinal cytomegalovirus infection in heart and heart-lung transplant recipients. Arch Intern Med 149:2095–2100
105. Keay S, Rasmussen L, Merigan TC (1988) Syngeneic monoclonal anti-idiotype antibodies that bear the internal image of a human cytomegalovirus neutralization epitope. J Immunol 140:944–948

106. Kerr LD, Inouve J, Davis N, Link E, Baeuerle PA, Bose HR, Verma IM (1991) The rel-associated pp40 protein prevents DNA binding of Rel and NF-κB: relationship with IκB-β and regulation by phosphorylation. Genes Dev 5:1464–1476
107. Kirmani N, Ginn RK, Mittal KK, Manischewitz JF, Quinnan GV Jr (1981) Cytomegalovirus-specific cytotoxicity mediated by non-T lymphocyte from peripheral blood of normal volunteers. Infect Immun 34:441–447
108. Klatt EC, Shibata D (1988) Cytomegalovirus infection in the acquired immunodeficiency syndrome. Clinical and autopsy finding. Arch Pathol Lab Med 112:340–344
109. Klemola E, Kaariainen L (1965) Cytomegalovir as a possible cause of a disease resembling infectious mononucleosis. Br J Med 2:1099–1102
110. Klemola E, Kaariainen L, von Essen R, Haltia K, Koivuniemi A, von Bonsdorff CH (1967) Further studies on cytomegalovirus mononucleosis in previously healthy individuals. Acta Med Scand 182:311–322
111. Klucher KM, Rabert DK, Spector DH (1989) Sequences in the human cytomegalovirus 2.7-promoter which mediate its regulation as an early gene. J Virol 63:5334–5343
112. Kowalik TF, McKnight KL, Huang ES (1990) Human cytomegalovirus can alter human papillomavirus gene expression and cellular transformation efficiency. Abstract 311, 15th international herpesvirus workshop, Georgetown, Washington. August 2–8, 1990
112a. Kowalik TF, Wing B, Haskill JS, Azikhan JC, Baldwin AS, Huang E-S (1993) Multiple mechanisms are implicated in the regulation of NF-κB activity during human cytomegalovirus infection. Proc Natl Acad Sci USA, in press
113. Kumar KL, Gold E, Nankervis GA (1975) Risk of acquired cytomegalovirus infection in infants of maternal CMV excretors. Pediatr Res 9:512
114. Kungu A, Gates DG (1981) Kaposi's sarcoma in Kenya: a retrospective clinicopathological study. Antibiot Chemother 29:38–55
115. Lang DJ, Hanshaw JB (1969) Cytomegalovirus infection and the post-perfusion syndrome: recognition of primary infections in four patients. N Engl J Med 280:1145–1149
116. Lang DJ, Kummer JF (1972) Demonstration of cytomegalovirus in semen. N Engl J Med 287:756–758
117. Larsen CG, Anderson AO, Appella E, Oppenheim JJ, Matsushima K (1989) The neutrophil-activating protein (NAP-1) is also chemotactic for T lymphocytes. Science 243:1464–1466
118. Lenardo MJ, Baltimore D (1989) NF-κB: a pleiotrophic mediator of inducible and tissue-specific gene control. Cell 58:227–229
119. Leonard JC, Tobin JO'H (1971) Polyneuritis associated with cytomegalovirus infections. Q J Med 40:435–442
120. Levin MJ, Rinaldo CR Jr, Leary PL, Zaia JA, Hirsh MS (1979) Immune response to herpes virus antigens in adults with acute cytomegalovirus mononucleosis. J Infect Dis 140:851–857
121. Levinsohn EM, Foy HM, Kenny GE, Wentworth BB, Grayston JT (1969) Isolation of cytomegalovirus from a cohort of 100 infants throughout the first year of life. Proc Soc Exp Biol Med 132:957–962
121a. Lin B, Stinski MF (1992) Human cytomegalovirus contains a tegument protein that enhances transcription from promoters with upstream ATF and AP-I cis-acting elements. J Virol 66:4434–4444
121b. Lindsley MD, Torpey DJ III, Rinaldo CR Jr (1986) HLA-DR-restricted cytotoxicity of cytomegalovirus-infected monocytes mediated by Leu-3-positive T cells. J Immunol 136:3045–3051
122. Lowenstein C (1907) Ueber protozoenartige Gebilde in den Organen von Kindern. Zentralbl Allg Pathol 18:513–518
123. Lowenthal JW, Ballard DW, Bohnlein E, Greene WC (1989) Tumor necrosis factor alpha induces proteins that bind specifically to kappa B-like enhancer elements and regulate interleukin 2 receptor alpha-chain gene expression in primary human T lymphocytes. Proc Natl Acad Sci USA 86:2331–2335

124. Lubon H, Ghazal P, Hennighausen L, Reynolds-Kohler C, Lochshin C, Nelson JA (1989) Cell-specific activity of the modulator region in the human cytomegalovirus major immediate early gene. Mol Cell Biol 9:1342–1345
125. Mach M, Stamminger T, Gerhard J (1989) Human cytomegalovirus: recent aspects from molecular biology. J Gen Virol 70:3117–3146
126. Macher AM, Reichert CM, Strau SE, Longo DL, Parrillo J, Lane HC, Fauci AS, Rook AH, Manischewitz JF, Quinnan GV Jr (1983) Death in the AIDS patient: role of cytomegalovirus. N Engl J Med 309:1454
127. Maddon PA, Dalgleish AG, McDougal JS (1986) The T4 gene encodes the AIDS virus receptor and is expressed in the immune system and the brain. Cell 47:333–348
128. Mar EC, Patel P, Huang ES (1981) Human cytomegalovirus-associated DNA polymerase and protein kinase activities. J Gen Virol 57:149–156
129. McCracken GJ Jr, Shinefield HR, Cobb K, Rausen AR, Dische MR, Eichenwald HF (1969) Congenital cytomegalovirus inclusion disease. A longitudinal study of 20 patients. Am J Dis Child 117:522–539
130. McKeating JA, Griffiths PD, Grundy JE (1986) Cytomegalovirus in urine specimens has host beta 2 microglobulin bound to the viral envelope: a mechanism of evading the host immune response? J Gen Virol 68:785:792
131. McKeating JA, Griffiths PD, Weiss RA (1990) HIV susceptibility conferred to human fibroblasts by cytomegalovirus-induced Fc receptor. Nature 343:659–661
132. Melnick JL, Lewis R, Wimberly I, Kaufman RH, Adams E (1978) Association of cytomegalovirus (CMV) infection with cervical cancer: isolation of CMV from cell cultures derived from cervical biopsy. Intervirology 10:115–119
133. Meyers JD, Spencer HC Jr, Watts JC, Gregg MB, Stewart JA, Troupin RH, Thomas ED (1975) Cytomegalovirus pneumonia after bone marrow transplantation. Ann Intern Med 82:181–188
134. Meyers JD, Flournoy N, Thomas ED (1986) Risk factors for cytomegalovirus infection after human marrow transplant. J Infect Dis 153:478–488
135. Michelson S, Tardy-Panit M, Barzu O (1984) Properties of a human cytomegalovirus-induced protein kinase. Virology 134:259–268
136. Miles SA, Martinez-Maza O, Rezai AR, Magpantay L, Kishimoto T, Nakamura S, Radka SF, Linsley PS (1992) Oncostatin M as a potent mitogen for AIDS-Kaposi's sarcoma-derived cells. Science 255:1432–1434
137. Miles SA, Rezai AR, Salazor-Gonzalez JF, Vander-Meyden M, Steven RH (1990) AIDS Kaposi sarcoma-derived cells produce and respond to interleukin 6. Proc Natl Acad Sci USA 87:4068–4072
138. Mintz L, Drew WL, Miner RC, Braff EH (1983) Cytomegalovirus infections in homosexual men: an epidemiological study. Ann Intern Med 99:326–329
138a. Mocarski ES jr (1991) Initial events involved in cytomegalovirus – cell interactions. Transplant Proc 23 [Suppl 3]:43–47
139. Morgello S, Cho ES, Nielsen S, Devinsky O, Petito CK (1987) Cytomegalovirus encephalitis in patients with acquired immunodeficiency syndrome: an autopsy study of 30 cases and a review of the literature. Hum Pathol 18:289–297
140. Mudryj M, Devato SH, Hilbert SW, Hunter T, Pines J, Nevins JR (1991) Cell cycle regulation of the E2F transcription factor involves an interaction with cyclin A. Cell 65:1243–1253
141. Nabel GJ, Baltimore D (1987) An inducible transcriptional factor activates expression of human immunodeficiency virus in T cells. Nature 326:711–713
142. Nelson JA, Fleckenstein B, Galloway DA, McDougall JK (1982) Transformation of NIH 3T3 cells with cloned fragments of human cytomegalovirus strain AD169. J Virol 43:83–91
143. Nelson JA, Groudine M (1986) Transcpritional regulation of the human cytomegalovirus major immediate-early gene is associated with induction of DNase 1-hypersensitive sites. Mol Cell Biol 6:452:461
144. Nelson JA, Reynolds-Kohler C, Oldstone MBA, Wiley CA (1988) HIV and HCMV coinfect brain cells in patients with AIDS. Virology 165:286–290

145. Nelson JA, Reynolds-Kohler C, Smith BA (1987) Negative and positive regulation by a short segment in the 5′ flanking region of the human cytomegalovirus major immediate-early gene. Mol Cell Biol 7:4125–4129
146. Nevins JR (1989) Mechanisms of viral-mediated trans-activation of transcription. Adv Virus Res 37:35–83
147. Nicholas J, Cameron KR, Honess RW (1992) Herpesvirus saimiri encodes homologues of G protein-coupled receptors and cyclins. Nature 355:362–365
148. Numazaki K, Goldman H, Wong I, Wainberg MA (1988) Viral infection of human islets of Langerhans. Replication of human cytomegalovirus in cultured human fetal pancreatic islets. Am J Clin Pathol 90:52–57
149. Numazaki Y, Yano N, Morizuka T, Takai S, Ishida N (1970) Primary infection with human cytomegalovirus: virus isolation from healthy infants and pregnant women. Am J Epidemiol 91:410–417
150. Osborn L, Kunkel S, Nabel GL (1989) Tumor necrosis factor alpha and interleukin 1 stimulate the human immunodeficiency virus enhancer by activation of the nuclear factor kappa B. Proc Natl Acad Sci USA 86:2336–2340
151. Pagano JS, Huang ES (1976) Application of RNA-DNA cytohybridization to viral diagnosis. In: Kurstak E, Morrisset T (eds) Comparative immunodiagnosis of viral infection. Academic, New York, pp 279–299
152. Pak CY, McArthur RG, Eun HM, Yoon JW (1988) Association of cytomegalovirus infection with autoimmune type 1 diabetes. Lancet 1:4
153. Pass RF, Dworsky ME, Whitely RJ, August AM, Stagno S, Alford CA Jr (1981) Specific lymphocyte blastogenic responses in children with cytomegalovirus and herpes simplex virus infections acquired early in infancy. Infect Immun 34:166–170
154. Pass RF, Stagno S, Britt WJ, Alford CA (1983) Specific cell mediated immunity and the natural history of congenital infection with cytomegalovirus. J Infect Dis 148:953–961
155. Peterson PK, Balfour HH Jr, Marker SC, Fryd DS, Howard RJ, Simmons RL (1980) Cytomegalovirus disease in renal allograft recipients: a prospective study of the clinical features, risk factors and impact on renal transplantation. Medicine (Baltimore) 59:283–300
156. Peveri P, Walz A, Dewald B, Baggiolini M (1988) A novel neutrophil-activating factor produced by human mononuclear phagocytes. J Exp Med 167:1547–1559
157. Pines J, Hunter T (1990) $p34^{cdc2}$: the S and M kinase? New Biologist 2:289–401
158. Pisano G (1910) Su di un reperto istologico raro in feto scleromatoso. Gazz Osp Clin 31:249–250
159. Rando RF, Srinivasan A, Feingold J, Gonczol E, Plotkin S (1990) Characterization of multiple molecular interactions between human cytomegalovirus (HCMV) and human immunodeficiency virus type 1 (HIV-1). Virology 176:87–97
160. Rapp F, Geder L, Murasko D, Laush R, Ladda R, Huang ES, Webber MM (1975) Long term persistence of cytomegalovirus genome in cultured human cells of prostatic origin. J Virol 16:982–990
161. Rasmussen LE (1991) Gene products of cytomegalovirus and their immunologic significance. In: Ho M (ed) Human cytomegalovirus: biology and infection, 2nd edn. Plenum, New York, pp 37–56
162. Rasmussen L, Resta S, Merigan T (1991) Human cytomegalovirus glycoprotein-receptor interaction. Transplant Proc 23 [Suppl 3]:60–63
163. Reynolds DW, Stagno S, Hostly TS, Tiller M, Alford CA Jr (1973) Maternal cytomegalovirus excretion and perinatal infection. N Engl J Med 289:1–5
164. Ribbert H (1904) Über protozoenartige Zellen in der Niere eines syphilitischen Neugeborenen und in der Parotis von Kindern. Zentralbl Allg Pathol Anat 15:945–948
165. Rifkind D (1965) Cytomegalovirus infection after renal transplantation. Arch Intern Med 116:554–558
166. Rinaldo CR Jr, Black PH, Hirsch MS (1977) Virus-leukocyte interactions in cytomegalovirus mononucleosis. J Infect Dis 136:667–678
167. Rinaldo CR Jr, Carney WP, Richter BS, Black PH, Hirsch MS (1980) Mechanism of immunosuppression in cytomegaloviral mononucleosis. J Infect Dis 141:488–495

168. Rinaldo CR Jr, Hamoudi WH, DiBaiasio RL, Rabin B, Hakala TR, Liebert M (1983) Cellular immune response and cytomegalovirus infection in renal transplant patients receiving cyclosporine. Transplant Proc 15:2775–2778
169. Riviere Y, Blank V, Kourilsky P, Israel A (1991) Processing of the precursor of NF-κB by the HIV-1 protease during acute infection. Nature 350:625–626
170. Robinson WE, Montefiori DC, Gillespie DH, Mitchell WM (1989) Complement-mediated, antibody-dependent enhancement of HIV-1 infection in vitro is characterized by increased protein and RNA synthesis and infectious virus release. AIDS 2:33–42
171. Roche JK, Cheng KS, Huang ES, Lang DL (1981) Cytomegalovirus: detection in human colonic and circulating mononuclear cells in association with gastrointestinal disease. Int J Cancer 27:659–667
172. Rook AH (1988) Interactions of cytomegalovirus with the human immune system. Rev Infect Dis 10:S460–467
173. Rosenberg ZF, Fauci AS (1990) Immunopathogenic mechanism of HIV infection: cytokine induction of HIV expression. Immunol Today 11:176–189
174. Rowe WP, Hartley JW, Waterman S, Turner HC, Huebner RJ (1956) Cytopathogenic agent resembling human salivary gland virus recovered from tissue cultures of human adenoids. Proc Soc Exp Biol Med 92:418–424
175. Rubin RH, Tolkoff-Rubin NE, Oliver D, Rota TR, Hamilton J, Betts RF, Pass RF, Hillis W, Szmuness W, Farrell ML, Hirsch MS (1985) Multicenter seroepidemiologic study of the impact of cytomegalovirus infection and renal transplantation. Transplantation 40:243–249
176. Safai B, Good R (1981) Kaposi's sarcoma: a review and recent developments. CA 31:2–12
177. Safai B, Diaz B, Schwartz J (1992) Malignant neoplasmas associated with human immunodeficiency virus infection. CA 42:74–95
178. Sanford EJ, Dagen JE, Geder L, Rohner JT, Rapp F (1977) Lymphocyte reactivity against virally transformed cells in patients with urologic cancer. J Urol 118:809–810
179. Sambucetti LC, Cherrington JM, Wilkinson GWG, Mocarski ES (1989) NF-κB activation of the cytomegalovirus enhancer is mediated by a viral transactivator and by T cell stimulation. EMBO J 8:4251–4258
180. Sawyer MH, Edwards DK, Spector SA (1987) Cytomegalovirus infection and bronchopulmonary dysplasia in premature infants. Am J Dis Child 141:303–305
181. Schmitz H, Enders G (1977) Cytomegalovirus as a frequent cause of Guillian-Barré syndrome. J Med Virol 1:21–27
182. Sen R, Baltimore D (1986) Multiple nuclear factors interact with the immunoglobulin enhancer sequences. Cell 46:705–716
183. Shelbourn SL, Kothari SK, Sissons JG, Sinclair JH (1989) Repression of human cytomegalovirus gene expression associated with a novel immediate early regulatory region binding factor. Nucleic Acids Res 17:9165–9171
184. Shirakawa F, Mizel SB (1989) In vitro activation and nuclear translocation of NF-κB catalyzed by cyclic AMP-dependent protein kinase and protein kinase C. Mol Cell Biol 9:2424–2430
185. Shirodka S, Ewen M, DeCaprio JA, Morgan J, Livingston DM, Chittenden T (1992) The transcription factor E2F interacts with the retinoblastoma gene product and a p107-cyclin A complex in a cell cycle-regulated manner. Cell 68:157–166
186. Singh N, Dummer JD, Kusne S, Breinig MK, Armstrong JA, Makowka L, Starzl TE, Ho M (1988) Infections with cytomegalovirus and other herpesviruses in 121 liver transplant recipients: transmission by donated organ and the effect of OKT3 antibodies. J Infect Dis 158:124–131
187. Skolnik PR, Kosloof BR, Hirsch MS (1988) Bidirectional interactions between human immunodeficiency virus type 1 and cytomegalovirus. J Infect Dis 157:508–514
188. Smith MG (1954) Propagation of salivary gland virus of mouse in tissue cultures. Proc Soc Exp Biol Med 86:435–440
189. Smith MG (1956) Propagation in tissue cultures of a cytopathogenic virus from human salivary gland virus (SGV) disease. Proc Soc Exp Biol Med 92:424–430

190. Spector DH, Klucher KM, Rabert DK, Wright DA (1990) Human cytomegalovirus early gene expression. Curr Top Microbiol Immunol 154:21–45
191. Spector DH, Shaw SB, Hock LT (1984) Association of human cytomegalovirus with Kaposi's sarcoma. In: Gottlieb MS, Groopman JE (eds) Acquired immune deficiency syndrome. Liss, New York, pp 109–126
192. Sprecher E, Becker Y (1988) Role of Langerhans cells and Thy. 1+ effector cells in herpes simplex-1 infection in the skin of newborn mice. Arch Virol 100:285–292
193. Sprecher E, Becker Y (1988) Role of epidermal Langerhans cell in viral infections. Arch Virol 103:1–14
194. Sprecher E, Becker Y (1989) Langerhans cell density and activity in mouse skin and lymph nodes affect herpes simplex type 1 (HSV-1) pathogenicity. Arch Virol 1989:191–205
195. Stagno S, Pass RF, Cloud G, Britt WJ, Henderson RE, Waltson PD, Veren DA, Page F, Alford CA (1986) Primary cytomegalovirus infection in pregnancy. Incidence, transmission to fetus and clinical outcome. JAMA 256:1904–1908
196. Stagno S, Reynolds DW, Huang ES, Thames SD, Smith RJ, Alford CA Jr (1977) Congenital cytomegalovirus: occurrence in an immune population. N Engl J Med 296:1254–1258
197. Stagno S, Reynolds DW, Lakeman A, Charamella LJ, Alford CA (1973) Congenital cytomegalovirus infection: consecutive occurrence due to viruses with similar antigenic compositions. Pediatrics 52:788–794
198. Starr JG, Bart RD, Gold E (1970) Inapparent congenital cytomegalovirus infection. Clinical and epidemiologic characteristics in early infancy. N Engl J Med 282:1075–1078
199. Starr SE, Tolpin MD, Friedman HM, Paucker K, Plotkin SA (1979) Impaired cellular immunity to cytomegalovirus in congenitally infected children and their mothers. J Infect Dis 140:500–505
200. Stern H, Elek SD, Booth JC, Fleck DG (1969) Microbial causes of mental retardation: the role of prenatal infections with cytomegalovirus, rubella virus, and toxoplasma. Lancet 2:443–448
201. Stern H, Tucker SM (1973) Prospective study of cytomegalovirus infection in pregnancy. Br Med J 2:268–270
202. Stingl G, Rappersberger K, Tschachler E, Gartner S, Groh V, Mann DL, Wolff K, Popovic M (1990) Langerhans cells in HIV-1 infection. J Am Acad Dermatol 22:1210–1217
203. Stinski MF (1990) Cytomegalovirus and its replication. In: Fields BN, Knipe DM et al. (eds) Virology, 2nd edn. Raven, New York, pp 1959–1980
204. Staprans SI, Spector DH (1986) 2.2-Kilobase class of early transcripts encoded by cell-related sequences in human cytomegalovirus strain AD169. J Virol 57:591–602
205. Takeda A, Tuazon CU, Ennis FA (1988) Antibody-enhanced infection of HIV via Fc receptor-mediated entry. Science 244:580–583
206. Tanaka S, Ihara S, Watanabe Y (1978) Human cytomegalovirus induces DNA-dependent RNA polymerases in human diploid cells. Virology 89:179–185
207. Taylor HP, Cooper NR (1989) Human cytomegalovirus binding to fibroblasts is receptor mediated. J Virol 63:3991–3998
208. Visser OH, Bos PJ (1986) Kaposi's sarcoma of the conjunctiva and CMV-retinitis in AIDS. Doc Ophthalmol 64:77–85
209. Vinters HV, Kwok MK, Ho HW, Anders KH, Tomiyasu U, Wolfson WL, Robert F (1989) Cytomegalovirus in the nervous system of patients with the acquired immune deficiency syndrome. Brain 112:245–268
209a. Wade M, Kowalik TF, Mudryj M, Huang E-S, Azizkhan JC (1992) E2F mediates dihydrofolate reductase promoter activation and multiprotein complex formation in human cytomegalovirus infection. Mol Cell Biol 12:4364–4374
210. Ward KP, Galloway WH, Auchterlonie IA (1979) A congenital cytomegalovirus infection and diabetes. Lancet 1:497

211. Webster A, Lee CA, Cook DG, Grundy JE, Emery VC, Kernoff PB, Griffiths PD (1989) Cytomegalovirus infection and progression towards AIDS in haemophiliacs with human immunodeficiency virus infection. Lancet ii:63–66
212. Weller TH (1971) The cytomegalovirus: ubiquitous agents with protean clinical manifestations. N Engl J Med 285:203–214, 267–274
213. Weller TH, Macauley JC, Craig JM, Wirth P (1957) Isolation of intranuclear inclusion producing agent from infants with illnesses resembling cytomegalic inclusion disease. Proc Soc Exp Biol Med 94:4–12
214. Whitely RJ, Brasfield DM, Reynolds DW, Stagno S, Tiller RE, Alford CA Jr (1976) Protracted pneumonitis in young infants associated with perinatally acquired cytomegalovirus infection. J Pediatr 89:16–22
215. Wildy P (1973) Herpes: history and classification. In: Kaplan AS (ed) The herpesvirus. Academic, New York, pp 1–22
215a. Wiley CA, Schrier RD, Denaro FJ, Nelson JA, Lampert PW, Oldstone MB (1986) Localization of cytomegalovirus proteins and genome during fulminant central nervous system infection in an AIDS patient. J Neuropathol Exp Neurol 45:127–139
216. Williams LL, Blakeslee Lee JR, Boldogh I, Haung ES (1980) Detection of cytomegalovirus genomes in human skin fibroblasts by DNA hybridization. J Gen Virol 51:435–438
217. Williams LL, Blakeslee Lee JR, Huang ES (1980) Isolation of a new strain of cytomegalovirus from explanted normal skin. J Gen Virol 47:529–523
218. Wingard JR, Chen DTH, Burns WH, Fuller DJ, Braine HG, Yeager AM, Kaiser H, Burke PJ, Graham ML, Santos GW (1988) Cytomegalovirus infection after autologous bone marrow transplantation with comparison to infection after allogenic bone marrow transplantation. Blood 71:1432–1437
219. Wingard JR, Mellits ED, Sostrin MB, Chen DY, Burns WH, Santos GW, Vriesendrop HM, Beschorner WE, Saral R (1988) Interstitial pneumonitis after allogeneic bone marrow transplantation. Medicine 67:175–186
220. Wright DA, Staprans SI, Spectro DH (1988) Four phosphoproteins with common amino termini are encoded by human cytomegalovirus AD169. J Virol 62:331–340
221. Wright HT Jr (1973) Cytomegalovirus. In: Kaplan AS (ed) The herpesviruses. Academic, New York, pp 353–388
222. Wyatt JP, Saxton J, Lee RS, Pinkerton H (1950) Generalized cytomegalic inclusion disease. J Pediatr 36:271–294
223. Yamanishi K, Rapp F (1979) Production of plasminogen activator by human and hamster cells infected with human cytomegalovirus. J Virol 31:415–419
224. Yeager AS, Grumet FC, Hafleigh EB, Arvin AM, Bradley JE, Prober CG (1981) Prevention of transfusion-acquired cytomegalovirus infections in newborn infants. J Pediatr 98:281–287
225. Yoshimura T, Matsushima K, Tanaka S, Robinson EA, Appella E, Oppenheim JJ, Leonard EJ (1987) Purification of a human monocyte-derived neutrophil chemotactic factor that has peptide sequence similarity to other host defense cytokines. Proc Natl Acad Sci USA 84:9233–9237
226. Zuelzer WW, Stulberg CS, Page RH, Teruya J, Brough AJ (1966) Etiology and pathogenesis of acquired hemolytic anemia. Transfusion 6:438–460

Chapter 2 Pathology of Human Cytomegalovirus Infection

Harry V. Vinters [1,2] and Jorge A. Ferreiro [1]

Summary

Cytomegalovirus (CMV) produces widely variable pathologic change in infected tissues, whether in the context of acquired immunodeficiency syndrome (AIDS) or another form of immunosuppression, e.g., that noted after organ or bone marrow transplantation. Characteristic cytomegalic cells may be present with minimal or absent inflammatory response in a given organ, or there may be extensive associated inflammation and necrosis with clinically significant dysfunction. This chapter discusses and illustrates the histologic manifestations of CMV infection in the context of their clinical presentation, and complements other chapters that discuss molecular mechanisms of CMV pathogenesis and neuropathogenesis.

Introduction and Historical Perspective

The cells which we now recognize in histologic sections as being characteristic, even diagnostic of infection of that tissue by cytomegalovirus (CMV) were first recognized in the early part of this century. At that time, however, their significance was not appreciated and the large cells were thought to represent evidence of a parasitic infection [116]. Initial reports were of cytomegalic cells found within the parotid and salivary glands, usually in children [116]. By the 1920s, the large intranuclear and somewhat smaller cytoplasmic inclusions (Fig. 1) were linked to viral infection. Soon thereafter, an appreciation of widespread cytomegalic inclusion disease (CID) evolved. Eventually, cytomegalic cells came to be discovered in sites other than the salivary glands. The term "cytomegalovirus" came into use approximately 30 years ago. Clearly, CID as a problematic nosologic entity was recognized long before the onset of the acquired immunodeficiency syndrome (AIDS) epidemic, although it is mainly in the context of this epidemic that CMV infection has come to be appreciated as a frequent and significant cause of morbidity and mortality.

[1] Department of Pathology and [2] Brain Research Institute, University of California, Los Angeles Medical Center, CHS Room 18-170, Los Angeles, CA 90024-1732, USA
Dr. Ferreiro's present address: Dept. of Pathology, Mayo Clinic, Rochester, MN, USA

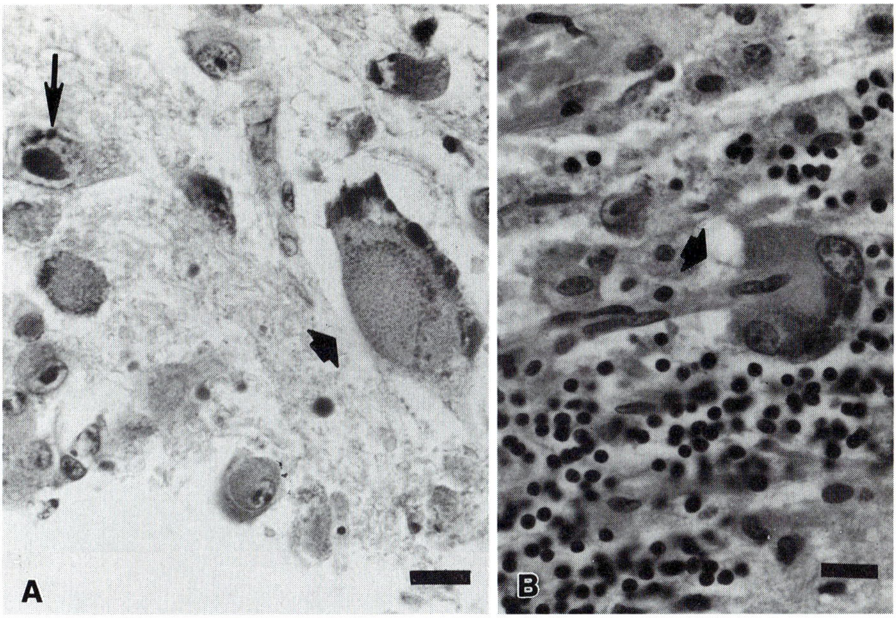

Fig. 1. **A** Characteristic cytomegalic cell (*arrowhead*) within brain, showing intranuclear and intracytoplasmic inclusions. Other cells (e.g., *arrow*) show nuclear inclusions only. H & E; *scale marker*, 20 µm. **B** Cerebellum from a patient with acquired immunodeficiency syndrome and cytomegalovirus encephalitis. Note cytomegalic cell with intracytoplasmic inclusions (*arrowhead*). H & E; *scale marker*, 20 µm

CMV is a ubiquitous organism that commonly infects man. Evidence for CMV infection is found in approximately 1% of live-born infants and 60%–80% of adults [7]. The incidence of CMV infection in adults increases with age [53]. Most CMV infections in healthy individuals are asymptomatic, and the virus then settles into a period of latency [7], possibly in the kidney and lymphocytes [7, 11, 71]. Reports of disseminated CMV in adults were infrequent in the literature until the advent of chemotherapy in the late 1940s and early 1950s [116]. The initial report of CMV infection in a cancer patient appeared in the 1950s [111]. By 1962, in a review of the literature, Wong and Warner [145] found just over 40 reported cases of CMV infection in adults. They described 14 cases from their own experience, most of them in patients with metastatic neoplasms. Although several reports of CID had appeared by the 1960s, the entity was felt to be rare [140, 145]. It was often described in immunosuppressed individuals with leukemia or lymphoma. The tendency for CMV to infect endothelial cells was noted [136], and this propensity has been reemphasized by the examination of tissues from individuals infected with the human immunodeficiency virus (HIV; Fig. 2). Even in the 1950s, CMV infection in adults was recognized as having important clinical and biologic differences from CMV infection in utero, or in the neonatal and juvenile period [101]. Excellent reviews pertaining to the early clinical, biologic, and diagnostic

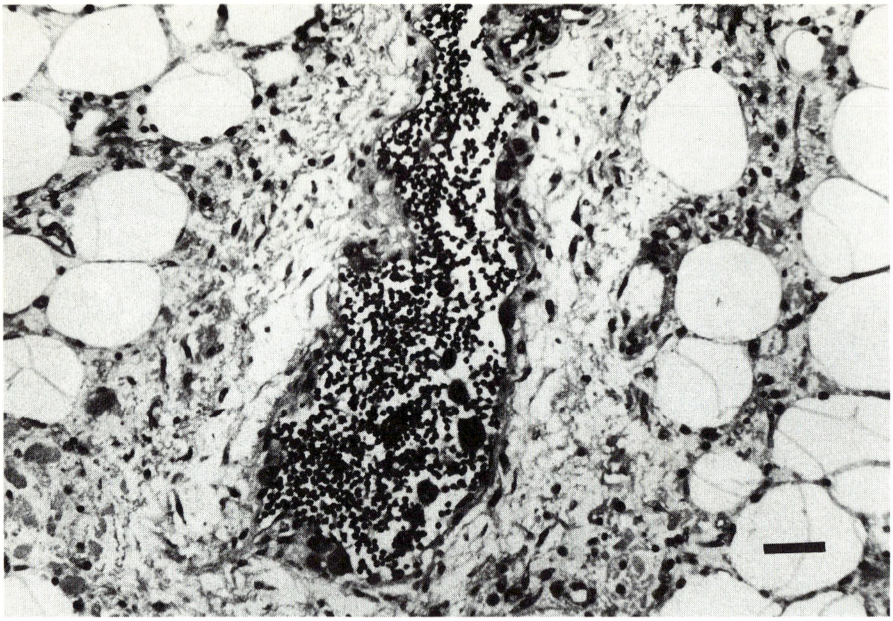

Fig. 2. Small blood vessel (*center of field*) running through connective tissue shows several cytomegalic endothelial cells. Large cells are also present within the lumen and may represent sloughed endothelium or circulating cytomegalovirus cells. H & E; *scale marker*, 50 μm

features of CID and cytomegalovirus infection in general have been published [106, 139]. The purpose of this chapter will be to indicate current morphological approaches to the diagnosis of CMV infection, as well as significant clinicopathologic features of CMV infection in both non-AIDS and AIDS patients. Molecular mechanisms described elsewhere in this book will not be reviewed, except insofar as they impinge on an understanding of morphological studies and techniques.

Morphological Approaches to the Diagnosis of CMV Infection

To a large extent, our current understanding of the complexities of CMV infection has evolved in parallel with the diagnostic armamentarium by which the virus can be detected in body fluids and tissue sections. Studies from the 1960s examined the ultrastructural morphology of infection by CMV, e.g., within renal tubular cells [32]. These investigations concluded that the virus forms in the cell nucleus and moves through the nuclear membrane to the cytoplasm, where viruses aggregate into a paracrystalline arrangement. By the 1970s, CMV and/or its antigens could be detected in many body fluids, including blood, saliva, urine, cervical secretions, and human semen [75]. Investiga-

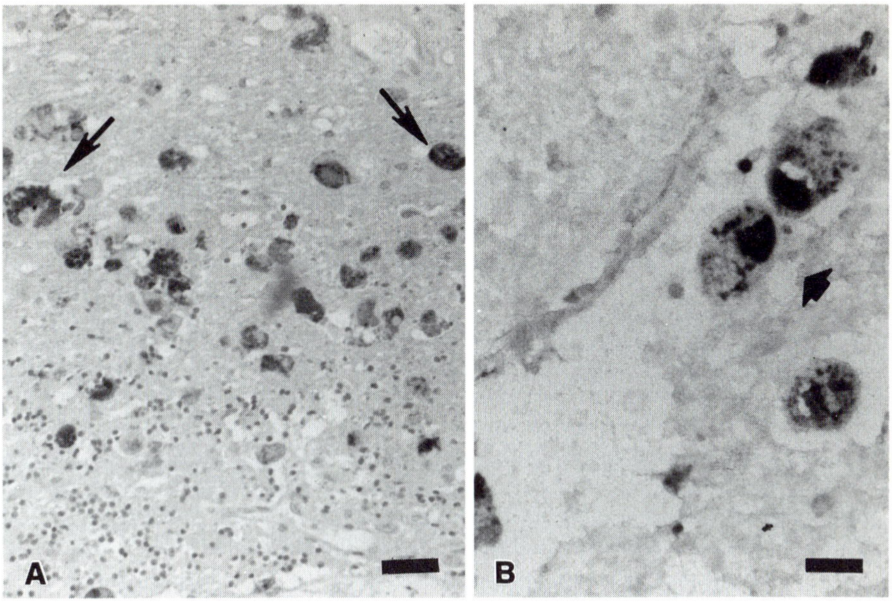

Fig. 3. A Cerebellum from a child with acquired immunodeficiency syndrome (AIDS) and cytomegalovirus (CMV) encephalitis. Immunoperoxidase stain using primary antibody (commercially available) to human CMV demonstrates many cytomegalic cells (e.g., *arrows*). Cerebellar granule cell layer is at the *bottom*. *Scale marker*, 50 µm. **B** In situ hybridization for CMV in brain of a patient with AIDS. For details of methods, see [135]. Note prominent nuclear and cytoplasmic labeling (*arrowhead*) by the chromogen. *Scale marker*, 20 µm

tors were able to correlate CMV morphology with the viral peptide composition [120]. Refinements in biochemical and molecular methods allowed for a detailed assessment of CMV infection by immunofluorescence microscopy, and strain variations within human and animal tissues could be analyzed [75]. Methods for the detection of CMV within various body fluids will not be reviewed here [25].

CMV antigen can be detected within tissue sections by standard immunofluorescence or multi-step immunoperoxidase techniques in conjunction with light microscopy [129]. Although somewhat superseded by techniques to be described below, immunohistochemistry still plays an important role in the rapid tissue diagnosis of CMV infection (Fig. 3). A quantum leap forward in our ability to study viral infections (including CMV) within human and animal tissues occurred with the development of morphological techniques which utilized the tools of molecular biology, viz. the methodology of in situ hybridization [18, 60, 80, 103, 133]. These techniques utilize radiolabeled, bromodeoxyuridine-labeled, biotinylated, or otherwise labeled nucleic acid probes to detect relatively low levels of virus genome within tissues suspected of harboring CMV infection (Fig. 3). They can be utilized in both autopsy- and biopsy-derived tissues. Probe studies can be carried out on archival material, thus increasing immensely their potential value in research on human viral (including CMV) infections. In addition to their value in research, the techniques of in situ hybridization have shown a practical use, e.g., in the assessment of CMV within bronchoalveolar lavage specimens from patients with AIDS [68]. Probe studies were found to be far more sensitive than conventional cytologic examination for CMV inclusions within lavage specimens. The authors concluded that direct in situ DNA hybridization is a useful and rapid method for CMV detection in such specimens. Recent studies indicate that hybridization for CMV can be carried out in plastic-embedded sections [23] and the methods have been refined to the point where ultrastructural localization of viral nucleic acids is a realistic possibility [144].

In situ hybridization for CMV has revealed that there may be widespread histologically occult CMV infection in organs that show little or no evidence of inflammatory or necrotic change that is routinely ascribed to the virus [95, 96]. Given the capability of CMV to produce latent infection, this is not surprising. Nevertheless, the use of such techniques to verify that CMV is frequently present when no reactive changes exist in a given tissue represented a significant advance in our understanding of the biology of CMV infection, especially in humans. Comparable hybridization studies have shown that CMV infection is an extremely heterogeneous phenomenon, especially within the lungs [95] but also in the nervous system (see below). Also, the sensitivity of in situ hybridization techniques is comparable to that of both viral culture and antigen detection in frozen sections when these techniques are employed to look for CMV pneumonia [95].

CMV Infection in Transplant Recipients

CMV infection is quite common in patients who have received organ or bone marrow transplants and in those who have been given multiple blood transfusions [22, 109]. CMV is the most frequently observed pathogen within the first 6 months posttransplantation, earning it the name "the troll of transplantation" [8]. The presence of CMV in patients after organ transplantation appears to be due to the immunosuppressive regimens used, since evidence of CID is found only in transplant patients receiving immunosuppressive drugs [78].

Renal Transplantation

The frequency of CMV infection in renal transplant patients does not appear to have changed since the introduction of cyclosporine [38a]. Kidney transplant recipients are the best-documented group in whom transplant-associated CID is a significant problem. Active CMV in patients after renal transplantation, defined by a fourfold rise in CMV antibody titer and/or recovery of the virus, is reported in 43%–92% of patients [53]. In these individuals, CMV may be shed in the urine or the oropharyngeal secretions. There appear to be two main sources for these infections: reactivation of a latent CMV infection, or a new primary infection [70]. The infection rate is generally higher in those patients seropositive for CMV before transplantation (88%) and lower in those who are seronegative (59%). This implies that infection is due mainly to reactivation rather than a de novo primary infection. Sources for primary CMV infection in renal transplant patients include blood products [46] and the donor organ itself [11, 71]. Ho et al. [71] found that CMV seronegative recipients who received kidneys from seronegative donors infrequently developed CMV infection, whereas the vast majority of seronegative recipients who received kidneys from seropositive donors became infected. Transfused blood did not appear to play a significant role unless a large number of units were transfused [71].

Most renal transplant-associated CMV infections are asymptomatic or manifest with only mild systemic effects [53]. Clinical syndromes characteristically occur in the first 4 months after transplant. The majority of CMV infections consist only of serologic changes of CMV antibody titers or asymptomatic viral shedding [53]. Approximately 30%–40% of CMV infections in renal transplant patients consist solely of fever, musculoskeletal pain, abnormal liver function tests, leukopenia, and respiratory symptoms [53]. Lymphocytosis, abdominal pain, and diarrhea may also occur. In most, the signs and symptoms are self-limited. In about 2%–3% of patients, the CMV infection is overwhelming and may be fatal [124]. Autopsy studies of renal transplant patients appearing from the 1960s onward have documented characteristic patterns of CID in these individuals [5, 29, 65, 69, 78, 91, 112, 113]. Millard et al. [91] described CMV infection either by the finding of characteristic inclusions or by viral culture in 42% of renal transplant patients.

The most common organ affected was the lung, which was involved by CMV in 38%–75% of cases [5, 29, 91, 113]. The histologic patterns of CID included diffuse panlobular interstitial pneumonia, focal interstitial pneumonitis, and scattered inclusion-bearing cells without an associated inflammatory response. Diffuse alveolar damage (DAD) with hyaline membranes was occasionally noted. Inclusions were found in the pneumocytes lining alveoli and in macrophages [29]. Other pathogens could be present but CMV in and of itself appeared to be a major source of injury to the lungs [91, 127]. The associated radiographic findings were varied and usually included evidence of patchy interstitial or alveolar infiltrates [45].

CMV infection of the gastrointestinal tract (GIT) is another important source of morbidity and mortality in renal transplant patients [2, 47, 91, 110, 124]. Foucar et al. [47] reported renal transplant recipients with colonic ulcerations and fatal lower gastrointestinal bleeding. Five patients showed either single or multiple ulcers that involved the ileocecal valve and/or colon. In some cases, ulcers extended to the anal region but the right side of the colon was predominantly affected. CMV inclusions were present in the lamina propria and muscularis mucosa, the colonic epithelial cells being rarely infected. All cases showed evidence of CMV vasculitis [47]. CMV infection associated with gastric, esophageal and small bowel ulcerations has also been described [2, 91, 124]. Press et al. [110] reported an unusual case of massive CMV infection of the myenteric plexus and lamina propria of the small bowel, colon, and appendix in association with an ulcer in the cecum. A single CMV inclusion in the base of the ulcer, as well as *Candida* hyphae, were noted. The epithelial cells were uninvolved by inclusions.

Hepatitis is a relatively common finding after renal transplantation and was seen in 45% of patients in one series [85]. Causes of hepatitis in these individuals are numerous but CMV has been implicated as an etiologic agent in a substantial number [2, 85]. Luby et al. [85] found the onset of hepatic dysfunction to be associated with CMV antibody seroconversion in a group of renal transplant patients without evidence of hepatitis B virus infection. Aldrete et al. [2] found hepatic dysfunction in 22% of a group of renal transplant recipients. Hepatic dysfunction was either mild, with only moderate liver function abnormalities in patients who remained asymptomatic (16%) or it was severe and often fatal (6%). Among the eight patients with fulminant and fatal hepatitis, the presence of CMV was documented in seven. Histologic findings have included periportal fibrosis, chronic inflammation, parenchymal necrosis, centrilobular fatty change and congestion with mild bile duct proliferation [2, 91]. Associated CMV inclusions were present.

CMV inclusions in renal transplant patients examined at necropsy have been noted in the adrenal glands, lymph nodes, salivary glands, thymus, parathyroids, spleen, prostate, and bladder [65, 113]. In general, these have been associated with little inflammatory response or tissue damage, but histologic descriptions have been sketchy. The kidneys themselves are infrequently infected in CID. Rifkind et al. [113] reported only one of five transplanted kidneys involved by CMV at autopsy despite the observation that 65% of the patients tested showed CMV viruria. Some authors have noted an association between CMV infection and rejection episodes [84]. Interpretations of this observation have included that either the virus triggers the rejection episode or the rejection episode activates a latent viral infection [84].

Ocular complications of renal transplantation include a 5% incidence of acute CMV retinitis [107]. CMV infection of the central nervous system (CNS) is seen in renal transplant recipients [33, 121]. Dorfman [33] reported evidence of CMV encephalitis in three renal transplant recipients examined at necropsy. Grossly, the brains were normal, but microscopically all patients showed microglial nodules (MGNs) scattered throughout all areas of the central neuraxis. Most of the MGNs were located in the gray matter. There was associated Alzheimer type II astrocytosis and rod cell proliferation. Sparse CMV inclusions were noted in two patients, sometimes associated with the MGNs. All patients had evidence of disseminated CMV. Schneck [121] reported evidence of CMV infection in 12 of 34 autopsied renal transplant patients with similar neuropathologic findings. The significance of MGNs will be described further below, in considering the CNS manifestations of CMV infection in AIDS.

Bone Marrow Transplantation

The average incidence of CMV infection in bone marrow transplantation (BMT) patients is approximately 50% [89]. Most CMV infections after BMT occur in the first 8–9 weeks after transplant. The incidence of CMV infection is higher in those seropositive for CMV before transplants than in those who are seronegative. Possible sources for CMV infection include reactivation of latent virus, blood products, and the donor marrow [89, 118]. CMV may be recovered from a number of sites, including the throat and the urine [89, 143].

The major complication of BMT is interstitial pneumonitis, which occurs in 50% of cases [24, 90, 98, 99]. This form of pneumonitis tends to occur 30–100 days posttransplant [24] and is fatal in approximately half of the patients [24, 98]. CMV is found in the lungs in 50% of patients who have pneumonitis [90]. In the remainder, no infectious agent is usually detected; however, *Pneumocystis carinii*, *herpes simplex*, and *herpes zoster* may be seen [142]. CMV-associated pneumonitis appears to be less frequent in autologous and syngeneic BMT recipients [100, 142]. At autopsy, the lungs have been described as showing varying degrees of pneumonitis and DAD [14]. Typical CMV inclusions are usually found within alveolar epithelial cells [90]. Beschorner et al. [10] described two major morphological patterns of CMV pneumonia: miliary and diffuse. Patients with the miliary pattern show multiple focal pulmonary lesions with necrosis, hemorrhage, and widespread CMV inclusions. All of these patients had a fulminant course. The other pattern consists of interstitial pneumonitis without alveolar cell hyperplasia, edema, lymphocytic infiltrate, and diffusely distributed CMV inclusions. The course in these patients was more indolent.

CMV-related gastrointestinal complications in BMT patients have included ulceration in all parts of the GIT [89, 128, 131]. Gastrointestinal symptoms may be the initial manifestation of CMV infection [131]. Tissues from these patients showed characteristic inclusions within capillary endothelial cells and stromal cells in the ulcer bed [131]. Grossly, the ulcers were multiple and varied in size, often with associated small hemorrhages.

Involvement of other organs (liver, pancreas, lymph nodes, adrenals, and kidneys) by disseminated CMV in BMT has been described, although detailed pathologic descriptions are lacking [14, 98].

CNS involvement by CMV is infrequent in BMT patients [93]. One autopsy series of 109 patients showed no cases with definite evidence of CMV infection of the brain, despite the fact that many patients had systemic CMV infection. One case of probable CMV encephalitis in a BMT case has been reported but pathologic confirmation was not available [28]. For unknown reasons, CMV infection of the CNS in BMT patients appears to be more infrequent than after kidney transplantation and in other immunosuppressed states.

Orthotopic Liver Transplantation

The incidence of CMV infection in orthotopic liver transplantation (OLT) patients ranges from 9% to 77% [17, 26, 49, 87, 125]. Those series with a higher incidence of CMV infection have relied on the finding of seroconversion as evidence for recent CMV infection [17, 125]. As with other organ transplants, CMV infection in these patients may be due to primary infection or reactivation of latent CMV. Reactivation accounts for the majority of infections [125]. The hepatic allograft is an important source of CMV infection in seronegative recipients [125]. In these patients, the lungs, GIT, CNS, and the liver allograft itself may be involved by CMV [3, 17, 26, 49, 87]. The incidence of interstitial pneumonitis in OLT patients appears significantly lower than in those who have received BMTs [26, 69].

GIT involvement by CMV in OLT patients has included esophagus, duodenum, stomach, and small bowel [3, 17], but the duodenum appears to be most commonly affected. Pathologic findings have included mucosal erythema, erosions, and ulcerations, with CMV inclusions in the ulcer craters. Curiously, CMV infection of the stomach has been associated with the presence of large antral folds [3].

Hepatic allograft involvement has been described in OLT [19, 31]. CMV hepatitis occurs in about 6% of OLT cases and has been associated with prolonged fever, increased total bilirubin, and elevated liver enzymes. Two morphological patterns seen include small clusters of neutrophils, with the portal areas relatively free of inflammation, and more extensive CMV inclusions, often associated with prominent lymphocytes in the portal areas. The inclusions are found almost entirely in hepatocytes, with less frequent involvement of the Kupffer cells, endothelium, and biliary epithelium.

CMV involvement of the CNS in OLT patients is infrequent, occuring in approximately 1% of patients [87]. MGNs are more common, occurring in about 15% of patients, but these in general are not associated with detectable cytomegalic inclusions.

Heart and Heart-Lung Transplantation

CMV infections have been found in 25%–100% of patients after heart transplant [20, 38, 38a, 58, 59, 72, 130]. Additionally, there is evidence that active CMV infection in cardiac transplants is associated with increased susceptibility to superinfection with other opportunistic pathogens [58]. CMV infection in these individuals can consist of a variety of CMV syndromes or pneumonitis [39]. In one series, 16% of cardiac transplant patients had CMV pneumonia and 75% of those with CMV pneumonitis died [39]. Another study found CMV to be the most common organism infecting the lungs of cardiac transplant patients, accounting for 37% of all cases of pneumonia [6]. Several series have documented disseminated CID involving the GIT, CNS, and retina [50, 72, 122]. Min et al. [92] recorded an unusual case of disseminated CMV infection involving the endothelium of coronary arteries of a cardiac transplant patient, with accompanying thrombosis and extensive myocardial necrosis.

CNS involvement by CMV in cardiac transplants has been noted in 6% of cases [122]. Anatomic regions involved have included the spinal ganglia, hippocampus, caudate, putamen, and thalamus. MGNs were noted in 33% of cases, but the vast majority of these nodules showed no inclusions.

Recipients of heart-lung transplants are also prone to CMV infections, infection rates varying from 63% to 100% [20, 39]. Patients who receive heart-lung transplants are more likely to develop CMV pneumonitis than patients with heart transplantation only [39]. Additionally, CMV pneumonitis in heart-lung transplant cases may be a significant risk factor for developing obliterative bronchiolitis [21].

CMV Infection in Miscellaneous Immunosuppressed (Non-transplant, Non-AIDS) Patients

CMV infection in patients with neoplastic disease is usually widely disseminated and occurs predominantly in those with lymphoreticular malignancies [117]. Rosen and Hajdu [117] found evidence of CMV infection in 19 of 5788 consecutive postmortem examinations carried out on cancer patients. Of the 19 individuals with CMV infection, 15 had lymphomas or leukemias and four had solid tumors. Those patients with solid tumors and CMV infection generally showed widespread metastases. CID is noted in children with leukemia [114]. Disseminated CMV infections also occur in immunocompromised individuals who lack evidence of malignancy (see below). Autopsy series of CMV infection in cancer patients have shown widespread inclusions in numerous organs, including the lungs, adrenal glands, kidneys, spleen, GIT, liver, pancreas, skin, thyroid, testis, and the brain [41, 83, 116, 117, 132, 145]. Despite the fact that CMV virus was histologically first detected and studied most extensively in the salivary glands and parotids, these organs seem rarely affected in adults [132]. Although CMV inclusions show a propensity for wide dissemination, the lungs, GIT, and adrenal glands are affected with disproportionate severity [117, 145].

The lung is the organ most commonly and severely affected in CID and the associated pneumonitis is a major cause of morbidity and mortality [116, 117, 145]. In three series, CMV inclusions were present in the lungs of 36 of 37 patients with cancer [13, 117, 145]. The gross features of CMV pneumonitis are nonspecific [116]. Microscopically, the CMV inclusions can be associated with pneumonitis or, more commonly, DAD. The typical inclusions can be found within endothelial cells, the alveolar septa, or within pneumocytes [41, 116]. Extensive hemorrhage and necrosis may be seen. In most cases (>70%) other pathogens are also identified in the lung, in particular *Pneumocystis carinii*, but CMV alone appears capable of causing a clinically significant pneumonitis [1].

Chest X-rays of patients with pure CMV chest infections can show either diffuse interstitial or alveolar infiltrates [1].

The adrenal glands are found to be the second most commonly affected organ in CID, when studied at autopsy [116, 117]. In two series the adrenals were affected in 5 of 9 and 7 of 19 patients, with widespread CID revealed at postmortem [117, 145]. The adrenals are usually grossly normal [116]. Microscopically, inclusions tend to involve the cortex rather than the medulla and can be associated with hemorrhage or focal necrosis. The necrosis is not usually extensive and cases of documented hypoadrenalism due to CMV in disseminated cancer have not been reported. Although the adrenals follow the lungs as the second most commonly affected organ, GIT lesions due to CMV tend to be clinically more significant.

Among cancer patients, the GIT in CID can be affected in one or more loci from the esophagus to the anus [56, 57, 66, 83, 97, 116]. CMV infection can be limited to one segment or may affect multiple sites. Ulcers, hemorrhage, diarrhea, colonic perforation, and vasculitis have all been reported as complications of CID. Ulcers due to CMV have been reported in the stomach, duodenum, jejunum, ileum, and colon [1, 13]. On gross inspection, they have ranged in size from small erosions to large serpiginous areas. Microscopically, CMV inclusions are typically found in the granulation tissue of the ulcer bed. In nonulcerated areas of mucosa the inclusions are present in the glandular mucosal cells and lamina propria. Fatal colonic perforation, apparently due to CMV, has been described [57]. Goodman and Porter [56] presented an unusual case of fatal colonic hemorrhage associated with vasculitis secondary to CMV.

The liver is commonly involved in CID and the infection can be associated with elevation of transaminases and alkaline phosphatase, although infection may be clinically silent [116, 145]. Henson et al. [67] reviewed 13 cases of CMV hepatitis and found focal mononuclear cell infiltrates in the liver lobules and mixed inflammatory infiltrates in the portal regions. CMV inclusions were present in all zones of the hepatic lobules but were commonly located in the hepatic cords with partial extrusion into the sinusoids. The portal areas were less frequently affected, but some inclusions were noted in vascular endothelial cells as well as in the bile duct epithelium. Bile stasis in CID of the liver is rarely reported [116].

Other organs are less frequently involved in CID [145]. CMV inclusions in the kidney are relatively uncommon despite the fact that many patients with CID show urinary excretion of the virus [40]. Inclusions in the kidney are more common in the glomerular capillaries than within tubular epithelium [145]. Bladder involvement in CID is unusual but was described in a case of hemorrhagic cystitis associated with cyclophosphamide treatment [55]. Splenic, thyroid, parathyroid, testicular, and lymph node involvement in CID have been described [41, 116, 117, 132, 145]. In most instances, CMV appeared to be unassociated with significant inflammation or tissue damage and most likely did not cause clinical signs or symptoms. Iwasaki et al. [76] reported necrotizing pancreatitis due to CMV. Most cases of CMV involvement of the pancreas, however, are unassociated with significant inflammation [117, 145].

Dermal involvement in disseminated CMV infection is rare [12, 43]. The clinical manifestations are relatively nonspecific and have included petechial, purpuric, morbilliform, and vesiculobullous lesions. Microscopically, most lesions show an uninvolved epidermis and a mixed inflammatory dermal infiltrate. Typically, CMV inclusions are noted within endothelial cells. Cardiac involvement in disseminated CMV infection is rare. Bodey et al. [13] reported one patient with CMV myocarditis associated with sudden pulmonary edema and a conduction defect that contributed to the patient's death. Most cases of myocarditis due to CMV have shown sparse numbers of inclusions associated with interstitial edema, myocyte necrosis, and interstitial inflammatory infiltrates [13, 115, 116].

In contrast to the situation with AIDS, a condition where up to 15%–25% of patients show some evidence of CMV in the CNS [4, 134], cancer patients rarely manifest CNS involvement by the virus. Rosen and Hajdu found no evidence of CNS CMV in more than 5700 consecutive autopsies performed on patients with neoplasms [117]. The case described by Goodman and Porter [56], of a large number of CMV inclusions in the cerebral cortex of a patient with malignant lymphoma, appears to be exceptional.

Disseminated CMV infection also occurs in immunosuppressed patients without metastatic neoplasms. The vast majority of these individuals have received cytotoxic agents and/or corticosteroids or have hypogammaglobulinemia. The underlying conditions are varied. CID has been reported in refractory anemia, uremia, Wegener's granulomatosis, thrombotic thrombocytopenic purpura, diabetes mellitus, empyema, lupoid hepatitis, burns, congenital immunologic deficiency, ulcerative colitis, and thymoma with associated immunoglobulin deficiency [42, 62, 74, 79, 102, 108, 115, 132, 145].

One case of CID with thymoma showed widespread CMV inclusions in the lungs and small intestine. The pathologic findings were similar to those reported in cases with disseminated cancer, with pneumonic consolidation and ulcers in the duodenum and ileum [62]. Another individual with CID associated with thymoma and immunoglobulin deficiency presented with numerous inclusions in the temporoparietal area characteristic of CMV encephalitis [79]. Since the number of cases of reported CID in thymoma/hypogammaglobulinemia is small, there may be a propensity for CNS involvement by CMV in this disorder.

CMV, apparently localized to the colon, has been reported in ulcerative colitis, Crohn's disease, and colitis of indeterminate etiology [27, 42, 62]. These patients are often treated with steroids and the diseases themselves are associated with impaired cell-mediated immunity [54]. Eyre-Brook and Dundas [42] found CMV inclusions in three of 26 cases of idiopathic inflammatory bowel disease. The inclusions did not appear to influence the course of the colitis and were not associated with progression to toxic megacolon, a possibility that has been suggested by others [27].

CMV Infection in AIDS

General Comments on CMV in AIDS

It is of historical interest to recall that early studies and reviews suggested that CMV may be not simply an opportunistic infection in patients with AIDS, but a major cause of the disorder. Immediately prior to the onset of the AIDS epidemic, the high prevalence of CMV infection in homosexual men was recognized by the finding that CMV could be cultured from the urine of 14 of 190 gay men but was not found in a single heterosexual man at a sexually transmitted disease clinic in San Francisco [36]. Significant CMV titers were present in almost 100% of gay men but in just over half of heterosexuals and in 43% of male blood donors. The following list provides a nonexhaustive summary of the known manifestations of CMV infection in patients with AIDS [35, 77, 146]:

1. Pulmonary
    - Pneumonitis
    - Diffuse alveolar damage
    - Usually other associated pathogens
2. Endocrine
    - Adrenalitis
    - "Incidental" infection of other endocrine glands
3. Gastrointestinal
    - Colitis, ileitis
    - Esophagitis
    - Gastritis
    - Hepatitis (rare)
    - Acalculous cholecystitis (rare)
4. Eyes
    - Chorioretinitis
    - Retinal detachment
    - Panuveitis
5. Skin
    - Localized infection, vasculitis
    - Association with Kaposi's sarcoma?
6. Central/Peripheral Nervous System
    - Encephalitis/ventriculitis
    - Polyneuropathy (including Guillain-Barré syndrome)

CMV can, in a given individual, produce extremely variable clinical and pathological manifestations, depending on the tissue or tissues infected. Clearly, immunosuppression – as seen in AIDS patients – can cause a latent infection to become active, even fulminant [77]. However, the most common clinical manifestation of CMV infection is either no overt disease or a nonspecific "viral" illness.

Clinical studies usually underestimate the frequency of CMV infection when compared with postmortem reviews [81]. As many as 70%–90% of AIDS patients show evidence of CMV infection in one or more organs at autopsy. A fraction of these individuals, variably estimated as 5%–25%, manifest significant morbidity and mortality as a direct function of the CMV infection. Pathologic findings related to CMV may be as variable as the clinical picture. The spectrum may range from CMV inclusions scattered throughout various organs to cytomegalic cells accompanied by extensive and very widespread necrosis, inflammation, and even hemorrhage. Klatt and Shibata [81] found evidence of CMV infection in approximately 50% of postmortem examinations performed on patients with AIDS. Organ failure that could be significantly attributed to CMV infection was seen in only one tenth of patients, however, and in almost all instances other pathogens were noted. In 62% of patients, multiple sites of CMV infection were present. The most common sites of infection, in decreasing order or frequency, were the adrenal glands, lungs, GIT, CNS, and eyes. Infants with AIDS can also develop widespread fulminant CMV infection, manifestations of which may include pancarditis, sialitis, and nephritis [16]. Some of the variability of the clinical and pathologic manifestations of CMV infection may relate to the existence of multiple strains of the virus within individual AIDS patients, a finding that has derived from elegant studies using highly specific probes in conjunction with Southern blot hybridization techniques [37, 126].

Ocular Manifestations

CMV chorioretinits is seen in 5%–10% of patients clinically and in almost one third of AIDS patients at autopsy [35, 73, 77, 105, 146]. When seen clinically, CMV retinitis portends a poor prognosis and often a rapidly fatal outcome of the AIDS syndrome. In a given individual, visual acuity may be relatively preserved if the macula is spared and inflammatory cells may be seen in the vitreous early in the course of the infection, but subsequently, as retinal atrophy develops, the inflammatory cells disappear. Lesions may be unilateral, but frequently involve both eyes. CMV chorioretinitis may be the first manifestation of disseminated CMV infection in an AIDS patient. Funduscopic examination of a patient with CMV retinitis shows multifocal yellow-white patches, variably associated with hemorrhage. Hemorrhagic necrosis may occur along vascular arcades with vascular sheathing. CMV retinitis may even develop in patients on appropriate ganciclovir therapy [104].

Many authors have emphasized the tendency of CMV to enter the endothelia of blood vessels (within the retina as elsewhere), with eventual progression from damaged vascular endothelium into adjacent retina [73, 105]. AIDS patients have also been shown to develop CMV panuveitis with infection of the corneotrabecular endothelium [30]. Virus has also been identified in the smooth muscle of the iris and ciliary body [30]. Specific endothelial changes have been ascribed to CMV inclusions within the cells lining blood vessels [123].

Pulmonary Manifestations

The isolation of CMV from the lungs or respiratory secretions of AIDS patients is a common occurrence, whereas clinically significant disease is somewhat less frequent [35, 77, 137, 138, 146]. Pulmonary infection by CMV is often seen in combination with other opportunistic pathogens, especially *Pneumocystis carinii,* which causes pneumoceptic pneumonia (PCP) [138]. Clinical manifestations of pneumonitis are relatively nonspecific, including nonproductive cough and dyspnea. Chest X-ray shows a picture similar to that noted with PCP, i.e., non-specific diffuse infiltrates within the lung fields [35, 77, 146]. In an autopsy study, almost three fourths of patients were found to have CMV documented by viral culture or the presence of characteristic light microscopic inclusions. Of those with CMV infection, 80% were felt to have pneumonitis, but frequently other pathologic findings were noted in the lungs [137]. However, in a small minority of patients, CMV was the only agent to which pulmonary changes could be ascribed.

CMV in the lung may produce extremely variable pathologic change. As in other organs, isolated CMV inclusions with no reactive change may be seen. Related pathologic findings vary from interstitial pneumonitis to diffuse alveolar damage, characterized as interstitial edema with hyaline membrane formation in the exudative phase or, eventually, a proliferative phase [137]. In terms of the diagnostic yield of pulmonary procedures for finding CMV, thoracotomy with sampling of lung tissue has the highest yield [137].

Gastrointestinal Tract

Virtually all parts of the GIT have been shown to harbor CMV infection in the context of AIDS [35, 77, 146]. Clinically, the most disabling infection is that which results in CMV colitis, estimated to occur in 5%–10% of patients. By clinical and endoscopic evaluation, CMV colitis may mimic Kaposi's sarcoma (KS). Clinical features include diarrhea, abdominal pain and hematochezia, anorexia, fever, and weight loss. Endoscopic features of CMV colitis include diffuse submucosal hemorrhages, erythema, and ulcers. Biopsy is usually diagnostic and frequently shows severe CMV vasculitis, with bowel necrosis [82, 88]. Clinically devastating consequences of CMV colitis include colonic perforation, hemorrhage, and peritonitis [48]. In the upper GIT, CMV may produce esophagitis and gastritis [9, 35, 77, 118a, 146]. Esophagitis may result in penetrating ulcers which are oval and of variable size, with projection into the esophageal lumen. When such lesions are seen on radiography, histologic verification of the diagnosis is imperative. CMV is an unusual cause of hepati-

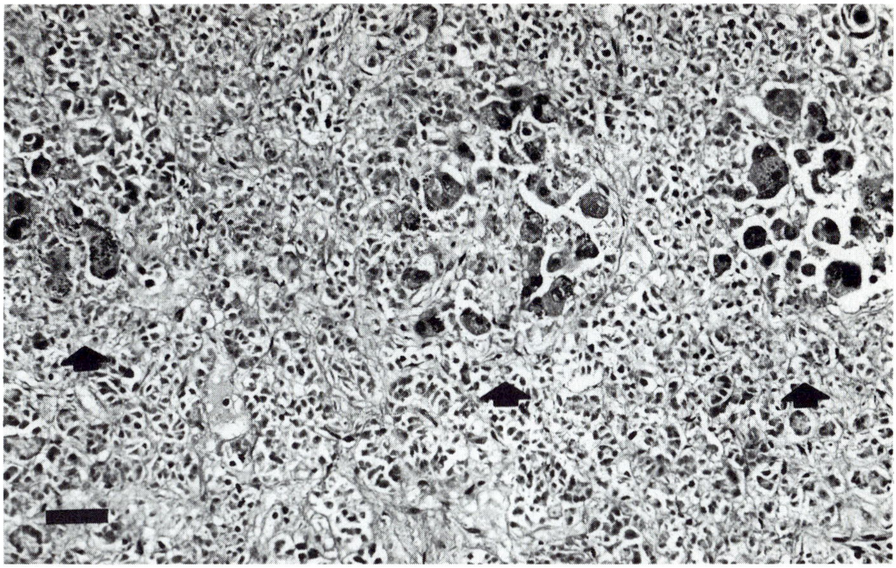

Fig. 4. Pancreas of a patient with widespread visceral cytomegalovirus. Note several clusters of cytomegalic cells (*arrowheads*). H & E; *scale marker*, 50 μm

tis [51]. Inclusions may be detected within the cytoplasm of Kupffer cells. There is a marked discrepancy between the finding of CMV inclusions and the presence of reactive and inflammatory change, i.e., single CMV inclusions may be noted in the absence of reactive, inflammatory or necrotic change within the tissues. In an autopsy series, CMV was detected in 2 of 42 specimens of liver examined [51]. CMV may also produce acalculous cholecystitis [119]. We have rarely observed CMV in the pancreas (Fig. 4).

Dermatologic Manifestations and KS

CMV may be seen as one of many pathogens within dermal abscesses in AIDS [15]. CMV has been hypothesized to be a significant pathogenetic cofactor in the development of KS associated with AIDS [34]. This hypothesis has recently been put to the test by the use of sensitive in situ hybridization techniques directed at CMV genome in KS lesions of individuals with or without AIDS.

In a study of 14 patients, CMV was assayed by in situ hybridization in 45 KS specimens, by the use of biotinylated CMV-DNA probes [63]. In half of the cases, small numbers of scattered CMV-positive cells were noted within lesions of KS, but most of the positive cells were not typical for KS, rather, were characteristic cytomegalic cells. All CMV-positive cases had at least some organs infected by CMV, with typical cytomegalic cells that contained nuclear and cytoplasmic inclusions (Fig. 5). The authors concluded that the hybridizations studies revealed only generalized CMV infection that was a function of

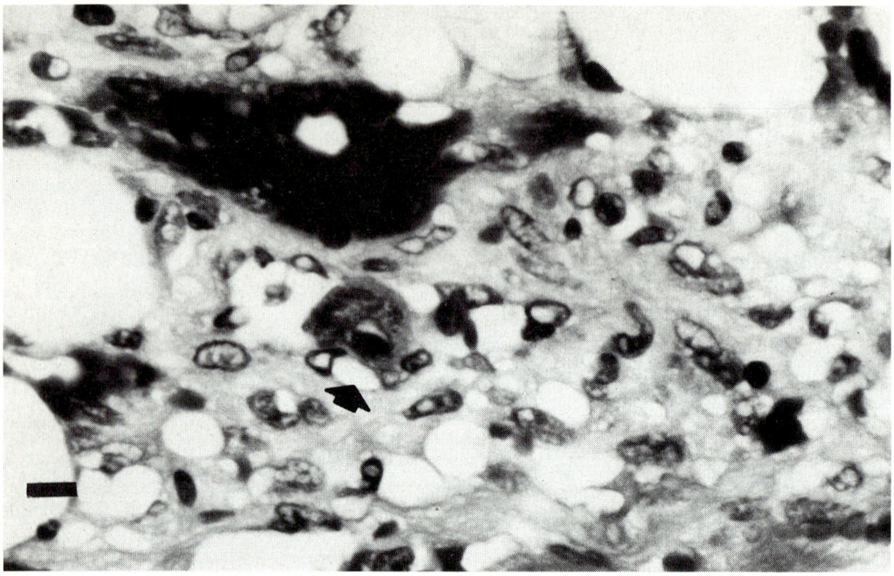

Fig. 5. Magnified view of a lesion of Kaposi's sarcoma, containing typical cytomegalic cell (*arrowhead*). H & E; *scale marker*, 10 μm

AIDS and failed to support the theory that CMV was a major *cause* of KS. In a study utilizing similar methodology, only one fifth of KS cases showed evidence of CMV involvement, and CMV-positive cells within KS lesions were rare and widely distributed [61]. Patients with "classic" (i.e., non-AIDS-related) KS showed no evidence of CMV infection by in situ hybridization or conventional light microscopy. In conclusion, there did not seem to be a strong etiologic association between KS and CMV, though the methods used as yet may not be sufficiently sensitive to detect a genuine association between the two entities.

CMV in Endocrine Glands

CMV inclusions or genome may be found in one or more of several endocrine glands of AIDS patients [35, 77, 146]. Clinically, the most significant infection is that of the adrenal gland, which may be accompanied by inflammation and necrosis of the gland [52]. CMV "adrenalitis" has been described in as many as 90% of AIDS patients. Medullary necrosis is especially pronounced when necrosis and inflammation are present. Patients may experience hypotension and sodium loss. CMV may also involve the pituitary gland (especially anterior pituitary), though this is rare, occurring in approximately 4%–5% of autopsies (random sections examined) [44]. CMV has not been found to cause a significant hypophysitis.

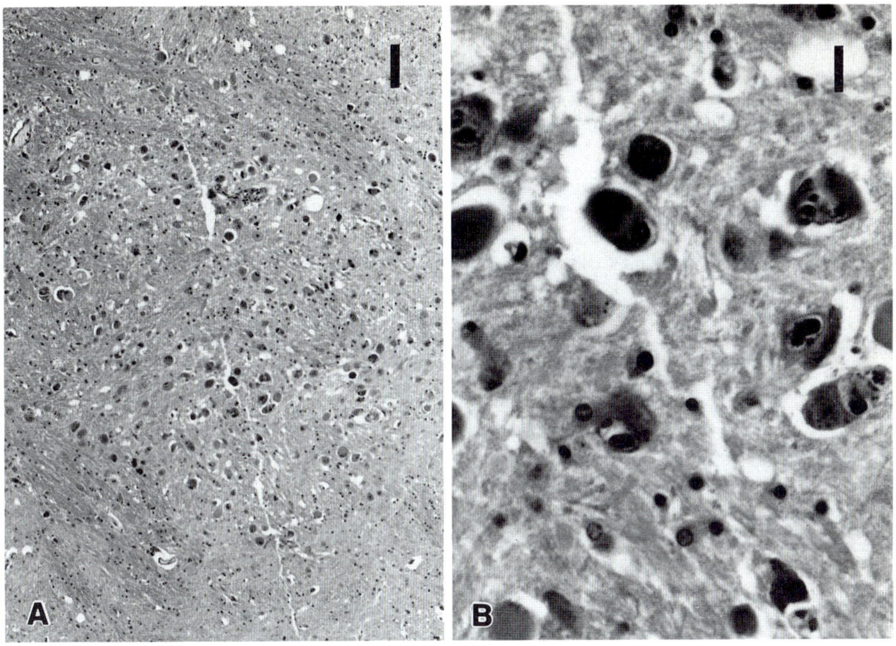

Fig. 6 A, B. Cytomegalovirus "encephalitis" in a patient with acquired immunodeficiency syndrome. **A** Field containing multiple inclusions but relatively minimal inflammation. H & E; *scale marker*, 50 μm. **B** Detail of cytomegalic cells. H & E; *scale marker*, 20 μm

Neurologic Manifestations (Central Nervous System and Peripheral Nervous System)

As in other organs, CMV in the CNS and peripheral nervous system (PNS) causes variable clinical and pathologic manifestations. CMV infection of the brain usually occurs only with widespread CMV infection throughout the rest of the body [135]. Lungs, retina, and adrenal glands are especially likely to be affected. Within the brain, CMV may be discovered as scattered cytomegalic cells in otherwise normal neural tissue (Fig. 6), or the virus may produce severe inflammatory and necrotizing change [64, 94, 135]. CMV probably gains access to the nervous system through the blood stream by way of the choroid plexus or the brain capillary endothelium (site of the blood-brain barrier). The virus has an apparent affinity for ependymal cells (Fig. 7), although it appears to be capable of infecting any neuroectodermal cell type as well as cerebral endothelium. Nevertheless, CMV may produce brisk ependymitis and ventriculitis at the ventricular surface. Elegant in situ hybridization and immunocytochemical studies show ventriculofugal spread of CMV virus from the ependymal lining into brain parenchyma [141]. The ventriculitis may be especially severe and necrotizing, causing virtual obliteration of the ventricular

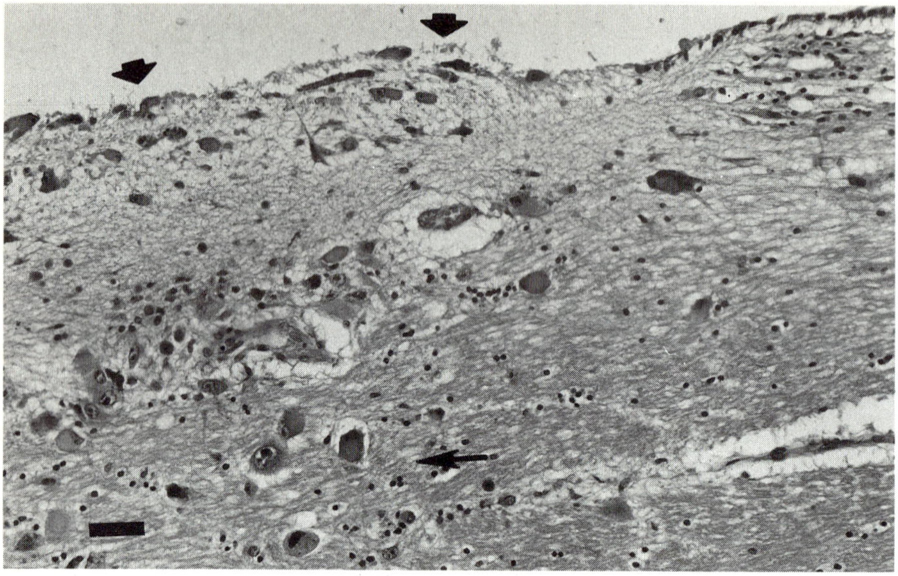

Fig. 7. Cytomegalovirus (CMV) "ependymitis". Ependymal and subependymal CMV (cytomegalic cells) in a patient with acquired immunodeficiency syndrome. Note focal loss of ependyma (*arrowheads*) and abundant inclusions in the subependymal neuropil (*arrow*). H & E; *scale marker*, 50 μm

lining (e.g., of the lateral ventricles) or it may be subtle, i.e., scattered CMV inclusions may be seen in rare foci along the ventricular system [135].

In brain parenchyma, CMV can produce a fulminant encephalitis with extensive acute and chronic inflammation with necrosis [135]. It has been suggested that CMV may produce demyelination in the white matter [134, 135]. CMV is frequently found to colocalize with HIV in the nervous system [135], and the two viruses may synergistically produce an especially severe encephalopathic picture (see Chap. 8 by M Fiala et al., this volume). Early in the course of the AIDS epidemic, CMV was associated with a low-grade MGN encephalitis, which is the most common histopathologic finding of the brain in patients with AIDS [134]. It appears that the MGN encephalitis may be associated with CMV and/or HIV infection, and is rarely present without either of the two pathogens being seen in the nervous system [134, 135].

In the peripheral nerve, CMV can produce an ascending polyradiculoneuropathy which presents clinically in a way similar to Guillain-Barré syndrome [134, 135]. In at least some instances of this entity, a major vascular component with microvascular thrombosis of vessels in the subarachnoid space and resultant necrosis of the nerve roots and even the peripheral spinal cord is noted. A more common scenario is to find cytomegalic cells within microvascular endothelium in and adjacent to skeletal muscle and peripheral nerve [134]. Peripheral neuropathies, however, are extremely common in AIDS, and the role of CMV infection in the pathogenesis of several of these is yet to be determined [86].

Conclusion

CMV can produce extremely heterogeneous pathologic change in AIDS and non-AIDS patients. The variability probably relates to the propensity of CMV to infect many different cell types and may reflect strain variations of the virus, even within a single individual. The role of CMV in many clinical entities, e.g., peripheral neuropathy in the context of AIDS, remains to be determined.

Acknowledgements. The final manuscript was prepared by Janet Railsback and Scott Brooks. Micrographs by courtesy of Stephen Kaufman. H.V. Vinters was supported in part by UCLA Multicenter AIDS Cohort Contract NO1-AI-72631.

References

1. Abdallah PS, Mark JBD, Merigan TC (1976) Diagnosis of cytomegalovirus pneumonia in compromised hosts. Am J Med 61:326–332
2. Aldrete JS, Sterling WA, Hathaway BM, Morgan JM, Diethelm AG (1975) Gastrointestinal and hepatic complications affecting patients with renal allografts. Am J Surg 129:115–124
3. Alexander JA, Cuellar RE, Fadden RJ, Genovese JJ, Gavaler JS, van Thiel DH (1988) Cytomegalovirus infection of the upper gastrointestinal tract before and after liver transplantation. Transplantation 46:378–382
4. Anders KH, Guerra WF, Tomiyasu U, Verity MA, Vinters HV (1986) The neuropathology of AIDS. UCLA experience and review. Am J Pathol 124:537–558
5. Andersen HK, Spencer ES (1969) Cytomegalovirus infection among renal allograft recipients. Acta Med Scand 186:7–19
6. Austin JHM, Schulman LL, Mastrobattista JD (1989) Pulmonary infection after cardiac transplantation: clinical and radiologic correlations. Radiology 172:259–265
7. Bale JF Jr (1984) Human cytomegalovirus infection and disorders of the nervous system. Arch Neurol 41:310–320
8. Balfour HH Jr (1979) Cytomegalovirus. The troll of transplantation. Arch Intern Med 139:279–280
9. Balthazar EJ, Megibow AJ, Hulnick D, Cho KC, Beranbaum E (1987) Cytomegalovirus esophagitis in AIDS: radiographic features in 16 patients. AJR 149:919–923
10. Beschorner WE, Hutchins GM, Burns WH, Saral R, Tutschka PJ, Santos GW (1980) Cytomegalovirus pneumonia in bone marrow transplant recipients: miliary and diffuse patterns. Am Rev Respir Dis 122:107–114
11. Betts RF, Freeman RB, Douglas RG Jr, Talley TE, Rundell B (1975) Transmission of cytomegalovirus infection with renal allograft. Kidney Int 8:385–392
12. Bhawan J, Gellis S, Ucci A, Chang T-W (1984) Vesiculobullous lesions caused by cytomegalovirus infection in an immunocompromised adult. J Am Acad Dermatol 11:743–747
13. Bodey GP, Wertlake PT, Douglas G, Levin RH (1965) Cytomegalic inclusion disease in patients with acute leukemia. Ann Intern Med 62:899–906
14. Bombi JA, Cardesa A, Llebaria C, Rives A, Carreras E, Granena A, Jimenez de Anta MT (1987) Main autopsy findings in bone marrow transplant patients. Arch Pathol Lab Med 111:125–129
15. Boudreau S, Hines HC, Hood AF (1988) Dermal abscesses with Staphylococcus aureus, cytomegalovirus and acid-fast bacilli in a patient with acquired immunodeficiency syndrome (AIDS). J Cutan Pathol 15:53–57

16. Brady MT, Reiner CB, Singley C, Roberts WH III, Sneddon JM (1988) Unexpected death in an infant with AIDS: disseminated cytomegalovirus infection with pancarditis. Pediatr Pathol 8:205–214
17. Breinig MK, Zitelli B, Starzl TE, Ho M (1987) Epstein-Barr virus, cytomegalovirus, and other viral infections in children after liver transplantation. J Infect Dis 156:273–279
18. Brigati DJ, Myerson D, Leary JJ, Spalholz B, Travis SZ, Fong CKY, Hsiung GD, Ward DC (1983) Detection of viral genomes in cultured cells and paraffin-embedded tissue sections using biotin-labeled hybridization probes. Virology 126:32–50
19. Bronsther O, Makowka L, Jaffe R, Demetris AJ, Breinig MK, Ho M et al. (1988) Occurrence of cytomegalovirus hepatitis in liver transplant patients. J Med Virol 24:423–434
20. Brooks RG, Hofflin JM, Jamieson SW, Stinson EB, Remington JS (1985) Infectious complications in heart-lung transplant recipients. Am J Med 79:412–422
21. Burke CM, Glanville AR, Macoviak JA, O'Connell BM, Tazelaar HD, Baldwin JC et al. (1986) The spectrum of cytomegalovirus infection following human heart-lung transplantation. J Heart Transplant 5:267–272
22. Campbell DA, Piercey JRA, Shnitka TK, Goldsand G, Devine RDO, Weinstein WM (1977) Cytomegalovirus-associated gastric ulcer. Gastroenterology 72:533–535
23. Cao M, Beckstead JH (1989) Localization of cytomegalovirus DNA in plastic-embedded sections by in situ hybridization. A methodologic study. Am J Pathol 134:457–463
24. Cardozo BL, Hagenbeek A (1985) Interstitial pneumonitis following bone marrow transplantation: pathogenesis and therapeutic considerations. Eur J Cancer Clin Oncol 21:43–51
25. Cockerill FR III (1985) Diagnosing cytomegalovirus infection. Mayo Clin Proc 60:636–638
26. Colonna JO II, Winston DJ, Brill JE, Goldstein LI, Hoff MP, Hiatt JR, Quinones-Baldrich W, Ramming KP, Busuttil RW (1988) Infectious complications in liver transplantation. Arch Surg 123:360–364
27. Cooper HS, Raffensperger EC, Jonas L, Fitts WT Jr (1977) Cytomegalovirus inclusions in patients with ulcerative colitis and toxic dilation requiring colonic resection. Gastroenterology 72:1253–1256
28. Cordonnier C, Feuilhade F, Vernant JP, Marsault C, Rodet M, Rochant H (1983) Cytomegalovirus encephalitis occurring after bone marrow transplantation. Scand J Haematol 31:248–252
29. Craighead JE (1971) Pulmonary cytomegalovirus infection in the adult. Am J Pathol 63:487–504
30. Daicker B (1988) Cytomegalovirus panuveitis with infection of corneo-trabecular endothelium in AIDS. Ophthalmologica 197:169–175
31. Demetris AJ, Lasky S, van Thiel DH, Starzl TE, Dekker A (1985) Pathology of hepatic transplantation. A review of 62 adult allograft recipients immunosuppressed with a cyclosporine/steroid regimen. Am J Pathol 118:151–161
32. Donnellan WL, Chantra-Umporn S, Kidd JM (1966) The cytomegalic inclusion cell. An electron microscopic study. Arch Pathol 82:336–348
33. Dorfman LJ (1973) Cytomegalovirus encephalitis in adults. Neurology (Minneap) 23:136–144
34. Drew WL (1986) Is cytomegalovirus a cofactor in the pathogenesis of AIDS and Kaposi's sarcoma? Mt Sinai J Med 53:622–626
35. Drew WL (1988) Cytomegalovirus infection in patients with AIDS. J Infect Dis 158:449–456
36. Drew WL, Mintz L, Miner RC, Sands M, Ketterer B (1981) Prevalence of cytomegalovirus infection in homosexual men. J Infect Dis 143:188–192
37. Drew WL, Sweet ES, Miner RC, Mocarski ES (1984) Multiple infections by cytomegalovirus in patients with acquired immunodeficiency syndrome: documentation by Southern blot hybridization. J Infect Dis 150:952–953

38. Dummer JS, Bahnson HT, Griffith BP, Hardesty RL, Thompson ME, Ho M (1983) Infections in patients on cyclosporine and prednisone following cardiac transplantation. Transplant Proc 15 (4) Suppl 1:2779–2781
38a. Dummer JS, Hardy A, Poorsattar A, Ho M (1983) Early infections in kidney, heart and liver transplant recipients on cyclosporine. Transplantation 36:259–267
39. Dummer JS, White LT, Ho M, Griffith BP, Hardesty RL, Bahnson HT (1985) Morbidity of cytomegalovirus infection in recipients of heart or heart-lung transplants who received cyclosporine. J Infect Dis 152:1182–1191
40. Duvall CP, Casazza AR, Grimley PM, Carbone PP, Rowe WP (1966) Recovery of cytomegalovirus from adults with neoplastic disease. Ann Intern Med 64:531–541
41. Evans DJ, Williams ED (1968) Cytomegalic inclusion disease in the adult. J Clin Pathol 21:311–316
42. Eyre-Brook IA, Dundas S (1986) Incidence and clinical significance of colonic cytomegalovirus infection in idiopathic inflammatory bowel disease requiring colectomy. Gut 27:1419–1425
43. Feldman PS, Walker AN, Baker R (1982) Cutaneous lesions heralding disseminated cytomegalovirus infection. J Am Acad Dermatol 7:545–548
44. Ferreiro J, Vinters HV (1988) Pathology of the pituitary gland in patients with the acquired immune deficiency syndrome (AIDS). Pathology 20:211–215
45. Fiala M, Payne JE, Berne TV, Moore TC, Henle W, Montgomerie JZ, Chatterjee SN, Guze LB (1975) Epidemiology of cytomegalovirus infection after transplantation and immunosuppression. J Infect Dis 132:421–433
46. Fine RN, Grushkin CM, Malekzadeh M, Wright HT Jr (1972) Cytomegalovirus syndrome following renal transplantation. Arch Surg 105:564–570
47. Foucar E, Mukai K, Foucar K, Sutherland DER, van Buren CT (1981) Colon ulceration in lethal cytomegalovirus infection. Am J Clin Pathol 76:788–801
48. Frank D, Raicht RF (1984) Intestinal perforation associated with cytomegalovirus infection in patients with acquired immune deficiency syndrome. Am J Gastroenterol 79:201–205
49. Fulginiti VA, Scribner R, Groth CG, Putnam CW, Brettschneider L, Gilbert S, Porter KA, Starzl TE (1986) Infections in recipients of liver homografts. N Engl J Med 279:619–626
50. Gentry LO, Zeluff BJ (1988) Nosocomial and other difficult infections in the immunocompromised cardiac transplant patient. J Hosp Infect 11 Suppl A:21–28
51. Glasgow BJ, Anders K, Layfield LJ, Steinsapir KD, Gitnick GL, Lewin KJ (1985) Clinical and pathologic findings of the liver in the acquired immune deficiency syndrome (AIDS). Am J Clin Pathol 83:582–588
52. Glasgow BJ, Steinsapir KD, Anders K, Layfield LJ (1985) Adrenal pathology in the acquired immune deficiency syndrome. Am J Clin Pathol 84:594–597
53. Glenn J (1981) Cytomegalovirus infections following renal transplantation. Rev Infect Dis 3:1151–1178
54. Glickman RM (1983) Inflammatory bowel disease. Ulcerative colitis and Crohn's disease. In: Petersdorf RG, Adams RD, Braunwald E, Isselbacher KJ, Martin JB, Wilson JD (eds) Harrison's principles of internal medicine, 10th edn. McGraw-Hill, New York, pp 1738–1752
55. Goldman RL, Warner NE (1970) Hemorrhagic cystitis and cytomegalic inclusions in the bladder associated with cyclophosphamide therapy. Cancer 25:7–11
56. Goodman MD, Porter DD (1973) Cytomegalovirus vasculitis with fatal colonic hemorrhage. Arch Pathol 96:281–284
57. Goodman ZD, Boitnott JK, Yardley JH (1977) Colonic perforation associated with cytomegalovirus infection. Lab Invest 36:339
58. Gorensek MJ, Stewart RW, Keys TF, McHenry MC, Babiak T, Goormastic M (1988) Symptomatic cytomegalovirus infection as a significant risk factor for major infections after cardiac transplantation. J Infect Dis 158:884–887
59. Green M, Wald ER, Fricker FJ, Griffith BP, Trento A (1989) Infections in pediatric orthotopic heart transplant recipients. Pediatr Infect Dis J 8:87–93

60. Grody WW, Cheng L, Lewin KJ (1987) In situ DNA hybridization in diagnostic surgical pathology. Hum Pathol 18:535–543
61. Grody WW, Lewin KJ, Naeim F (1988) Detection of cytomegalovirus DNA in classic and epidemic Kaposi's sarcoma by in situ hybridization. Hum Pathol 19:524–528
62. Gupta S, Saverymuttu SH, Gibbs JSR, Evans DJ, Hodgson HJF (1985) Watery diarrhea in a patient with myasthenia gravis, thymoma, and immunodeficiency. Am J Gastroenterol 80:877–881
63. Hashimoto H, Müller H, Müller F, Schmidts HL, Stutte HJ (1987) In situ hybridization analysis of cytomegalovirus lytic infection in Kaposi's sarcoma associated with AIDS. A study of 14 autopsy cases. Virchows Arch [A] 411:441–448
64. Hawley DW, Schaefer JF, Schulz DM, Muller J (1983) Cytomegalovirus encephalitis in acquired immunodeficiency syndrome. Am J Clin Pathol 80:874–877
65. Hedley-Whyte ET, Craighead JE (1965) Generalized cytomegalic inclusion disease after renal homotransplantation. Report of a case with isolation of virus. N Engl J Med 272:473–475
66. Henson DE (1972) Cytomegalovirus inclusion bodies in the gastrointestinal tract. Arch Pathol 93:477–482
67. Henson DE, Grimley PM, Strano AJ (1974) Postnatal cytomegalovirus hepatitis. An autopsy and liver biopsy study. Hum Pathol 5:93–103
68. Hilborne LH, Nieberg RK, Cheng L, Lewin KJ (1987) Direct in situ hybridization for rapid detection of cytomegalovirus in bronchoalveolar lavage. Am J Clin Pathol 87:766–769
69. Hill RB Jr, Rowlands DT Jr, Rifkind D (1964) Infectious pulmonary disease in patients receiving immunosuppressive therapy for organ transplantation. N Engl J Med 271:1021–1027
70. Ho M (1977) Virus infections after transplantation in man.Brief review. Arch Virol 55:1–24
71. Ho M, Suwansirikul S, Dowling JN, Youngblood LA, Armstrong JA (1975) The transplanted kidney as a source of cytomegalovirus infection. N Engl J Med 293:1109–1112
72. Hofflin JM, Potasman I, Baldwin JC, Oyer PE, Stinson EB, Remington JS (1987) Infectious complications in heart transplant recipients receiving cyclosporine and corticosteroids. Ann Intern Med 106:209–216
73. Holland GN, Pepose JS, Pettit TH, Gottlieb MS, Yee RD, Foos RY (1983) Acquired immune deficiency syndrome. Ocular manifestations. Ophthalmology 90:859–873
74. Hoyer JR, Cooper MD, Gabrielsen AE, Good RA (1968) Lymphopenic forms of congenital immunologic deficiency: clinical and pathologic patterns. Birth Defects 4:91–103
75. Huang E-S, Kilpatrick BA, Huang Y-T, Pagano JS (1976) Detection of human cytomegalovirus and analysis of strain variation. Yale J Biol Med 49:29–43
76. Iwasaki T, Tashiro A, Satodate R, Sata T, Kurata T (1987) Acute pancreatitis with cytomegalovirus infection. Acta Pathol Jpn 37:1661–1668
77. Jacobson MA, Mills J (1988) Serious cytomegalovirus disease in the acquired immunodeficiency syndrome (AIDS). Clinical findings, diagnosis, and treatment. Ann Intern Med 108:585–594
78. Kanich RE, Craighead JE (1966) Cytomegalovirus infection and cytomegalic inclusion disease in renal homotransplant recipients. Am J Med 40:874–882
79. Kauffman CA, Linnemann CC Jr, Alvira MM (1979) Cytomegalovirus encephalitis associated with thymoma and immunoglobulin deficiency. Am J Med 67:724–728
80. Keh WC, Gerber MA (1988) In situ hybridization for cytomegalovirus DNA in AIDS patients. Am J Pathol 131:490–496
81. Klatt EC, Shibata D (1988) Cytomegalovirus infection in the acquired immunodeficiency syndrome. Clinical and autopsy findings. Arch Pathol Lab Med 112:540–544
82. Knapp AB, Horst DA, Eliopoulos G, Gramm HF, Gaber LW, Falchuk KR, Falchuk ZM, Trey C (1983) Widespread cytomegalovirus gastroenterocolitis in a patient with acquired immunodeficiency syndrome. Gastroenterology 85:1399–1402

83. Levine RS, Warner NE, Johnson CF (1964) Cytomegalic inclusion disease in the gastro-intestinal tract of adults. Ann Surg 159:37–48
84. Lopez C, Simmons RL, Mauer SM, Najarian JS, Good RA, Gentry S (1974) Association of renal allograft rejection with virus infections. Am J Med 56:280–289
85. Luby JP, Burnett W, Hull AR, Ware AJ, Shorey JW, Peters PC (1974) Relationship between cytomegalovirus and hepatic function abnormalities in the period after renal transplant. J Infect Dis 129:511–518
86. Mah V, Vartavarian LM, Akers MA, Vinters HV (1988) Abnormalities of peripheral nerve in patients with human immunodeficiency virus infection. Ann Neurol 24:713–717
87. Martinez AJ, Estol C, Faris AA (1988) Neurologic complications of liver transplantation. Neurol Clin 6:327–348
88. Meiselman MS, Cello JP, Margaretten W (1985) Cytomegalovirus colitis. Report of the clinical, endoscopic, and pathologic findings in two patients with the acquired immune deficiency syndrome. Gastroenterology 88:171–175
89. Meyers JD (1984) Cytomegalovirus infection following marrow transplantation: risk, treatment, and prevention. Birth Defects 20:101–117
90. Meyers JD, Spencer HC Jr, Watts JC, Gregg MB, Stewart JA, Troupin RH, Thomas ED (1975) Cytomegalovirus pneumonia after human marrow transplantation. Ann Intern Med 82:181–188
91. Millard PR, Herbertson BM, Nagington J, Evans DB (1973) The morphological consequences and the significance of cytomegalovirus infection in renal transplant patients. Q J Med 42:585–596
92. Min KW, Wickemeyer WJ, Chandran P, Shadur CA, Gervich D, Phillips SJ, Zeff RH, Song J (1987) Fatal cytomegalovirus infection and coronary arterial thromboses after heart transplantation: a case report. J Heart Transplant 6:100–105
93. Mohrmann RL, Mah V, Vinters HV (1990) Neuropathologic findings after bone marrow transplantation: an autopsy study. Hum Pathol 21:630–639
94. Morgello S, Cho E-S, Nielsen S, Devinsky O, Petito CK (1987) Cytomegalovirus encephalitis in patients with acquired immunodeficiency syndrome: an autopsy study of 30 cases and a review of the literature. Hum Pathol 18:289–297
95. Myerson D, Hackman RC, Meyers JD (1984) Diagnosis of cytomegaloviral pneumonia by in situ hybridization. J Infect Dis 150:272–277
96. Myerson D, Hackman RC, Nelson JA, Ward DC, McDougall JK (1984) Widespread presence of histologically occult cytomegalovirus. Hum Pathol 15:430–439
97. Nakoneczna I, Kay S (1967) Fatal disseminated cytomegalic inclusion disease in an adult presenting with a lesion of the gastrointestinal tract. Am J Clin Pathol 47:124–128
98. Neiman P, Wasserman PB, Wentworth BB, Kao GF, Lerner KG, Storb R, Buckner CD, Clift RA, Fefer A et al. (1973) Interstitial pneumonia and cytomegalovirus infection as complications of human marrow transplantation. Transplantation 15:478–485
99. Neiman PE, Reeves W, Ray G, Flournoy N, Lerner KG, Sale GE, Thomas ED (1977) A prospective analysis of interstitial pneumonia and opportunistic viral infection among recipients of allogeneic bone marrow grafts. J Infect Dis 136:754–767
100. Neiman PE, Thomas ED, Reeves WC, Ray CG, Sale G, Lerner KG, Buckner CD et al. (1976) Opportunistic infection and interstitial pneumonia following marrow transplantation for aplastic anemia and hematologic malignancy. Transplant Proc 8:663–667
101. Nelson JS, Wyatt JP (1959) Salivary gland virus disease. Medicine (Baltimore) 38:223–241
102. Ng JWD, Chan AYT (1987) Severe hemorrhage from cytomegalovirus rectal ulcers in a burned adult. Am J Gastroenterol 82:695–698
103. Niedobitek G, Finn T, Herbst H, Bornhoft G, Gerdes J, Stein H (1988) Detection of viral DNA by in situ hybridization using bromodeoxyuridine-labeled DNA probes. Am J Pathol 131:1–4

104. O'Donnell JJ, Jacobson MA, Mills J (1987) Development of cytomegalovirus (CMV) retinitis in a patient with AIDS during ganciclovir therapy for CMV colitis. N Engl J Med 316:1607–1608
105. Pepose JS, Holland GN, Nestor MS, Cochran AJ, Foos RY (1985) Acquired immune deficiency syndrome. Pathogenic mechanisms of ocular disease. Ophthalmology 92:472–484
106. Plummer G (1973) Cytomegaloviruses of man and animals. Prog Med Virol 15:92–125
107. Porter R, Crombie AL, Gardner PS, Uldall RP (1972) Incidence of ocular complications in patients undergoing renal transplantation. Br Med J 3:133–136
108. Powell RD, Warner NE, Levine RS, Kirsner JB (1961) Cytomegalic inclusion disease and ulcerative colitis. Report of a case in a young adult. Am J Med 30:334–340
109. Preiksaitis JK, Brown L, McKenzie M (1988) The risk of cytomegalovirus infection in seronegative transfusion recipients not receiving exogenous immunosuppression. J Infect Dis 157:523–529
110. Press MF, Riddell RH, Ringus J (1980) Cytomegalovirus inclusion disease. Its occurrence in the myenteric plexus of a renal transplant patient. Arch Pathol Lab Med 104:580–583
111. Reinhard EH, Good JT, Martin E (1950) Chemotherapy of malignant neoplastic diseases. JAMA 142:383–390
112. Rifkind D, Starzl TE, Marchioro TL, Waddell WR, Rowlands DT Jr, Hill RB Jr (1964) Transplantation pneumonia. JAMA 189:808–812
113. Rifkind D, Goodman N, Hill RB Jr (1967) The clinical significance of cytomegalovirus infection in renal transplant recipients. Ann Intern Med 66:1116–1128
114. Rinker CT, McGraw JP (1967) Cytomegalic inclusion disease in childhood leukemia. Cancer 20:36–39
115. Robson GS, Mackay IR (1969) Generalized cytomegalovirus infection in a patient with lupoid hepatitis. Australas Ann Med 18:147–150
116. Rosen PP (1978) Cytomegalovirus infection in cancer patients. Pathol Annu 13:175–208
117. Rosen PP, Hajdu S (1971) Cytomegalovirus inclusion disease at autopsy of patients with cancer. Am J Clin Pathol 55:749–756
118. Rubin RH, Russell PS, Levin M, Cohen C (1979) Summary of a workshop on cytomegalovirus infections during organ transplantation. J Infect Dis 139:728–734
118a. St Onge G, Bezahler GH (1982) Giant esophageal ulcer associated with cytomegalovirus. Gastroenterology 83:127–130
119. Saraux J-L, Lenoble L, Toublanc M, Smiejan J-M, Dombret M-C (1987) Acalculous cholecystitis and cytomegalovirus infection in a patient with AIDS. J Infect Dis 155:829
120. Sarov I, Abady I (1975) The morphogenesis of human cytomegalovirus. Isolation and polypeptide characterization of cytomegalovirions and dense bodies. Virology 66:464–473
121. Schneck SA (1965) Neuropathological features of human organ transplantation. I. Probable cytomegalovirus infection. J Neuropathol Exp Neurol 24:415–429
122. Schober R, Herman MM (1973) Neuropathology of cardiac transplantation. Survey of 31 cases. Lancet 1:962–967
123. Severin M, Hartmann C (1988) Endothelial alterations in AIDS with cytomegalovirus infection. Ophthalmologica 196:7–10
124. Simmons RL, Matas AJ, Rattazzi LC, Balfour HH Jr, Howard RJ, Najarian JS (1977) Clinical characteristics of the lethal cytomegalovirus infection following renal transplantation. Surgery 82:537–546
125. Singh N, Dummer JS, Kusne S, Breinig MK, Armstrong JA, Makowka L, Starzl TE, Ho M (1988) Infections with cytomegalovirus and other herpesviruses in 121 liver transplant recipients: transmission by donated organ and the effect of OKT3 antibodies. J Infect Dis 158:124–131
126. Spector SA, Hirata KK, Neuman TR (1984) Identification of multiple cytomegalovirus strains in homosexual men with acquired imunodeficiency syndrome. J Infect Dis 150:953–956

127. Spencer ES (1974) Clinical aspects of cytomegalovirus infection in kidney-graft recipients. Scand J Infect Dis 6:315–323
128. Spencer GD, Shulman HM, Myerson D, Thomas ED, McDonald GB (1986) Diffuse intestinal ulceration after marrow transplantation: a clinicopathologic study of 13 patients. Hum Pathol 17:621–633
129. Sternberger LA (1986) Immunocytochemistry, 3rd edn. Wiley, New York
130. Stinson EB, Bieber CP, Griepp RB, Clark DA, Shumway NE, Remington JS (1971) Infectious complications after cardiac transplantation in man. Ann Intern Med 74:22–36
131. Strayer DS, Phillips GB, Barker KH, Winokur T, DeSchryver-Kecskemeti K (1981) Gastric cytomegalovirus infection in bone marrow transplant patients: an indication of generalized disease. Cancer 48:1478–1483
132. Symmers WSC (1960) Generalized cytomegalic inclusion-body disease associated with Pneumocystis pneumonia in adults. A report of three cases, with Wegener's granulomatosis, thrombotic purpura, and Hodgkin's disease as predisposing conditions. J Clin Pathol 13:1–21
133. Unger ER, Budgeon LR, Myerson D, Brigati DJ (1986) Viral diagnosis by in situ hybridization. Description of a rapid simplified colorimetric method. Am J Surg Pathol 10:1–8
134. Vinters HV, Anders KH (1990) Neuropathology of AIDS. CRC, Boca Raton
135. Vinters HV, Kwok MK, Ho HW, Anders KH, Tomiyasu U, Wolfson WL, Robert F (1989) Cytomegalovirus in the nervous system of patients with the acquired immune deficiency syndrome. Brain 112:245–268
136. Vogel FS (1958) Enhanced susceptibility of proliferating endothelium to salivary gland virus under naturally occurring and experimental conditions. Am J Pathol 34:1069–1079
137. Wallace JM, Hannah J (1987) Cytomegalovirus pneumonitis in patients with AIDS. Findings in an autopsy series. Chest 92:198–203
138. Wallace JM, Hannah JB (1988) Pulmonary disease at autopsy in patients with the acquired immunodeficiency syndrome. West J Med 149:167–171
139. Weller TH (1971) The cytomegaloviruses: ubiquitous agents with protean clinical manifestations. II. N Engl J Med 285:267–274
140. Weller TH, Hanshaw JB (1962) Virologic and clinical observations on cytomegalic inclusion disease. N Engl J Med 266:1233–1244
141. Wiley CA, Schrier RD, Denaro FJ, Nelson JA, Lampert PW, Oldstone MBA (1986) Localization of cytomegalovirus proteins and genome during fulminant central nervous system infection in an AIDS patient. J Neuropathol Exp Neurol 45:127–139
142. Wingard JR, Chen D Y-H, Burns WH, Fuller DJ, Braine HG, Yeager AM, Kaiser H, Burke PJ et al. (1988) Cytomegalovirus infection after autologous bone marrow transplantation with comparison to infection after allogeneic bone marrow transplantation. Blood 71:1432–1437
143. Winston DJ, Gale RP, Meyer DV, Young LS (1979) Infectious complications of human bone marrow transplantation. Medicine (Baltimore) 58:1–31
144. Wolber RA, Beals TF, Lloyd RV, Maassab HF (1988) Ultrastructural localization of viral nucleic acid by in situ hybridization. Lab Invest 59:144–151
145. Wong T-W, Warner NE (1962) Cytomegalic inclusion disease in adults. Report of 14 cases with review of literature. Arch Pathol 74:403–422
146. Yarrish RL (1987) Cytomegalovirus infections in AIDS. In: Wormser GP, Stahl RE, Bottone EJ (eds) AIDS-acquired immune deficiency syndrome and other manifestations of HIV infection. Noyes, Park Ridge, pp 478–517

Chapter 3 Cytomegalovirus Infection and Neonatal Hepatitis

Mei-Hwei Chang and Chin-Yun Lee

Summary

Neonatal hepatitis is an inflammatory disease of the liver found in early infancy presenting with intrahepatic cholestasis. The etiologies remain unknown in about one half to two thirds of patients. Cytomegalovirus is an important etiologic agent of neonatal hepatitis. Either congenital or perinatal infection by cytomegalovirus can cause neonatal hepatitis. However, the role of cytomegalovirus may be underestimated. An extensive search for evidence of cytomegalovirus in patients with neonatal hepatitis, including urine or saliva culture, serology, immunocytochemistry, and molecular biology studies, may show that the proportion of patients with idiopathic neonatal hepatitis is less than is currently believed.

Neonatal Hepatitis

Neonatal hepatitis is an inflammatory disease of the liver, characterized by intrahepatic cholestasis. Occurring in neonates of up to 2 months of age, the neonatal hepatitis syndrome includes infectious, metabolic, toxic, and other causes of hepatitis during their early days [25]. In a more narrow sense, the syndrome is used to refer to neonatal infectious hepatitis only [3, 32]. In many instances, it is very difficult to differentiate infectious from metabolic causes of neonatal hepatitis when similar clinical manifestations occur in different etiologies. The etiology of neonatal hepatitis often remains undetermined, despite major research efforts. As used in this paper, neonatal hepatitis refers to intrahepatic cholestasis in infancy, with its onset before 60 days of life; excluded are bacterial infections, liver disease induced by parenteral nutrition, paucity of interlobular bile ducts, and extrahepatic biliary anomalies.

Prolonged intrahepatic cholestasis is the main clinical manifestation of neonatal hepatitis. It may appear in the first week of life as neonatal hyperbilirubinemia, with persistence of jaundice beyond two weeks of life, or it may

Department of Pediatrics, College of Medicine, National Taiwan University, Taipei, Taiwan, Republic of China recur after neonatal hyperbilirubinemia disappers. In some cases, it may appear later in the neonatal period, without neonatal hyperbilirubinemia. Stool color may range from clay color to light yellow to normal color.

Among the known infectious causes of neonatal viral hepatitis, including CMV, herpes simplex virus, rubella virus, Coxsackie B virus, adenovirus type 2, reovirus type 3, varicella-zoster virus, parainfluenza virus, and ECHO viruses, CMV is the virus most commonly related to neonatal hepatitis [12].

Hepatitis A virus and hepatitis B virus are not etiologic agents of neonatal hepatitis [5]. Acute or fulminant hepatitis B virus infections occur mainly in infants of hepatitis B e antibody positive, hepatitis B surface antigen (HBsAg) carrier mothers, with a minimum incubation period of 2 months [9, 33]. Thus, the symptoms of acute hepatitis B will not appear until the third month of life. Although about 85%–90% of infants of hepatitis B e antigen positive mothers may become HBsAg carriers [6], these infants usually remain asymptomatic for as long a period of time as several years.

The role of reovirus type 3 in neonatal hepatitis is controversial. Glaser et al. [18] suggested that reovirus type 3 infection may be related to biliary atresia and neonatal hepatitis. Dussaix et al. [15] and Brown et al. [8] both denied the role of reovirus type 3 in these diseases. There was no difference in either serologic level or tissue antigen display of reovirus type 3 between infants with neonatal hepatitis and the control group.

The proportion of cases said to be accounted for by idiopathic neonatal hepatitis depends upon the facilities available for etiologic investigations. About one half to two thirds of neonatal hepatitis in infancy was idiopathic in most reports [12, 25, 29]. Unknown metabolic or infectious disease may acount for the idiopathic neonatal hepatitis. A study in Taiwan revealed the important role of CMV in the pathogenesis of neonatal hepatitis after careful search for evidence of CMV infection in cholestatic infants [10]. Extensive investigations into the etiology of neonatal hepatitis are needed to show that a lower proportion of cases are idiopathic than is currently thought.

CMV and Hepatitis

CMV causes hepatitic diseases. Hanshaw et al. [19] demonstrated that 39% of children with hepatomegaly or chronic liver diseases had evidence of CMV infection. In their study, an association of liver abnormalities in 28 of 29 children with acquired CMV infection suggests that chronic CMV infection may be clinically significant and that CMV is localized in the liver. Abnormal liver function was six times more frequent in virus-positive than in control children. Culture of the liver tissues can occasionally isolate CMV. In disseminated CMV infection, inclusion-bearing giant cells, characteristic of cytomegalic inclusion disease, can be found in the liver [16]. However, in most instances, no inclusion body, either intranuclear or intracytoplasmic, can be demonstrated in the liver in the nonimmunocompromised host, although clinical evidence of liver involvement is present [34].

In congenital infection, CMV can cause hepatitis and possibly cirrhosis in infants [35]. In addition to infants, CMV hepatitis can be observed in adults, especially in immunocompromised hosts. Henson [20] first discovered CMV inclusions in the nucleus and cytoplasm of hepatocytes in an adult who had had juvenile-onset diabetes mellitus. CMV can cause some common histologic changes of the liver. The light microscopic findings include portal and sinusoidal infiltrations of mononuclear cells, increased mitosis of hepatocytes, and minimal hepatocellular necrosis. The less common features were granuloma formation [7, 30], bile duct epithelial damage, fatty change, fibrosis, and bile stasis. Bile duct damage was found in three of the six cases of CMV liver disease reported by Snover et al. [34] as evidenced by epithelial necrosis, nuclear atypia and cytoplasmic vacuolation. These changes are very similar to those found in graft-versus-host disease [26].

Cytomegalic inclusion bodies were rarely found in the liver tissues in immunocompetent hosts infected with CMV. However, they were frequently seen in salivary glands, kidneys, lungs [21], and occasionally in the liver of CMV-infected neonates and immunocompromised hosts. Immunoperoxidase or immunofluorescent antibody often fails to demonstrate CMV in the liver tissues in immunocompetent hosts. Snover et al. [34] conducted specific immunoperoxidase staining for CMV, using high-titer human anti-CMV antibody, with negative results in five of six patients. In a normal host, the cellular immune response may be able to destroy and clear the infected cells very rapidly, leading to a state of such a minimal amount of virus in liver tissues that it is very difficult to detect the virus antigen.

Sacks [31] showed direct evidence for CMV viral antigens by an indirect fluorescence technique using monoclonal antibodies against CMV antigens. Both nuclear and cytoplasmic inclusions were demonstrated using two different monoclonal antibodies simultaneously, but biopsy specimens of the liver failed to grow CMV or show viral inclusions.

CMV and Neonatal Hepatitis

CMV as an Etiologic Agent of Neonatal Hepatitis

The neonatal hepatitis caused by CMV could be either isolated hepatitis or part of generalized CMV disease [32]. In infants with symptomatic CMV infection, either congenitally or perinatally infected, acute liver involvement was frequently found [24]. Jaundice, clay-colored or light-yellowish stools, and hepatosplenomegaly are the main clinical manifestations.

The time of infection in CMV hepatitis could be intrauterine or perinatal. The symptoms of onset in infants of intrauterine CMV infection usually begin between 48 h and the third week of age [28]. Progressive jaundice and hepatosplenomegaly are the main indications. Serum bilirubin level may rise to 20–30 mg/dl or even higher. Thrombocytopenia, hemolytic anemia, choreoretinitis, microcephaly, and low birth weight are frequent accompanying findings in severe cases. McCracken et al. [24] followed 20 infants with CMV hepatitis for up to 9 years. Among them, 18 of the 20 had congenital CMV infection, 18 had hepatomegaly, and ten had abnormal liver function up to 21 months of age. In perinatal infection by CMV, jaundice and hepatosplenomegaly are also the main clinical manifestations. Symptoms are usually mild; however, fulminant hepatic failure may occur in rare cases.

Diagnosis can be made from clinical hepatitis and rising CMV antibody titers or positive IgM antibody in spite of absence of inclusion bodies in the liver tissues or failure to demonstrate CMV antigens in the liver by immunoperoxidase or immunofluorescent staining. Liver histology shows deranged lobular structure, variable inflammation, giant cell transformation, ballooning or necrosis of hepatocytes, cholestasis, and, occasionally, large intranuclear inclusions. Isolation of virus from fresh urine is frequently positive. Positive cultures were reported from liver biopsy specimens.

Alagille [2] reported that 5 of 224 patients had neonatal hepatitis caused by cytomegalic inclusion disease, while in 169 patients the disease was idiopathic. Mowat [25] reported that 3 cases of the disease in 142 infants with neonatal hepatitis were caused by CMV infection, while 91 were idiopathic. A study of an Australian group of 130 infants showed that 13 cases of neonatal hepatitis came from CMV infection, while 88 were idiopathic [12]. In a study from Africa, none of the 107 cases of neonatal hepatitis were due to CMV infection, while 52 were idiopathic [29]. Due to the diagnostic difficulty in demonstrating CMV in liver tissues, CMV-induced neonatal hepatitis might be underdiagnosed. A more sensitive method is needed to detect CMV in the liver.

Prognosis for CMV neonatal hepatitis is good in general. McCracken et al. [24] followed up 12 of 18 congenitally or perinatally infected infants with hepatomegaly for periods of from 1 to 8 years. No evidence of severe liver disease was found by clinical, chemical, or biopsy criteria during this follow-up period [31]. Deutsch et al. [13] reported that in neonatal hepatitis of infectious origin, CMV caused a particularly benign form of hepatitis, but was a frequent cause of brain damage or other disabilities [2]. None of 21 infants with CMV neonatal hepatitis died before 12 months of age, and only one died from liver disease after 12 months of age. In contrast, infants with neonatal hepatitis from other infectious causes, such as toxoplasmosis, adenovirus, Coxsackie virus, and rubella virus had poorer prognosis (6 of 15 died within the first year of life). However, fulminant hepatic failure and biliary cirrhosis may be the outcome of severe CMV neonatal hepatitis [35]. Dick and Mowat [14] reported a high mortality rate in patients with neonatal hepatitis caused by systemic viral infection in contrast to the more favorable outcome of CMV neonatal hepatitis reported by Danks et al. [12].

CMV Infection in Neonatal Hepatitis in Taiwan

CMV infection is very common in Taiwan. The infection occurs early in life, mainly during infancy and early childhood. A seroepidemiologic survey in

Taipei city in 1984 using enzyme-linked immunosorbent assay showed a 40%–50% seropositive rate in children of 1–2 years of age and a 50%–60% positive rate in children aged between 3 and 5 years. This reached 70% after 9 years of age. The seroepidemiologic study done in 1989, in the same city, showed that seropositive rates remained at 41%–51% for ages 2–10 years, with a rise to 74% at the age of 11.

In Taiwan, 70%–90% of pregnant women were seropositive for CMV. The overall isolation rate of CMV from the uterine cervix was 28% in a longitudinal study of 33 women [11]. CMV was found in the cervix in 53% of the patients in whom local antibody was 1:64 or higher.

CMV is closely associated with neonatal hepatitis in Taiwan. The virus was recovered from the urine culture of 43.2% of 81 infants with neonatal hepatitis, 14.3% of 14 infants with biliary atresia, and 11.4% of 70 control infants with bronchiolitis [23]. In a recent study, evidence of CMV infection, including CMV-positive urine culture and/or positive results of serologic tests, was found in 22 (49%) of 45 infants with neonatal hepatitis [10]; eight patients were both virus-culture- and serologically positive, six were serologically positive only, and eight were virus-culture-positive only. Both serologic tests and urine culture gave negative results in 23 cases (51%).

The prognosis of CMV neonatal hepatitis in Taiwan is not different from neonatal hepatitis of unknown etiologies [23]. Of the 22 CMV-infected patients with long-term follow-up, four died, four recovered but were suffering from psychomotor retardation, and fourteen recovered without sequelae. Four patients had severe giant cell hepatitis with hemolytic anemia. All four had CMV infection and glucose-6-phosphate dehydrogenase deficiency. Three of them died from fulminant hepatic failure and one is living without liver disease but with hearing impairment. Of the 23 patients without evidence of CMV infection by serologic examination of urine culture, four died, three recovered but had psychomotor retardation, and sixteen recovered without sequelae.

Molecular Biology Studies of CMV in Neonatal Hepatitis

Detection of CMV in Liver Tissues of Infants with Neonatal Hepatitis by In Situ Hybridization

In 22 infants with neonatal hepatitis, diagnosed by clinical and histologic liver examinations, in situ hybridization in liver tissue revealed that 12 had evidence of CMV infection. In ten, both urine cultures and serologic tests were positive for CMV; in one, urine culture only was positive; and in one, results of serologic tests only were positive. CMV DNA probes were prepared from plasmids containing CMV DNA fragments and were separated from the vector DNA. Of the 22 infants with neonatal hepatitis, 11 showed positive results of in situ hybridization for CMV. The correlation between the results of serologic tests/urine culture and in situ hybridization study was good.

Detection of CMV in Liver Tissues of Infants with Neonatal Hepatitis by Polymerase Chain Reaction

The copy number of CMV in the liver tissue of infants with neonatal hepatitis is possibly too small to be demonstrated in patients with neonatal hepatitis by immunofluorescent stain unless there are inclusion bodies in the hepatocytes or biliary epithelium.

Using polymerase chain reaction (PCR), the genome of CMV can be amplified to at least 10^5 times. Forty-six infants with neonatal hepatitis were studied for CMV in liver tissues by PCR using two pairs of primers, one located at the immediate early gene region one, the other at the immediate early gene two (the latter was provided by Professor Eng-Shang Huang). Both products of the PCR were 240 bp DNA. Forty-six percent of the 46 infants with neonatal hepatitis showed positive results of PCR for CMV. Fifty percent of these 46 infants had evidence of CMV infection with either positive urine culture or positive serology (positive for immunoglobulin M or rising titers of complement fixation antibody). None of the liver tissues from 30 infants without clinical evidence of cholestasis and CMV infection showed positive result for CMV by PCR.

The PCR results indicate that the relationship between CMV and neonatal hepatitis is become closer and more direct.

CMV Infection and Paucity of the Interlobular Bile Ducts

Besides neonatal hepatitis, CMV infection was also reported to be a possible cause of paucity of interlobular bile ducts (intrahepatic biliary hypoplasia). CMV is bile duct tropic. Oppenheimer et al. [27] reported a CMV-infected black male neonate with paucity of intrahepatic bile ducts. The infant died at 5 days old due to complications from surgery for the relief of meconium peritonitis. Characteristic inclusion bodies were noted in numerous bile ducts, but were not seen in parenchymal cells [27]. There was bile stasis, extramedullary hematopoiesis, mild portal inflammatory infiltration, and an apparent decrease in the number of bile ducts. No multinucleated giant cells were found.

Finegold and Carpenter [17] also reported a fetus at 24 weeks' gestation with ascites and calcification of the abdomen. Pathologic examination revealed disseminated CMV infection with inclusions in the lung, pancreas, kidney, and liver. There were no bile ducts in most portal areas. In other portal areas, there was a combination of inclusion in epithelial cells of the remaining interlobular bile ducts and intense duct-oriented inflammation.

Paucity of interlobular bile ducts was found also with intrahepatic cholestasis in early infancy, which should be differentiated from neonatal hepatitis. It can be divided into syndromic and nonsyndromic type. The former has a familial tendency associated with multiple associated anomalies including characteristic facies, peripheral pulmonary artery stenosis, vertebral arch defect, and posterior embryotoxon of the eyes [4]. The nonsyndromic paucity of the interlobular bile ducts may be caused by several pathogens. CMV is one of the important etiologic agents. As proposed by Finegold and Carpenter [17], CMV may cause inflammatory destruction of intrahepatic bile ducts, leading to paucity of the intrahepatic bile ducts. In patients with acquired immunodeficiency syndrome, CMV infection has also caused progressive mucosal irregularities of the intrahepatic ducts with ultimate duct destruction [1].

Future Prospect

CMV is an important etiologic agent of neonatal hepatitis. The diagnostic sensitivity may be increased by extensive research using serologic tests, virus culture, immunocytochemistry, and molecular biologic methods such as in situ hybridization and PCR. Bile duct inflammation and destruction by CMV can very likely lead to bile duct anomalies during the fetal or neonatal period.

Because normal subjects can also have saliva or urine cultures positive for CMV, further investigations may be needed to clarify the role of CMV in neonatal hepatitis and biliary anomalies. The concept of "infantile obstructive cholangiopathy" is plausible [22]. The timing and the target of CMV infection, i.e., hepatocytes or bile duct epithelial cells, may affect the outcome.

References

1. Agha FP, Nostrant TT, Abrams GD, Mazanec M, Van Moll L, Gumucio JJ et al. (1986) Cytomegalovirus cholangitis in a homosexual man with acquired immune deficiency syndrome. Am J Gastroenterol 81:1068–1072
2. Alagille D (1972) Clinical aspects of neonatal hepatitis. Am J Dis Child 123:287–291
3. Alagille D, Odievre M (1979) Liver and biliary tract disease in children. Wiley, New York
4. Alagille D, Estrada A, Hadchouel M, Gautler M, Odievre M, Dommergues JP (1987) Syndromic paucity of interlobular bile ducts (Alagille syndrome or arteriohepatic dysplasia): review of 80 cases. J Pediatr 110:195–200
5. Balistreri WF, Tabor E, Gerety RJ (1980) Negative serology for hepatitis A and B viruses in 18 cases of neonatal cholestasis. Pediatrics 66:269–271
6. Beasley RP, Trepo C, Stevens CE, Szmuness W (1977) The e antigen and vertical transmission of hepatitis B surface antigen. Am J Epidemiol 105:94–98
7. Bonkowsky HL, Lee RV, Klatskin G (1975) Acute granulomatous hepatitis – occurrence in cytomegalovirus mononucleosis. JAMA 232:1284–1288
8. Brown WR, Sokol RJ, Levin MJ, Silverman A, Tamaru T, Lilly JR, Hall RJ, Cheney M (1988) Lack of correlation between infection with reovirus 3 and extrahepatic biliary atresia or neonatal hepatitis. J Pediatr 113:670–676
9. Chang MH, Lee CY, Chen DS, Hsu HC, Lai MY (1987) Fulminant hepatitis in children in Taiwan: the important role of hepatitis B virus. J Pediatr 111:34–39
10. Chang MH, Hsu HC, Lee CY, Wang TR, Kao CL (1987) Neonatal hepatitis: a follow-up study. J Pediatr Gastroenterol Nutr 6:203–207

11. Chiang WT, Chen HM, Hsieh CY, Tsai WS, Wei PY, Alexander ER (1981) Cytomegalovirus infection of the uterine cervix: local cervical infection and antibody response. Int J Gynaecol Obstet 19:177–180
12. Danks DM, Campbell PE, Jack I, Rogers J, Smith AL (1977) Studies of the aetiology of neonatal hepatitis and biliary atresia. Arch Dis Child 52:360–367
13. Deutsch J, Smith AL, Danks DM, Campbell PE (1985) Long term prognosis for babies with neonatal liver disease. Arch Dis Child 60:447–451
14. Dick MC, Mowat AP (1985) Hepatitis syndrome in infancy – an epidemiologic survey with 10 year follow up. Arch Dis Child 60:512–516
15. Dussaix E, Hadchouel M, Tardieu M, Alagille D (1984) Biliary atresia and reovirus type 3 infection. N Engl J Med 310:658
16. Embil JA, Krause VW, Haldane EV, Easterbrook KB, Crosby JM (1969) Congenital cytomegalovirus infection: clinical, pathological and virological studies of two fetal cases. Can Med Assoc J 101:697–705
17. Finegold MJ, Carpenter RJ (1982) Obliterative cholangitis due to cytomegalovirus: a possible precursor of paucity of intrahepatic bile ducts. Hum Pathol 13:662–665
18. Glaser JH, Balistreri WF, Morecki R (1984) Role of reovirus type 3 in persistent infantile cholestasis. J Pediatr 105:912–915
19. Hanshaw JB, Betts RF, Simon G, Boynton RC (1965) Acquired cytomegalovirus infection – association with hepatomegaly and abnomal liver-function tests. N Engl J Med 272:602–609
20. Henson D (1969) Cytomegalovirus hepatitis in an adult – an autopsy report. Arch Pathol 88:199–203
21. Ho M (1982) Cytomegalovirus-biology and infection. Plenum, New York
22. Landing BH (1974) Considerations of the pathogenesis of neontatal hepatitis, biliary atresia and choledochal cyst – the concept of infantile obstructive cholangiopathy. Prog Pediatr Surg 6:113–139
23. Lee CY (1979) Cytomegalovirus as an important cause of neonatal hepatitis in Taiwan. Acta Paediatr Sin 20:271–272
24. McCracken GH, Shinefield HR, Cobb K, Rausen AR, Dische MR, Eichenwald HF (1969) Congenital cytomegalic inclusion disease – a longitudinal study of 20 patients. Am J Dis Child 117:552–539
25. Mowat AP (1987) Liver disorders in childhood. Butterworth, London
26. O'Grady JG, Alexander GJM, Sutherland S, Donaldson PT, Harvey F, Potmann B, Calne RY, Williams R (1988) Cytomegalovirus infection and donor/recipient HLA antigens: interdependent co-factors in pathogenesis of vanishing bile-duct syndrome after liver transplantation. Lancet 2:302–305
27. Oppenheimer EH, Esterly JR (1973) Cytomegalovirus infection: a possible cause of biliary atresia. Am J Pathol 71:2a
28. Panjvani ZFK, Hanshaw JB (1981) Cytomegalovirus in the perinatal period. Am J Dis Child 135:56–60
29. Pretorius PJ, Roode H (1974) Obstructive jaundice in early infancy. S Afr Med J 48:811
30. Reller LB (1973) Granulomatous hepatitis associated with acute cytomegalovirus infection. Lancet 2:20–22
31. Sacks SL (1984) Cytomegalovirus hepatitis. Evidence for direct hepatic viral infection using monoclonal antibodies. Gastroenterology 86:346–350
32. Silverman A, Roy CR (1983) Pediatric clinical gastroenterology. Mosby, St Louis
33. Sinatra FR, Shah P, Wessman JY, Thomas DW, Merritt RJ, Tong MJ (1982) Perinatal transmitted acute icteric hepatitis B in infants born to hepatitis B surface antigen-positive and antihepatitis B e-positive carrier mothers. Pediatrics 90:557–559
34. Snover DC, Horwitz CA (1984) Liver disease in cytomegalovirus mononucleosis. A light microscopical and immunoperoxidase study of six cases. Hepatology 4:408–412
35. Wyatt JP, Saxton J, Lee RS, Pinkerton H (1950) Generalized cytomegalic inclusion disease. J Pediatr 36:271–294

Chapter 4 Human Cytomegalovirus and Atherogenesis *

Joseph L. Melnick [1], Ervin Adam [1], and Michael E. DeBakey [2]

Summary

The frequent finding of cytomegalovirus (CMV) antigens and nucleic acid sequences in arterial smooth muscle cells suggests that infection of the arterial wall may be common in patients with atherosclerosis. Immunosuppressive treatment of heart transplant patients often leads to CMV infection. As an apparent consequence, severe atherosclerosis develops in the transplanted organ. In seroepidemiologic studies, high levels of CMV antibodies were found to be associated with atherosclerotic disease, suggesting the occurrence of a periodically activated latent infection. Since CMV DNA, but not infectious virus, is found in arterial cells, the artery itself might be the site of latency and contribute to the initiation of atherogenesis. Furthermore, as a working hypothesis, it seems that the biological properties of CMV are consistent with pathogenic involvement of the virus at several levels of the atherogenic process.

Introduction

In 1988, in Vol. 35 of *Progress in Medical Virology*, we reviewed in some detail work of the past 15 years on the possible role of viruses in the pathogenesis of atherosclerosis. Beyond our own studies, little had been published on the association of virus with human atherosclerosis. Since then, a number of significant articles have appeared which strengthen the hypothesis for a role of cytomegalovirus (CMV) in this widespread and serious disease.

Atherosclerotic plaques consist of the complex accumulations produced by arterial smooth muscle cells, which have been stimulated to proliferate excessively at the site of plaque formation. This abnormal cellular proliferation may

[1] Division of Molecular Virology and
[2] Department of Surgery, Baylor College of Medicine, Texas Medical Center, One Baylor Plaza, Houston, TX 77030, USA

* This article is based on a presentation made by one of the authors (J.L.M.) at the meeting of the European Society Against Viral Disease, held in Groningen, The Netherlands, June 18, 1989

be initiated by an injury to the endothelial lining of the artery, which results in exposure of underlying smooth muscle cells to hormones, low-density lipoproteins, and various growth-promoting factors associated with serum and platelets. There may also be a transforming event that causes arterial smooth muscle cells to begin dividing and form a focus of proliferating cells.

The possibility that virus infection plays a role in the pathogenesis of atherosclerosis is compatible with the hypotheses described above, since viruses may cause cell destruction, alter cellular metabolism, or induce transformation of infected cells. Recent work in this area has been stimulated by the finding that atherosclerotic lesions, strikingly similar to those in human disease, were reproducibly induced in chickens by an avian herpesvirus. Viral antigens were identified by immunofluorescence in smooth muscle cells within the developing lesions, further substantiating a viral etiology for atherosclerosis in chickens.

The above considerations have prompted us to search for evidence of involvement of CMV and herpes simplex virus (HSV), in human arterial disease. These viruses are very common and cause primary infections in infants and young children in every country. Particularly in the case of CMV, viremia is associated with such infections, thus exposing cells of the blood vessels to the virus early in life.

No markers of HSV infection were found in the arterial samples we studied. However, CMV-infected cells were detected in a number of lesions taken from patients with atherosclerosis, and also in biopsies of apparently uninvolved aorta taken from such patients [9, 16, 20]. Infectious virus was not recovered, but CMV antigen and viral DNA were detected. In addition, epidemiological studies were conducted in which viral antibodies were measured in patients with atherosclerosis and in matched controls [1, 21]. High levels of antibodies to CMV were associated with clinically manifest atherosclerotic disease. The recently discovered characteristics of the infection of arterial cells by CMV are consistent with the biological properties of the virus, and offer a hypothesis for the pathogenic involvement of CMV at several points in the atherogenic process. This view has been supported by a number of recent publications, which are reviewed below.

Animal Model Systems

Strong support for a viral etiology of atherosclerosis comes from the Fabricants' experiments showing that atherosclerotic plaques can be reproducibly induced in chickens by the Marek's disease virus, an avian herpesvirus which previously had been known to cause cells to proliferate and to produce a fatal lymphoma in chickens [5]. The plaques, strikingly similar to those seen in human atherosclerosis, were characterized by extensive proliferation of smooth muscle cells within the intima. In contrast, uninfected chickens did not develop atherosclerotic plaques, regardless of their blood cholesterol level. Avian herpesvirus antigens were identified by immunofluorescence in smooth muscle cells within the developing lesions, and virus nucleic acid sequences were subsequently detected in arteries of infected chickens, by use of in situ hybridization methods. Prior immunization with a related herpesvirus of turkeys prevented virus-induced atherosclerosis [6].

A second avian model system for herpesvirus-related atherosclerosis is provided by the Japanese quail. Strains of quail were extensively inbred by Shih et al. [23], and selected for either susceptibility or resistance to atherosclerosis induced by dietary cholesterol. Dot hybridization experiments using a library of viral DNA probes showed that DNA extracted from arteries or from embryos of susceptible quail contained sequences related to the avian herpesvirus, whereas DNA from tissues of resistant quail did not.

The mechanism of virus-induced atherogenesis was investigated by infecting smooth muscle cells cultured from normal chicken arteries with the virus [4]. Virus-infected cells contained more cholesterol and cholesteryl esters than did mock-infected cells. In addition, arterial tissue of infected chickens was analyzed and showed an increase in total lipids, especially cholesterol, cholesteryl esters, and phospholipid [10].

Herpesviridae Associated with Atherosclerosis in Humans

Many characteristics of the human herpesviruses, and of CMV in particular, are consistent with a role in atherogenesis. All are widely distributed in the population, and childhood infections are common. For example, in the United States the prevalence of antibodies to CMV is about 10%–15% in the adolescent population, rises to more than 50% by age 35, and exceeds 70% in adults over age 65, a pattern similar to the incidence of atherosclerosis. Herpesviruses can establish both chronic persistent and latent infections, with nervous tissue the site of latency for HSV and varicella-zoster virus (VZV), and lymphocytes for Epstein-Barr virus (EBV), another member of the human herpesvirus family. The site of latency for CMV is unknown, although this virus has been isolated from a variety of tissues and cells throughout the body, including lymphocytes, which have prolonged contact with cells lining the blood vessel walls. Because of features of these viruses relating to latency and transformation, it has been speculated that infection of arterial smooth muscle cells by CMV or other human herpesviruses might stimulate these cells to proliferate and thereby contribute to the formation of atherosclerotic plaques.

The experiments demonstrating herpesvirus-mediated atherosclerosis in chickens, together with the current knowledge concerning human herpesviruses, influenced several research groups to look for evidence of possible herpesvirus involvement in human atherosclerosis. These studies are summarized in the following paragraphs.

In our studies [1, 16, 20, 21], immunocytochemical techniques (immunofluorescence and immunoperoxidase) were used to screen arterial tissues for evidence of infection with HSV1, HSV2, and CMV. This approach was based on the premise that cells which are abortively or persistently infected with a virus may express one or more proteins coded by the viral genome, even if little or no infectious virus is produced. Atherosclerotic plaque tissues were obtained primarily from patients undergoing endarterectomy to relieve stenosis of the carotid arteries, and hence represented an advanced stage of the disease. A few plaque tissues from abdominal aortas, iliac arteries, and femoral arteries also were obtained. In addition, punch biopsies of the ascending aortas were obtained from patients undergoing coronary artery bypass surgery. These "uninvolved" tissues showed minimal atherosclerotic changes upon histological examination. By direct electron microscopic examination of biopsy specimens from the proximal aorta of patients with atherosclerosis, virions of the *Herpesviridae* family could be detected, but only after a painstaking, meticulous search [9]. Observed in smooth muscle cells in uninvolved areas in 10 of 60 patients examined, they had the features of incomplete virions. The virions were relatively few in number, but when present they were often present in a cluster. Sections from more than 300 plaque tissues and 60 "uninvolved" aortic punch biopsies were reacted with hyperimmune antisera to HSV1, HSV2, and CMV. None of these tissues reacted with any of the viral antisera.

Production of viral proteins is often higher in actively growing cells than in quiescent cells such as those in differentiated tissue. Therefore, explant cultures were established from both the plaque tissues and the "uninvolved" aortic tissues of the above patients. Smooth-muscle-like cells were successfully grown from finely minced pieces of 54 arterial samples. These cells were tested during their first or second passage in culture for both CMV and HSV1 antigens, and in some cases for HSV2 antigens. Of the 54 arterial outgrowths, 20 yielded cells containing CMV-specific proteins, whereas none contained HSV1 or HSV2 proteins. If CMV is indeed a direct cause of atherosclerosis, it may seem somewhat surprising that a higher percentage of cultures from the "uninvolved" aorta tissues (52%) contained CMV antigens than did cultures from advanced atherosclerotic plaques (29%). However, in the virus-infected chickens discussed above, viral antigens were found in smooth muscle cells of the media during the early stages of pathogenesis. But in advanced disease, viral antigens were found only in smooth muscle cells at the periphery of atherosclerotic plaques, never in the lesions themselves. Thus, CMV may be an initiating factor that is no longer active in advanced complex plaques. These plaques contain few viable cells (as indicated by the low rate of success in establishing explant cultures), and it is likely that the cells that did grow were derived from tissue peripheral to the necrotic areas of the plaques.

Seventeen of the cell cultures were also examined for the presence of CMV and HSV nucleic acids by the method of in situ hybridization using viral DNA probes [20]. The results were similar to those described above, except that some cultures that were negative for CMV antigens proved positive for CMV nucleic acids, reflecting the greater sensitivity of the in situ hybridization reaction.

The in situ hybridization technique was used by Benditt et al. [2] to look for nucleic acid sequences specific for HSV2, CMV, and EBV in small pieces of ascending aortic tissue removed during coronary bypass surgery. In the initial series of experiments, HSV sequences were detected in 11 of 160 tissue samples. In most cases there was little intimal thickening, and positive cells were scattered in the media. In the second series of experiments, four tissue samples were selected because they contained abnormally thickened intima. Sections cut from these tissues were hybridized with DNA probes for HSV2, CMV, and EBV. Two tissues reacted with the HSV2 probe; none reacted with any of the other probes. The cells containing HSV nucleic acid sequences were located in discrete foci of increased cellularity within or adjacent to the intima.

A subsequent study conducted by Yamashiroya et al. [28] demonstrated the presence of HSV and CMV genomic sequences and antigens in the coronary arteries and thoracic aortas of 20 young trauma victims between 15 and 35 years of age. Each had been in good health prior to being killed in an accident. Fresh arterial tissue was removed at autopsy and studied by in situ DNA hybridization and by immunoperoxidase methods.

Among the 20 subjects, either HSV or CMV latency was detected in the coronary arteries of 8 subjects, and in the thoracic aortas of 7 subjects. None of the specimens were positive for EBV. It is noteworthy that the positive HSV/CMV findings were often present in areas of the arterial wall showing early atheromatous changes: focal areas of intimal thickening with smooth muscle proliferation and lymphocytic infiltration. No complete infectious virus could be detected, in keeping with our earlier studies.

In recent investigations, carried out in the Netherlands by Hendrix et al. [11, 12], femoral or abdominal arterial samples were obtained (1) from 44 patients undergoing vascular surgery (mean age, 66 years) and (2) from an autopsy-control group of 34 patients (mean age, 69 years), who died from non-atherosclerosis-associated diseases and in whom abdominal aorta specimens were removed 12 h postmortem. Demonstration of sequence homology to CMV nucleic acid in smooth muscle cells in the arterial media was achieved by use of an immediate early 7-kb fragment as well as a 2.9-kb fragment from the late genomic region. Initially, both in situ hybridization and homology by dot-blotting with extracted DNA were used in the Bruggeman laboratory [11]. Subsequently, the more sensitive polymerase chain reaction was added in an extended study [12].

The dot-blot DNA hybridization detected viral genome in a low percentage (18%–29%) of samples, regardless of whether an early or late viral DNA probe was used, and regardless of the source of the tissue specimen. These findings are similar to those made by other laboratories [16, 20, 28]. The in situ DNA hybridization technique demonstrated viral nucleic acid in about half of both groups of patients using the early probe, but only in 12%–15% with the late probes. As shown in Table 1, only the more sensitive polymerase chain reaction (PCR) permitted differences to be detected between the two groups of patients by demonstrating CMV DNA in 90% of arterial tissues of the surgical patients as compared to 53% of the autopsy-control group. Identical case-control differences were found using both immediate early and late sequence primers, as both sequences were found in all the samples that were positive by

Table 1. Results of dot-blot and in situ DNA hybridization with probes derived from immediate early (Es fragment) and late (BH fragment) genomic regions and of the polymerase chain reaction with primers reactive with immediate early (IE primers) and late (LA primers) genomic sequences (from [12])

	Arteries of atherosclerosis patients			Arteries of control patients		
	Samples tested (*n*)	Positive results *n*	Positive results %	Samples tested (*n*)	Positive results *n*	Positive results %
Dot-blot hybridization						
Early viral gene sequence	44	11	25	33	7	21
Late viral gene sequence	14	4	29	23	4	18
In situ hybridization						
Early viral gene sequence	41	18	44	33	19	58
Late viral gene sequence	41	5	12	33	5	15
Polymerase chain reaction						
Early viral gene primers	30	27	90	34	18	53
Late viral gene primers	30	27	90	34	18	53

the PCR. As in studies by other investigators [1, 2, 16, 28], no infectious virus was isolated from the arterial specimens.

In the studies that had been conducted in Houston and in Chicago, the CMV probe consisted of a mixture of late sequences of DNA of the Towne strain of CMV. In the Dutch study, in addition to a late sequence, an immediate early 7-kb fragment (of AD169 strain) was selected, because the investigators felt it would be more apt to detect transcripts present not only during reproductive viral cycles but also during latent infection (as is the case with HSV latency in neurons).

Recently, the PCR with primers reactive with late genomic frequencies has been used in Houston for studies of 135 frozen tissue specimens obtained during vascular surgery. The PCR products were then analyzed by electrophoretic bands of viral DNA in gels. A positive result was obtained in 81% of the specimens. The dot-blot hybridization method gave a similar result, with 78% of the specimens positive for CMV DNA (Melnick et al. 1991, unpublished data). These results are similar to 90% positives obtained from atherosclerotic lesions by the Dutch investigators [12].

With the early probes, use of the in situ DNA hybridization technique resulted in an increase in the percentage of CMV DNA-positive specimens relative to the dot-blot technique, which the Dutch investigators [3] believe is largely due to the formation of RNA-DNA hybrids. A similar phenomenon was not observed when the late probe was used. When both techniques were used – with the early probe or with the late probe – no significant differences were observed between the group with severe atherosclerosis and the control group. However, the highly sensitive PCR detected viral DNA in 90% of the vessel wall samples derived from atherosclerotic patients, using either early or late primer, while in the control group only 53% were positive – a difference supporting the possible role of CMV in the pathogenesis of atherosclerosis. Since no differences were found with the sensitive polymerase chain reaction, using the early or the late primer, the suggestion was made that the whole CMV genome was present in the arterial wall.

Seroepidemiologic Studies

In another approach to the problem, the association of infections by CMV, HSV1, and HSV2 with atherosclerosis was studied in a group of patients who underwent surgery for atherosclerotic vessel disease and a control group with high cholesterol levels but with no clinical evidence of disease [1, 21]. The surgical patients were pair-matched by age, sex, race, and socioeconomic status with control subjects who were participants in a lipid research program extending over a period of 5 years. Blood samples for determination of antibody levels were taken both from the atherosclerosis patients before surgery, and from the control subjects at the end of the 5-year study period.

Two pair-matched male case-control groups were followed: Group A included 134 pairs of patients who underwent cardiovascular surgery and controls who did not have clinical signs of atherosclerosis disease. Group B consisted of 46 pairs in which the surgical patients were matched with controls who, during the 5-year observation period, developed myocardial infarction, suffered events compatible with myocardial infarction, or actually required cardiovascular surgery.

As shown in Table 2, the prevalence of antibodies to HSV1 and HSV2 was similar among the surgical cases and the control groups, but differences in CMV antibody were noted, particularly in the rates of high levels of CMV antibody in surgical patients as compared with their matched controls. In group A, the 134 patients (70% with high antibody levels) differed significantly ($p<0.001$) from their matched group A controls (43% with high levels), none of whom had experienced a cardiovascular event. However, in group B the 46 surgical patients did not differ in the rate of high levels of CMV antibody (80%) from that of their matched controls (72%) – those who had developed a diagnosed cardiovascular event in the 5-year observation period. Another group, in this instance 69 female patients who had cardiovascular surgery, did not differ significantly in prevalence of high levels of CMV antibody (76%) from 69 matched male surgical patients (70%), but they had a significantly greater frequency ($p<0.001$) of high antibody levels than 69 male control patients free of cardiovascular disease (46%). Like the male patients, the female patients with atherosclerosis showed no difference in antibody levels when compared with the group B controls (72%), all of whom had developed myocardial infarction or cardiovascular symptoms compatible with coronary insufficiency, during the 5 years of observation.

Table 2. Prevalence of high levels of CMV antibodies in pairs of male surgical patients with atherosclerosis and their matched controls, and in female surgical patients matched with male controls

Group	Patients	Positive for CMV antibodies		*p*	
	(*n*)	(*n*)	(%)	Control A	Control B
A Male surgical	134	94	70	<0.001	>0.9
Control	134	58	43		
B Male surgical	46	37	80	<0.001	>0.5
Control	46	33	72		
Female surgical	69	52	76	<0.001	>0.8

In group A matched pairs the controls did not have any recorded cardiovascular event. In group B matched pairs the controls developed myocardial infarction during the observation period, or suffered events compatible with myocardial infarction, or actually required cardiovascular surgery

Atherosclerosis in Transplanted Hearts

It is becoming apparent that coronary artery disease may be the leading cause of death in patients who have received heart transplants. Several revealing studies have been reported.

Loebe et al. [13] in Germany studied the association of CMV infection with accelerated graft atherosclerosis in transplanted hearts of 30 long-term survivors. Six of nine patients (67%) with graft atherosclerosis, diagnosed by coronary angiography, had acquired CMV infection, while only 5 of 21 patients (24%) without such pathologic findings acquired CMV infection. In a later follow-up [14], postoperative CMV infection was detected in 77% of 26 patients who developed atherosclerosis in the transplanted heart within 1–4 years, as opposed to 25% of 24 patients who did not develop atherosclerotic changes.

In an independent study at Stanford [8], a large number of patients received heart transplants and were treated by immunosuppression. They were followed systematically for CMV infection and development of late graft atherogenesis in the transplanted organ. If CMV infection occurred at the time of the heart transplant or soon thereafter, there was a high correlation with the subsequent development of atherosclerosis in the transplanted heart. A follow-up report [7] included 387 cardiac transplant recipients who were given immunosuppressive therapy between 1980 and 1989. During this period CMV infection was detected in 122 patients (33%) as determined by a fourfold rise in IgG antibody to CMV, isolation of CMV in human fibroblast cultures, or appearance of CMV inclusion bodies in tissue. Most of the CMV infections occurred within the first 3 months after transplantation. These 122 patients were compared with 265 transplant patients who remained free of CMV.

Atherosclerosis occurred in the transplanted heart more frequently and earlier in the CMV group. By 5 years after transplantation: (1) only 32.2% of CMV-positive patients survived, in contrast to 68.3% of CMV-negative patients; (2) the rate of graft loss due to atherosclerosis (which led to death or retransplantation) was 68.8% in the CMV-positive patients but only 36.8% in the CMV-negative patients; and (3) 7.6% of CMV-positive patients died with more than 50% luminal obstruction in their coronary arteries, in contrast to only 0.8% of CMV-negative patients.

In another study, in Minneapolis [15], all of 102 immunosuppressed patients who had received a cardiac transplant between 1983 and 1987 and who survived for at least 1 year were included in this study, which is summarized as follows: (1) 31.3% of the 32 CMV-positive patients developed coronary artery disease in the graft, in contrast to 8.6% of the 70 CMV-negative patients. (2) Of the CMV-positive patients, 68% had a probability of remaining free of severe atherosclerosis at 2 years posttransplant and only 55% at 3 years, in contrast to 90% at 2 years for the CMV-negative patients.

Even though CMV infection has been associated in heart transplant patients with graft occlusion and ischemic injury, the precise mechanism has not been established. Pober [22] has indicated that the affected arteries exhibit concentric accumulation of smooth muscle cells and extracellular matrix, but they lack the foam cells and extracellular lipid accumulation of typical atherosclerosis. He suggests graft arteriosclerosis is a more descriptive term for the nature of the lesion – perhaps brought on by the effect of CMV on the drug-suppressed immune system. However, as described in the following section, CMV may directly affect the biology of the arteries.

Cytomegalovirus Infection of Endothelial Cells

The fact that CMV and HSV imprints were detected in arterial tissues that showed minimal atherosclerotic changes suggests that virus infection could be an early event in the atherosclerotic process, particularly since one of the features reported for CMV infection is the accumulation of cholesterol within the host cells. Another important property of CMV is its capacity to infect but not kill endothelial cells [24, 25, 27]. Viral glycoproteins appear at the surface of the infected endothelial cells, which then demonstrate a great increase in adherence of polymorphonuclear leukocytes. Thus, the inflammatory type of response in the endothelial intima set off by a viral blood-borne infection may be the initiating event in atherogenesis [24, 25]. In many respects, the biological properties of CMV are compatible with an atherogenic potential [26]. In contrast, herpesvirus type 1 and herpesvirus type 2 cause rapid cytolytic infections in human endothelial and smooth muscle cell cultures.

Further support comes from a study by Myerson et al. [19], who identified and enumerated cells which appeared normal morphologically but were found to have a latent CMV infection. In patients with disseminated CMV infection, typical cytomegalic cells were present in lungs and other organs, and virus was isolated from lungs and kidneys. However, by use of biotin-labeled viral DNA probes, occult (latent) virus was detected in many tissues, particularly in scattered foci of endothelial cells of the blood vessels. In spite of this, the cells containing the latent CMV infection appeared normal. There was hardly any local tissue destruction, but hyperplasia was sometimes found.

Conclusions

There is solid evidence that a member of the herpesvirus family can cause atherosclerosis in chickens. In vitro experiments as well as studies of arteries from infected birds suggest that a virus-induced alteration of cellular metabolism, which results in the accumulation of cholesterol and cholesteryl esters, may be the primary mechanism in development of viral atherosclerosis. In addition, the fact that the same virus induces a malignant lymphoma suggests that it may also have the potential to stimulate the proliferation of arterial smooth muscle cells, a prominent feature of atherogenesis.

The evidence for involvement of one or more members of the herpesvirus family in human atherosclerosis is much more circumstantial, but it is increasing. The findings of CMV and HSV antigens and nucleic acid sequences in arterial smooth muscle cells suggest that virus infection of the arterial wall may be common in patients with severe atherosclerosis. Although certainly suggestive, these findings by themselves do not demonstrate a viral role in the patho-

Table 3. Hypothesis of CMV initiation and development of atherosclerosis

1. Systemic CMV infection
2. Infection of arterial endothelium. Viral glycoproteins appear at the surface of infected cells
3. Polymorphonuclear leukocyte adherence (inflammatory response) leading to damaged endothelium
4. Leakage of CMV from infected endothelial cells and exposure of neighboring smooth muscle cells within the arterial wall
5. Latent and persistent infections of smooth muscle cells, detected by tracing viral genes or antigens
6. Cell-to-cell spread of CMV within scattered foci along the blood vessels
7. CMV may transform cells and cause smooth muscle cells to proliferate locally, without destroying them, and may induce changes in cellular metabolites, including accumulation of cholesterol
8. At sites of CMV latency, the arterial lesion may be periodically activated, followed by viral infection of the intimal endothelial cells. This would result in another bout of adherence of polymorphonuclear leukocytes. Virus from the damaged endothelial cells leads to proliferation of surrounding smooth muscle cells. This benign transformation may lead to the formation of atheroma and, when coupled with risk factors such as hypercholesterolemia, to an increase in the size of the lesion and ultimately to clinically apparent atherosclerosis

genesis of atherosclerosis. However, they lead to an attractive working hypothesis of the steps involved (Table 3).

Of special importance are the recent findings that heart transplant patients who are immunosuppressed and become infected with CMV are particularly prone to develop severe atherosclerosis in the transplanted organ.

In seroepidemiologic studies, high levels of CMV antibodies were found to be associated with clinically manifest atherosclerotic disease, suggesting that a periodically activated latent infection or continuously active infection is present in patients with atherosclerosis. Since CMV DNA, but not infectious virus, is found in arterial cells, the artery itself might be the site of latency.

In summary, several recent studies show that infection of arterial wall cells by CMV may have occurred in cardiovascular patients. The biological properties of CMV are consistent with pathogenic involvement at several levels of the atherogenic process, as listed in Table 3. Many of these properties are shared by other herpesviruses, and data linking CMV to atherosclerosis by no means exclude the possible involvement of other herpesviruses. Rather, the studies reviewed here should provide a basis for further investigation of the role of viruses in human atherogenesis, and of their control by means of vaccination or chemotherapy.

References

1. Adam E, Melnick JL, Probstfield JL, Petrie BL, Burek J, Bailey KR, McCollum CH, DeBakey ME (1987) High levels of cytomegalovirus antibody in patients requiring vascular surgery for atherosclerosis. Lancet 2:291–293
2. Benditt EP, Barrett T, McDougall JK (1983) Viruses in the etiology of atherosclerosis. Proc Natl Acad Sci USA 80:6386–6389
3. Bruggeman CA, van Dam-Mieras MCE (1991) The possible role of cytomegalovirus in atherogenesis. Prog Med Virol 38:1–26
4. Fabricant CG, Fabricant J (1985) Marek's disease virus-induced atherosclerosis and evidence for a herpesvirus role in the human vascular disease. In: Calnek BW, Spencer JL (eds) International Symposium on Marek's disease, American Association on Avian Pathology, pp 391–407
5. Fabricant CG, Fabricant J, Litrenta MM, Minick CR (1978) Virus-induced atherosclerosis. J Exp Med 148:335–340
6. Fabricant CG, Fabricant J, Minick CR, Litrenta MM (1983) Herpesvirus-induced atherosclerosis in chickens. Fed Proc 42:2476–2479
7. Grattan MT (1991) Accelerated graft atherosclerosis following cardiac transplantation: clinical perspectives. Clin Cardiol 14 Suppl 2:II-16–II-20
8. Grattan MT, Moreno-Cabral CE, Starnes VA, Oyer P, Stinson EB, Shumway NE (1989) Cytomegalovirus infection is associated with cardiac allograft rejection and atherosclerosis. JAMA 261:3561–3566
9. Gyorkey F, Melnick JL, Guinn GA, Gyorkey P, DeBakey ME (1984) Herpesviridae in the endothelial and smooth muscle cells of the proximal aorta in arteriosclerotic patients. Exp Mol Pathol 40:328–339
10. Hajjar DP, Fabricant CG, Minick CR, Fabricant J (1986) Virus-induced atherosclerosis: herpesvirus infection alters aortic cholesterol metabolism and accumulation. Am J Pathol 122:62–70

11. Hendrix MGR, Dormans PHJ, Kitslaar P, Bosman F, Bruggeman CA (1989) The presence of cytomegalovirus nucleic acids in arterial walls of atherosclerotic and nonatherosclerotic patients. Am J Pathol 134:1151–1157
12. Hendrix MGR, Salimans MMM, van Boven CPA, Bruggeman CA (1990) High prevalence of latently present cytomegalovirus in arterial walls of patients suffering from grade III atherosclerosis. Am J Pathol 136:23–28
13. Loebe M, Schuler S, Zais O, Warnecke H, Hetzer R (1989) The role of cytomegalovirus (CMV) infection for the development of coronary artery disease (CAD) in the transplanted heart (Abstr). J Heart Transplantation 8:104
14. Loebe M, Schuler S, Spiegelsberger S, Warnecke H, Fleck E, Hetzer R (1990) Cytomegalievirusinfektion und Koronarsklerose nach Herztransplantation. Dtsch Med Wochenschr 115:1266–1269
15. McDonald JL, Rector RS, Braunlin EA, Kubo SH, Olivari MT (1989) Association of coronary artery disease in cardiac transplant recipients with cytomegalovirus infection. Am J Cardiol 64:359
16. Melnick JL, Petrie BL, Dreesman GR, Burek J, McCollum CH, DeBakey ME (1983) Cytomegalovirus antigen within human arterial smooth muscle cells. Lancet 2:644–647
17. Melnick JL, Adam E, DeBakey ME (1990) Possible role of cytomegalovirus in atherogenesis. JAMA 263:2204–2207
18. Melnick JL, Adam E, DeBakey ME (1991) Accelerated graft atherosclerosis following cardiac transplantation: do viruses play a role? Clin Cardiol 14 Suppl 2:II-21–II-26
19. Myerson D, Hackman RC, Nelson JA, Ward DC, McDougall JK (1984) Widespread presence of histologically occult cytomegalovirus. Hum Pathol 15:430–439
20. Petrie BL, Melnick JL, Adam E, Burek J, McCollum CH, DeBakey ME (1987) Nucleic acid sequences of cytomegalovirus in cells cultured from human arterial tissue. J Infect Dis 155:158–159
21. Petrie BL, Adam E, Melnick JL (1988) Association of herpesvirus/cytomegalovirus infections with human atherosclerosis. Prog Med Virol 35:21–42
22. Pober JS (1991) Immunologic basis of cardiovascular disease: an overview. Clin Cardiol 14 Suppl 2:II-1–II-2
23. Shih JCH, Pullman EP, Kao KJ (1983) Genetic selection, general characterization, and histology of atherosclerosis-susceptible and -resistant Japanese quail. Atherosclerosis 49:41–53
24. Smiley ML, Mar E-C, Huang E-S (1988) Cytomegalovirus infection and viral-induced transformation of human endothelial cells. J Med Virol 25:213–226
25. Span AHM, van Boven CPA, Bruggeman CA (1989) The effect of cytomegalovirus infection on the adherence of polymorphonuclear leucocytes to endothelial cells. Eur J Clin Invest 19:542–548
26. Tumilowicz JJ, Gawlik ME, Powell BB, Trentin JJ (1985) Replication of cytomegalovirus in human arterial smooth muscle cells. J Virol 56:839–845
27. Visser MR, Jacob HS, Goodman JL, McCarthy JB, Furcht LT, Vercellotti GM (1989) Granulocyte-mediated injury to herpes simplex virus-infected human endothelium. Lab Invest 60:296–403
28. Yamashiroya HM, Ghosh L, Yang R, Robertson AL Jr (1988) Herpesviridae in the coronary arteries and aorta of young trauma victims. Am J Pathol 130:71–79

Chapter 5 Cytomegalovirus as a Sexually Transmitted Disease

W. Lawrence Drew

Summary

In the developed nations, one of the important mechanisms of CMV transmission is sexual contact. This has been demonstrated to occur between heterosexual men and women and between homosexual men. Sexual intercourse, including anal receptive intercourse, is a risk for this transmission but salivary exchange, i.e., kissing may also facilitate cross infection. Reinfection by additional strain(s) of CMV may occur as a result of sexual transmission. Condoms, tested in laboratory simulations of sexual intercourse, reduce transmission of CMV and may be useful in clinical practice.

In the developed or industrialized nations, approximately one half of the adult population is seronegative for cytomegalovirus (CMV) antibody. This is in marked contrast to the age-related prevalence of CMV antibody in the underdeveloped countries of the world where >90% of the population is seropositive by the age of 2 years. The probable explanations for this are that in the underdeveloped countries the living conditions are more crowded, there is more close and repeated contact with infected urine, and more frequent breast feeding of infants. Thus, in the developed countries, there is a large pool of uninfected adults who then acquire this virus at a slow rate, i.e., approximately 1%–2% seroconversions per year. It appears that these seroconversions result from close contact with virus-positive individuals. Such contact may be sexual with exchange of body fluids, including saliva, but other types of close contact may bring about transmission. For example, adults may be infected during maternal or paternal contact with a virus-positive child, or by blood transfusion or organ transplantation. In this chapter we will concentrate on evidence supporting the role of sexual transmission as an effective means of spreading the virus. In so doing we will consider the evidence in two different settings, heterosexual and homosexual.

Departments of Laboratory Medicine and Medicine, Mount Zion Medical Center of the University of California, 1600 Divisadero Street, San Francisco, CA 94120, USA

CMV as a Heterosexually Transmitted Infection

In the United States only 10%–15% of adolescents are seroimmune to CMV. However, during young adulthood the rate of seropositivity rapidly increases so that by age 35 approximately 50% show serologic evidence of past infection [1]. The evidence that many of these infections are sexually transmitted may be summarized as follows:

1. The virus does not spread readily among adults by ordinary, nonsexual, person-to-person contact [2], even during prolonged exposure to individuals known to be excreting the virus [3, 4]. For example, among military recruits living in close contact with a recently infected index case, no seroconversions occurred. Also, among health care workers in close contact with actively infected patients, few, if any, seroconversions can be attributed to their nursing functions [4–6].
2. The prevalence of CMV antibody more than doubles during the years of beginning sexual activity (ages of 15–35 years) [1, 7].
3. CMV has been isolated from the cervix of 13% [8]–23% [9] of women attending clinics for suspected venereal disease. Knox et al. [10] found that the prevalence of CMV shedding in the genital tract of inner city women with high rates of infection in adolescence decreased steadily with age, from a peak of 15% at 11–14 years of age to an undetectable level at age 31. Most likely these results reflect the age at acquisition, i.e., women acquiring the virus at age 30 would probably excrete the virus for the same duration as a newly infected adolescent.
4. CMV has been isolated from semen [11]; the prevalence of CMV in semen among random donors for artificial insemination was 0.4% [12].
5. Active CMV infection (virus recovered from the cervix and a positive CMV IgM antibody titer) was described in the female sexual partner of a man whose semen had been virus positive during the preceding 5 months. In addition, Chretien et al. [13] reported CMV mononucleosis in two men after sexual contact with a woman whose cervix and urine were CMV positive. Evidence of recent CMV infection was also found in another female sexual contact of one of the two male patients, whereas roommates of these patients who were not their sexual partners had negative CMV complement fixation (CF) antibody titers.
6. Cytomegalovirus proctitis has been reported in a woman who had "vigorous receptive anal intercourse for 4 consecutive days" [14]. One week later she developed symptoms of proctitis and colonic biopsy revealed inclusions characteristic of CMV, while cultures were negative for herpes simplex and *Neisseria gonorrhoe*. Serologic results were consistent with acute CMV infection. She had both vaginal and anal intercourse with an additional three to four different men during the preceding 6 months, so the exact source of infection was not clear.

Evidence of Reinfection with CMV Among Heterosexuals

Analysis of different strains of CMV cannot be accomplished in a practical manner by study of antigenic variation. Instead, analysis of genomic variation using restriction endonuclease cleavage reveals that no two viruses have identical DNA fingerprints when multiple enzyme digests are compared. The exceptions are strains recovered from (1) different sites in the same individual, (2) sexual partners and (3) mother-child pairs.

Huang et al. [15] were the first to show that reinfection with a different strain of CMV may occur. Two different strains of CMV were recovered from infants born of the same mother. Recently Chandler et al. [16] studied cultures from the cervix, urine, and throat of eight women attending a sexually transmitted disease (STD) clinic. Four of the eight women were infected with more than one strain of CMV, two concurrently from different sites and two serially.

CMV as an STD Among Homosexual Men

The initial documentation of high rates of CMV infection in homosexual men resulted from prevalence studies performed at the San Francisco City Clinic in 1979 [17]. Urinary excretion of CMV was noted in 14 of 90 (7.4%) homosexual men but in none of 101 heterosexual men attenting the same STD clinic ($P<0.005$). Similarly, antibody to CMV was detected in 130 of 139 (93.5%) homosexual men but in only 38 of 70 (54.3%) heterosexual men ($P<0.005$).

In a subsequent prospective study [18] of 237 homosexual men participating in the Western Study Group Hepatitis Vaccine Trial at the San Francisco City Clinic, a high prevalence of CMV IgG serum antibody (206 of 237, 86.9%) was noted. Of the 31 men lacking CMV antibody on initial testing, 22 experienced seroconversion within 9 months of follow-up, for an attack rate of 71% during this time period. During a mean follow-up period of 14.3 months (range, 2–20) 66 of the 206 initially seropositive men (32%) excreted CMV in their urine on one or more occasions. Both a urine and a semen specimen were obtained during a single visit from 52 of the homosexual men. CMV was recovered from 18 of the semen specimens but from only 3 of the 18 corresponding urine samples. Specimens from a single individual grew CMV from the urine but not from the semen. Semen therefore appears to be nearly five times as sensitive as urine in detecting the presence of CMV. Clearly, the widespread occurrence of CMV viruria and "virusemenia" in this population makes exposure to the virus all but inevitable and accounts for the extraordinarily high attack rate of CMV infections among seronegative homosexual men. Among the men who were seropositive on initial testing, those who excreted CMV during the study period were significantly younger (mean age, 26.6 years) than those who did not (mean age, 32.7 years; $P<0.01$). A Seattle study has reported that, on a single visit, 36% of homosexual men were culture positive for CMV, most commonly from semen. They estimated the mean duration of semen positivity to be 22 months versus 9 months for urine [19].

Table 1. Prevalence of CMV antibody among homosexual and heterosexual men

Group	Men	Positive	
	(*n*)	*n*	%
1 Homosexual men: passive anal intercourse	59	57	96.6
2 Homosexual men: no passive anal intercourse	19	14	73.7
3 Heterosexual men	70	38	54.3

1 vs 2, $P<0.01$
1 vs 3, $P<0.01$
2 vs 3, not statistically significant

In the San Francisco study questionnaires concerning demographic data, clinical histories, and sexual practices were completed by 78 subjects (54 of whom were initially seropositive and 24 of whom were initially seronegative, including 17 of the 22 seroconverters and 7 of the 9 who remained persistently seronegative).

Information was obtained regarding the frequency of participation in the following sex practices: kissing, oral-anal contact (oral role), oral-anal contact (anal role), fellatio (oral role), fellatio (genital role), anal intercourse (active role), and anal intercourse (passive role) [18]. Only passive anal intercourse correlated with the initial presence of anti-CMV antibody or with seroconversion to this virus during the course of the study. Of 59 men who engaged in passive anal intercourse, CMV antibody was present in 96.6%, but of the 19 men who did not engage in this practice, antibody was present in only 73.7% ($P<0.01$; Table 1). The latter figure does not differ significantly from the prevalence of CMV antibody among heterosexual men attending a venereal disease clinic. These data suggest that exposure of the anorectal mucosa to CMV-infected semen constitutes the major route of acquisition of CMV infection by homosexual men.

Reinfection with CMV in Homosexual Men

Data on the prevalence of CMV IgM antibody suggests that homosexual men experience repeated episodes of CMV infection. CMV IgM antibody was detected on one or more occasions in the sera of more than 90% of the homosexual men and tended to appear, disappear, and reappear over time [18]. In contrast, IgM antibody to CMV was detected in only 3.8% of 103 serum specimens randomly collected from volunteer male blood donors. CMV IgM antibody was detected in a significantly ($P<0.05$) higher proportion of serum samples from the 206 initially seropositive men (67% of 1136 samples) than in the postconversion samples obtained from the 22 seroconverters (53% of 86 samples). These data are summarized in Table 2. The higher prevalence of CMV IgM antibody in long-standing seropositive men than in recent sero-

Table 2. Presence of CMV IgM antibody in 237 prospectively studied homosexual men

Group	Subjects positive			Serum samples positive		
	No. tested	n	%	No. tested	n	%
Seronegative	9	0	0	54	0	0
Seropositive	206	196	95	1136	765	67
Seroconverts	22	20	91	86	46	53 [a]

[a] Samples obtained after seroconversion

converters suggests that the former group is continually being reexposed to (and probably reinforced with) exogenous strains of the virus. Since CMV infection alone, i.e., in the absence of concomitant human immunodeficiency virus (HIV) infection, can cause sustained suppression of CD4 to CD8 ratios [20], multiple exogenous reinfections of homosexual men with differing strains of CMV may result in protracted suppression of host immunity. In addition, CMV infection or reinfection in HIV positive men may activate latent HIV infection [21, 22].

To determine whether more than one CMV infection actually occurs in homosexual men, we analyzed multiple virus isolates from autopsy tissues of each of four AIDS patients by use of a Southern blot method for comparing the genetic relatedness of clinical isolates of CMV. This method had the distinct advantage of not requiring purification of virus or viral DNA and requires only relatively small numbers of infected cells from which total DNA is extracted. Each of the four patients we studied had at least two different strains of CMV as determined by *Bam*HI restriction site polymorphisms revealed by Southern blot analysis.

Similar multiple CMV infections in AIDS patients have been documented by Spector et al. [23]. These results indicate that double infections with CMV do occur in patients with AIDS but may represent terminal CMV superinfections in patients already immunocompromised. Others have shown that reinfection with CMV can occur in immunocompromised patients. For example, Chou [24] showed that CMV-seropositive renal transplant recipients can acquire CMV infection from donor kidneys. To determine whether CMV might contribute to the early pathogenesis of HIV infection, it is necessary to determine whether exogenous reinfection with CMV occurs in homosexual men prior to the development of AIDS.

To answer this question, we have investigated a cohort of homosexual men without AIDS for the excretion of more than one strain of CMV. Isolates were obtained at intervals from urine or semen and compared for molecular relatedness by the Southern blot method described above. Among 17 men followed for an average of 7 months, 8 excreted more than one strain. Two of these individuals were HIV antibody negative indicating that more than one strain of CMV can be acquired by homosexual men even in the absence of HIV infection. This should not be surprising given the high titer of virus in semen and the frequency of anal receptive intercourse among homosexual men. In effect, anal receptive intercourse may be equivalent to an intravenous injection of virus given the potential for multiple bleeding points in the traumatized anorectal mucosa.

In a recent report from Seattle, serial isolates from 11 homosexual men were available for restriction fragment analysis [19]. Five subjects were seronegative for HIV, and six were seropositive for HIV. Subsequently, two seronegative subjects developed antibody to HIV. Four of the 11 subjects shed more than one strain of CMV. Three subjects, all HIV antibody positive, shed two different strains. Four different strains of CMV were evident in the one HIV-seronegative subject, two of which persisted over time. At the initial visit a single strain was isolated from semen; 15 months later, a different strain was isolated from his throat. A urine isolate, 17 months after his first isolate, contained a mixture of the two previously isolated strains; throughout the genome, all bands present in both the previous isolates were seen. CMV was isolated from both semen and urine 24 months after the initial visit.

This study provides additional evidence that infection with multiple strains of CMV is a relatively common occurrence among homosexual men with and without HIV infection and is not restricted to severely immunosuppressed individuals.

Prevention of Sexual Transmission

Vaccine

An effective vaccine to prevent infection would be desirable for population groups at high risk for acquiring CMV. However, as discussed above, infection with "wild" CMV may not prevent infection with additional strains of CMV. Multiple reinfections with wild virus strains may be extraordinary in that they may reflect infection of anorectal mucosa in homosexual men and by multiple partners in both homosexual men and heterosexual women. Possibly vaccines would be efficacious among heterosexuals experiencing sexual contact with a limited number of partners. (Vaccines are discussed elsewhere in this volume.)

Condoms

We performed a study to evaluate the possible utility of condoms to prevent CMV transmission by semen [25]. Five different types of latex condoms were used. The strain of CMV used was AD-169 at a median log 10 TCID50 titer of 4.5 as determined by Reed-Meunch titration. A 2-ml portion of virus suspension was placed in a rinsed condom, which was then stretched all of the way over the shaft of a disposable plastic 35-cc syringe container. The condom was then sealed at its open end with tape. A 2-ml portion of Eagle's minimal essential medium (MEM) containing 10% fetal calf serum was then placed in a second rinsed condom. This second condom was placed over the CMV-containing condom, unrolled three quarters of the way up the syringe container shaft, and sealed with tape, to serve as a potential receptacle for any CMV transmitted across the barrier provided by the first (inner) condom.

In the first part of the experiment three such test devices were assembled and incubated at 37 °C for 15, 30, and 60 min, respectively. After incubation the solutions in the inner and outer condoms were pipetted and cultured separately. Twelve repetitions of this procedure were completed using different types of condoms. CMV was recovered in all cultures taken from inner condoms and from none of the outer condoms, indicating that no transmission occurred across the condom membranes (Table 3).

The second set of experiments served as an attempt to more closely mirror in vivo condom use by simulating the trauma associated with sexual intercourse. While imposing an external force on the condoms, the test device was thrust up and down 100 times in 5 min. The solutions from the inner and outer condoms were then cultured as above. Five repetitions of this procedure were completed, again using different types of condoms.

CMV was recovered in all cultures taken from the inner condoms (Table 4), except for one specimen which was toxic in tissue culture. No virus was recovered from any of the outer condoms. (The time elapsed before detection of viral cytopathogenic effect (CPE) in each culture is recorded in the Tables 3 and 4 so as to provide a semiquantitative assessment of the relative virus titer in the samples.)

These results suggest that condoms might effectively block the sexual transmission of CMV. Even after applying trauma simulating sexual intercourse, no virus leaked from the inner condom. Although the experimental procedure

Table 3. Failure of transmission of CMV across condoms

Trial	Initial log 10 TCID50 titer	Results of culture (days to detection) of inner/outer condoms after incubation period of		
		15 min	30 min	60 min
1	ND	+(17)/−	ND/ND	+(21)/−
2	ND	+(12)/−	+(5)/−	ND/ND
3	3.5	+(6)/−	+(6)/−	+(6)/−
4	5.2	+(7)/−	+(7)/−	+(7)/−
5	ND	+(6)/−	+(6)/−	+(7)/−
6	ND	+(6)/−	+(6)/−	+(6)/−
7	4.5	+(7)/−	+(7)/−	+(7)/−
8	4.5	+(7)/−	+(7)/−	+(7)/−
9	4.5	+(7)/−	+(7)/−	+(7)/−
10	ND	+(6)/−	+(6)/−	+(6)/−
11	ND	+(6)/−	+(9)/−	+(9)/−
12	ND	+(6)/−	+(6)/−	+(9)/−

ND, not done

Table 4. Failure of transmission of CMV across condoms after simulated intercourse and subsequent incubation for 30 min

Trial	Cultures			
	from inner condom		from outer condom	
	CMV	Days to detection	CMV	Days to detection
1	+	8	–	NA
2	Toxic		–	NA
3	+	7	–	NA
4	+	7	–	NA
5	+	15	–	NA

NA, not applicable

used in this investigation does not fully reproduce the act of sexual intercourse, the similarity is sufficient to make it an acceptable simulation for an in vitro model.

References

1. Wentworth BB, Alexander ER (1971) Seroepidemiology of infections due to members of the herpesvirus group. Am J Epidemiol 94:496–507
2. Wenzel RP, McCormick DP, Davies JA et al. (1973) Cytomegalovirus infection: a seroepidemiologic study of recruit population. Am J Epidemiol 97:410–414
3. Betts RF, Cestero RVM, Freeman RB et al. (1979) Epidemiology of cytomegalovirus infection in end stage renal disease. J Med Virol 4:89–96
4. Tolkoff-Rubin NE, Rubin RH, Keller EE et al. (1978) Cytomegalovirus infection in dialysis patients and personnel. Ann Intern Med 89:625–628
5. Dworsky ME, Welch K, Cassady G et al. (1983) Occupational risk for primary cytomegalovirus infection among pediatric health-care workers. N Engl J Med 309:950–953
6. Gerberding JL, Bryant-LeBlanc CE, Nelson K et al. (1987) Risk of transmitting the human immunodeficiency virus, cytomegalovirus, and hepatitis B virus to health care workers exposed to patients with AIDS and AIDS-related conditions. J Infect Dis 156:1–8
7. Stern H, Elek SD (1985) The incidence of infection with cytomegalovirus in a normal population. A serological study in greater London. J Hyg (Camb) 63:79–87
8. Jordan MC, Rousseau WE, Noble GR et al. (1973) Association of cervical cytomegalovirus with venereal disease. N Engl J Med 288:932–934
9. Wentworth BB, Bonin P, Holmes KK et al. (1973) Isolation of viruses, bacteria and other organisms from venereal disease clinic patients: methodology and problems associated with multiple isolations. Health Lab Sci 10:75–81
10. Knox GE, Pass RF, Reynolds DW et al. (1979) Comparative prevalence of subclinical cytomegalovirus and herpes simplex virus infections in the genital and urinary tracts of cytomegalovirus mononucleosis. J Infect Dis 170:419–422
11. Lang DJ, Kummer JF, Hartley DP (1974) Cytomegalovirus in semen: persistence and demonstration in intracellular fluids. N Engl J Med 291:121–123

12. Tjiam KH, van Heijst BY, Polak-Vogelzang AA et al. (1987) Sexually communicable micro-organisms in human semen samples to be used for artificial insemination by donor. Genitourinary Med 63:116–118
13. Chretien JH, McGuinniss OG, Muller A (1977) Venereal causes of cytomegalovirus mononucleosis. JAMA 238:1644–1645
14. Rabinowitz M, Bassan I, Robinson MJ (1988) Sexually transmitted cytomegalovirus proctitis in a woman. Am J Gastroenterol 83:885–887
15. Huang E-S, Alford CA, Reynolds DW et al. (1980) Molecular epidemiology of cytomegalovirus infections in women and their infants. N Engl J Med 303:958–962
16. Chandler SH, Handsfield HH, McDougall JK (1987) Isolation of multiple strains of cytomegalovirus from women attending a clinic for sexually transmitted diseases. J Infect Dis 155:655–660
17. Drew WL, Mintz L, Miner RC et al. (1981) Prevalence of cytomegalovirus infections in homosexual men. J Infect Dis 143:188–192
18. Mintz L, Drew WL, Miner RC et al. (1983) Cytomegalovirus infection in homosexual men. An epidemiological study. Ann Intern Med 99:326–329
19. Collier AC, Chandler SH, Handsfield HH et al. (1989) Identification of multiple strains of cytomegalovirus in homosexual men. J Infect Dis 159:123–126
20. Drew WL, Mills J, Levy JA et al. (1985) Cytomegalovirus infection and abnormal T-lymphocyte subset ratios in homosexual men. Ann Intern Med 103:61–63
21. Webster A, Lee CA, Cook DG et al. (1989) Cytomegalovirus infection and progression towards AIDS in hemophiliacs with human immunodeficiency virus infection. Lancet 2:63–66
22. Hirsch MS, Schooley RT, Ho DD et al. (1984) Possible viral interactions in the acquired immunodeficiency syndrome. Rev Infect Dis 6:726–731
23. Spector SA, Rua JA, Spector DH et al. (1984) Detection of human cytomegalovirus in clinical specimens by DNA-DNA hybridization. J Infect Dis 150:121–126
24. Chou S (1986) Acquisition of donor strains of cytomegalovirus by renal transplant recipients. N Engl J Med 314:1418–1423
25. Katznelson S, Drew WL, Mintz L (1984) Efficacy of the condom as a barrier to the transmission of cytomegalovirus. J Infect Dis 150:155–157

Chapter 6 Cytomegalovirus and Macrophage Interaction

Stephen Haskill, Lindsay Dudding, and Eng-Shang Huang

Summary

Infection of human promyelocytic cells or monocytes with human cytomegalovirus (HCMV) results in transcriptional enhancement of many important inflammatory mediator genes. These include IL-1β, TNF-α, CSF-1, and IL-8/NAP-1. Housekeeping genes and constitutively expressed genes such as lysozyme were not influenced. While IL-1β messenger RNA (mRNA) levels were elevated for at least 4 days postinfection, apparent translational activity was more transient. In situ hybridization techniques were used to demonstrate that a low but significant proportion of monocytes persistently expressed high levels of IL-1β mRNA, similar to that observed immediately after infection. Transfection studies using chloramphenicol acetyltransferase (CAT) constructs of the pro-IL-1β promoter in combination with various HCMV intermediate early (IE) gene region DNA fragments confirmed that the IE region products, particularly region 2, were capable of transactivating inflammatory mediator genes such as IL-1β. Thus a significant proportion of monocytes are persistently modified to express important cytokines that can profoundly modulate systemic immunity.

Introduction

Infection of monocytes appears to be a critical factor in the immunosuppression that accompanies persistent cytomegalovirus (CMV) infections [6, 13, 25, 26, 35, 36]. The emphasis of this review article is on two aspects of this phenomenon which are as yet not totally understood. These are the apparent overall suppressive effects observed in the face of what appears to be only limited infection, and the low frequency of cells expressing human CMV (HCMV) gene products [13, 16, 25, 26, 35, 36]. We will discuss recent data from our own studies and those of others that appear to shed light on these problems.

Departments of Obstetrics and Gynecology, Microbiology and Immunology, Medicine, and Comprehensive Cancer Center, The University of North Carolina at Chapel Hill, Chapel Hill, NC 27599-7295, USA

HCMV infection of monocytes appears to be limited to the synthesis of the immediate early (IE) and early gene products and it is presumed that these play the decisive factor in the immunosuppression that accompanies infection [6, 13, 16, 25, 26, 35, 36]. Recently it has been reported that inactivated HCMV and Epstein-Barr virus (EBV) proteins can indirectly activate cytokine production by monocytes [9], suggesting an alternative or additional mechanism of regulation of systemic immunity following virus exposure. Indeed, internalization or interaction with intact virus may not be required to produce clinically significant symptoms, as at least some viruses need only shed proteins which subsequently bind, as with the gp120 molecule of human immunodeficiency virus (HIV-1) to the CD4 molecule, to trigger signal transduction processes [40].

Macrophages derived from different body sites or isolated at different stages of differentiation, are unlikely to be equally responsive to infection with diverse viruses. This is at least in part due to the fact that macrophages are end cells that do not proliferate further (except for the myeloid cell lines) and they remain responsive to numerous cytokine signals, thus presenting a potentially changing target for the virus. It is likely, therefore, that such cells, on exposure to virus, will vary in their ability to bind, internalize, degrade or permit viral replication, or establish a state of latency to virus. Interpretation of all these studies is complicated by the consistent observation that the fraction of monocytes expressing the IE product ranges from 0%–5% depending upon the strain of virus and the cell type used [13, 16, 25, 26, 35, 36]. In spite of the low frequency of infection and the lack of a full cycle of replication in cells of the mononuclear phagocyte series, dramatic influences on macrophage function have been reported [6, 13, 25, 26, 35, 36].

Major systemic effects of virus infection could readily arise if a significant proportion of exposed cells responded by secretion of various important cytokines, such as interleukin-1β (IL-1β) and tumor necrosis-factor alpha (TNF-α), which have important local and systemic effects [11], as well as mediators such as colony-stimulating factor 1 (CSF-1) which have more selective influences on macrophages including enhanced responsiveness to HIV-1 infection [19]. Functional studies have indicated that HCMV infection results in reduced production of IL-1β 3 days postinfection [26], and others have shown that virus also induces production of an IL-1β inhibitor [36], suggesting that the apparent immunosuppression in a high frequency of macrophages might result from production of factors that would inactivate important macrophage functions such as antigen presentation.

In order to address several aspects of the problems outlined above, we have recently studied the effects of HCMV infection of human macrophages regarding induction of several key cytokines as well as the frequency of monocytes which show long-term influences of exposure to virus [14]. These results lead to the conclusion that a significant but small fraction of monocytes are persistently modified to express high levels of cytokines which have the ability to profoundly modulate systemic immunity.

Materials and Methods

Preparation and Culture of Human Monocytes

Normal human monocytes were obtained from donors who were seronegative for HCMV, as determined by the enzyme-linked immunosorbent assay (ELISA). The mononuclear cells were first isolated by Ficoll-Hypaque separation [3]. These cells were allowed to adhere at 37 °C for 30 min. After removal of nonadherent cells, the remaining adherent cells, which were more than 95% peroxidase-positive mononuclear cells, were cultured in Roswell Park Memorial Institute medium (RPMI 1640) supplemented with 5% AB serum for 18h at 37 °C. After overnight incubation, adherent monocytes were recovered in cell suspension by repeated pipetting with cold Versene solution (Gibco, Grand Island, NY, USA).

Culture of ML-3 Cells and Induction of Cell Differentiation

ML-3 promyelocytic cells were grown in endotoxin-free RPMI 1640 (Cellgro, Mediatech, USA) supplemented with 10% fetal calf serum (FCS; Hyclone, Logan, UT, USA). For induction of cell differentiation, ML-3 cells were cultured in complete RPMI 1640 containing phorbol myristate acetate (PMA, 5 ng/ml) for 20 h and then washed once with RPMI 1640.

Virus

HCMV Towne strain, passages 39 and 40, was used for all experiments. Virus was grown in WI-38 human fibroblasts and used for infection when the titer was $5 \times 10^6 - 10^7$ plaque-forming units (pfu) per milliliter in fibroblasts.

HCMV Infection of Monocytes and ML-3 Cells

Cells were infected by adding virus to loose cell pellets at a ratio of 2:5 pfu/cell in conical polypropylene centrifuge tubes. Virus was allowed to adsorb to cells at 37 °C for 90 min with gentle mixing every 15 min. Nonadsorbed virus was removed by washing the cells twice in RPMI 1640. Cells were mock-infected with supernatant from uninfected fibroblast cultures.

Monocytes were resuspended to a concentration of 1×10^6 cells per milliliter in RPMI 1640 supplemented with 5% AB serum, and ML-3 cells were resuspended to the same concentration in RPMI 1640 supplemented with 10% FCS and cultured for varying numbers of days postinfection.

Northern Blot Analysis of mRNA Expression

Total cellular RNA was isolated from ML-3 cells by guanidine isothiocyanate extraction [7] followed by cesium chloride density gradient centrifugation [20]. RNA (15 μg/lane) was applied to formaldehyde gels for northern transfer analysis and hybridized as previously described [14].

Dot-Blot Analysis of Monocyte mRNA Expression

Dot-blot analysis of IL-1β mRNA levels in monocytes was performed as described by White and Bancroft [42]. Total cellular RNA was isolated from 2×10^6 viable monocytes per data point.

Western-Blotting Analysis of Cell-Associated IL-1β

Western transfer analysis was carried out on approximately 5×10^6 monocytes or ML-3 cells as described by Laemmli [27] and Dudding et al. [14]. After transferring proteins to the nitrocellulose, IL-1β molecules were visualized by using rabbit antihuman IL-1β (Cistron Biotechnology, Pine Brook, NJ, USA) as the first antibody and goat antirabbit immunoglobulin conjugated with horseradish peroxidase as the second antibody [34].

Plasmid DNA

A plasmid containing putative human pro-IL-1β gene regulatory regions was derived by insertion of the fragment derived from the BDC-454 clone described by Clark et al. [8] located between positions -512 and $+12$ (fragment AT) into the pSVCAT-3M plasmid described by Laimins et al. [28]. This fragment contains a TATA sequence at position -31 as well as other features that have been described elsewhere [2].

Plasmids containing various HCMV IE gene regions – pHD101SV1, pHD101SV2, and 10142 (equivalent to 101-4) [10] – were used to study the interaction between HCMV IE gene products and the IL-1β promoter. In pHD101SV1, region 1 and region 2 of the HCMV IE region are under control of the HCMV IE promoter with the simian virus 40 (SV40) enhancer located further upstream. Plasmid pHD101SV2 is identical to pHD101SV1 except that the 5.5-kb *Bam*HI fragment containing region 2 has been deleted. Plasmid 10142 has the exon sequence of region 1 deleted.

Gene Transfer into ML-3 Cells

DNA was introduced into PMA-stimulated or unstimulated ML-3 cells by electroporation with a Zapper electroporation unit at 1300 V (University of

Wisconsin Medical Electronics Lab, Madison, WI, USA). Approximately 10^7 cells were transfected in 0.5 ml of growth medium with 10 μg of the plasmid 3M-AT and varying amounts of HCMV IE region plasmid DNA. After voltage was applied to the samples, the cells were diluted into 10 ml medium and incubated at 37 °C in an atmosphere of 5% CO_2 to 95% air for 48 h.

Assay of Chloramphenicol Acetyltransferase

Chloramphenicol acetyltransferase (CAT) assays were performed 48 h after transfection. Cell extracts were prepared and assayed as described [21].

Results

HCMV Enhances Expression of Many but not All Inflammatory Mediator-Associated Genes in ML-3 Promyelocytes

Macrophage precursor cell lines are routinely used to investigate a variety of macrophage-dependent aspects of inflammation, including response to virus infections. In the present study, we initially investigated the influence of HCMV on expression of steady-state levels of several important inflammatory response genes in the promyelocytic cell line ML-3 [14]. Control studies indicated that induction of the macrophage phenotype by the phorbol ester PMA was required prior to and not post-exposure to virus in order to be effective [14]. In these experiments, we employed probes for IL-1β, TNF-α, and CSF-1, all genes previously reported to be rapidly induced in monocytes following adherence to both matrix components and endothelial cells and fibroblasts [15, 23, 24]. In addition, we used lysozyme as an example of a gene that is rapidly downregulated by adherence and actin as a control for normalization of RNA levels [15]. As shown in Fig. 1, HCMV had a long-lasting stimulatory influence on steady-state mRNA levels for the inflammatory mediator genes. This was apparent 24 h postinfection but was most prominent 48 and 72 h later. In contrast to previous adherence studies [15] HCMV failed to downregulate lysozyme. We also examined whether HCMV could enhance expression or was acting as an inducer of steady-state RNA by examining the alterations in expression of a series of novel complementary DNA (cDNA) clones representative of additional inflammation-associated genes derived from adhered monocytes [39]. Three of these, MAD-2 (a homologue of the *gro* gene [1]), MAD-9, apparently identical to IL-8/NAP-1 [29, 33, 43], and MAD-6 (a cDNA showing no apparent homology to known genes) were examined in a study similar to the first. IL-1β was employed as a control probe. As shown in Fig. 2, IL-1β was elevated by exposure to HCMV in PMA-treated ML-3 cells. A similar observation was made for MAD-9. However, for those genes not induced by PMA, MAD-2 and MAD-6, HCMV failed to have an apparent

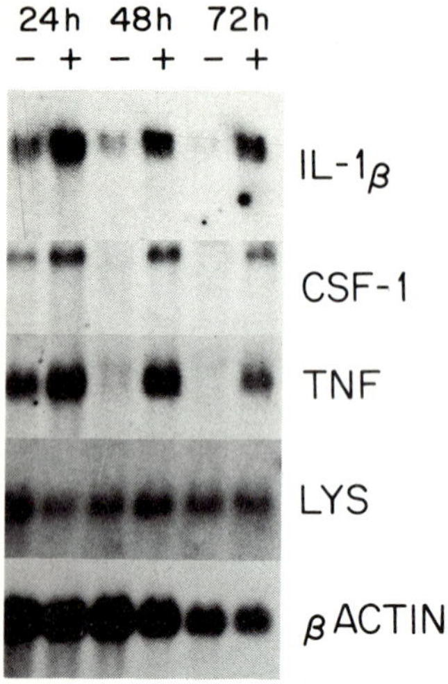

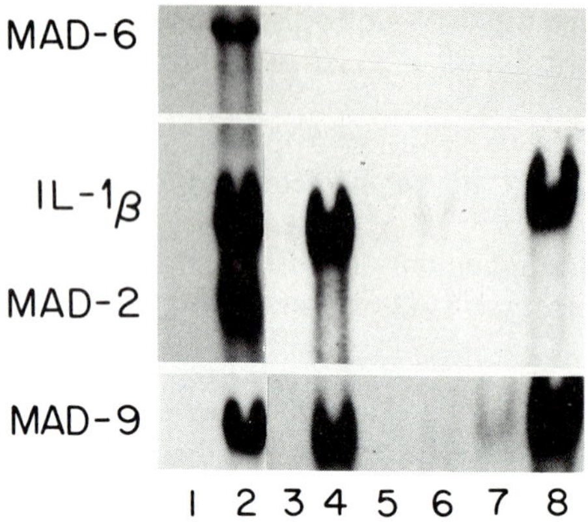

Fig. 1 (left). Northern transfer analysis demonstrating that human cytomegalovirus (HCMV) infection modulates expression of IL-1β, TNF-α, and CSF-1 in ML-3 cells induced to differentiate along the monocytic pathway before infection. Autorads were exposed overnight for IL-1β, TNF-α, and CSF-1; for 2 days for lysozyme (LYS) and β-actin. +, HCMV infected; −, uninfected. (From [14])

Fig. 2 (right). Not all monocyte-associated inflammatory gene expression is upregulated by exposure to human cytomegalovirus (HCMV) in ML-3 cells inducted to differentiate by phorbol myristate acetate (PMA). *Lane 1*, human monocytes isolated by percoll gradient separation; *lane 2*, monocytes adhered to plastic for 30 min.; *lane 3*, ML-3 cells before exposure to PMA; *lane 4*, cultured with PMA for 8 h; ML-3 cells cultured for 2 days; *lane 5*, in the absence of PMA or HCMV; *lane 6*, cultured with HCMV; *lane 7*, cultured with PMA; *lane 8*, exposed to both HCMV and PMA. (From [14])

influence, suggesting that the virus effect was one of apparent transcriptional enhancement rather than transcriptional activation.

In order to confirm that the observations made with cell lines were applicable to freshly isolated monocytes as well, monocytes were exposed to HCMV, with or without lipopolysaccharide (LPS), as well as LPS alone in order to detail the potential differences in response that might be derived from these different but biologically important stimuli. As seen in Fig. 3, monocytes adhered in the absence of additional stimuli, show little steady-state mRNA for IL-1β 24 h post culture. In contrast, LPS sustained a longer response which was amplified by the addition of HCMV. Infection, with virus alone, provided the longest sustained response. These data then confirmed the general nature of the enhancing effect by virus on both cell lines and fresh monocytes.

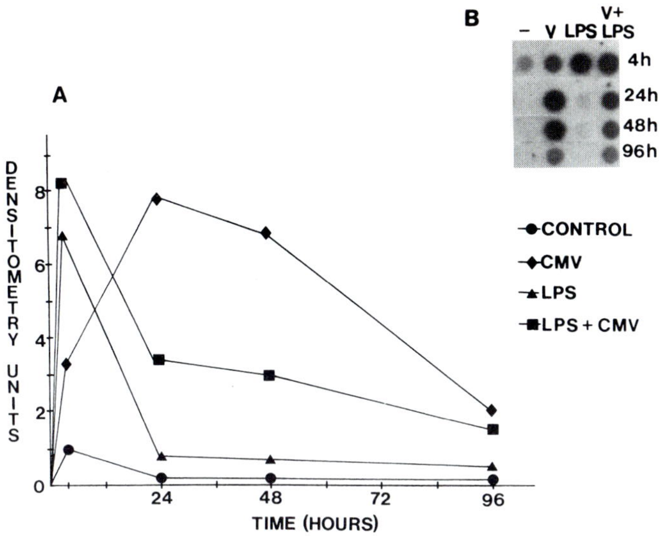

Fig. 3A, B. Total cytoplasmic dot-blot analysis demonstrating that IL-1β expression in monocytes is enhanced and prolonged by infection with human cytomegalovirus (HCMV) more than is obtained under conditions of lipopolysaccharide (LPS) stimulation. Densitometric analysis (**A**) was derived from analysis of the dot-blots in part (**B**). It is intended as an approximation of the kinetics of the response rather than an exact quantitation. (From [4])

Persistent Expression of High Levels of IL-1β mRNA by a Subpopulation of HCMV-Infected Monocytes

As HCMV exposure is usually reported to result in a generalized depression of immunity, we were interested in determining if all monocytes were similarly effected or if only a minor population of cells expressed sustained and elevated levels of steady-state mRNA. In order to evaluate these possibilities, we used in situ hybridization to examine the frequency of monocytes expressing IL-1β transcripts at various times postexposure to virus. An example of this approach is given in Fig. 4. The number of autoradiographic grains per monocyte was determined for monocytes cultured 1, 2, and 4 days in the presence and absence of HCMV. One day postexposure, most cells were shown to have above control levels of grains per cell. (Controls were hybridized with the sense RNA riboprobe.) However, both at 2 and 4 days postexposure, a significant proportion of monocytes retained levels of grains as high as were observed 1 day postexposure. A similar observation was made with two other donors [14]. This indicates that the general elevation in steady-state mRNA is a result of low proportion of monocytes expressing persistently high levels of message. This fraction ranged from 1%–8% of the total depending upon the donor. Thus, it seems probable that a generalized enhancement of IL-1β expression

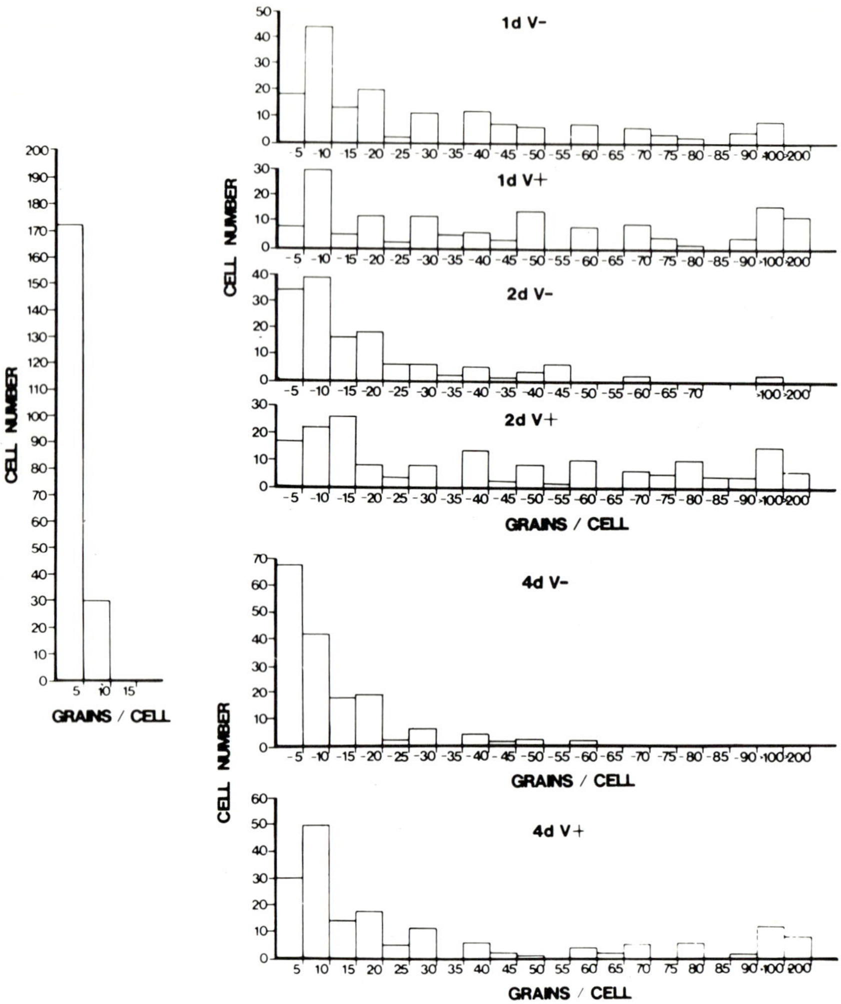

Fig. 4. IL-1β-mRNA expression in human cytomegalovirus-(HCMV)-infected and uninfected peripheral blood monocytes analyzed by in situ hybridization using [^{35}S]-labeled antisense RNA probes specific for IL-1β. Background staining was revealed by hybridizing cells to [^{35}S]-labeled IL-1β sense RNA sequences. Grain counts and numbers of positive cells were determined by counting approximately 200 cells per slide. IL-1β-mRNA expression is shown 1, 2, and 4 days postinfection with (+) and without (−) virus. (From [14])

results from selective stimulation of a subpopulation of cells. As this is of similar magnitude to the proportion of monocytes reported to express the IE genes following exposure to laboratory strains of HCMV [13, 16, 25, 26, 35, 36], it will be important to determine if the IL-1β-positive cells are the same cells which show expression of IE genes.

HCMV Infection Results in Transient IL-1β Translation in Spite of Long-Term Transcription

We have previously demonstrated that high levels of steady-state mRNA for IL-1β, TNF-α, and CSF-1 may be induced in monocytes following adherence, but this fails to result in significant translational activity [23]. A second stimulus such as LPS was required for both translation and secretion to occur. We, therefore, were interested in determining if HCMV enhancement of steady-state mRNA was a sufficient signal for translation. This was of additional significance as it has been reported that an IL-1β inhibitor may be released following exposure to virus [36]. Western transfer analysis indicated that while significant levels of the pro-IL-1β protein could be detected in monocytes 24 h after exposure to either live or killed virus, in PMA-treated ML-3 cells pro-IL-1β protein was only detected 24 h postexposure to live virus (Fig. 5).

These data are in contrast to the high mRNA levels, indicating that an uncoupling of transcription and translation had apparently occurred (see Figs. 1, 3). Thus, decreased levels of IL-1β in response to virus infection need not result from coexpression of an IL-1β inhibitor.

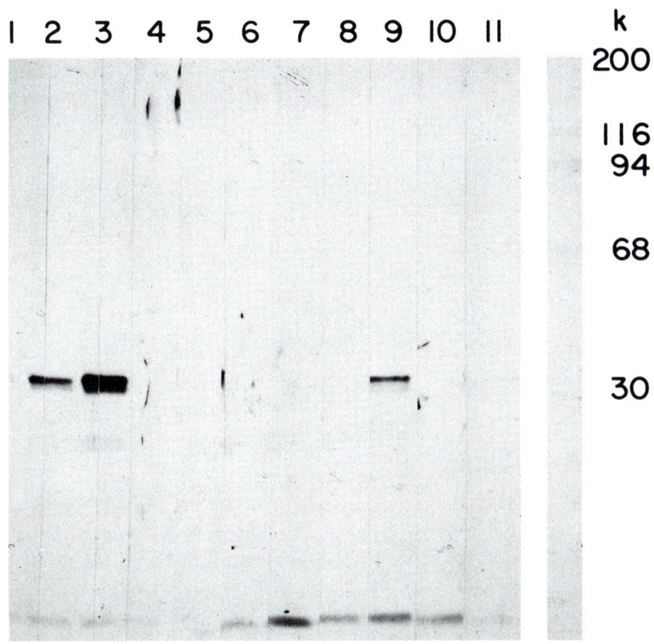

Fig. 5. Western transfer analysis of IL-1β translation products in monocytes (*lanes 1–5*) or ML-3 cells (*lanes 6–11*). *Lane 1*, uncultured monocytes, and *lane 6*, untreated ML-3 cells; cells treated for 24 h with heat-inactivated (*lanes 2* and *8*), infectious virus (*lanes 3* and *9*), 72 h with heat-inactivated (*lanes 4* and *10*), or infectious human cytomegalovirus (*lanes 5* and *11*). (From [14])

The Product of Region 2 of the Immediate Early Gene of HCMV Can Transactivate the IL-1β Gene

Infection of macrophages with laboratory strains of HCMV seldom leads to a complete replication cycle. Rather, if any virus genes are detected they are limited to those designated IE [16, 35]. We were, therefore, interested in determining if the enhanced expression of IL-1β seen in macrophages resulted from transactivation of the IL-1β gene by the IE gene products. We examined this possibility, in collaboration with B. D. Clark and P. E. Auron [14]. Chimeric CAT constructs containing the pro-IL-1β promoter were transfected into ML-3 cells together with various HCMV IE gene constructs. Results shown in Fig. 6 indicate that when plasmid 3M-AT DNA containing 524 bp of pro-IL-1β genomic DNA was transfected with HCMV IE region 1 and 2 expression plasmid, pHD101SV1, it stimulated activity of the IL-1β promoter. In contrast, the HCMV construct containing region 1 (pHD101SV2) stimulated to a lesser extent, while the region 2 construct (pHD10142) was fully active. As was observed in the early experiments with HCMV infection of ML-3 cells, prior induction of differentiation with PMA was required in order to detect activity. This, and the earlier results shown in Fig. 1, suggest that a state of

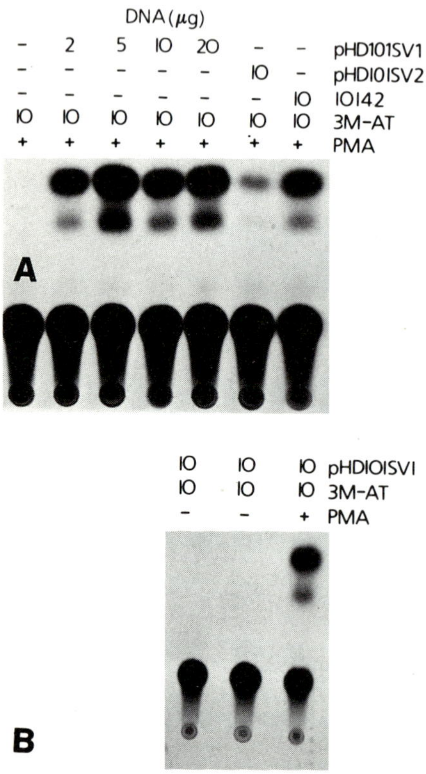

Fig. 6 A, B. Effect of human cytomegalovirus immediate early (HCMV-IE) region gene products on the IL-1β gene in phorbol myristate acetate-(PMA)-differentiated (**A**) and undifferentiated (**B**) ML-3 cells. Cells were transfected singly with IL-1β-CAT plasmid DNA (3M-AT), or cotransfected with various HCMV-IE region expression plasmids, pHD101SV1 (IE regions 1 and 2), pHD101SV2 (IE region 1), or pHD10142 (IE region 2). (From [14])

competence, already established with blood monocytes, is required prior to a successful HCMV effect in ML-3 cells.

Discussion

There is increasing evidence for macrophages playing an important role in not only host defense against virus infection but also for the opposite role, that of a "silent" host harboring virus and awaiting the appropriate challenge before breaking out of the latent state [4]. While it has been difficult to demonstrate a complete round of virus replication in macrophages, several groups have shown that the IE gene product(s) can be detected in a low percentage of cells. This is especially true when clinical isolates of the virus have been used [13, 16, 25, 26, 35, 36]. When established stocks passed in fibroblasts are used, the frequency is too low to detect the IE by immunofluorescence [16]. Nonetheless, several groups have demonstrated that such cells can have severely depressed function. For example, Kapasi and Rice [25] were able to show significant depression of respiratory burst activity (>90%), especially with clinical isolates, although no more than 3% of the cells could be shown to express the IE gene product. Rice et al. [35] demonstrated that monocytes were the major cells to be infected in peripheral blood. These authors found that no more than 10% of the cells expressed the IE gene but found high levels of immunosuppression with these cells. Once again, the clinical isolates were superior in inducing suppression and in expressing the IE gene product. Rodgers et al. [36] employed the AD169 strain to demonstrate induction of an IL-1β inhibitor. This appeared rapidly (within 2–8 h) yet was not accompanied by the appearance of IE protein. A possible explanation for the apparent immunosuppression observed has been recently reported by two different groups. Buchmeier und Cooper [5], as well as Scott et al. [38], have observed that there is negligible immunosuppression in normal mononuclear cells when mycoplasma-free virus preparations are employed. Both groups concluded that HCMV by itself does not seem to be capable of producing immuno-unresponsiveness. This is more in keeping with our observations that HCMV transcriptionally activates many important inflammatory mediator genes and would seem to infer that mycoplasma may interfere with the overall pathway of subsequent macrophage functional development.

The state of activity and differentiation of the host cell are likely to be of utmost importance when macrophages are infected. An often overlooked complexity in this issue is the highly variable state of differentiation/activation that cells of the mononuclear phagocyte series may exhibit and the influence that this may have on the outcome of virus exposure. Promyelocytic cell lines such as HL-60 and ML-3 as well as the monocytic lines U937 and THP-1 all possess some macrophage-like characteristics but require exposure to differentiating agents to exhibit most macrophage traits [22]. In spite of these provisos, cell lines such as U937 have provided much valuable information with regard to virus–macrophage interactions. For example, Weinshenker et al. [41] have been able to produce a full round of CMV infection in the THP-1 cell line. Petit et al. [32] have also been able to infect the U937 cell line with HIV demonstrating the viruses ability to downregulate HLA class II genes. Folks et al. [17] have also reported inducing persistent but apparently latent HIV infection in U937 cells. In this case, the authors were able to demonstrate that this was sufficient to induce enhanced levels of the IL-1β gene, which was accompanied by increased production of IL-1β protein. The state of macrophage activation/differentiation can profoundly influence susceptibility to infection. Thus, an as yet uncharacterized state of competence must exist prior to virus exposure in order to permit infection. Weinshenker et al. [44], for example, have reported that one monocytic cell line THP-1 could be productively infected but only following induction of differentiation with the phorbol ester PMA, suggesting that a state of competence had to be established prior to infection. We have reported that lung macrophages appear to be quite resistant to infection with HIV-1, whereas most samples of peritoneal macrophages showed extremely rapid fusion and often lyse [31]. Monocytes demonstrated intermediate responses that were in general unaffected by differentiation in culture [31]. In contrast, visna virus infection of sheep monocytes proceeded more efficiently with monocytes that had been cultured under conditions which favored the more mature phenotype [18]. Our data clearly indicate that fresh monocytes can be infected with CMV to the extent that enhanced expression of certain host cell genes is observed. In particular, the only genes showing this response are those which must be induced in the ML-3 cell line with PMA (this chapter), or can be induced in nonadhered monocytes in response to PMA stimulation (data derived with a series of cDNA clones that are specifically induced in a rapid response to adherence; submitted for publication) [39]. Genes that are constitutively expressed, such as lysozyme or HLA-DR, were unaffected by virus. It appears then, that there is a direct relationship between the induction of these genes and enhancement by the IE gene product of HCMV.

Infection with HCMV also leads to enhanced translational activity in the ML-3 cells and monocytes, although the effect is transient and does not continue in parallel with the prolonged expression of steady-state mRNA levels. In addition, heat-killed virus appeared to be capable of inducing a significant but lower level of the pro-IL-1β precursor protein in adherent monocyte cultures, but not in the PMA-treated ML-3 cells. Further studies are required to determine if the lack of stimulation by heat-killed virus in ML-3 cells is a detection problem or is a genuine lack of stimulation. Although IL-1β, TNF-α, and CSF-1 expression are rapidly induced following adherence of monocytes, little if any protein is secreted in the absence of a second signal as is usually produced following exposure to LPS [23]. The present data indicate that heat-inactivated HCMV can probably also serve that role, indicating that interactions in addition to direct influences on transcription by abortive infections may be important. Finally, the data derived from flow cytometric analysis indicates that the majority of macrophages have enhanced levels of IL-1β protein [14], suggesting, in agreement with others [26], that the effect of virus is manifested on the majority of the population.

The present studies have indirectly addressed one of the fundamental questions of macrophage–HCMV interactions. Why is such a high frequency of cells altered when such a low number actually are infected sufficiently to express IE genes? One explanation may be that the level of expression is just too low to detect in macrophages by indirect immunofluorescence. Indeed, Nelson et al. [30] have demonstrated that the frequency of double-infected cells in CNS specimens was highly underestimated when immunocytochemical assessment was carried out (1%), in contrast to the 26% figure that was obtained when in situ hybridization methods were used. Recently, it has also been reported that use of the polymerase chain reaction (PCR) permits detection of a far higher frequency of HIV-1 positive lymphocytes in most AIDS patients than the prior 0.1%–1% estimate derived from immunocytochemistry [37]. While a true estimate of the frequency of IE-gene-expressing monocytes cannot at present be given, the observation that as high as 10% may "chronically" express very high levels of IL-1β transcripts, and by analogy other mediator genes as well, suggests that the effective level of HCMV expression from in vitro exposure to laboratory adapted strains is unlikely to exceed 10%. Additional data derived from flow cytometric analysis of HCMV infected monocytes indicated that virtually all cells contained above background levels of IL-1β, indicating that there may be two sets of responding monocytes: one population that expresses IE gene products, resulting in "chronic" enhancement, and a second that shows a more transient elevation, perhaps resulting from secondary response to secreted cytokines or ingestion/bindung of the stimulatory HCMV proteins. The possibility that a general elevation in cytokine expression results from a paracrine response by monocytes is highly likely as monocytes have been shown to rapidly respond to many of their own cytokines, including IL-1β and TNF-α.

References

1. Anisowicz A, Bardwell L, Sager R (1987) Constitutive over-expression of a growth-regulated gene in transformed Chinese hamster and human cells. Proc Natl Acad Sci USA 84:7188–7192
2. Auron PE, Clark BD, Fenton MJ, Rey JL, Webb AC (1989) Regulation of human prointerleukin 1β gene transcription. Colloq INSERM 179:61–69
3. Boyum A (1968) Isolation of mononuclear cells and granulocytes from human blood. Scand J Clin Lab Invest 21 Suppl 97:77–89
4. Brautigam AR, Dutko FJ, Olding LB, Oldstone MBA (1979) Pathogenesis of murine cytomegalovirus infection: the macrophage as a permissive cell for cytomegalovirus infection, replication and latency. J Gen Virol 44:349–359
5. Buchmeier NA, Cooper NR (1989) Suppression of monocyte functions by human cytomegalovirus. Immunology 66:278–283
6. Carney WP, Hirsch MS (1981) Mechanisms of immunosuppression in CMV mononucleosis. II. Virus–monocyte interactions. J Infect Dis 144:47–54
7. Chirgwin JM, Przybyla AE, MacDonald RJ, Rutter WJ (1979) Isolation of biologically active ribonucleic acid from sources enriched in ribonuclease. Biochemistry 18:5294–5299

8. Clark BD, Collins KL, Gandy MS, Webb AC, Auron PE (1986) Genomic sequence for human prointerleukin 1 beta: possible evolution from a reverse transcribed prointerleukin 1 alpha gene. Nucleic Acids Res 14:7897–7914
9. Clouse KA, Robbins PB, Fernie B, Ostrove JM, Fauci AS (1989) Viral antigen stimulation of the production of human monokines capable of regulating HIV1 expression. J Immunol 143:470–475
10. Davis MG, Kenney SC, Kamine J, Pagano JS, Huang E-S (1987) Immediate-early gene region of human cytomegalovirus transactivates the promoter of human immunodeficiency virus. Proc Natl Acad Sci USA 84:8642–8646
11. Dinarello CA (1984) Interleukin-1. Rev Infect Dis 6:51–95
12. Dinarello CA, Cannon JG, Wolff SM, Bernheim HA, Beutler B, Cerami A, Figari IS, Palladino Jr MA, O'Connor JV (1986) Tumor necrosis factor (cachectin) is an endogenous pyrogen and induces production of interleukin 1. J Exp Med 163:1433–1450
13. Dudding LR, Garnett HM (1987) Interaction of strain AD169 and a clinical isolate of cytomegalovirus with peripheral monocytes: the effect of lipopolysaccharide stimulation. J Infect Dis 155:891–896
14. Dudding LR, Haskill S, Clark BD, Auron PE, Sporn S, Huang E-S (1989) Cytomegalovirus infection stimulates expression of monocyte-associated mediator genes. J Immunol 143:3343–3352
15. Eierman DF, Johnson CE, Haskill JS (1989) Human monocyte inflammatory gene expression is selectively regulated by adherence substrates. J Immunol 142:1970–1976
16. Einhorn L, Ost A (1988) Cytomegalovirus infection of human blood cells. J Infect Dis 149:207–214
17. Folks TM, Justement J, Kinter A, Dinarello CA, Fauci AS (1987) Science 238:800–802
18. Gendelman HE, Narayan O, Kennedy-Stoskopf S, Kennedy PFE, Ghotbi Z, Clements JE, Stanley J, Pezeshkpour G (1986) Tropism of sheep lentiviruses for monocytes: susceptibility to infection and virus gene expression increase during maturation of monocytes to macrophages. J Virol 58:67–74
19. Gendelman HE, Orenstein JM, Martin MA, Ferrua C, Mitra R, Phipps T, Wahl LA, Lane HC, Fauci AS, Burke DS, Skillman D, Meltzer MS (1988) Efficient isolation and propagation of human immunodeficiency virus on recombinant colony-stimulating factor 1-treated monocytes. J Exp Med 167:1428–1441
20. Glisin V, Crkvenjakav R, Byus C (1974) Ribonucleic acid isolated by cesium chloride centrifugation. Biochemistry 13:2633–2637
21. Gorman CM, Moffat LF, Howard BH (1982) Recombinant genomes which express chloramphenicol acetyltransferase in mammalian cells. Mol Cell Biol 2:1044–1051
22. Harris P, Ralph P (1985) Human leukemic models of myelomonocytic development. A review of the HL-60 and U937 cell lines. J Leuk Biol 37:407–422
23. Haskill S, Johnson C, Eierman D, Becker S, Warren K (1988) Adherence induces selective mRNA expression of monocyte mediators and proto-oncogenes. J Immunol 140:1690–1694
24. Johnson CE (1989) Characterization of inflammatory gene expression in monocytes and in vascular and connective tissue cells. Thesis, University of North Carolina, Chapel Hill
25. Kapasi K, Rice GPA (1986) The role of the monocyte in cytomegalovirus-mediated immunosuppression in vitro. J Infect Dis 154:881–884
26. Kapasi K, Rice GPA (1988) Cytomegalovirus infection of peripheral blood mononuclear cells: effects on interleukin-1 and -2 production and responsiveness. J Virol 62:3603–3607
27. Laemmli UK (1970) Cleavage of structural proteins during the assembly of the head of bacteriophage T4. Nature 227:680–685
28. Laimins LA, Gruss P, Pozzatti R, Khoury G (1984) Characterization of enhancer elements in the long terminal repeat of Moloney murine sarcoma virus. J Virol 49:183–189
29. Larsen CG, Anderson AO, Appella E, Oppenheim JJ, Matsushima K (1989) The neutrophil-activating protein (NAP-1) is also chemotactic for T lymphocytes. Science 243:1464–1466

30. Nelson JA, Reynolds-Kohler C, Oldstone MBA, Wiley CA (1988) HIV and HCMV coinfect brain cells in patients with AIDS. Virology 165:286–290
31. Olafsson K, Smith MS, Marshburn P, Carter S, Haskill S (1991) Variation of HIV infectibility of macrophages as a function of donor, stage of differentiation, and site of origin. J Acquir Immune Defic Syndr 4:154–164
32. Petit AJC, Tersmette M, Terpstra FG, de Goede REY, van Lier RAW, Miedema F (1988) Decreased accessory cell function by human monocytic cells after infection with HIV. J Immunol 140:1485–1489
33. Peveri P, Walz A, Dewald B, Baggiolini M (1988) A novel neutrophil-activating factor produced by human mononuclear phagocytes. J Exp Med 167:1547–1559
34. Renart J, Reiser J, Stark GR (1979) Transfer of proteins from gels to diazobenzyloxymethyl-paper and detection with anti-sera: a method for studying antibody specificity and antigen structure. Proc Natl Acad Sci USA 76:3116–3120
35. Rice GPA, Schrier RD, Oldstone MBA (1984) Cytomegalovirus infects human lymphocytes and monocytes: virus expression is restricted to immediate-early gene products. Proc Natl Acad Sci USA 81:6134–6138
36. Rodgers GC, Scott DM, Mundin J, Sissons JGP (1985) Monocyto-derived inhibitor or interleukin 1 induced by human cytomegalovirus. J Virol 55:527–532
37. Schnittman SM, Psallidopoulos MC, Lane HC, Thompson L, Baseler M, Massari F, Fox CH, Salzman NP, Fauci AS (1989) The reservoir for HIV-1 in human peripheral blood is a T cell that maintains expression of CD4. Science 245:305–308
38. Scott DM, Rodgers BC, Freeke C, Buiter J, Sissons JGP (1989) Human cytomegalovirus and monocytes: limited infection and negligible immunosuppression in normal and mononuclear cells infected in vitro with mycoplasma-free virus strains. J Gen Virol 70:685–694
39. Sporn SA, Eierman DF, Johnson DE, Martin G, Ladner M, Haskill S (1990) Monocyte adherence results in selective induction of novel genes sharing homology with mediators of inflammation and tissue repair. J Immunol 144:4434–4441
40. Wahl SM, Allen JB, Gartner S, Orenstein JM, Popovic M, Chenoweth DE, Arthur LO, Farrar WL, Wahl LM (1989) HIV-1 and its envelope glycoprotein down-regulate chemotactic ligand receptors and chemotactic function of peripheral blood monocytes. J Immunol 142:3553–3559
41. Weinshenker BG, Wilson S, Rice GPA (1988) Phorbol ester-induced differentiation permits productive human cytomegalovirus infection in a monocytic cell line. J Immunol 140:1625–1631
42. White BA, Bancroft FC (1982) Cytoplasmic dothybridization: simple analysis of relative RNA levels in multiple small cell or tissue samples. J Biol Chem 257:8569–8572
43. Yoshimura T, Matsushima K, Tanaka S, Robinson EA, Appella E, Oppenheim JJ, Leonard EJ (1987) Purification of a human monocyte-derived neutrophil chemotactic factor that has peptide sequence similarity to other host defense cytokines. Proc Natl Acad Sci USA 84:9233–9237

Section II Human Cytomegalovirus Infections and the Immuncompromised Host

Chapter 7 Role of Cytomegalovirus Infection in Neurologic Abnormalities of Acquired Immunodeficiency Syndrome

Clayton A. Wiley [1] and Jay A. Nelson [2]

Summary

Neurologic disease in acquired immunodeficiency syndrome (AIDS) patients is frequently mediated by viral infections. In this review the role of cytomegalovirus (CMV) in the encephalopathy and neuropathy of AIDS is placed in the context of other viral infections. The implications of the histopathology on the pathogenesis of CMV infection of the nervous system are discussed.

Introduction

Incidence of Neurologic Abnormalities in Acquired Immunodeficiency Syndrome

A wide variety of neurologic abnormalities have been observed in patients with acquired immunodeficiency syndrome (AIDS) [1]. Between 10% and 25% of patients with AIDS present with neurologic disease, while three quarters will develop neurologic symptoms during the course of their disease [2, 3]. Neuropathology will be found in over three quarters of the autopsies of AIDS patients [1, 4, 5].

Clinical symptoms

Both central and peripheral neurologic symptoms are noted in patients infected with human immunodeficiency virus (HIV). Central neurologic symptoms range from focal lesions to a more diffuse encephalopathy. While the focal lesions are observed more frequently, the diffuse encephalopathy found in a smaller subset of AIDS patients can be the most debilitating and difficult to treat [2, 3]. The most frequently observed encephalopathy found in AIDS

---

[1] Department of Pathology, University of California San Diego, La Jolla CA 92093, USA
[2] Department of Microbiology and Immunology, Oregon Medical Center, L-220, 3181 SW Som Jackson Park Road, Portland, Oregon, 97201-3098, USA

patients has been variously termed "subcortical dementia" or "AIDS dementia complex" [2].

Clinical Signs

As defined by Navia et al. [2], AIDS dementia complex entails impaired memory and concentration, psychomotor slowing, and is frequently accompanied by motor and behavioral disturbances. A variety of clinical studies have observed this complex in up to one third of AIDS patients, with some studies suggesting that the complex is a presenting symptom of AIDS in as many as 10% of cases [6].

Radiologic findings

Focal neurologic symptoms are usually associated with focal radiologic findings. Depending upon the nature of the pathologic process (see below), computed tomography (CT) and magnetic resonance imaging (MRI) will identify lesions throughout the central nervous system (CNS). As has been observed in many disease processes, MRI has the greatest sensitivity in detecting focal abnormalities, however. CT is critical in distinguishing brain edema from the primary lesion and precisely localizing regions for biopsy [7].

The radiologic correlate of nonfocal CNS abnormalities is less well defined. Cerebral atrophy (central greater than peripheral) has been noted by CT and MRI in most demented patients. Additionally, many of these patients have demonstrated diffuse deep white and gray matter high-intensity signals on MRI [7].

Laboratory Findings

Serologic evaluation has been of limited utility in the evaluation of CNS symptoms. However, because of the high frequency of cerebral toxoplasmosis, patients with multiple focal lesions who gave positive results for toxoplasmosis from serologic tests are given a trial of chemotherapy for this agent before initiating a more extensive and invasive evaluation. Cerebrospinal fluid studies can be important in defining eukaryotic and prokaryotic infections, however, their utility in diagnosing CNS parenchymal lesions, particularly those due to viral infections, are severely limited in both sensitivity (e.g. cytomegalovirus, CMV) and specificity (e.g. human immunodeficiency virus, HIV) [8].

Neuropathology of Viral Encephalitis

The wide spectrum of neuropathology observed in AIDS replaces tuberculosis and syphilis as the paradigm disease for teaching the brain's reaction to infectious and neoplastic (e.g., primary lymphoma) processes. Many excellent reviews exist on this topic [1, 4], however, here we will focus on those processes caused by viral infections in general and CMV in particular.

Viral Encephalitis

Human immunodeficiency virus

Encephalitis due to HIV infection has been noted in up to one third of patients who die with AIDS [4, 9–11]. Initially this diagnosis was dependent upon identification of multinucleated giant cells, however, more recently direct identification of HIV antigens by immunocytochemistry or HIV nucleic acids by in situ hybridization have been considered the gold standard in the diagnosis of HIV encephalitis [10–13] (Fig. 1). Whether any of these techniques really delineate the true extent of HIV infection within the CNS, or simply represent the proverbial tip of the iceberg, awaits future study. Nevertheless, when HIV is detected, it is found most frequently within multinucleated giant cells and macrophages and less frequently within endothelial cells of the deep white and gray matter [10–13].

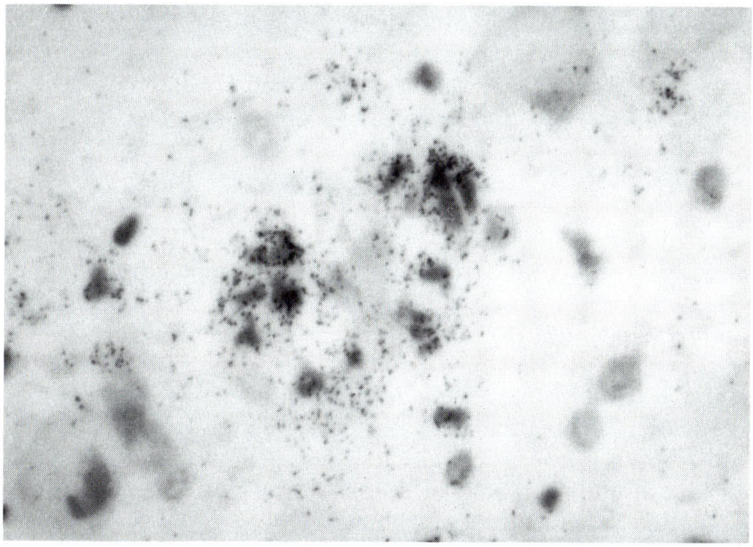

Fig. 1. Section of brain tissue from an acquired immunodeficiency syndrome patient, hybridized with a radioactive nucleic acid probe to human immunodeficiency virus and counterstained with hematoxylin. Numerous emulsion grains are noted above infiltrating inflammatory cells

JC Virus

As noted in other immunocompromised patients, patients with AIDS can develop progressive multifocal leukoencephalopathy. Between 2% and 5% of AIDS patients will develop this JC virus infection of oligodendroglia followed by destructive demyelination [14].

Herpesvirus

Both types of herpes simplex viruses (HSV) have been detected in destructive lesions of the CNS of AIDS patients [15]. Surprisingly, given the incidence of systemic HSV infection, CNS infection by these agents has not been significantly more frequent than the non-AIDS population. Varicella-zoster infection of the CNS has rarely been noted in AIDS patients [16, 17]. Epstein-Barr virus (EBV) has been recovered from the cerebrospinal fluid (CSF) cells of non-AIDS patients, however, to our knowledge it has not been recovered from AIDS patients. Nevertheless, several investigators have found evidence implicating EBV in the pathogenesis of the most frequent neoplasm involving the CNS of AIDS patients, primary CNS lymphoma [18, 19].

Cytomegalovirus

In contrast to the other herpesvirus infections, CMV infection of the CNS of AIDS patients is quite common [5]. In our experience one third of AIDS patients have some form of CMV encephalitis [14]. Two thirds of these patients have concurrent CNS infection by HIV, raising the possibility of biological and molecular cooperativity between the viruses.

Subacute Encephalitis

By far the most frequently observed form of CMV encephalitis in AIDS patients is a subacute encephalitis pathologically similar to that noted in immunosuppressed patients in the pre-AIDS era. This encephalitis consists of a diffuse peppering of the white and gray matter by microglial nodules (Fig. 2). The frequency and distribution of these nodules is consistent with the distribution of the microvasculature of the CNS (i.e., gray matter more than white matter). This distribution is consistent with a hematogenous dissemination of CMV to the CNS, but unlike embolic infections of the CNS where microorganisms or neoplasms lodge at the gray-white junction, CMV disseminates according to the distribution of *micro*vessels [14]. This distribution is consistent with a primary endothelial cell infection. This has been documented morphologically on numerous occasions. After infection of the endothelial cell, CMV rapidly extends into the CNS where it grows readily within neurons

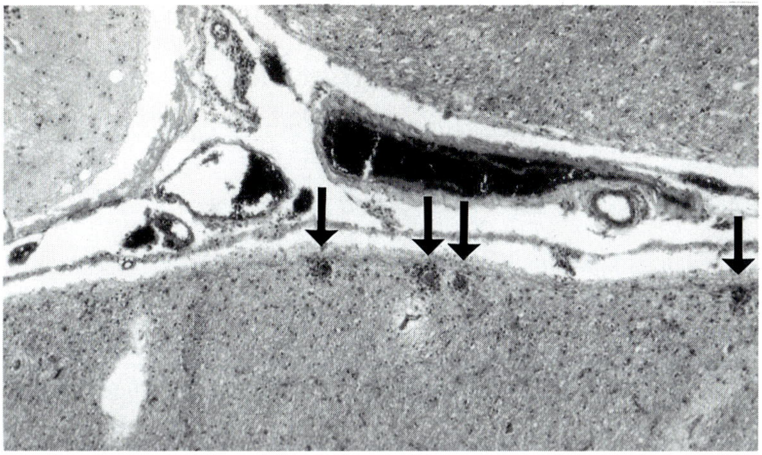

Fig. 2. Section of brain tissue, from an acquired immunodeficiency syndrome patient, stained with hematoxylin and eosin. Several microglial nodules are noted along the surface (*arrows*)

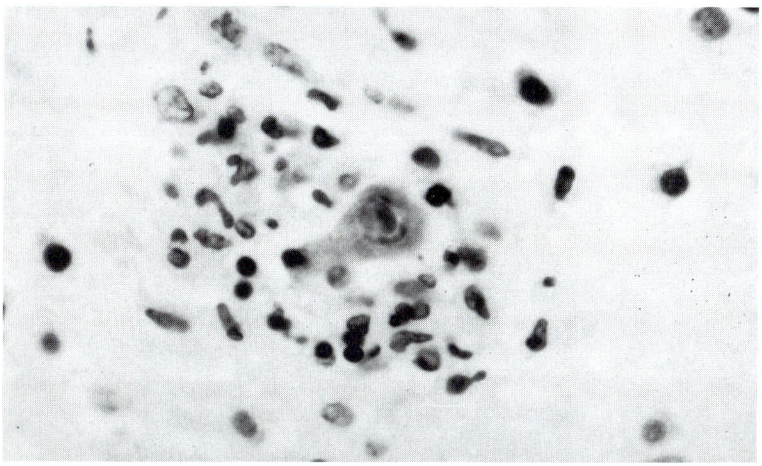

Fig. 3. Section of brain tissue, from an acquired immunodeficiency syndrome patient, stained with hematoxylin and eosin. A central neuron shows early cytomegalic change with a Cowdry type A inclusion. The neuron is surrounded by microglial cells

and glia. These sites are then surrounded by microglial cells and form a distinctive microglial nodule (Fig. 3).

CMV Infarction

Occasionally, possibly depending upon the size or morphology of the involved vessel, CMV infection will focally spread in a nidus of infarction [10]. It is not clear whether CMV has secondarily colonized a previously infarcted region of CNS tissue or whether CMV infection of endothelial cells resulted in tissue infarction. These regions can become quite large and when involving the brain stem can result in significant morbidity or mortality.

CMV Ventriculitis

In a rarer, but nevertheless significant proportion of terminal AIDS patients (approximately 10% [20] in our and other series), CMV infection is diffusely disseminated throughout the surfaces of the brain in contact with the CSF. Particularly within the lateral ventricles and spinal cord (see below), these cases of CMV encephalitis demonstrate rapid viral growth by direct extension into the CNS parenchyma (Fig. 4). In the ventricular regions this growth demonstrates a ventriculofugal pattern with a wave of infection extending into the CNS tissue. The cascade replicative process of CMV is mimicked in the tissue by expression of immediate early genes at the leading edge of the infectious wave, with expression of the late genes in the trailing edge [20].

As noted above, a high percentage of AIDS patients with CMV encephalitis also have HIV infection of the CNS. In that subgroup of patients with CMV ventriculitis we have noted coinfected of individual cells by CMV and HIV; it remains to be determined whether this documented coinfection plays a significant role in the more common subacute encephalitis of AIDS.

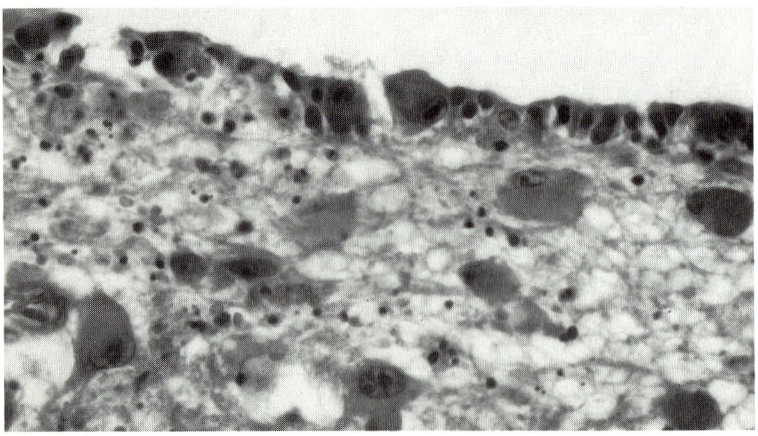

Fig. 4. Section of brain tissue, from an acquired immunodeficiency syndrome patient, stained with hematoxylin and eosin. Ependymal surface is infected by cytomegalovirus, and shows spread into deeper brain regions

Neuropathology of Peripheral Neuropathy

The incidence of peripheral neuropathy in AIDS has not been carefully studied [1, 5]. Depending upon whether one defines the disease on the basis of symptoms, clinical signs, or histopathology, estimates of peripheral neuropathy in AIDS range from 5% to 50% [1, 21–25].

Definition

Virtually the entire spectrum of neuropathies have been described in AIDS. These can occur at any time after infection and can involve any region of the peripheral nervous system. Clinically these diseases have been categorized on the basis of: course of infection, region of the peripheral nervous system involved, presence or absence of inflammation, and involvement of myelin, axons, or neurons.

Pathology

The peripheral nervous system is notoriously difficult to assess pathologically. Dysesthesias occurring in the foot could have a pathologic cause occurring anywhere along the course of the nerve. Despite the inherent sampling difficulties, a spectrum of axonal and demyelinating neuropathies have been documented in AIDS patients. While axonal loss has been described [25], the most common neuropathologic finding in peripheral nerves of AIDS patients is an acute or chronic inflammatory infiltrate. This infiltrate has been demonstrated within dorsal root ganglia and within vessel walls of peripheral nerve, but chronic inflammation within the nerve parenchyma is found more commonly.

Pathogenesis

In several cases CMV has been implicated in the etiology of the peripheral nerve inflammation. We [26] and others [27] have shown cytomegalic cells within several cases of peripheral neuritis. These cells contain CMV antigens when immunocytochemically stained. On the basis of double-label immunocytochemistry for S-100 and CMV antigens, and on the basis of cell morphology many of these cells have been classified as Schwann cells (the cells that form and maintain the myelin sheath in the peripheral nervous system). Lysis or immune destruction of these cells would explain the demyelinating neuropathy observed clinically. Intense infections, with prominent inflammation, might result in significant peripheral nerve edema and pressure which could lead to axonal loss. We have observed several cases of polyradiculopathy where CMV infection of the nerve roots has resulted in an intense inflammatory infiltrate and complete axonal loss from nerve roots.

CMV may enter the peripheral nerve by a variety of mechanisms. One mechanism is suggested by the findings of Vinters and associates who recently demonstrated CMV infection of the endothelial cells within chronically inflamed nerves [27]. Such a hematogenous dissemination followed by breaching of the blood–nerve barrier and rapid growth within peripheral nerve elements is highly reminiscent of what has been noted in the CNS.

Conclusions

CMV commonly infects the nervous system of AIDS patients. On an incidence basis CMV infection is second only to HIV as a cause of CNS viral encephalitis and is probably the primary cause of peripheral neuritis. In contrast to other herpesviruses, CMV appears to disseminate to the nervous system by hematogenous infection of the vascular endothelial cells. Productive infection of these cells leads to a breech in the blood–nerve or – brain barriers followed by rapid growth within the nervous system tissue.

Acknowledgments. This study was supported by a grant from the University of California AIDS Task Force, NIH grants NS-25178 and NS-27417, a Teacher Investigator Development Award from NIH NS-00928 to C. A. Wiley, and NIMH grants 1 P50 MH45294 and 5 RO1 MH43298. J. Nelson is the recipient of a Faculty Award from the American Cancer Society and NIH awards AI24178 and AI21640.

References

1. Levy RM, Bredesen DE, Rosenblum M (1985) Neurological manifestations of the acquired immunodeficiency syndrome (AIDS): experience at UCSF and review of the literature. J Neurosurg 62:475–495
2. Navia BA, Jordan BD, Price RW (1986) The AIDS dementia complex: I. Clinical features. Ann Neurol 19:517–524
3. Price RW, Brew B, Sidtis J, Rosenblum M, Scheck AC, Cleary P (1988) The brain in AIDS: central nervous system HIV-1 infection and AIDS dementia complex. Science 239:586–592
4. Anders KH, Guerra WF, Tomiyasu U, Verity MA, Vinters HV (1986) The neuropathology of AIDS. UCLA experience and review. Am J Pathol 124:537–558
5. Snider WD, Simpson DM, Nielsen S, Gold JWM, Metroka CE, Posner JB (1983) Neurological complications of acquired immune deficiency syndrome: analysis of 50 patients. Ann Neurol 14:403–418
6. Levy JA, Shimabukuro J, Hollander H, Mills J, Kaminsky L (1985) Isolation of AIDS-associated retroviruses from cerebrospinal fluid and brain of patients with neurological symptoms. Lancet 2:586–588
7. Post MJ, Tate LG, Quencer RM, Hensley GT, Berger JR, Sheremata WA, Maul G (1988) CT, MR, and pathology in HIV encephalitis and meningitis. AJR 151:373–380
8. Ho DD, Rota TR, Schooley R, Kaplan JC, Allan JD, Groopman JE, Resnick L, Felsenstein D, Andrews CA, Hirsch M (1985) Isolation of HTLV-III from cerebrospinal fluid and neural tissues of patients with neurologic syndromes related to the acquired immunodeficiency syndrome. N Engl J Med 313:1493–1497

9. Navia BA, Cho ES, Petito CK, Price RW (1986) The AIDS dementia complex: II. Neuropathology. Ann Neurol 19:525–535
10. Wiley C, Nelson JA (1988) Role of human immunodeficiency virus and cytomegalovirus in AIDS encephalitis. Am J Pathol 133:73–81
11. Wiley C, Schrier RD, Nelson JA, Lampert PW, Oldstone MB (1986) Cellular localization of human immunodeficiency virus infection within the brains of acquired immune deficiency syndrome patients. Proc Natl Acad Sci USA 83:7089–7093
12. Gabuzda DH, Ho DD, de la Monte SM, Hirsch M, Rota TR, Sobel RA (1986) Immunohistochemical identification of HTLV-III antigen in brains of patients with AIDS. Ann Neurol 20:289–295
13. Eilbott DJ, Peress N, Burger H, LaNeve D, Orenstein J, Gendelman HE, Seidman R, Weiser B (1989) Human immunodeficiency virus type 1 in spinal cords of acquired immunodeficiency syndrome patients with myelopathy: expression and replication in macrophages. Proc Natl Acad Sci USA 86:3337–3341
14. Wiley C, Grafe MR, Kennedy C, Nelson JA (1988) Human immunodeficiency virus (HIV) and JC virus in acquired immune deficiency syndrome (AIDS) patients with progressive multifocal leukoencephalopathy. Acta Neuropathol (Berl) 76:338–346
15. Pepose JS, Hilborne LH, Cancilla PA, Foos RY (1984) Concurrent herpes simplex and cytomegalovirus retinitis and encephalitis in the acquired immune deficiency syndrome (AIDS). Ophthalmology 91:1669–1677
16. Rostad SW, Olson K, McDougall J, Shaw CM, Alvord EC Jr (1989) Transsynaptic spread of varicella zoster virus through the visual system: a mechanism of viral dissemination in the central nervous system [published erratum appears in Hum Pathol 1989 Aug; 20(8):820]. Hum Pathol 20:174–179
17. Gilden DH, Murray RS, Wellish M, Kleinschmidt-DeMasters BK, Vafai A (1988) Chronic progressive varicella-zoster virus encephalitis in an AIDS patients. Neurology 38:1150–1153
18. Patchell RA (1988) Primary central nervous system lymphoma in the transplant patient. Neurol Clin 6:297–303
19. Rosenblum M, Levy RM, Bredesen DE, So YT, Wara W, Ziegler JL (1988) Primary central nervous system lymphomas in patients with AIDS. Ann Neurol 23:S13–S16
20. Wiley C, Schrier RD, Denaro FJ, Nelson JA, Lampert PW, Oldstone MB (1986) Localization of cytomegalovirus proteins and genome during fulminant central nervous system infection in an AIDS patient. J Neuropathol Exp Neurol 45:127–139
21. So YT, Holtzman DM, Abrams DI, Olney RK (1988) Peripheral neuropathy associated with acquired immunodeficiency syndrome. Prevalence and clinical features from a population-based survey. Arch Neurol 45:945–948
22. Janssen RS, Saykin AJ, Kaplan JE, Spira TJ, Pinsky PF, Sprehn GC, Hoffman JC, Mayer WB Jr, Schonberger LB (1988) Neurological complications of human immunodeficiency virus infection in patients with lymphadenopathy syndrome. Ann Neurol 23:49–55
23. Fiala M, Cone LA, Cohen N, Patel D, Williams K, Casareale D, Shapshak P, Tourtelotte W (1988) Responses of neurologic complications of AIDS to 3′-azido-3′-deoxythymidine and 9-(1,3-dihydroxy-2-propoxymethyl) guanine I. Clinical features. Rev Infect Dis 10:250–256
24. Smith T, Jakobsen J, Gaub J, Helweg-Larsen S, Trojaborg W (1988) Clinical and electrophysiological studies of human immunodeficiency virus-seropositive men without AIDS. Ann Neurol 23:295–297
25. Mah V, Vartavarian LM, Akers MA, Vinters HV (1988) Abnormalities of peripheral nerve in patients with human immunodeficiency virus infection. Ann Neurol 24:713–717
26. Grafe MR, Wiley C (1989) Spinal cord and peripheral nerve pathology in AIDS: the roles of cytomegalovirus and human immunodeficiency virus. Ann Neurol 25:561–566
27. Vinters HV, Kwok MK, Ho HW, Anders KH, Tomiyasu U, Wolfson WL, Robert F (1989) Cytomegalovirus in the nervous system of patients with the acquired immune deficiency syndrome. Brain 112:245–268

Chapter 8 Role of Cytomegalovirus Infection in Acquired Immunodeficiency Syndrome, with Emphasis on Neurological and Ophthalmological Complications

Milan Fiala [1,2], Michael C. Graves [1], Wayne W. Grody [3], and Harry V. Vinters [4]

Summary

Cytomegalovirus (CMV), by virtue of its immunosuppressive and transactivating properties, is ideally suited as a cofactor in acquired immunodeficiency syndrome (AIDS). CMV enhances human immunodeficiency virus (HIV) replication in CD4+ lymphoblasts, monocytes, and astrocytes, and, conversely, HIV potentiates replication of some CMV strains in lymphoblasts and macrophages.

CMV viremia, demonstrated by culture or polymerase chain reaction (PCR) and CMV retinitis are the most useful indices of disseminated infection. Although still considered an opportunistic pathogen of terminally ill patients, the evidence is mounting that CMV plays an essential role in the progression of immune deficiency and relase of HIV p24 antigen into the blood stream. In the nervous system, CMV is synergistic with HIV as a cause of severe AIDS encephalopathy, polyradiculoneuropathy, and peripheral neuropathy. AIDS dementia complex complicated by CMV encephalopathy (ACE) is distinguished from pure AIDS dementia complex (ADC) by CMV viremia with a high virus titer, intra-blood-brain barrier CMV antibody production, seizures, coma, and rapid demise. In AIDS patients, disseminated CMV infection also involves, with variable intensity, the lungs, gastrointestinal tract, adrenal glands, and other organs, sometimes without typical cytopathology which renders the diagnosis of CMV infection a challenge for hybridization and immunocytochemistry technologies.

[1] Department of Neurology, University of California Medical Center, Los Angeles, CA 90024-1732, USA
[2] Department of Medicine, University of California (Irvine) School of Medicine, Orange, CA 92668, USA
[3] Department of Pathology, Molecular Pathology, and Medical Genetics, University of California, Medical Center, Los Angeles, CA 90024-1732, USA
[4] Department of Neuropathology, University of California Medical Center, Los Angeles, CA 90024-1732, USA

Pathogenesis of Cytomegalovirus Role in Acquired Immunodeficiency Syndrome: Cytomegalovirus Aggravates the Course of Acquired Immunodeficiency Syndrome by Immunosuppressing the Host and Transactivating Human Immunodeficiency Virus

Patients suffering from acquired immunodeficiency syndrome (AIDS) as a result of infection with human immunodeficiency (HIV) are severely immunodeficient, particularly in the function of CD4+ lymphocytes, monocytes, and neutrophils [102], and consequently become infected with a multiplicity of opportunistic pathogens. In the general population, depending on the social class [58], asymptomatic CMV infection is very common (50%–80%), and it is even more frequent in homosexual men [26]. Cytomegalovirus (CMV) is a well-known opportunistic pathogen of iatrogenically immunosuppressed allograft recipients [32].

The role of CMV in AIDS has been previously regarded as that of an opportunistic pathogen which may become disseminated preterminally [64]. However, unlike nonviral opportunists, some herpes viruses, including Epstein-Barr virus, CMV, and human herpesvirus-6, may infect, replicate, and damage immune cells. In vitro, CMV infects lymphoblasts in a restricted fashion [94, 111] and its replication is enhanced by interleukin-2 [12]. In vivo, CMV is found in granulocytes (as infectious virus [32]) and mononuclear cells (as viral DNA [98]). CMV infection causes immune suppression, especially during primary infection. CMV interferes with certain functions of lymphocytes and monocytes, including the release of and responsiveness to interleukin-1 and -2 by T cells [53, 95, 106], HLA-DR expression, and antigen presentation by monocytes (Garnett, personal communication), and bacterial phagocytosis [2, 104]. Whereas, in heterosexual subjects, CMV mononucleosis is accompanied by a temporary increase in the OKT8+ lymphocyte subset, in homosexual men primary CMV infection causes prolonged abnormalities in the CD4+ to CD8+ ratio [27] and a decrease in CD4+ cells [20]. The concentration of CMV DNA in the blood cells of HIV-infected persons increases with the progression of their disease [40], as does the titer of CMV viremia [34].

Zidovudine may decrease the frequency of CMV viremia and thus retard the progression to AIDS [101]. In AIDS patients, coinfection of a single leukocyte with both CMV and HIV is probably an exceptional event but, when it occurs, could result in enhanced yields of both viruses. We have made the following observations regarding CMV and HIV coinfection of a lymphoblastoid cell line [14]: cultures infected with both viruses ultimately showed complete lysis, whereas in cultures infected with HIV alone only 30% of the cells died. When observed by electron microscopy, those cells displaying only retroviral particles were morphologically intact; all those cells comprising herpes virions and dense bodies intracellularly and retroviral particles extracellularly, adjacent to the remnants of the cell membrane, were lysed. Bidirectional enhancement of CMV by HIV and of HIV by CMV was observed in another

CD4+ lymphoblastoid cell line [107]. CMV and herpes simplex virus type 1 transactivate transcription of sequences in the long terminal repeat region of HIV which are distinct from the TAR region [72, 73, 81, 92]. The bidirectional interactions between CMV and HIV observed in vitro and in vivo are based on molecular and immunological mechanisms, which are likely to operate in a variety of cells and tissues and may include glial cells and neurons [29, 78, 116]. Additionally, HIV coinfection of monocytes may render these ubiquitous cells permissive for CMV replication (Schrier RD et al. 1990, personal communication; Baldwin GC et al. 1991, in preparation).

Seroepidemiological studies [21, 113] as well as prospective studies of patients with CMV viremia [34], suggest that HIV-infected patients with active CMV infection are at a greater risk of progression to AIDS, especially when involving neurological complications, than CMV-uninfected patients. Primary CMV infection alone may lead to inversion of the CD4+ to CD8+ ratio, a hallmark of AIDS [27]. Our recent data show that disseminated CMV infec-

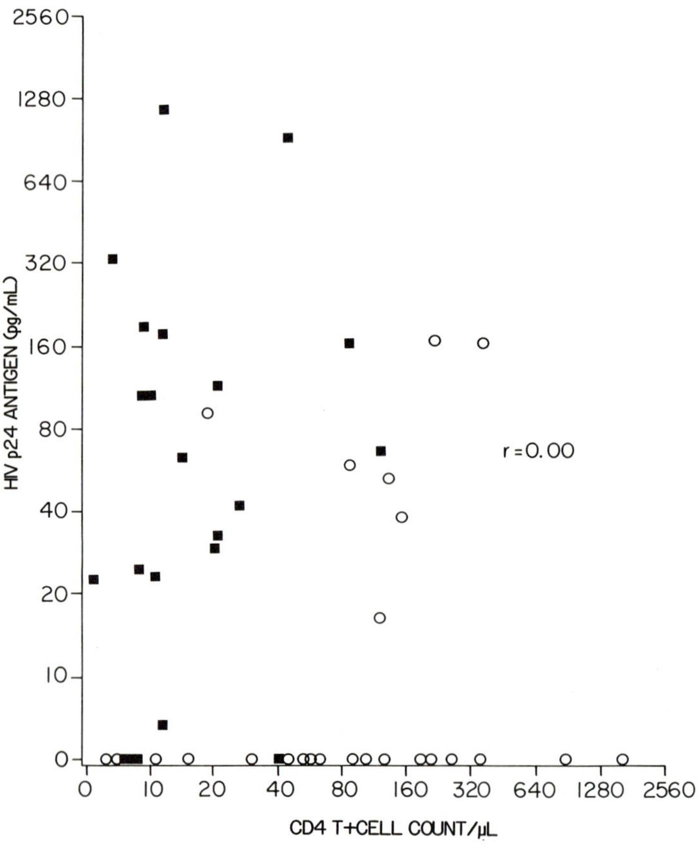

Fig. 1. Relationship of p24 antigenemia to CD4+ and cytomegalovirus (CMV) retinitis. *Full squares,* AIDS patients with CMV retinitis; *open circles,* AIDS patients without CMV retinitis

tion with retinitis is associated with HIV p24 antigenemia and severe immune deficiency (Fig. 1), whereas HIV p24 antigenemia is by itself not correlated with depression of the CD4+ cell count. In a late stage of AIDS, when CD4+ cell count has decreased below 0.050×10^9 cells/l and CD8+ below 0.400×10^9 cells/l, CMV frequently causes disseminated infection with retinitis and encephalitis [36].

Diagnosis of CMV Infection in AIDS Patients

CMV viremia is a hallmark of a recent or disseminated CMV infection [32, 98], unlike virus shedding in the urine, throat, etc. in chronically infected individuals. CMV viremia is detected in over 90% of patients with AIDS by culture of polymorphonuclear (PMN) leukocytes, but less often by culture of mononuclear leukocytes [36, 98], although the reason for lower infectivity of mononuclear leukocytes is obscure. The existence of "lymphocytotropic" CMV strains (growing less vigorously in fibroblasts than in lymphocytes) or a restricted nature of CMV infection in lymphocytes could result in such a discrepancy. We have observed limited genomic differences between two CMV strains, one strain isolated from PMN leukocytes and the other from mononuclear leukocytes separated from a single blood specimen of an AIDS patient (Fig. 2). Although we did not study biological behavior of the former strain, the latter strain infected CD4+ lymphoblasts after preinfection with HIV [14].

The detection of CMV in bronchoalveolar lavage specimens is accelerated by staining the cell culture with fluorescein-conjugated monoclonal CMV antibody [31, 65] or by in situ hybridization [45]. These techniques have been widely applied to the diagnosis of CMV infection in the lungs but, due to their high sensitivity, often lead to identification of CMV in specimens where it has no pathogenic role. The bone marrow responds to CMV infection by an outpouring of PMN leukocytes, including immature forms; a predominance of PMN leukocytes in the cerebrospinal fluid (CSF) has also been suggestive of CMV infection [19].

Virus culture of peripheral blood leukocytes in human fibroblasts (the fibroblasts should be in a low passage and seeded in plastic trays) is the golden yardstick of CMV viremia. The leukocytes should be removed 24–48 h after inoculation, and the media changed every 7 days. For maximum sensitivity, the incubation time of this assay should be extended to 6 weeks [32]. The long incubation period delays the results of the technique. For this reason alone, nucleic acid hybridization techniques have long been needed because of their rapidity, sensitivity (which approaches or surpasses that of the infectious assay) and applicability to various problems. Nucleic acid hybridization, either DNA–DNA or RNA–DNA, has been performed for diagnostic purposes employing the dot-blot technique [100, 109]. Using a cloned CMV DNA fragment (AD169 strain, *Hin*dIII DNA fragment "L," 11.7 KB), without homology to human DNA, as either a DNA probe or as a template for an RNA

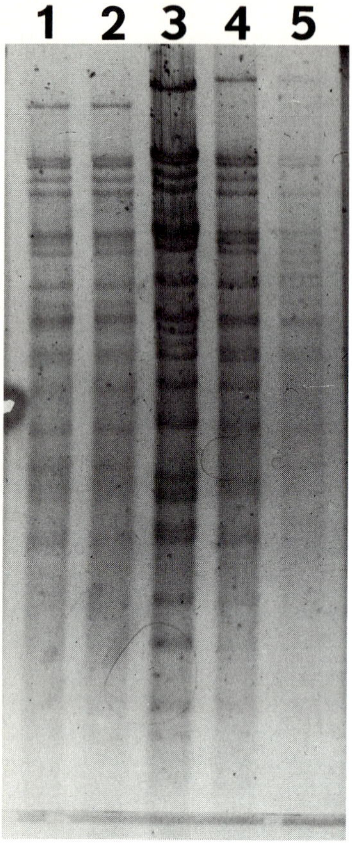

Fig. 2. Restriction enzyme analysis of genomic DNA of two cytomegalovirus (CMV) strains: One strain was isolated from polymorphonuclear leukocytes and a second strain from mononuclear leukocytes – both fractions were separated from the same blood specimen of an acquired immunodeficiency syndrome (AIDS) patient. Viral DNA was digested by *Eco*RI, run on 0.5% agarose gel, and stained with ethidium bromide. *Lanes 1 and 2:* genomic DNA of the strain from mononuclear cells; *lane 1,* 6th passage in cell culture; *lane 2,* 29th passage. *Lanes 3, 4 and 5:* DNA of the strain from polymorphonuclear leukocytes; *lane 3,* 6th passage; *lane 4,* 29th passage; *lane 5,* 32nd passage

probe, a minimum of 3 pg of CMV DNA was detected. Schuster et al. [100] compared the hybridization technique with virus isolation from urine and found a sensitivity of 83% and a specificity of 92%. CMV DNA comprises sequences homologous to human DNA [39, 96], including sequences resembling the gene of class I major histocompatibility molecule HLA-A2 [6]. For this reason, the hybridization assays demonstrating CMV DNA in Kaposi's sarcoma tissues have to be interpreted with proper attention given to the choice of the probe and the ubiquitous presence of CMV viremia in AIDS patients [3, 24, 97]. Recently, sensitivity of the hybridization assay for CMV DNA has been increased enormously by amplifying viral DNA, using a PCR [105]. Using the PCR technique for CMV DNA in lymphocytes belonging to different subsets, we have obtained preliminary evidence that certain viremic AIDS patients have CMV DNA in a substantial proportion (perhaps as high as 10^{-2}–10^{-3}) of CD4+, CD8+, and B1+ subsets, and of PMN leukocytes (Fig. 3).

In the area of histopathology, the advances in recombinant DNA technology have made possible the use of specific DNA and RNA probes which will

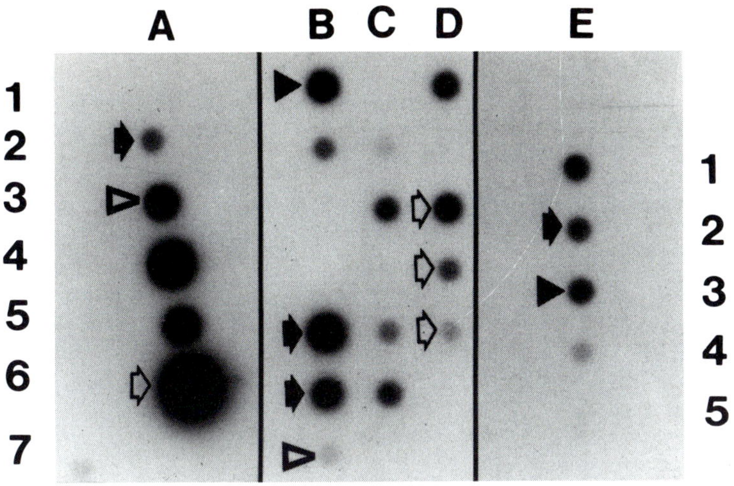

Fig. 3. Quantitative evaluation of cytomegalovirus (CMV) DNA in leukocytes by polymerase chain reaction (PCR). Increasing numbers of leukocytes belonging to different subsets were used as the starting material for PCR and dot-blot hybridization. The lymphocyte subsets were separated using monoclonal antibodies and immunomagnetic beads. The minimum numbers of leukocytes in the starting material which produced a positive reaction were:

Patient	CD4+	CD8+	B1+	PMN	Monocyte
JV	250	1000	neg	300	neg
GS	20	80	20	260	690

Open arrowheads, D3, 4500 polymorphonuclears (PMNs); D4, 750 PMNs; D5, 150 PMNs. *Closed arrowheads,* B5, 12000 PMNs; B6, 2400 PMNs. *Triangles,* A3, 20 CD4+; B7, 1500 CD4+

hybridize to endogenous CMV nucleic acid sequences in pathologic specimens in situ. Because the hybridization reaction involves complementary base pairing, through the formation of hydrogen bonds, to a target sequence hundreds or thousands of nucleotides long, the technique is also highly specific and usually not subject to the same background problems of immunological reagents, which recognize epitopes as short as 5–10 amino acids [115]. Furthermore, hybridization techniques are capable of detecting the presence of viral gene sequences, even if the encoded proteins are not being synthesized at a level sufficient for immunological detection. In situ hybridization in tissue sections may be helpful to distinguish a latent from an active infection. DNA and RNA remain intact and accessible to DNA probe hybridization, even after fixation in formalin and embedding in hot paraffin [41]. This procedure can be performed using either radiolabeled or biotin-labeled probes. The probe is labeled by incorporation of a biotinylated nucleotide derivative, through either nick translation or random priming [61], and detected by an avidin-alkaline phosphatase complex, which generates a blue precipitate at the site of hybridization. This technique is useful for early diagnosis of CMV pneumoni-

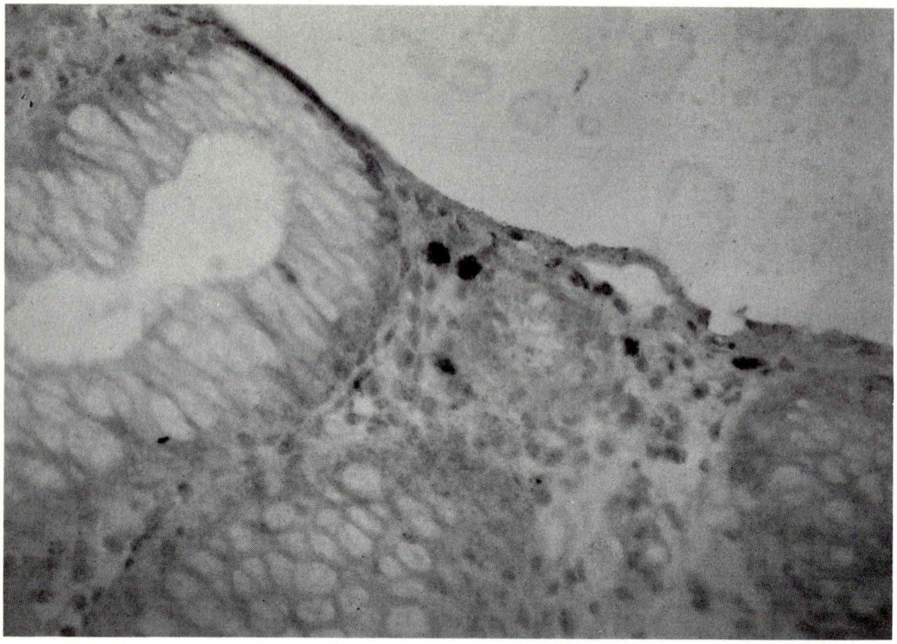

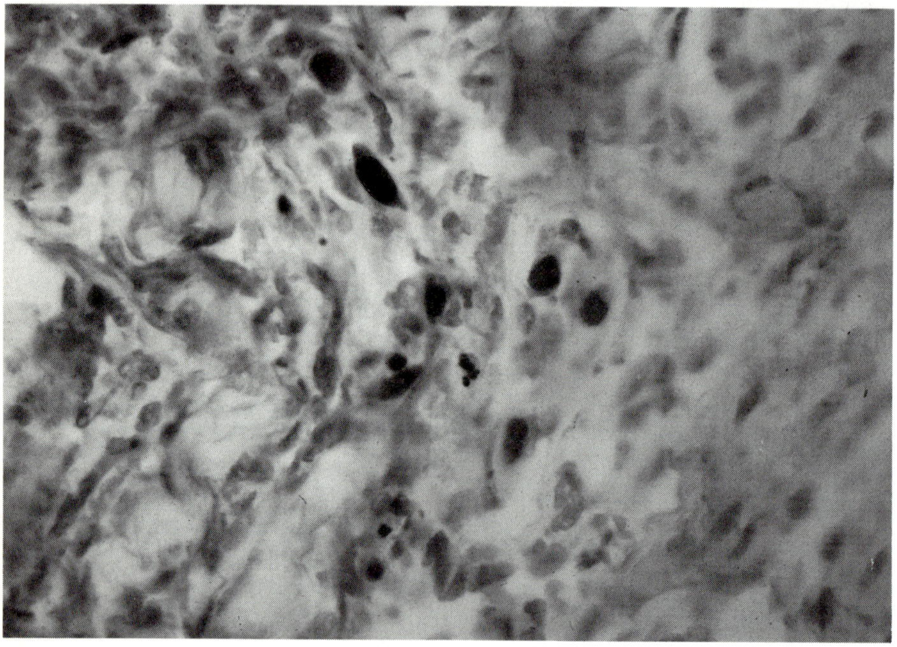

Fig. 4 (*above*). Cytomegalovirus (CMV) DNA detected by in situ hybridization in epithelial cells of the rectal mucosa. Note lack of cytomegalic intranuclear inclusions in cells positive for CMV DNA

Fig. 5 (*below*). Cytomegalovirus DNA detected by in situ hybridization in typical spindle-shaped cells in Kaposi's sarcoma tissue. Intranuclear inclusion is surrounded by a halo at the *top*

tis in AIDS patients, on either lung biopsy sections or bronchoalveolar lavage smears, allowing semiquantitation of virus load. It will also demonstrate disseminated CMV infection in a variety of other tissues obtained by biopsy or autopsy from AIDS patients, such as kidney, adrenal, esophagus, and rectum (Fig. 4), as well als within Kaposi's sarcoma lesions (Fig. 5) [42]. Importantly, it will detect CMV in many cells which lack classic cytomegalic inclusions (for example, see Fig. 4) and thus would have been missed on routine histologic screening [76].

Serologic evaluation has been used in epidemiologic studies delineating the pathogenesis of primary and secondary CMV infections in transplant patients [15] as well as in AIDS encephalopathy (see below). Serology has been, however, of little diagnostic value in AIDS patients, since past CMV infection is extremely common in homosexual individuals, and CMV IgM antibody is only rarely demonstrable in AIDS patients with viremic infection. Recently, IgM antibodies to CMV polypeptides have been found surprisingly often in asymptomatic HIV-infected patients [60].

CMV Infection of the Nervous System in AIDS

CMV infects the central nervous system (CNS) of immunologically "normal" adults, but this is a rare phenomenon [16, 86]. Conversely, fetuses and neonates are frequently infected by CMV following in utero exposure and CNS manifestations commonly result [118]. Some of these may be subtle and manifest only as delayed mental development later in life. CMV is frequently seen in the brains of patients who are immunosuppressed because of intercurrent illness or who have experienced iatrogenic immunosuppression (e.g., after organ or bone marrow transplantation [23, 54]). The most severe and pathologically varied cases of CMV infection of the nervous system are found among patients with AIDS. Two animal models of CMV infection are relevant. A disseminated form of CMV infection (involving brain as well as other organs) has been described in rhesus monkeys experimentally infected with lentivirus SIV/delta [5]. Microglial nodule encephalitis was observed in the brains of non-immunosuppressed guinea pigs infected with CMV [10]. In live AIDS patients, the diagnosis of CMV encephalitis or meningoencephalitis [112] is difficult to make and depends upon: intra-blood – brain barrier CMV antibody synthesis, CMV isolation from blood and spinal fluid, and detection of CMV DNA in the CSF after amplification by PCR. Although such techniques are being applied to this problem, in hospital practice the primary difficulty revolves around the fact that CMV lesions may be extremely varied [71] and difficult to detect by neuroimaging methods. Diffuse subependymal enhancement around the lateral ventricles is the most distinct radiological presentation [89]. To compound these difficulties, AIDS patients may have infection of the CNS or peripheral nervous system (PNS) by one or several of the other opportunistic pathogens and are also prone to developing CNS lymphomas [4]. CMV has a wide range of susceptible cells in the CNS, including neurons, astroglial cells, endothelial cells, ependymal cells (Fig. 6), and choroid plexus epithelium; whereas, HIV infects mainly macrophages. CMV is notoriously difficult to isolate from CSF [30, 35, 36, 112].

CMV can cause a remarkable morphological variety of CNS and PNS lesions. In AIDS patients that were studied at UCLA [4, 112], as well as in other series, the neuropathologic findings range from scattered rare inclusion-bearing cells, which are surrounded by minimal or totally absent inflammation (changes that have probably not contributed to overt neurologic signs and symptoms), to severe multifocal necrotizing ventriculoencephalitis that may be the major cause of neurologic morbidity. Observation of the neuropathology in routine tissue sections leads to a conclusion that the heterogeneous and highly variable effects of CMV on the nervous system reflect the ability of the virus to actively infect several cell types within the nervous system, including neurons, astrocytes, vascular endothelium, ependymal cells, and choroid plexus epithelium. CMV may cause occult infection of many cell types with negligible effects on the cytologic appearance of a given cell [76]. In situ hybridization has shown that, within the brains of patients with AIDS examined at necropsy, even CMV-antigen-negative cells that appear morphologically normal (neurons and glia) may contain CMV DNA [76, 78]. The affinity of CMV for ventricular and aqueductal ependymal surfaces, and the tendency for the virus to spread from the ventricles out into brain parenchyma, have

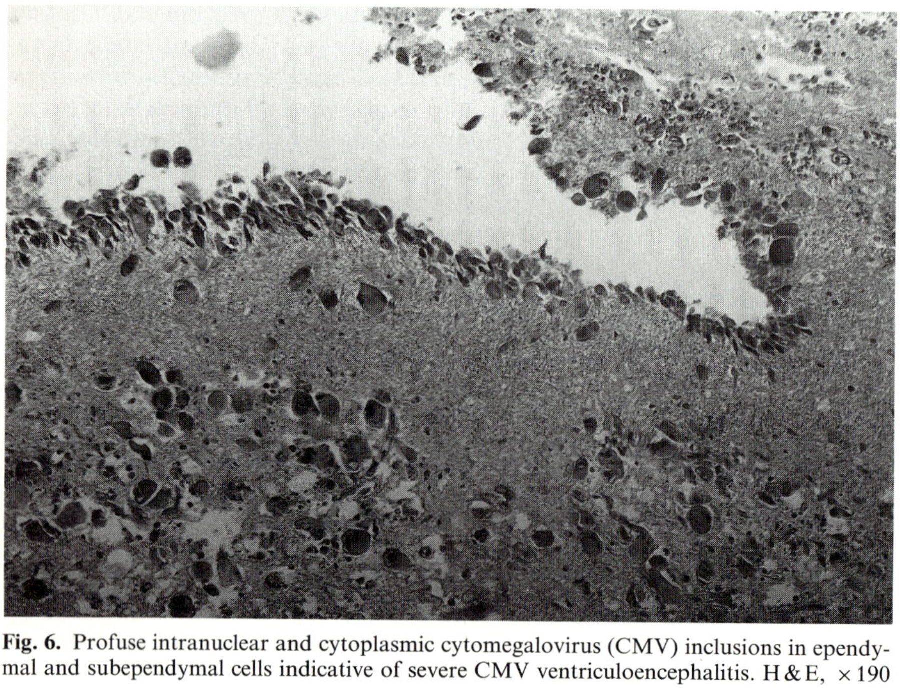

Fig. 6. Profuse intranuclear and cytoplasmic cytomegalovirus (CMV) inclusions in ependymal and subependymal cells indicative of severe CMV ventriculoencephalitis. H&E, ×190

been documented by immunocytochemistry and hybridization methodologies [44, 117]. Current studies suggest that, in AIDS patients, CMV enters the brain from the blood and then is disseminated further by the CSF prior to subsequent movement into the brain parenchyma [117] (Fig. 6). CSF production, flow, and dynamics may be altered by the presence of CMV within epithelial cells of the choroid plexus [112]. However, in our experience, the involvement of the choroid plexus has been rare and, when present, CMV inclusions are seen in only a few epithelial cells of the structure. The inclusions are occasionally surrounded by rare mononuclear inflammatory cells. CMV has been associated with demyelinization of both CNS and PNS structures, but the extent to which this occurs, in the absence of overt tissue necrosis, has not been extensively assessed [74]. CMV may produce a syndrome clinically identical to ascending polyradiculoneuropathy (Guillain-Barré syndrome) by involvement of the spinal cord nerve roots [7, 112].

CMV has been incriminated as a cause of a clinically distinct peripheral neuropathy (painful peripheral neuropathy) caused by dorsal root ganglionitis [38]. A specific syndrome of neuroradiculopathy of the lower lumbar and sacral segments with incontinence and weakness has also been associated with CMV infection. Miller et al. [70] reported seven patients with this clinical presentation, four of whom had CMV cultured from CSF, and five of whom had autopsy findings of CMV inclusions in sacral ganglia. Two patients, who were treated with ganciclovir soon after diagnosis, did improve. Although the outcome is poor in most cases, the clinical recognition of this syndrome is possible, and will be important as new treatments for CMV become available [7, 110].

The pathogenesis of the neuropathies associated with CMV is not completely understood but may involve two different but related mechanisms: infection of the Schwann cell and induction of autoimmunity. In contrast to the herpes simplex and zoster viruses, CMV probably does not establish a latency in neurons. Plotkin et al. [87], however, isolated human CMV from two of 20 human thoracic ganglion explants, suggesting that latent CMV may be present in peripheral nerves of asymptomatic individuals. CMV inclusions were found in Schwann cells of some AIDS patients with inflammatory neuropathies [18, 69, 82, 110]. The state of viral expression in the Schwann cell depends upon two factors: the state of cellular differentiation of the infected cell and the immune status of the host. Schwann cells replicate and become permissive for CMV following injury to the nerve in vitro and possibly in vivo. Immune suppression is capable of reactivating CMV in the clinical context of transplantation or in patients with AIDS. Autoimmune mechanisms may be engendered by anti-idiotypic-antibodies against CMV receptor on peripheral nerve cells several weeks after CMV infection (Graves, unpublished data).

In AIDS patients, coinfection of the brain by CMV and HIV is demonstrable by combined in situ hybridization and immunocytochemistry [8, 78]. Colocalization of CMV and HIV within the same brain cells is also suggested by morphological criteria, i.e., presence of Cowdry A inclusions in the nuclei of multinucleated giant cells (the former is characteristic of CMV and the latter of HIV) [112]. Recent findings in brain explant cultures suggest that CMV alone may reproduce histopathological findings attributed to HIV [90]. Microglial nodules (a nonspecific histologic finding within the brain of an AIDS patient, but associated with both CMV and HIV infection in the older literature) appear to colocalize more commonly with HIV than with CMV lesions, as assessed by classical light microscopic criteria. Within the brain, CMV infection produces a higher proportion of defective viral particles than in its effects on the lung [75].

CMV encephalitis usually develops in the presence of a widespread CMV infection in many organs [114], coexisting with other opportunistic infections (including *Pneumocystis carinii* pneumonia, esophageal candidiasis, cryptococcal meningitis, disseminated *Mycobacterium avium-intracellulare* infection) and malignancies. Disseminated CMV infection is usually, but not invariably, accompanied by chorioretinitis (Fiala et al., J Neurol, in press). In our experience with 25 patients afflicted by CMV retinitis, 69% had severe AIDS encephalopathy complicated by CMV infection of the CNS. The respective roles of CMV and HIV in AIDS encephalopathy are suggested by the criteria in Table 1. The relationship of CMV to AIDS progression is explained by the propensity of CMV to transactivate HIV as well as the opposite transactivation of CMV by HIV. In an individual case, the role of CMV in encephalitis is highlighted by: intensive viremia in patients with retinitis and encephalitis; increased ratio of CMV antibodies in the spinal fluid IgG and the plasma IgG; isolation of CMV from the spinal fluid in severe cases; and temporary improvement of symptoms and signs by antiviral therapy with ganciclovir (Table 1) [35, 36]. Neuropathological examination of three patients with ACE, who were part of our original clinically defined group, revealed severe CMV ventriculoencephalitis accompanied by ependymitis (Fig. 6). Although without neuropathological examination or positive virological test results in the spinal fluid, the respective roles of CMV and HIV in each case may remain something of an enigma, in patients with a lesser degree of immunodeficiency (CD4+ count above 0.200×10^9 cells/per liter) HIV is usually alone in causing "AIDS dementia complex (ADC)" [77]; whereas, in patients with severe immune deficiency, CMV in synergy with HIV appears to be a cause of "AIDS dementia complex complicated by CMV encephalopathy (ACE)" (Fiala et al., J Neurol, in press). Magnetic resonance imaging usually does not differentiate between HIV and CMV-complicated HIV encephalitis; in both entities, large bilateral high-signal areas within the white matter may be observed (cf Fig. 2 in [35]). Although not seen frequently, subependymal enhancement around lateral ventricles reflects ependymitis, which is characteristic of CMV encephalitis.

CMV Retinitis

The incidence of CMV retinitis varies in literature between 5.7% [49, 50] and 29% [48]. Our experience is derived from 60 patients admitted to Eisenhower

Table 1. Clinical and laboratory findings in patients with AIDS encephalopathy suggestive of pathogenetic roles of HIV alone or CMV in synergy with HIV (Fiala et al., J Neurol, in press)

Finding	Evidence	
	HIV only (AIDS dementia complex)	CMV with HIV (AIDS/CMV encephalopathy)
CD4+ cell count ($\times 10^9$/l)	>0.100	<0.100
Clinical course	Slowly progressive to dementia	Rapidly progressive to coma
CMV retinitis	Absent	Present
Salient neurologic findings	Progressive dementia with memory loss, apathy, and motor dysfunction	Repetitive seizures, altered sensorium, and coma
CMV viremia	At a low titer	Constant and at high titer (10^{-5}–10^{-3} PFU per leukocyte)
Infectious CMV in the spinal fluid	Absent	Present (in severe cases)
Ratio of CMV antibodies in the spinal fluid IgG and the plasma IgG	A low ratio (1.0–3.0)	A high ratio (>6.0)
Ratio of HIV antibodies in the spinal fluid IgG and the plasma IgG	Elevated	Elevated
HIV p24 antigenemia	Usually absent	Almost always present
Ganciclovir therapy	Not appropriate	Transitory improvement
Zidovudine therapy	Long-lasting improvement	No effect
Suggestive MRI findings	High-signal areas in the white matter, and brain atrophy	Subependymal enhancement around lateral ventricles (seen rarely)
Neuropathology	Multinucleated giant cells	Cytomegalic cells with intranuclear Cowdry type A inclusions in enlarged neurons, ependymal cells, glial cells and endothelial cells

PFU, plaque-forming units

Medical Center between July 1985 and April 1987, the era before zidovudine was widely available. Of these patients, 24 (40%) ultimately developed CMV retinitis as detected by direct ophthalmoscopy screening. Since the introduction of zidovudine, the incidence in the same hospital has decreased (from 70% in 1985 to 40% in 1986 and 17% in 1987 and thereafter). Nevertheless, some patients have developed retinitis while receiving zidovudine, but with a longer incubation period since the onset of AIDS. Retinal disease in AIDS progresses through the stages of ischemia, cotton-wool spots, exudates, and hemorrhages along vascular arcades [47, 85]; however, only the latter two manifestations define CMV retinitis. Although cotton-wool spots are found in a variety of diseases with ischemia of the retina and focal axonoplasmic stasis, in AIDS and AIDS-related complex (ARC) patients these spots frequently herald CMV retinitis [47].

Nonetheless, histopathologic and immunocytochemical studies have failed to identify CMV in cotton-wool spots. The cotton-wool spots are foci of retinal ischemia with axonoplasmic stasis and may be related to HIV-induced retinal endothelial changes [80], as well as immune complex deposition and embolic occlusion by CMV-infected leukocytes [33]. Early lesions of CMV retinitis may resemble cotton-wool spots but are smooth edged, unlike feather-edged spots. The retinitis involves the whole thickness of the retina. Choroiditis and vitreitis may be present concurrently with retinitis. Exudative retinal detachment and hemorrhage are serious complications leading to blindness. Overall, CMV retinitis is characterized by an acute inflammatory reaction in over 50% of patients [85]. CMV retinitis frequently begins peripherally, which makes a follow-up by direct ophthalmoscopy less sensitive than the indirect technique (Fig. 7). CMV has been demonstrated in the retina by immunocytochemistry and in situ hybridization [56, 84, 108]. Single cells in the retina may be coinfected with CMV and HIV [108].

Intravenous ganciclovir has been the antiviral choice for initial and maintenance therapy of disseminated CMV infections [119], but recently come CMV strains have acquired ganciclovir resistance (ED50 greater than 6 μM) while continuing to be susceptible to foscarnet (ED50 less than or equal to 300 μM). Although foscarnet has been effective as initial and maintenance therapy for CMV retinitis, with presumably less hematological toxicity than ganciclovir (neutropenia is usually not severe, although anemia may develop), associated renal insufficiency, mineral and electrolyte problems render the use of foscar-

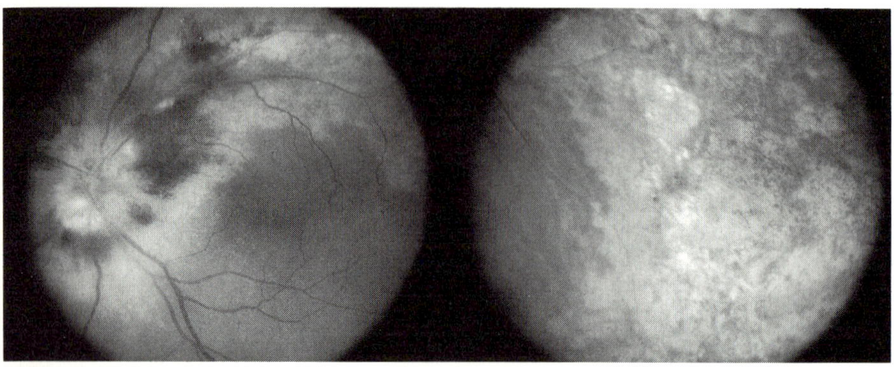

Fig. 7. Cytomegalovirus retinitis in previously untreated acquired immunodeficiency syndrome patient. Acute peripapillary retinitis had been preceded by peripherally located retinitis

net more demanding compared to ganciclovir [62]. Foscarnet may be effective in ganciclovir-resistant cases of retinitis [28, 51]. A randomized trial sponsored by the United States National Institutes of Health was terminated in October 1991 because the median survival for patients treated with foscarnet was 12 months, 4 months longer than for those treated with ganciclovir [120]. The reason for longer survival of patients receiving foscarnet is not clear, although it is suspected to be related to more effective anti-retroviral suppression in the foscarnet group.

Role of CMV in Pulmonary Complications

Pneumocystis carinii is the most important pathogen in diffuse interstitial pneumonia in AIDS. Many patients with *Pneumocystis carinii* pneumonia also have concurrent CMV viremia; on biopsy their lungs frequently reveal typical cytomegalic inclusions. CMV, as a principal or contributory cause of pneumonia, was found at autopsy in 93% of patients [83], but before death CMV pneumonia is diagnosed surprisingly rarely. Recent clinical studies have not found differences in the course of patients either with or without CMV in bronchoalveolar lavage [11, 67] or with or without anti-CMV therapy [11]. CMV impairs the function of the alveolar macrophage [25] and the production of interleukin-1 [53] and may be able to interfere with clearing of *Pneumocystis carinii* as well as other pathogens, such as *Candida* and *Pseudomonas aeruginosa*, from the lungs of viremic patients, as was shown in transplant recipients [15]. In AIDS, the pulmonary involvement represents a plurimicrobial process, although its pathogenesis may also involve autoimmune mechanisms. In bone marrow graft recipients, CMV pneumonitis occurs exclusively in the recipients of allogeneic transplants. This is believed to occur as a result of a graft-versus-host reaction complicated by viral infection [103]. Pulmonary involvement by CMV occurs in a focal or diffuse manner [17]. Necrotizing tracheitis or bronchiolitis may also develop with CMV inclusions on biopsy. The severity of CMV involvement in the lungs appears to depend upon the residual immune function. Although a London group caring for recipients of allogeneic bone marrow transplants has emphasized the role of immunopathogenic mechanisms [68], CMV is terminally a cytopathic virus per se, as demonstrated by autopsy studies [83].

Role of CMV in Gastrointestinal Complications

In different geographical areas, CMV appears to have a variable propensity to cause complications in the respiratory, gastrointestinal, urological, and ophthalmological systems. CMV infection has been observed to be present in the cells or tissues coinfected with another pathogen, such as mycobateria (*M.*

avium-intracellulare) [59], *Cryptosporidium* [52], or *Toxoplasma* [88]. Although the direction of enhancement is not clear, CMV infection could enhance the replication of another intracellular pathogen by interference with the function of the monocyte/-macrophage; on the other hand certain parasitic and bacterial pathogens could also increase CMV replication.

CMV infection may involve the whole length of the gastrointestinal tract from the gingiva to the anus, although the colon, especially the right colon, is most severely affected. The virus infects productively mesenchymal and endothelial cells and causes an inflammatory reaction with mononuclear and PMN leukocytes. CMV vasculitis with severe inflammatory reaction results in ulcerative lesions leading to thrombosis, hemorrhage and perforation, especially in the right colon [46, 66]. The manifestations include prolonged guaiac-positive diarrhea, which is associated with weight loss and anemia. Radiographic appearance mimics ulcerative colitis with features such as nodularity due to pseudomembranes, aphthous ulcerations, or large ulcerations appearing as thumb printing, and skip areas [37]. The patient with upper gastrointestinal tract involvement may have bleeding gums, odynophagia, pharyngeal ulcers, nausea, anorexia, or abdominal pain. Other microorganisms, such as parasites, *Candida albicans*, mycobacteria, and salmonellae, also cause diarrhea in AIDS patients, although at endoscopy only CMV is associated with deep colonic ulcerations and cytomegalic inclusions [93]. In addition, CMV may cause cholecystitis [55], papillary stenosis [99], sclerosing cholangitis [99], hepatitis [63], and probably pancreatitis [35]. Pancreatitis is a well-known cause of abdominal pain related to antiretroviral drugs. In AIDS patients with CMV viremia, pancreatitis appears to be related to CMV, as it had been observed even before the use of reverse transcriptase inhibitors and its onset followed closely the onset of CMV viremia [35]. We have also observed unusu-

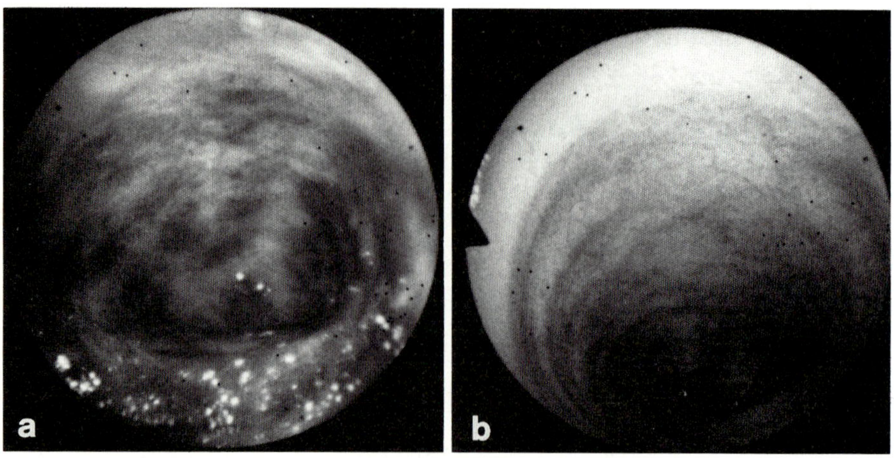

Fig. 8a, b. Colonoscopic appearance of cytomegalovirus colitis before (**a**) and after (**b**) ganciclovir therapy. (Courtesy of Dr. D. Dieterich)

ally high levels of circulating immune complexes and depressed C3 and CH100 levels in another patient with pancreatitis, AIDS, and CMV viremia. Although during life the gastrointestinal involvement may appear isolated, at autopsy CMV is found to involve the lungs, adrenal glands, liver, retina, pancreas, brain, lymph nodes, spleen, heart, pericardium kidneys, and other organs. In situ hybridization, with biotinylated CMV DNA probes, has revealed that CMV may involve cells which appear normal by light microscopy [76]. These cells are widely present in many organs infected with CMV, such as the lungs, liver, gastrointestinal tract, kidney, and even the female reproductive tract [13]. The gastrointestinal involvement is favorably influenced by treatment with antiviral drugs, such as ganciclovir [22] (Fig. 8) or foscarnet [79], which may prolong survival [66].

Other Manifestations of AIDS Possibly Related to CMV

The experience in immunosuppressed transplant patients suggests that CMV infection becomes disseminated via the blood stream in phagocytic leukocytes, granulocytes, and monocytes [32], with a predilection for the retina, brain, lung, and gastrointestinal tract, wherein severe symptoms result. Many patients with ARC or AIDS suffer from low blood pressure, tachycardia, and a protosystolic gallop. CMV could be causing these symptoms by involvement of the adrenal gland and the myocardium. The wasting syndrome, a characteristic manifestation of AIDS, may be also related to CMV as ganciclovir therapy appears to replete the body mass [57].

Although the bone marrow depression of AIDS patients is commonly thought to be due to HIV infection of the blood cell progenitors, it is likely that CMV, in addition to HIV, contributes to leukopenia by involvement of the stromal cells. CMV osteomyelitis may be encountered in AIDS [9]. Skin lesions described as epithelioid angiomatosis are related to simultaneous infection with CMV and cat-scratch disease bacillus [1]. In the reproductive tract, CMV may infect the endometrium [13], prostate, epididymis [91], and testis.

Acknowledgements. We thank Dr. Gary Holland for helpful comments regarding CMV retinitis, Dr. Douglas T. Dieterich for providing photographs of CMV colitis, Sandra Champagne-Fiala and Diana Sanderson for essential editorial assistance.

References

1. Abrams J, Farhood AI (1989) Infection-associated vascular lesions in AIDS patients. Hum Pathol 20:1025–1026
2. Abramson JS, Mills EL (1988) Depression of neutrophil function induced by viruses and its role in secondary microbial infections. Rev Infect Dis 10:326–341

3. Ambinder RF, Newman C, Hayward GS et al. (1987) Lack of association of cytomegalovirus with endemic African Kaposi's sarcoma. J Infect Dis 156:193–197
4. Anders KH, Guerra WF, Tomiyasu U, Verity MA, Vinters HV (1986) The neuropathology of AIDS. UCLA experience and review. Am J Pathol 124:537–558
5. Baskin GB (1987) Disseminated cytomegalovirus infection in immunodeficient rhesus monkeys. Am J Pathol 67:345–352
6. Beck S, Barrell BG (1988) Human cytomegalovirus encodes a glycoprotein homologous to MHC class-1 antigens. Nature 331:269–272
7. Behar R, Wiley C, McCutchan JA (1987) Cytomegalovirus polyradiculoneuropathy in acquired deficiency syndrome. Neurology 37:557–561
8. Belec L, Gray F, Mikol J et al. (1990) Cytomegalovirus (CMV) encephalomyeloradiculitis and human immunodeficiency virus (HIV) encephalitis: presence of HIV and CMV coinfected multinucleated giant cells. Acta Neuropathol (Berl) 81:97–104
9. Berhan S, Jensen J (1990) Cytomegalovirus-induced osteomyelitis in a patient with the acquired immunodeficiency syndrome. South Med J 83:1231–1232
10. Booss J, Dann PR, Griffith BP, Kim JH (1988) Glial nodule encephalitis in the guinea pig: serial observations following cytomegalovirus infection. Acta Neuropathol (Berl) 75:465–473
11. Bower M. Barton SE, Nelson MR et al. (1990) The significance of the detection of cytomegalovirus in the bronchoalveolar lavage fluid in AIDS patients with pneumonia. AIDS 4:317–320
12. Braun RW, Reiser HC (1986) Replication of human cytomegalovirus in human peripheral blood T cells. J Virol 60:29–36
13. Brodman M, Deligdisch L (1986) Cytomegalovirus endometritis in a patient with AIDS. Mt Sinai J Med 53:673–675
14. Casareale D, Fiala M, Chang CM, Cone LA, Mocarski E (1989) Cytomegalovirus enhances lysis of HIV-infected T lymphoblasts. Int J Cancer 44:124–130
15. Chatterjee SN, Fiala M, Weiner J, Stewart JA, Warner N (1978) Primary cytomegalovirus and opportunistic infection. JAMA 240:2446–2449
16. Cohen JI, Corey GR (1985) Cytomegalovirus infection in the normal host. Medicine (Baltimore) 64:100–114
17. Craighead JD (1971) Pulmonary cytomegalovirus infection in the adult. Am J Pathol 63:487–504
18. Dalakas MC, Pezeshkpour GH (1988) Neuromuscular diseases associated with human immunodeficiency virus infection. Ann Neurol 23 Suppl:38–48
19. De Gans J, Tiessens G, Portegies P et al. (1990) Predominance of polymorphonuclear leukocytes in cerebrospinal fluid of AIDS patients with CMV polyradiculomyelitis. J Acquir Immune Defic Syndr 3:1155–1160
20. Detels R, Visscher BR, Fahey JL et al. (1984) The relation of cytomegalovirus and Epstein-Barr virus antibodies to T-cell subsets in homosexually active men. JAMA 251:1719–1722
21. Detels R, Visscher BR, Fahey JL et al. (1987) Predictors of clinical AIDS in young homosexual men in a high-risk area. Int J Epidemiol 16:271–276
22. Dieterich DT, Rahmin M (1991) Cytomegalovirus colitis in AIDS: presentation in 44 patients and a review of the literature. J Acquir Immune Defic Syndr 1 Suppl: 529–535
23. Dorfman LJ (1973) Cytomegalovirus encephalitis in adults. Neurology (Minneap) 23:136–144
24. Drew WL, Huang ES (1988) Etiology and role of cytomegalovirus in Kaposi's sarcoma. In: Ziegler JL, Dorfman RF (eds) Kaposi's sarcoma: pathophysiology and clinical management. Dekker, New York
25. Drew WL, Mintz L, Hoo R, Finley TN (1979) Growth of herpes simplex and cytomegalovirus in cultured human alveolar macrophages. Am Rev Respir Dis 119:287–291
26. Drew WL, Mintz L, Miner RC et al. (1981) Prevalence of cytomegalovirus infection in homosexual men. J Infect Dis 143:188–192

27. Drew WL, Mills J, Levy J, Dylewski J et al. (1985) Cytomegalovirus infection and abnormal T-lymphocyte subset ratios in homosexual men. Ann Intern Med 103:61–63
28. Drew WL, Miner RC, Busch DF et al. (1991) Prevalence of resistance in patients receiving ganciclovir for serious cytomegalovirus infection. J Infect Dis 163:716–719
29. Duclos H, Elfassi E, Michelson S, Arenzan-Seisdedos F, Munier A, Virelizier JL (1989) Cytomegalovirus infection and transactivation of HIV-1 and HIV-2 LTR's in human astrocytoma cells. AIDS Res Hum Retroviruses 5:217–224
30. Edwards RH, Messing RL, McKendall RR (1985) Cytomegalovirus meningoencephalitis in a homosexual man with Kaposi's sarcoma: isolation of CMV from CSF cells. Neurology 35:560–562
31. Emanuel D, Pepard J, Stover D, Gold J, Armstrong D, Hammerling U (1986) Rapid immunodiagnosis of cytomegalovirus pneumonia by bronchoalveolar lavage using human and murine monoclonal antibodies. Ann Intern Med 104:476–481
32. Fiala M, Payne JE, Berne TV et al. (1975) Epidemiology of cytomegalovirus infection after transplantation and immunosuppression. J Infect Dis 132:421–433
33. Fiala M, Chatterjee SN, Poolsawat S et al. (1977) Cytomegalovirus retinitis secondary to chronic viremia in phagocytic leukocytes. Am J Ophthalmol 84:567–573
34. Fiala M, Cone LA, Chang CM, Mocarski ES (1986) Cytomegalovirus viremia increases with progressive immune deficiency in patients infected with HTLV-III. AIDS Res 2:175–181
35. Fiala M, Cone LA, Cohen N et al. (1988) Responses of neurologic complications of AIDS to 3'azido-3'deoxy-thymidine and 9-(1,3'dihydroxy-2-propoxymethyl) guanine. I. Clinical features. Rev Infect Dis 10:250–256
36. Fiala M, Cone LA, Gornbein JA et al. (1991) Human immunodeficiency virus type 1 antigenemia is enhanced in patients with disseminated cytomegalovirus infection and deficient T lymphocytes. Res Immunol 142:815–819
37. Frager DH, Frager JD, Wolf EL et al. (1986) Cytomegalovirus colitis in acquired immune deficiency syndrome: radiologic spectrum. Gastrointest Radiol 11:241–246
38. Fuller GN, Jacobs JM, Guiloff RJ (1989) Association of painful peripheral neuropathy in AIDS with cytomegalovirus infection. Lancet 2:937–941
39. Gelmann EP, Clanton DJ, Jariwalla RJ, Rosenthal LJ (1983) Characterization and location of myc homologous sequences in human cytomegalovirus DNA. Proc Natl Acad Sci USA 80:5107–5111
40. Gnann JW, Schrier RD, Truax AB, Oldstone MBA, Nelson JA (1986) Differential expression of cytomegalovirus in peripheral blood cells from AIDS patients detected by in situ hybridization. 11th International Herpes Virus Workshop, Leeds
41. Grody WW, Cheng L, Lewin KJ (1987) In situ viral DNA hybridization in diagnostic surgical pathology. Hum Pathol 18:535–543
42. Grody WW, Lewin KJ, Naeim F (1988) Detection of cytomegalovirus DNA in classic and epidemic Kaposi's sarcoma by in situ hybridization. Hum Pathol 19:524–528
43. Gross JG, Bozzette SA, Mathews WC et al. (1990) Longitudinal study of cytomegalovirus retinitis in AIDS. Ophthalmology 97:681–686
44. Hawley DA, Schaefer JF, Schulz DM, Muller J (1983) Cytomegalovirus encephalitis in acquired immunodeficiency syndrome. Am J Clin Pathol 80:874–877
45. Hilborne LH, Nieberg RK, Cheng L, Lewin KJ (1987) Direct in situ hybridization for rapid detection of cytomegalovirus in broncho-alveolar lavage. Am J Clin Pathol 87:766–769
46. Hinnant KL, Rotterdam HZ, Bell ET, Tapper ML (1986) Cytomegalovirus infection of the alimentary tract: a clinicopathological correlation. Am J Gastroenterol 81:944–950
47. Holland GN, Pepose JS, Pettit TH, Gottlieb MS, Yee RD, Foos RY (1983) Acquired immune deficiency syndrome. Ocular manifestations. Ophthalmology 90:859–873
48. Jabs D, Enger C, Bartlett JG (1989) Cytomegalovirus retinitis and acquired immunodeficiency syndrome. Arch Ophthalmol 107:75–80
49. Jacobson MA, Mills J (1988) Serious cytomegalovirus disease in the acquired immunodeficiency syndrome. Ann Intern Med 108:585–594

50. Jacobson MA, O'Donnell JJ, Porteous D, Brodie H, Feigal D, Mills J (1988) Retinal and gastrointestinal disease due to cytomegalovirus in patients with the acquired immune deficiency syndrome: prevalence, natural history, and response to ganciclovir therapy. Q J Med 254:473–486
51. Jacobsen MA, Drew WL, Feinberg J et al. (1991) Foscarnet therapy for ganciclovir-resistant cytomegalovirus retinitis in AIDS. J Infect Dis 163:1348–1351
52. Kahn DG, Garfinkle JM, Klonoff DC, Pembrook LJ, Morrow DJ (1987) Cryptosporidial and cytomegaloviral hepatitis and cholecystitis. Arch Pathol Lab Med 111:879–881
53. Kapasi K, Rice GPA (1988) Cytomegalovirus infection of peripheral blood mononuclear cells: effects on interleukin-1 and -2 production and responsiveness. J Virol 62:3603–3607
54. Kauffman CA, Linnemann CC Jr, Alvira MM (1979) Cytomegalovirus encephalitis associated with thymoma and immunoglobulin deficiency. Am J Med 67:724–728
55. Kavin H, Jonas RB, Chowdhury L, Kabins S (1986) Acalculous cholecystitis and cytomegalovirus infection in the acquired immunodeficiency syndrome. Ann Intern Med 104:53–54
56. Kennedy PG, Newsome DA, Hess J, Narayan O, Suresch DL, Green WR, Gallo RC, Polk BF (1986) Cytomegalovirus but not human T lymphocytic virus type III/lymphadenopathy associated virus detected by in situ hybridization in retinal lesions in patients with the acquired immune deficiency syndrome. Br Med J 293:162–164
57. Kotler DP, Tiernay AR, Altilio D et al. (1989) Body mass repletion during ganciclovir treatment of cytomegalovirus infections in patients with AIDS. Arch Intern Med 149:901–905
58. Krech U, Jung M, Jung F (1971) Cytomegalovirus infections of man. Karger, Basel
59. Kwan TH, Kaufman HW (1986) Acid-fast bacilli with cytomegalovirus and herpesvirus inclusions in the skin of an AIDS patient. Am J Clin Pathol 85:236–238
60. Landini MP, Mirolo G, Re MC, Ripalti A, LaPlaca M (1989) Antibody reactivity to cytomegalovirus structural polypeptides in subclinical and clinical human HIV infections. Eur J Clin Microbiol Infect Dis 8:159–163
61. Langer PR, Waldrop AA, Ward DC (1981) Enzymatic synthesis of biotin-labeled polynucleotides: novel nucleic acid affinity probes. Proc Natl Acad Sci USA 78:6633–6637
62. Lehoang P, Girard B, Robinet M et al. (1989) Foscarnet in the treatment of cytomegalovirus retinitis in AIDS. Ophthalmology 96:865–873
63. Lobdell DH (1987) "Ring" granulomas in cytomegalovirus hepatitis. Arch Pathol Lab Med 111:881–882
64. Macher AM, Reichert CM, Straus SE et al. (1983) Death in the AIDS patient. Role of cytomegalovirus. N Engl J Med 309:1454
65. Martin WJ II, Smith TF (1986) Rapid detection of cytomegalovirus in bronchoalveolar lavage specimens by a monoclonal antibody method. J Clin Microbiol 23:1006–1008
66. Meiselman MS, Cello JP, Margaretten W (1985) Cytomegalovirus colitis. Report of the clinical, endoscopic, and pathologic findings in two patients with the acquired immune deficiency syndrome. Gastroenterology 88:171–175
67. Miles PR, Baughman RP, Linnemann CC Jr (1990) Cytomegalovirus in the bronchoalveolar lavage fluid of patients with AIDS. Chest 97:1072–1076
68. Millar AB, Paton G, Miller RF et al. (1990) Cytomegalovirus in the lungs of patients with AIDS. Respiratory pathogen or passenger? Am Rev Respir Dis 141:1474–1477
69. Miller RG, Parry GJ, Phaeffl W, Lang W, Lippert R, Kiprov D (1988) The spectrum of peripheral neuropathy associated with ARC and AIDS. Muscle and Nerve 11:857–863
70. Miller RG, Storey JR, Greco CM (1990) Ganciclovir in the treatment of progressive AIDS-related polyradiculopathy. Neurology 40:569–574
71. Morgello S, Cho ES, Nielsen S, Devinski D, Petito CK (1987) Cytomegalovirus encephalitits in patients with acquired immunodeficiency syndrome: an autopsy study of 30 cases and a review of the literature. Hum Pathol 18:289–297

72. Mosca JD, Bednarik DP, Raj NB et al. (1987) Herpes simplex virus type 1 can reactivate transcription of latent human immunodeficiency virus. Nature 325:67–70
73. Mosca JD, Bednarik DP, Raj NBK et al. (1987) Activation of the human immunodeficiency virus by herpes virus infection: Identification of a region within the long terminal repeat that responds to a trans-acting factor encoded by herpes simplex virus. 1. Proc Natl Acad Sci USA 84:7408–7412
74. Moskowitz LB, Gregorios JC, Hensley GT, Berger JR (1984) Cytomegalovirus-induced demyelination associated with acquired immune deficiency syndrome. Arch Pathol Lab Med 108:873–877
75. Munoz DG, Perl DP, Pendlebury WW, Highland RA (1987) Comparison of cytomegalovirus infection of brain and lung in a patient with subacute encephalopathy of acquired immunodeficiency syndrome. Arch Pathol Lab Med 111:234–237
76. Myerson D, Hackman RC, Nelson JA, Ward DC, McDougall JK (1984) Widespread presence of histologically occult cytomegalovirus. Hum Pathol 15:430–439
77. Navia BA, Jordan BD, Prace RW (1986) The AIDS dementia complex. I. Clinical features. Ann Neurol 19:517–524
78. Nelson JA, Reynolds-Kohler C, Oldstone MBA, Wiley CA (1988) HIV and CMV co-infect brain cells in patients with AIDS. Virology 165:286–290
79. Nelson MR, Connolly GM, Hawkins DA, Gazzard BG (1991) Foscarnet in the treatment of cytomegalovirus infection of the esophagus and colon in patients with the acquired immune deficiency syndrome. Am J Gastroenterol 86:876–881
80. Newsome DA, Green WR, Miller ED et al. (1984) Microvascular aspects of acquired immune deficiency syndrome retinopathy. Am J Ophthalmol 98:590
81. Ostrove JM, Leonard J, Weck KE, Rabson AB, Gendelman HE (1987) Activation of the human immunodeficiency virus by herpes simplex virus type 1. J Virol 61:3726–3732
82. Parry GJ (1988) Peripheral neuropathies associated with human immunodeficiency virus infection. Ann Neurol 23 Suppl:49–53
83. Pass HI, Potter DA, Macher AM et al. (1984) Thoracic manifestations of the acquired immune deficiency syndrome. J Thorac Cardiovasc Surg 88:654–658
84. Pepose JS, Hilborne LH, Cancilla PA, Foos RY (1984) Concurrent herpes simplex and cytomegalovirus retinitis and encephalitis in the acquired immune deficiency syndrome (AIDS). Ophthalmology 91:1669–1677
85. Pepose GN, Holland GN, Nestor MS, Chochran AJ, Foos RY (1985) Acquired immune deficiency syndrome. Pathogenic mechanisms of ocular disease. Ophthalmology 92:472–484
86. Phillips CA, Fanning WL, Gump DW, Phillips CF (1977) Cytomegalovirus encephalitis in immunologically normal adults. Successful treatment with vidarabine. JAMA 238:2299–2300
87. Plotkin SA, Stein S, Snyder M, Immesoete P (1977) Attempts to recover varicella virus from ganglia. Ann Neurol 2:249
88. Pomeroy C, Jordan MC, Filice GA (1989) Murine cytomegalovirus induces reactivation of dormant Toxoplasma gondii infection: lymphocyte subsets and function. Second International Cytomegalovirus Workshop, 27–30 March, San Diego
89. Post MJ, Hensley GT, Moskowitz LB, Fischl M (1986) Cytomegalic inclusion virus encephalitis in patients with AIDS: CT, clinical, and pathologic correlation. AJNR 7:275–280
90. Pulliam L (1991) Cytomegalovirus preferentially infects a monocyte derived macrophage/microglial cell in human brain cultures: Neuropathology differs between strains. J Neuropath Exp Neurol 50:432–440
91. Randazzo RF, Hulette CM, Gottlieb MS, Rajfer J (1986) Cytomegaloviral epididymitis in a patient with acquired immune deficiency syndrome. J Urol 136:1095–1097
92. Rando RF, Pellett PE, Luciw PA et al. (1987) Transactivation of human immunodeficiency virus by herpes viruses. Oncogenes 1:13–18
93. Rene A, Marche C, Chevalier T et al. (1988) Cytomegalovirus colitis in patients with acquired immunodeficiency syndrome. Dig Dis Sci 33:741–750

94. Rice GPA, Schrier RD, Oldstone MBA (1984) Cytomegalovirus infects human lymphocytes and monocytes: virus expression is restricted to immediate-early gene products. Proc Natl Acad Sci USA 81:6134–6138
95. Rinaldo CR Jr, Ho M, Hamoudi WH et al. (1983) Lymphocyte subsets and natural killer cell responses during cytomegalovirus mononucleosis. Infect Immun 40:472–477
96. Rüger R, Bornkamm GW, Fleckenstein B (1984) Human cytomegalovirus DNA sequences with homologies to the cellular genome. J Gen Virol 65:1351–1364
97. Rüger R, Colimon R, Fleckenstein B (1984) Search for DNA sequences of human cytomegalovirus in Kaposi's sarcoma tissues with cloned probes. Antibiot Chemother 32:43–47
98. Saltzman RL, Quirk MR, Jordan MC (1988) Disseminated cytomegalovirus infection. Molecular analysis of virus and leukocyte interactions in viremia. J Clin Invest 81:75–81
99. Schneiderman DJ, Cello JP, Laing FC (1987) Papillary stenosis and sclerosing cholangitis in the acquired immunodeficiency syndrome. Ann Intern Med 106:546–549
100. Schuster V, Matz B, Wiegand H, Traub B, Kampa D, Neumann-Haeflin D (1986) Detection of human cytomegalovirus in urine by DNA–DNA and RNA–DNA hybridization. J Infect Dis 154:309–314
101. Segondy M, Atoui N, Reynes J et al. (1990) Cytomegalovirus viremia in HIV-infected patients treated with zidovudine. Scand J Infect Dis 22:653–657
102. Seligmann M, Pinching AJ, Rosen FS et al. (1987) Immunology of human immunodeficiency virus infection and the acquired immunodeficiency syndrome. Ann Intern Med 107:234–242
103. Shanley JD, Jordan MC (1986) Viral pneumonia in the immunocompromised patient. Semin Respir Infect 1:193–201
104. Shanley JD, Persanti EL (1980) Replication of murine cytomegalovirus in lung macrophages: effect on phagocytosis of bacteria. Infect Immun 29:1152–1159
105. Shibata D, Martin JW, Appleman MD, Causey DM, Leedom JM, Arnheim N (1988) Detection of cytomegalovirus DNA in peripheral blood of patients infected with human immunodeficiency virus. J Infect Dis 158:1185–1192
106. Sing GK, Garnett HM (1984) The effects of human cytomegalovirus challenge in vitro on subpopulations of T cells from seronegative donors. J Med Virol 14:363–371
107. Skolnik PR, Kosloff BR, Hirsch MS (1988) Bidirectional interactions between human immunodeficiency virus type 1 and cytomegalovirus. J Infect Dis 157:508–513
108. Skolnik PR, Pomerantz RJ, de la Monte SM et al. (1989) Dual infection of retina with human immunodeficiency virus type-1 and cytomegalovirus. Am J Ophthalmol 107:361–372
109. Spector SA, Rua JA, Spector DH, McMillan R (1984) Detection of human cytomegalovirus in clinical specimens by DNA–DNA hybridization. J Infect Dis 150:121–126
110. Storey JR, Greco C, Bolan R, Calanchini P, Denys E, Parry G, Miller R (1988) Electrodiagnostic findings in cytomegalovirus radiculomyelopathy related to acquired immunodeficiency syndrome. Muscle Nerve 11:971
111. Tocci MJ, St Jeor SC (1976) Susceptibility of lymphoblastoid cells to infection with human cytomegalovirus. Infect Immun 23:418–423
112. Vinters HV, Kwok MK, Ho HW, Anders KH, Tomiyasu U, Wolfson WL, Robert F (1989) Cytomegalovirus in the nervous system of patients with acquired immune deficiency syndrome. Brain 112:245–268
113. Webster A, Lee CA, Cook DG et al. (1989) Cytomegalovirus infection and progression towards AIDS in haemophiliacs with human immunodeficiency virus infection. Lancet 2:63–65
114. Welch K, Finkbeiner W, Alpers CE, Blumenfeld W, Davis RL, Smucker EA, Beckstead A (1984) Autopsy findings in the acquired immune deficiency syndrome. JAMA 252:1152–1159

115. Westhof E, Altschuh D, Moras D, Bloomer AC, Mondragon A, Klug A, van Regenmortel MHV (1984) Correlation between segmental mobility and the location of antigenic determinants in proteins. Nature 311:123–126
116. Wiley CA, Nelson JA (1988) Role of human immunodeficiency virus and cytomegalovirus in AIDS encephalitis. Am J Pathol 133:73–81
117. Wiley CA, Schrier RD, Denaro FJ, Nelson JA, Lampert PW, Oldstone MBA (1986) Localization of cytomegalovirus proteins and genome during fulminant central nervous system infection in an AIDS patient. J Neuropathol Exp Neurol 45:127–139
118. Zaia JA, Lang DJ (1984) Cytomegalovirus infection of the fetus and neonate. Neurol Clin 2:387–410
119. Collaborative DHPG treatment study group (1986): Treatment of serious cytomegalovirus infections with 9-(1,3-dihydroxy-2-propoxymethyl)guanine in patients with AIDS and other immunodeficiencies. New Engl J Med 314:801–805
120. Meinert CL et al. (1992) Mortality in patients with the acquired immunodeficiency syndrome treated with either foscarnet or ganciclovir for cytomegalovirus retinitis. New Engl J Med 326:213–220

Chapter 9 Cytomegalovirus and Blood Transfusion

John D. Hamilton

Summary

This chapter summarizes the evidence that cytomegalovirus is present in certain cells in whole blood in both the active and latent state and that the virus can be transmitted in its latent state to a susceptible host by transfusion. Normal and immunosuppressed adults and newborn infant recipients are discussed as well as some methods of prevention.

Introduction

Cytomegalic cells in autopsy specimens from children were first reported in the early 1900s [32, 41, 61], and later, similar cells were identified in the salivary glands of mice [47]. The virus responsible for these unique cells in mice was isolated in 1954 by Smith [70], and the human salivary gland virus was isolated in 1956 [63, 71, 83]. Subsequently named cytomegalovirus (CMV), a further association with human disease was not recognized until 1965 when Klemola et al. described a mononucleosis-like illness as a possible consequence of CMV [35]. Implication of blood transfusions as the vector for these infections was reported in 1966 by Kaariainen et al. [33]. This chapter is a brief review of the current concepts about the relationship of CMV and blood. Summary monographs and papers should be consulted for more detailed consideration of specific points [1, 26, 29, 80].

Background

There is no doubt that viremia is an important element in the pathogenesis of CMV infection and is attended by serious morbidity and mortality [8, 25, 29, 55, 60, 65, 66, 68, 74, 86]. What is less clear is how that explains the ability of

---

Department of Medicine, Duke University Medical Center and Department of Veterans Affairs Medical Center, 508 Fulton Street, Durham, NC 27705, USA blood transfusions from normal donors to transmit this virus to a recipient. Blood donors are, generally, well and certainly not expected to be viremic. It was this apparent paradox which prompted the interest of many investigators and which has resulted in better understanding of the concept of latent infection, a characteristic of CMV and other herpesviruses. Central to this concept is that CMV has at least two distinguishable phases of growth. The first is active viral replication, when the virus is actively proliferating, has definite effects on the cells and tissues that it has infected, and is generally accompanied by a clinical disease. The second phase is inactive replication (latent), when the virus, though present as viral DNA, is not infectious and is not attended by demonstrable cellular abnormalities or disease. Recognition of these phases of viral replication provided a link with the clinical observations once it was learned that the latent virus could be reactivated.

Although capable of infecting many cell types, CMV has the propensity to infect cells with a primarily immune function, a feature with important ramifications not only for the infected host but also for the spread of virus. Of the cells in blood capable of being infected, most of the reported studies identify the polymorphonuclear leukocytes and, to a lesser extent, the circulating mononuclear cells, including certain T lymphocyte subsets, as likely targets [4, 19, 21, 23, 24, 46, 62, 66]. Saltzman et al. concluded, after comparison of standard culture with dot-blot hybridization of the DNA from fractionated peripheral blood leukocytes, that infectious virus resides in the granulocytes while the peripheral blood mononuclear cell is more likely to contain viral DNA in the absence of whole, infectious virus [66].

Certainly, CMV has been isolated from the blood of normal, healthy hosts [19, 22, 27, 36, 39], but this is considered to be rare [9, 10, 53]. Thus, it now appears that some proportion of previously infected individuals retain the virus in some circulating blood cells, which can be transfused to a susceptible recipient. Just how many previously infected individuals retain the latent virus is not clear because of the difficulty both of detection of the original infection and of the technical difficulties in identifying latent virus. Nonetheless, using seropositivity to CMV as the marker of prior infection in blood donors and susceptible recipients (seronegative) as the indicators, a substantial proportion of previously infected individuals retain latent virus which can be reactivated long after their initial infection. Using more sensitive techniques such as nucleic acid hybridization and the polymerase chain reaction (PCR), persistent viral DNA, which presumably reflects the presence of latent virus, can be detected. In nearly all of those who remain seropositive [67, 73, 75] viral DNA is found, but not all seropositive individuals have detectable viral DNA [31]. In addition, of course, there are likely to be many variables which alter the efficiency of conversion of a latent infection into an active infection. In one study, of ten seronegative individuals, five were found to be PCR positive, suggesting that antibody may not be a sufficiently sensitive or durable indicator of prior exposure to CMV [75]. Tolpin et al. [82] demonstrated identical restriction enzyme profiles of viral DNA isolated from two infant recipients and their single blood donor as a further verification that blood is the source of virus.

It therefore appears that more data will be required to establish the certainty that a prior infection eventually leads to a permanent latent infection.

Clinical Diseases

Rubin [64] summarized the clinical consequences of CMV for the allograft recipient, but these might be applied to the normal host as well. They are: (1) unique viral syndromes such as heterophile-negative infectious mononucleosis; (2) increased susceptibility to opportunistic pathogens as a result of virus-induced immune suppression; (3) distinctive forms of allograft rejection in the actively infected organ transplant recipients; (4) associations with particular types of malignancy; and (5) new reports of possible links with atherosclerosis. While these consequences are of great importance to the particular infected individual, whether derived from a blood transfusion or another source, I will not discuss them further except in those instances where they relate more directly to the issue of blood and/or blood product transfusion and CMV. There is no reason to believe that CMV from different sources has different clinical implications for the infected person.

Clinical Studies

Much of the information about CMV and blood is derived from studies of specific patient populations. The postperfusion syndrome, as it became known subsequently, prompted much of the early interest in the transmission of CMV to the normal host. That a virus was the cause of the mononucleosis-like syndrome was first suggested by Wheeler et al. [84] in 1962. Klemola and Kaariainen [35] implicated CMV, and Kaariainen et al. [33] suggested that transfused blood was the vector. The contribution of the extracorporeal circulation (heart-lung machine) for open heart surgery is now felt to be incidental to the more important variables, including the volume and serologic status of the blood used. Nonetheless, because of the circumstances of the clinical situation, the syndrome was named the postperfusion syndrome.

Following the recognition of the postperfusion syndrome, many investigators directed their attention to the study of the variables that could be important. These included the serologic status of the donor and recipient, the type of blood or blood product used, the processing of the particular blood component, the volume of blood, and the age and underlying disease or treatment of the recipients. In the next section I will discuss those situations where a seronegative individual is the recipient of blood and/or blood products from a seropositive donor, since that is perhaps the purest measure of the contribution of the blood itself. Further, I will discuss, in separate sections, the results of studies in the "normal," immunocompetent adult; the immunoincompetent adult; and the very young.

Immunocompetent Recipients

Transfusions to these "normal" recipients constitute the majority, but the studies differ in several important respects such as the underlying disease and indications for transfusion, the volume and method of processing of blood, and the age and serologic status of the recipients. Table 1 summarizes the 19 published studies since 1966 [3, 5, 7, 15, 20, 22, 28, 33, 34, 36, 37, 40, 44, 48, 51, 54, 56, 57, 59, 85]. Most of the series are in patients who have had open heart surgery, but some are representative of a variety of medical indications as well.

Each patient had a mean of 5–6 transfusions. Among all recipients there was a range of posttransfusion CMV of 0.9%–67%. Over these 22 years, the percentage of all patients infected has declined, a finding mirrored among those "primarily" infected but not among those with "recurrent" infection. Assuming the transfusion of latent CMV in blood is the route by which patients are primarily infected and reactivation of latent endogenous virus is the mechanism of recurrent infection, these data suggest a secular change in the donor pool, the blood processing procedures, the age/susceptibility of recipients, or all of these. Since the mean number of units transfused per

Table 1. Incidence of primary and recurrent cytomegalovirus infections in immunocompetent transfusion recipients (modified from [80])

Source	Year	Total patients			Seronegative patients			Seropositive patients		
		Transfused (*n*)	Infected *n*	Infected %	Transfused (*n*)	Infected *n*	Infected %	Transfused (*n*)	Infected *n*	Infected %
Kaariainen et al.	1966 [33, 34]	21	9	43	6	6	100	15	3	20
Paloheimo et al.	1968 [54]	63	19	30	17	10	59	36	9	25
Embil et al.	1968 [20]	16	7	44	15	6	40	1	1	100
Foster and Jack	1969 [22]	9	6	67	1	0	0	8	6	7
Klemola et al.	1969 [36]	24	14	58	24	14	58	0		
Henle et al.	1970 [28]	152	53	35	61	36	59	91	17	19
Prince et al.	1971 [59]	152	30	20	93	17	18	59	13	22
Caul et al.	1971 [15]	55	21	38	21	7	33	34	14	41
Luthardt et al.	1971 [44]	73	12	16	35	8	23	38	4	11
Med. Res. Council	1974 [48]	712	37	5	270	24	9	442	13	3
Monif et al.	1976 [51]	207	19	9	140	16	11	67	3	4
Armstrong et al.	1976 [5]	119	15	13	93	9	10	26	6	23
Bayer	1977 [7]	159	5	3	30	1	3	129	4	3
Lang et al.	1977 [40]	10	5	50	6	4	67	4	1	25
Kumar et al.	1980 [37]	29	5	17	10	2	20	19	3	16
Adler et al.	1985 [3]	94	12	12.8	0			94	12	12.8
Preiksaitis et al.	1985 [56]	68	1	1.5	68	1	1.5	0		
Wilhelm et al.	1986 [85]	595	7	1.2	595	7	1.2	0		
Preiksaitis et al.	1988 [57]	637	6	0.9	637	6	0.9	0		

patient is the same in those series before 1972 and those after 1972, the volume of blood does not seem to be a variable. As to the other possible explanations, screening out of blood with surrogate markers for CMV, e.g., hepatitis B virus, (HBV) and human immunodeficiency virus (HIV), and self-selection of the donor pool in the 1970s and, particularly, in the 1980s when blood borne disease was better understood, would seem to be the most likely [76]. In any case, the current incidence of posttransfusion CMV is very low (<2%) when noncommercial blood is used in the seronegative patient. In the seropositive recipient, one would expect a continuing low level of recurrent infection that is likely to be something less than 10%. In addition, it is of great importance that the frequency of disease attending these infections is very low. In fact, in the series just reviewed, 12% of those with an infection had a demonstrable disease. Most (two thirds) of those with disease had a primary infection. Because CMV infection and its accompanying disease are so infrequent and generally mild, it is not considered necessary to impose any additional preventive measures for the normal recipient.

Immunocompromised Recipients

In immunocompromised patients, however, there are many incentives to avoid the occurrence of CMV infection and, therefore, it is reasonable to assess the contribution of transfusions. Two separate categories of immunocompromised patients are frequently transfused: organ allograft recipients of, e.g., kidney, liver and heart; and allogeneic bone marrow transplant recipients. Each will be considered separately, since the circumstances and consequences of each are different.

Organ Allograft Recipients

The indications for use of transfusions in renal transplant patients have evolved over the years. Previously, it was usual for patients with chronic renal failure, especially if they were on dialysis, to be transfused because of their low hemoglobin. With the recognition of the hazards of transfusion from hepatitis B and non-A, non-B hepatitis (HCV), however, that policy was modified. However, transfused blood that is first screened for the blood-borne viruses such as HBV, HCV, and HIV is now routinely administered to prolong graft survival. The types of immunosuppressive therapy have also changed, and this may have had an impact on the occurrence of posttransfusion and posttransplantation CMV.

Most agree that the major source of CMV in renal allograft recipients is the organ itself, but infection was observed in 17%–24% of the seronegative recipients of a kidney from a seronegative donor. These patients received an average of 2.4 units of unscreened whole blood [65]. Another study found no cases of CMV attributable to transfusion [17]. While one report demonstrated a correlation of the increased occurrence of CMV infections with a simultaneous increase in transfusions [14], four others showed either no or a very weak correlation [13, 16, 30, 43].

In recipients of cardiac and liver transplants, CMV infections are common, but the contributions of pre-, peri-, or posttransplant transfusions have not been quantitated. Since studies suggest that the organs themselves are the major source of latent virus, as with kidney transplantation, the role of transfusions has been felt to be insufficient to justify a major modification of the policy to administer blood that has not been screened for CMV to any of the recipients of whole organ transplants.

Allogeneic Bone Marrow Transplant Recipients

Among recipients of allogeneic bone marrow transplants, the incidence of CMV infection is high (36% in seronegative patients and 69% in seropositive patients), and CMV pneumonia occurs in as many as 15%, with a case-fatality rate of 15% [50]. The complexity of determining the source of CMV in these patients is increased because of the several unique forms and amounts of "blood" that are administered to these patients. In addition to large amounts of platelets and, to a lesser extent, red blood cells (RBCs), these patients may receive granulocyte transfusions to prevent infection, and, of course, they are infused with the donor marrow. Studies designed to detect the contribution of these possible sources have concluded that the serologic status of the bone marrow donor constitutes the major risk for future CMV in the seronegative recipient (relative risk 2.3). Prophylactic granulocyte transfusions, however, more than double (relative risk 2.5) the risk of posttransplant CMV infection if the bone marrow donor is seronegative [50]. Blood products, including whole blood and platelets, seem to be of somewhat lesser importance. Bowden et al. demonstrated a reduction in posttransplant CMV from 8/25 (33%) to 1/32 (3.1%) in seronegative recipients of seronegative bone marrow donors who either received unscreened blood or screened, seronegative blood products, respectively [11]. These benefits of CMV seronegative blood have been confirmed [45]. If the marrow donor or the recipient are seropositive, however, the benefits are lost. One approach, discussed elsewhere in this volume, suggests that prophylactic immune globulin is either not effective [11] or only partially effective [18, 49, 87] in the protection against posttransplant CMV. The consensus seems to be that CMV infection should be avoided if possible and that use of seronegative blood and blood products should be used.

Infants

Several studies in the late 1970s and early 1980s suggested serious morbidity and mortality in newborn recipients of whole blood [6, 72, 88]. The CMV diseases that accompanied these infections included atypical lymphocytosis, hepatosplenomegaly, gray pallor, respiratory distress, and death. The infected children were recognized chiefly in nurseries for high-risk or premature infants or among low birth weight babies. The common denominator linking these three categories of newborns was that they all received substantial amounts of whole blood, and it quickly became apparent that the serologic status of potential donors should be taken into account, at least in certain subsets of newborns. Other risk factors included seronegativity of the newborn and receipt of greater than 50 ml of blood. Follow-up studies then began to address the problem in a more quantitative manner [2, 89]. Like the declining incidence of CMV after transfusions in the normal host, there is a similar decline in incidence of CMV in infants from 32% in the 1981 study to 2% in the 1988 study [38, 58, 69, 78]. In the course of these studies, the value of seronegative blood was confirmed as was the particular vulnerability of the premature and low birth weight infant. What was not understood was why the previously high incidences of posttransfusion CMV infection seemed to be disappearing. Many procedures have changed in the collection, processing, storage, and administration of blood over the past 10 years, and probably the best that can be said is that changes in the selection of donors, reductions in the volumes of blood administered, and some inadvertent processing procedures have conspired to reduce the transmission of CMV. That the risk seems to have dramatically fallen casts an entirely different light on the need for screened, seronegative blood in all but a few selected circumstances. Opinions seem to vary, but most agree that, if used at all, seronegative blood is most indicated for premature and low birth weight infants.

Impact of Blood Processing

Interest in this approach was perhaps initiated by the report of Lang et al. [40], who demonstrated that the incidence of CMV infection declined from 50% to 20% in recipients of cardiac surgery patients who had received blood transfusions depleted of leukocytes. Tegtmeier [80] discussed the evidence supporting various procedures for preparation of blood transfusions as well as the contrary evidence. Although benefits in the decreased incidence of posttransfusion CMV have been documented in many clinical studies, including those with seronegative citrated whole blood [11, 45, 79, 89], leucocyte-depleted blood (washed RBCs) [40, 42], frozen deglycerolized red cells [12, 77, 81], and filtration [52], the incidence of infection and disease in the normal recipient is considered to be too low to justify the effort and resources except in a selected population. The method of choice in the few instances where the incentive for "safe" blood is greater, such as the prevention of CMV in the low birth weight newborn, or the allogeneic bone marrow transplant recipient who is seronegative, is the provision of CMV-antibody-negative blood.

Conclusion

Blood and blood products have become extraordinarily important elements in today's therapeutic armamentarium and will almost surely continue to be. Although substitutes of nonhuman origin are being developed, it is very unlikely that products will soon be available that are free of human infectious agents such as CMV. In the meantime, appropriate concern and interventive measures have succeeded in keeping this important treatment option free of serious liabilities except under certain defined conditions.

References

1. Adler SP (1983) Transfusion-associated cytomegalovirus infections. Rev Infect Dis 5:977–993
2. Adler SP, Chandrika T, Lawrence L, Baggett J (1983) Cytomegalovirus infections in neonates acquired by blood transfusions. Pediatr Infect Dis 2:114–118
3. Adler SP, Baggett J, McVoy M (1985) Transfusion-associated cytomegalovirus infections in seropositive cardiac surgery patients. Lancet 2:743–747
4. Armstrong D, Ely M, Steger L (1971) Post-transfusion cytomegaloviremia and persistence of cytomegalovirus in blood. Infect Immun 3:159–163
5. Armstrong JA, Tarr GC, Youngblood LA et al. (1976) Cytomegalovirus infection in children undergoing open-heart surgery. Yale J Biol Med 49:83–91
6. Ballard RA, Drew WL, Hufnagle KG et al. (1979) Acquired cytomegalovirus infection in preterm infants. Am J Dis Child 133:442–448
7. Bayer WL (1977) The effect of frozen blood on the relationship of cytomegalovirus and hepatitis virus to infection and disease. In: Dawson RB, Barnes A Jr (eds) Clinical and practical aspects of the use of frozen blood. American Association of Blood Banks, Washington, pp 133–145
8. Betts RF (1982) Cytomegalovirus infection in transplant patients. Prog Med Virol 28:44–64
9. Betts RF, Freeman RB, Douglas RG Jr, Talley TE, Rundell B (1975) Transmission of cytomegalovirus infection with renal allograft. Kidney Int 8:385–392
10. Betts RF, Cestero RVM, Freeman RB, Douglas RC Jr (1979) Epidemiology of cytomegalovirus infection in end stage renal disease. J Med Virol 4:89–96
11. Bowden RA, Sayers M, Flournoy N et al. (1986) Cytomegalovirus immune globulin and seronegative blood products to prevent primary cytomegalovirus infection after marrow transplantation. N Engl J Med 314:1006–1010
12. Brady MT, Milam JD, Anderson DC et al. (1984) Use of deglycerolized red blood cells to prevent posttransfusion infection with cytomegalovirus in neonates. J Infect Dis 150:334–339
13. Braun WE, Nankervis G, Banowsky LH, Protiva D, Biekert E, McHenry MC (1976) A prospective study of cytomegalovirus infections in 75 renal allograft recipients. Proc Clin Dial Transplant Forum 6:8–12
14. Brautigam AR, Dutko FJ, Olding LB, Oldstone MBA (1979) Pathogenesis of murine cytomegalovirus infection: the macrophage as a permissive cell for cytomegalovirus infection, replication and latency. J Gen Virol 44:349–359
15. Caul EO, Clarke SKR, Mott MG et al. (1971) Cytomegalovirus infections after open heart surgery. Lancet 1:777–781

16. Chou S, Kim DY, Norman DJ (1987) Transmission of cytomegalovirus by pretransplant leukocyte transfusions in renal transplant candidates. J Infect Dis 155:565–567
17. Chou SW, Norman DJ (1988) The influence of donor factors other than serologic status on transmission of cytomegalovirus to transplant recipients. Transplantation 46:89–93
18. Condie RM, O'Reilly RJ (1984) Prevention of cytomegalovirus infection by prophylaxis with an intravenous, hyperimmune, native, unmodified cytomegalovirus globulin: randomized trial in bone marrow transplant recipients. Am J Med 76:134–141
19. Diosi P, Moldovan E, Tomescu N (1969) Latent cytomegalovirus infection in blood donors. Br Med J 4:660–662
20. Embil JA, Folkins DF, Haldane EV et al. (1968) Cytomegalovirus infection following extra-corporeal circulation in children: a prospective study. Lancet 2:1151–1155
21. Fiala M, Chatterjee S (1982) The role of lymphocytes in infections due to Epstein-Barr virus and cytomegalovirus (Letter). J Infect Dis 146:300–301
22. Foster KM, Jack I (1969) A prospective study of the role of cytomegalovirus in post-transfusion mononucleosis. N Engl J Med 280:1311–1316
23. Gadler H, Tillegard A, Groth CG (1982) Studies of cytomegalovirus infection in renal allograft recipients. I. Virus isolation. Scand J Infect Dis 14:81–87
24. Garnett HM (1982) Isolation of human cytomegalovirus from peripheral blood T cells of renal transplant patients. J Lab Clin Med 99:92–97
25. Gentry LO, Zeluff BJ (1986) Diagnosis and treatment of infection in cardiac transplant patients. Surg Clin North Am 66:459–465
26. Hamilton JD (1982) Cytomegalovirus and immunity, vol. 12. Karger, Basel
27. Harnden DG, Elsdale TR, Young DE, Ross A (1967) The isolation of cytomegalovirus from peripheral blood. Blood 30:120–125
28. Henle W, Henle G, Scriba M et al. (1970) Antibody responses to the Epstein-Barr virus and cytomegalovirus after open-heart and other surgery. N Engl J Med 282:1068–1074
29. Ho M (1982) Cytomegalovirus – biology and infection. Plenum, New York
30. Ho M, Suwansirikul S, Dowling JN, Youngblood LA, Armstrong JA (1975) The transplanted kidney as a source of cytomegalovirus infection. N Engl J Med 293:1109–1112
31. Jackson JB, Orr HT, McCullough JJ, Jordan MC (1987) Failure to detect human cytomegalovirus DNA in IgM-seropositive blood donors by spot hybridization. J Infect Dis 156:1013–1016
32. Jesionek A, Kiolemenoglou B (1904) Über einen Befund von protozoenartigen Gebilden in den Organen eines hereditär-luetischen Fötus. MMW 51:1905–1907
33. Kaariainen L, Klemola E, Paloheimo J (1966) Rise of cytomegalovirus antibodies in an infectious-mononucleosis-like syndrome after transfusion. Br Med J 1:1270–1272
34. Kaariainen L, Paloheimo J, Klemola E et al. (1966) Cytomegalovirus-mononucleosis: isolation of virus and demonstration of subclinical infections after blood transfusion in connection with open-heart surgery. Ann Med Exp Biol Fenn 44:297–301
35. Klemola E, Kaariainen L (1965) Cytomegalovirus – a possible cause of a disease resembling infectious mononucleosis. Br Med J 2:1099–1102
36. Klemola E, von Essen R, Paloheimo J, Furuhjelm U (1969) Cytomegalovirus antibodies in donors of fresh blood to patients submitted to open-heart surgery. Scand J Infect Dis 1:137–140
37. Kumar A, Nankervis GA, Cooper AR et al. (1980) Acquisition of cytomegalovirus infection in infants following exchange transfusion: a prospective study. Transfusion 20:327–331
38. Lamberson HV Jr, McMillian JA, Weiner LB et al. (1988) Prevention of transfusion-associated cytomegalovirus (CMV) infection in neonates by screening blood donors for IgM to CMV. J Infect Dis 157:820–823
39. Lang DJ, Hanshaw JB (1969) Cytomegalovirus infection and the postperfusion syndrome. N Engl J Med 280:1145–1149
40. Lang DJ, Ebert PA, Rodgers BM, Boggess HP, Rixse RS (1977) Reduction of postperfusion cytomegalovirus-infections following the use of leukocyte depleted blood. Transfusion 17:391–395

41. Lowenstein C (1907) Über protozoenartige Gebilde in den Organen von Kindern. Zentralbl Allg Pathol Pathol Anat 18:513–518
42. Luban NL, Williams AE, MacDonald MG, Mikesell GT, Williams KM, Sacher RA (1987) Low incidence of acquired cytomegalovirus infection in neonates transfused with washed red blood cells. Am J Dis Child 141:416–419
43. Luby JP, Burnett W, Hull AR, Ware AJ, Shorey JW, Peters PC (1974) Relationship between cytomegalovirus and hepatic function abnormalities in the period after renal transplant. J Infect Dis 129:511–518
44. Luthardt T, Siebert H, Losel I et al. (1971) Cytomegalievirus-Infektionen bei Kindern mit Blutaustauschtransfusion im Neugeborenenalter. Klin Wochenschr 49:81–86
45. Mackinnon S, Burnett AK, Crawford RJ, Cameron S, Leask BG, Sommerville RG (1988) Seronegative blood products prevent primary cytomegalovirus infection after bone marrow transplantation. J Clin Pathol 41:948–950
46. Martin DC, Katzenstein DA, Yu GSM, Jordan MC (1984) Cytomegalovirus viremia detected by molecular hybridization and electron microscopy. Ann Intern Med 100:222–225
47. McCordock HA, Smith MG (1936) The visceral lesions produced in mice by the salivary gland virus of mice. J Exp Med 63:303–310
48. Medical Research Council (MRC) Working Party on Post-Transfusion (1974) Hepatitis report to the MRC Blood Transfusion Research Committee: Post-transfusion hepatitis in a London hospital: results of a two-year prospective study. J Hyg (Lond) 73:173–188
49. Meyers JD, Leszczynski J, Zaia JA et al. (1983) Prevention of cytomegalovirus infection by cytomegalovirus immune globulin after marrow transplantation. Ann Intern Med 98:442–446
50. Meyers JD, Flournoy N, Thomas ED (1986) Risk factors for cytomegalovirus infection after human marrow transplantation. J Infect Dis 153:478–488
51. Monif GRG, Daicoff GI, Flory LL (1976) Blood as a potential vehicle for the cytomegaloviruses. Am J Obstet Gynecol 126:445–448
52. Murphy MF, Grint PC, Hardiman AE, Lister TA, Waters AH (1988) Use of leucocyte-poor blood components to prevent primary cytomegalovirus (CMV) infection in patients with acute leukaemia (Letter). Br J Haematol 70:253–254
53. Nankervis GA (1976) Cytomegalovirus infections in the blood recipient. Yale J Biol Med 49:13–15
54. Paloheimo JA, von Essen R, Klemola E, Kaariainen L, Siltanen P (1968) Subclinical cytomegalovirus infections and cytomegalovirus mononucleosis after open heart surgery. Am J Cardiol 22:624–630
55. Preiksaitis JK, Rosno S, Grumet C, Merigan TC (1983) Infections due to herpesviruses in cardiac transplant recipients: role of the donor heart and immunosuppressive therapy. J Infect Dis 147:974–981
56. Preiksaitis JK, Grumet FC, Smith WK, Merigan TC (1985) Transfusion-acquired cytomegalovirus infection in cardiac surgery patients. J Med Virol 15:283–290
57. Preiksaitis JK, Brown L, McKenzie M (1988) The risk of cytomegalovirus infection in seronegative transfusion recipients not receiving exogenenous immunosuppression. J Infect Dis 157:523–529
58. Preiksaitis JK, Brown L, McKenzie M (1988) Transfusion-acquired cytomegalovirus infection in neonates. A prospective study. Transfusion 28:205–209
59. Prince AM, Szmuness W, Millian SJ et al. (1971) A serologic study of cytomegalovirus infections associated with blood transfusions. N Engl J Med 284:1125–1131
60. Quinnan GV Jr, Masur H, Rook AH et al. (1984) Herpesvirus infections in the acquired immune deficiency syndrome. JAMA 252:72–77
61. Ribbert H (1904) Über protozoenartige Zellen in der Niere eines syphilitischen Neugeborenen und in der Parotis von Kindern. Zentralbl Allg Pathol Pathol Anat 15:945–948
62. Rinaldo CRJ, Black PH, Hirsch MS (1977) Interaction of cytomegalovirus with leukocytes from patients with mononucleosis due to cytomegalovirus. J Infect Dis 136:667–678

63. Rowe WP, Hartley JW, Waterman S, Turner HE, Huebner RJ (1956) Cytopathogenic agent resembling human salivary gland virus recovered from tissue cultures of human adenoids. Proc Soc Exp Biol Med 92:418–424
64. Rubin RH (1989) The indirect effects of cytomegalovirus infection on the outcome of organ transplantation. JAMA 261:3607–3609
65. Rubin RH, Tolkoff-Rubin NE, Oliver D et al. (1985) Multicenter seroepidemiologic study of the impact of cytomegalovirus infection on renal transplantation. Transplantation 40:243–249
66. Saltzman RL, Quirk MR, Jordan MC (1988) Disseminated cytomegalovirus infection. Molecular analysis of virus and leukocyte interactions in viremia. J Clin Invest 81:75–81
67. Schrier RD, Nelson JA, Oldstone MBA (1985) Detection of human cytomegalovirus in peripheral blood lymphocytes in a natural infection. Science 230:1048–1051
68. Singh N, Dummer JS, Kusne S et al. (1988) Infections with cytomegalovirus and other herpesviruses in 121 liver transplant recipients: transmission by donated organ and the effect of OKT3 antibodies. J Infect Dis 158:124–131
69. Smith D Jr, Wright P, Estes W et al. (1983) Posttransfusion cytomegalovirus infection in neonates weighing less than 1250 grams (Abstr). Transfusion 23:420
70. Smith MG (1954) Propagation of salivary gland virus of the mouse in tissue cultures. Proc Soc Exp Biol Med 86:435–440
71. Smith MG (1956) Propagation in tissue cultures of a cytopathogenic virus from human salivary gland virus (SGV) disease. Proc Soc Exp Biol Med 92:424–430
72. Spector SA, Schmidt K, Ticknor W et al. (1979) Cytomegaloviruria in older infants in intensive care nurseries. J Pediatr 95:444–446
73. Spector SA, Rua JA, Spector DH, McMillan RM (1984) Detection of human cytomegalovirus in clinical specimens by DNA–DNA hybridization. J Infect Dis 150:121–126
74. Stagno S, Pass RF, Dworsky ME et al. (1982) Congenital cytomegalovirus infection: the relative importance of primary and recurrent maternal infection. N Engl J Med 306:945–949
75. Stanier P, Taylor DL, Kitchen AD, Wales N, Tryhorn Y, Tyms AS (1989) Persistence of cytomegalovirus in mononuclear cells in peripheral blood from blood donors. Br Med J 299:897–898
76. Surgenor D, Wallace E, Hao S, Chapman R (1990) Collection and transfusion of blood in the United States, 1982–1988. N Engl J Med 322:1646–1651
77. Taylor BJ, Jacobs RF, Baker RL, Moses EB, McSwain BE, Shulman G (1986) Frozen deglycerolyzed blood prevents transfusion-acquired cytomegalovirus infections in neonates. Pediatr Infect Dis 5:188–191
78. Tegtmeier GE (1985) Cytomegalovirus and blood transfusion. In: Dodd RY, Barker LF (eds) Infection immunity and blood transfusion. Liss, New York, pp 175–199
79. Tegtmeier GE (1986) Transfusion-transmitted cytomegalovirus infections: significance and control. Vox Sang 51 Suppl 1:22–30
80. Tegtmeier GE (1989) Posttransfusion cytomegalovirus infections. Arch Pathol Lab Med 113:236–245
81. Tolkoff-Rubin NE, Rubin RH, Keller EE (1978) Cytomegalovirus infection in dialysis patients and personnel. Ann Intern Med 89:625–628
82. Tolpin MD, Stewart JA, Warren D et al. (1985) Transfusion transmission of cytomegalovirus confirmed by restriction endonuclease analysis. J Pediatr 107:953–956
83. Weller TH, Mccauley JC, Craig JM, Wirth P (1957) Isolation of intranuclear inclusion producing agents from infants with illnesses resembling cytomegalic inclusion disease. Proc Soc Exp Biol Med 94:4–12
84. Wheeler EO, Turner JD, Scannell JG (1962) Fever, splenomegaly and atypical lymphocytes. N Engl J Med 266:454–456
85. Wilhelm JA, Matter L, Schopfer K (1986) The risk of transmitting cytomegalovirus to patients receiving blood transfusions. J Infect Dis 154:169–171
86. Winston DJ, Gale RP, Meyer DV, Young LS, Group UBMT (1979) Infectious complications of human bone marrow transplantation. Medicine (Baltimore) 58:1–31

87. Winston DJ, Ho WG, Lin C, Budinger MD, Champlin RE, Gale RP (1984) Intravenous immunoglobulin for modification of cytomegalovirus infections associated with bone marrow transplantation. Am J Med 76:128–133
88. Yeager AS (1974) Transfusion-acquired cytomegalovirus infection in newborn infants. Am J Dis Child 128:478–483
89. Yeager AS, Grumet FC, Hafleigh EB, Arvin AM, Bradley JS, Prober CG (1981) Prevention of transfusion-acquired cytomegalovirus infections in newborn infants. J Pediatr 98:281–287

Chapter 10 Cytomegalovirus Infection After Solid Organ Transplantation

M. Ho

Summary

Cytomegalovirus (CMV) infection is usually latent and subclinical. In the transplant recipient, immunodeficiency and allograft reactions modify infections such that they become clinically significant. Primary infection and reinfections by CMV largely transmitted by the transplanted organ or tissue may be more symptomatic than reactivation infections. Immunopathology, perhaps influenced by allograft reactions, may further exacerbate the clinical picture, as in the example of CMV pneumonitis in marrow and lung recipients. More precise diagnosis of modalities of infection are essential because effective preventive and therapeutic measures for CMV are within reach.

Introduction

Significant advances have been made in solid organ transplantation since the introduction of cyclosporine in the United States in 1981 [89]. Before then, the major solid organ transplanted was the kidney. Since then, significant inroads have been made in the transplantation of other major organs. For example, in 1981 at the University of Pittsburgh there were 107 transplantations, mostly kidneys. In 1986, there were 703 patients who received transplants. The specific organs transplanted were 314 livers, 271 kidneys, 102 hearts, and 16 heart-lungs.

The nature of cytomegalovirus (CMV) infection had been largely studied in renal transplant recipients before 1981 [44]. In this chapter we will review the important principles of CMV infection in transplant patients established in earlier studies, bring them up to date, and also determine how they apply to other types of organ transplantation.

Department of Infectious Diseases and Microbiology, Graduate School of Public Health, and Departments of Medicine and Pathology, School of Medicine, University of Pittsburgh, Pittsburgh, PA 15261, USA

Biology of CMV Infection

CMV infects most humans but usually does not cause disease. It is clinically innocuous in most immunocompetent subjects. However, the human organism is not completely successful in coping with infection by this virus. This may be seen from two phenomena. Firstly, the majority of seropositive transplant recipients, that is, those individuals who were previously infected and supposedly immune at the time of transplantation, will show evidence of infection after transplantation. A large proportion of such infections represent reactivations of latent infection present prior to transplantation. Secondly, CMV is efficiently transmitted by kidneys from seropositive donors to immunologically naive or seronegative recipients [5, 45]. These two observations suggest that CMV is a highly successful parasitic virus. Once the host is infected, the virus cannot be totally eradicated and remains latent but potentially infective. Latent virus in tissues or transmitted by transplanted organs can be reactivated when the host is immunosuppressed.

Which tissues or cells are latently infected by CMV? The evidence is accummlating that many types of tissues, perhaps all tissues, are latently infected. In all types of visceral transplantation that have been carefully studied, i.e., kidney, heart, and bone marrow [55, 68, 69], and more recently liver [84], the transplanted organ has been found capable of transmitting the virus. Whether this is because the site of latency is latently infected white blood cells distributed by blood to all tissues, or whether there are multiple tissue sites of latency is unknown. Abortive lymphocyte infection by CMV has been demonstrated by monoclonal antibodies against early antigens [28, 74]. Using in situ hybridization and a nucleic acid probe of immediate early (IE) antigen, lymphocytes of healthy seropositive individuals have been reported to harbor CMV RNA transcripts [78]. Polymorphonuclear leukocytes have also been shown to be abortively infected [98]. Therefore, there is some support for the thesis that blood is a common carrier of CMV. However, several considerations make it unlikely that latently infected blood cells are the vehicle of transmission of CMV by transplanted tissues. Firstly, there may not be enough infected blood cells in tissues to transmit infection. The precise amount of blood needed to transmit is not known, but the probability that a unit of CMV-seropositive blood can transmit CMV to a seronegative recipient is probably not higher than 3% [44]. The transmission frequency is considerably lower ($<1\%$) in more recent studies in which large numbers of seronegative transfusion recipients (>500) were studied [70, 98].

Secondly, there is now evidence that many other types of tissue cells may be latently infected in the body besides blood cells. In autopsy studies of normal subjects who died of trauma, Toorkey and Carrigan [92] found tissue cells in the brain, kidney, spleen, lung, and liver which were positive for the IE antigen of CMV. No virus was demonstrated by cultural means. These abortively or latently infected cells may be the source of viral transmission.

How CMV latency is modulated and activated, and the role of the recipient in this process are important unsolved problems. More knowledge about the molecular biology of latency, the mechanism of viral activation, and the role of host immunity in latency is required.

What determines whether a CMV infection will be asymptomatic or will produce a symptomatic pathologic reaction, organ dysfunction, and disease? The answer to this question is also incomplete. Disease and inflammatory response are associated with the presence of the virus in large numbers. But the presence of the virus or virus-infected cells alone is not enough to produce disease. Complete or lytic CMV can be carried asymptomatically in the tubules of the kidney, in the uterine cervix, spleen, blood cells, and upper respiratory tract with impunity. The modulation of host responses may be the key.

While host immunity is inadequate to eradicate a CMV infection, it does have the important function of limiting viral replication and providing for recovery from CMV disease. The following themes will run through our discussion of CMV infection and disease: (1) When there is immunologic deficiency, disease can occur after either primary or secondary infection. It is usually more severe after primary or de novo infection. (2) The more severe the immundeficiency the more likely a secondary infection may become symptomatic. Severe immune depression may obscure the difference in severity of disease due to primary and secondary CMV infections. In bone marrow transplantation or in renal transplantation in which antilymphocyte globulin (ATG) was used, the greater severity of primary infection was earlier not recognized [51, 53]. Now, in bone marrow transplantation it is also recognized that primary infection is more severe, that prior immunity provides some protection against CMV pneumonia, and administration of ATG is a risk factor for the development of pneumonia [55].

CMV Infection, Immune Response, and Allograft Reactions

CMV infection itself is immunosuppressive. CMV infection in immunocompetent as well as in transplant patients is associated with decreased helper to suppressor T lymphocyte ratios [12] and depression of cellular immunity as measured by specific as well as nonspecific tests such as the lymphocyte proliferation test [62, 68, 76]. Such suppression may be clinically significant in transplant patients. After development of primary CMV infection in transplant recipients, the frequency of both bacterial and fungal infections is increased [14, 36, 71].

The relationship between CMV infection and the rejection reaction is a complex one. Which is cause and which is effect is difficult to sort out in patients because both occur so frequently in the first few months after transplantation. While there is no evidence that CMV infection suppresses rejection, it is difficult to determine whether CMV infection is a cause of rejection or if rejection facilitates infection. There is ample evidence from animal work that both phenomena occur. We showed that allograft reactions, i.e., both host-vs-graft (HvG) and graft-vs-host (GvH) reactions may lead to enhancement of CMV infection [23, 103]. More recently, it was found that in the mouse model a GvH reaction can facilitate the production of interstitial pneumonia [37], and conversely the presence of CMV infection in the host can accentuate a GvH reaction produced by allogeneic spleen cells [37, 93]. The fact that human cadaveric transplant recipients, who have a higer frequency of rejection than recipients of organs from living related donors, have more CMV infections is presumptive evidence that allograft reactions may also increase frequency of CMV infections in man [42, 61].

There is both theoretical and circumstantial evidence in man that CMV infection may increase rejection episodes or accentuate pathology associated with rejection. CMV infection has been found to upregulate the expression of class II HLA antigens in kidney cells, presumably on the basis of gamma interferon production [94]. This may explain how CMV infection might enhance rejection. That such enhancement actually occurs in renal transplant patients has been suspected since 1970 [32, 50, 83], even if evidence for it has been limited.

Betts et al. [6] studied a series of younger patients, who received organs from living related donors a significant proportion of whom were CMV-seronegative. This population made it possible to study the effect of primary CMV infection with enough controls who had no rejection episodes. Rejection occurred in 4 out of 16 patients with primary infection, while 24 seronegative recipients who did not develop primary infection had no rejection ($p < 0.05$). More recently, Grattan et al. [36] reported on the effects of CMV infection on 301 cardiac transplant recipients. As determined largely by serologic methods 91 patients (30%) had CMV infection. Their frequency of graft rejection, graft loss, and mortality were all significantly higher than the uninfected group. One criticism of this paper is that the rate of CMV infection was unusually low. One suspects that mild infections may have been overlooked; hence, the "infected" population may have consisted of selected patients with higher morbidity. It was interesting, however, that long-term follow-up showed that death due to coronary atherosclerosis was significantly greater in the infected population, which provides some support for the hypothesis that CMV infection plays a role in the pathogenesis of atherosclerosis [52, 104].

There are several other phenomena illustrating the bidirectional relationships between CMV infection and allograft reaction: (1) There is a strong association between GvH reaction and the frequency of CMV interstitial pneumonia in recipients of allogeneic marrow transplants. The frequency of CMV pneumonia in patients who received autologous marrow transplants was strikingly low [63, 99]. The pathogenesis of this type of pneumonia is assumed to have a strong immunopathologic component (see below) even though so far the role of the GvH reaction has not been explained. (2) CMV infection has been shown to be a risk factor for the pathogenesis of the vanishing bile duct syndrome after liver transplantation [58]. This syndrome is a variant of chronic graft rejection after liver transplantation. It is also seen in patients with a complete mismatch for HLA-A/-B antigens and paradoxically with one to two matches for HLA-DR antigens [21]. (3) There are a number of isolated observations which suggest that the grafted organ may be particularly prone to

CMV and other viral infections. One may assume that the graft is the site of active allograft reactions. Richardson et al. [75] described a peculiar glomerular lesion which was thought to be due to CMV (see below). CMV hepatitis is a fairly common complication after liver transplantation [9, 84] (see below). The grafted liver is also prone to herpes simplex hepatitis [49]. Patients with heart-lung transplants were more prone to develop CMV pneumonitis than patients with kidney, liver, or heart transplants [24, 27].

The Effect of Immunosuppression on CMV Infection

CMV infections were observed to occur with the routine use of azathioprine and prednisone as the standard immunosuppressive agents after transplantation. These agents were the single most important cause of the development of CMV infection. We arrived at this conclusion in 1977 [42], based largely on our observations that 56% of CMV-seropositive patients with connective tissue disorders treated with cytotoxic immunosuppressants such as cyclophosphamide reactivated [22]. The frequency of infection by CMV in the azathioprine era is shown in Table 1. In most series, the rate of secondary or reactivation infection was close to 100%. While it is impossible in large series to distinguish between reinfection and reactivation infection, the degree of immunosuppression required for graft survival was sufficient to activate the majority of all latent infections.

The morbidity, however, may vary greatly despite the high frequency of active CMV infection, even in the same institution. For example, in 1978, the Minnesota group [64] reported that in a group of 141 consecutive transplant patients *overt* CMV disease was found in 59 (42%). Of the 59 symptomatic patients, 25 (42%) or 13% of the total group had evidence of pulmonary infiltrates. In 1983, Peterson et al. [65] reported that, from 1980 to 1982, out of 273 renal transplant patients 24 or 8.8% developed CMV pneumonia.

Table 1. CMV infection in transplant patients before 1981 (from [44])

	Type of transplant			
	Kidney	Marrow	Heart	Liver
Primary infection				
Seronegative (*n*)	542	485	44	37
Infected (%)	52	35	64	46
Secondary infection				
Seropositive (*n*)	734	485	53	56
Infected (%)	84	55	100	67
All subjects (*n*)	1276	970	97	93
Infected (%)	70	44	85	53

There are a number of studies comparing the older and new immunosuppressive regimens after the introduction of cyclosporine. Bia et al. [7] compared 24 renal patients on cyclosporine with 40 on azathioprine. The number of symptomatic CMV infections were comparable (58% and 48% respectively). Both groups also received steroids and some received ATG. Excluding patients on azathioprine who received ATG for acute rejections reduced the frequency of symptomatic CMV infection to 24%.

At the University of Pittsburgh, we undertook a comparison of infections occurring in renal patients on traditional azathioprine-prednisone combination with the cyclosporine-prednisone combination [25]. No ATG was used. The frequency of CMV infection was similar; the amount of symptomatic disease was also similar. It may be illustrated by the amount of CMV pneumonia in two such groups: There were three cases in each group of 138 and 131 transplant recipients (2.2% and 2.3%) [27, 43].

Najarian et al. [57] compared 230 renal recipients on cyclosporine-prednisone with 109 on azathioprine-prednisone-ATG. Symptomatic CMV infection during the first year after transplantation was only 9% in the cyclosporine group but 28% in the azathioprine group. However, the cyclosporine group did not routinely get 14 days of antilymphocyte serum (ALS) or ATG; hence, the two groups were not strictly comparable.

The effect of ATG on CMV infection was also vividly demonstrated by Rubin et al. [77] in a survey of 1245 renal transplant recipients from 46 transplant centers. They found that twice as many deaths occurred in cadaveric transplant recipients who received ATG than in those who did not receive ATG (19% vs 6%). Interestingly, the mortality of patients with no evidence of CMV was not affected by the use of ATG (4%). The higher mortality is assumed to be due to CMV infection which was exacerbated by ATG.

Andreone et al. [2] from Minnesota reported a reduction of infections in heart transplant recipients after institution of low-dose "triple" drug immunotherapy. Before 1983, when ALS, prednisone, and azathioprine were used, there were 1.3 episodes of infection per patient. After 1983, when high-dose cyclosporine (blood level 250–300 ng/ml by high-pressure liquid chromatography) was substituted for azathioprine, there were 1.6 episodes of infection per patient. In the third era, low-dose cyclosporine (blood level, 150–200 ng/ml), azathioprine and prednisone, but no ALS, was used; there were only 0.6 infections per patient. Deaths from infections during the three periods were 2/11, 3/16, and 2/35, or 18%, 19%, and 6% respectively. The most striking reduction was in symptomatic CMV infections. During the first two time periods the frequency of symptomatic CMV infection was 8/27 or 30%, with three deaths due to CMV. During the third era, only 1/35 or 3% symptomatic CMV infections were recorded without any deaths due to CMV. This is quite comparable to the morbidity from CMV infection in renal transplant recipients who did not receive ALS or ATG immunosuppression (see above).

The last immunosuppressive regime was also associated with higher actuarial survival rate and lower rejection rates. Two additional measures may have helped reduce the rate of CMV morbidity, particularly from primary infection.

One was the use of CMV-negative blood for seronegative recipients, and the second was the administration of CMV-hyperimmune globulin. It is not clear which of these three measures contributed most to the reduction of morbidity due to CMV.

More recently, an immunosuppressant similar in biological action to cyclosporine, FK-506, has been widely tested. Reportedly, CMV infections are lower following its use [1], but this has not been proven. Whether this is due to the direct effect of the drug, or to less rejection, is unclear.

The more modern ALSs are also suspected of enhancing CMV infections. Singh et al. [84] studied the effect of OKT3 serum used for rejections in 121 liver transplant recipients. Patients who received OKT3 had significantly more episodes of disseminated CMV infection (five out of a total of six cases) and more episodes of oral and genital herpes than those who did not.

In summary, the type of immunosuppression had a profound effect on infectious complications, in particular on morbidity due to CMV infection. While essential immunosuppressants such as azathioprine, cyclosporine, or FK-506 may account for different frequencies of CMV infections, the dosages used may even be more important. The determinants of morbidity due to CMV are ever more complex. One culprit is ALS and antithymocyte serum. Newer monoclonal ALSs are also suspect, although they have not been studied as carefully as ALS or ATG. It is fair to conclude, however, that no immunosuppressant has yet been found which can avoid the CMV problem.

Primary and Secondary (Reinfection and Reactivation) Infections

Since primary infections are clinically more severe and by definition such infections are caused by an exogenous agent, its source is an important concern. In 1975, we found that patients not previously infected with CMV were at much greater risk to develop primary CMV infection if they were engrafted with a kidney from a seropositive donor [45]. This seroepidemiologic observation has since been found not only for renal transplantation [5] but has been extended to heart [55, 68] and more recently liver transplantation [33, 84].

Weir et al. [97] reported a series of 167 renal transplant patients from Baltimore who received cyclosporine and prednisone immunosuppression. There were 15 cases of symptomatic CMV disease, 12 of these, or 80%, occurred among the 20 seronegative recipients who received organs from seropositive donors. Only three cases of CMV disease occurred among 142 seropositive recipients.

Smiley et al. [85] studied a series of 153 patients from Philadelphia who were on azathioprine-prednisone immunosuppression. There were 23 CMV-seronegative patients who received kidneys from seropositive donors and 14 (61%) developed CMV disease. This group had the highest mean point score of disease severity and also the greatest number of major complications (26%). Only one patient developed CMV disease among 49 seronegative recipients who received kidneys from seronegative donors.

They also separated their CMV-seropositive recipients' groups into subgroups who received either a seropositive or a seronegative donor. This is a crude way to separate reinfection from reactivation. There were 41 seropositive recipients who received kidneys from seropositive donors (first group) and 40 seropositive recipients who received kidneys from seronegative donors (second group). The frequency of CMV disease in these two groups was similar, 10:41 (24%) and 8:40 (20%). However, the first group had more severe disease as measured by the point score, and more severe major complications. This is presumptive evidence that reinfections may produce more disease syndromes than reactivation infections. Of course, the actual proportion of reinfections versus reactivation infections in the first group was unknown, while the second group may have represented mostly reactivation infections.

Recently, the precise nature of secondary infections has received additional attention. Reinfections of immune individuals have been shown to occur in various population groups, such as sexually highly active heterosexual women or homosexual men. Chandler et al. [13] found that reinfections of the uterine cervix with different strains of CMV in "immune" women may be identified by restriction fragment polymorphism. Similarly, Spector et al. [87] cultured different strains of CMV from buffy coat, lung, and urine from individual gay men with AIDS, which could only be explained by multiple reinfections. Similar results have been obtained by others [91]. Restriction fragment polymorphism has conclusively shown that reinfections may occur in renal [15, 39], heart [16], and marrow recipients [101].

Grundy et al. [40] addressed the question of whether patients who are reinfected are more symptomatic than patients who reactivate a latent infection. Reinfection may be positively identified if an infecting strain in a CMV-seropositive recipient was found to be identical to a donor strain transmitted by the other kidney to another recipient. Of five seropositive recipients who were superinfected with such donor strains, three had symptomatic disease. Four seropositive recipients received kidneys from seronegative donors, developed active infection, and hence presumably reactivated, but none was symptomatic. Chou [17] found, in a similar study of renal transplant recipients, that symptomatic CMV disease was identified in 21 of 25 primary infections, 2 of 16 reinfections, and 1 of 4 reactivations. These data suggested that secondary infections are less symptomatic than primary infections, but they do not support the findings of Grundy et al. [40] that morbidity after reinfection is higher than after reactivation. Admittedly the numbers from both studies are too small from which to draw definite conclusions. Winston et al. [101] confirm the assumption that in the severely immunosuppressed marrow recipient a reactivated infection may be symptomatic and even lethal. Two out of four seropositive recipients developed CMV interstitial pneumonia. These four had identical isolates in the urine before transplantation and after transplantation as identified by restriction polymorphism identical. The strains associated with the pneumonias were identical to those found at other sites. However, the extreme morbidity of secondary infections is a special case of the severely immunosuppressed, such as the patient with a marrow transplant or with acquired immunodeficiency syndrome (AIDS). The question still remains as to whether reinfections with CMV in solid organ recipients is a serious clinical problem. It is an important question because potential prophylactic measures are available.

CMV Disease and the Type of Transplantation

In Pittsburgh we have noticed that despite the use of similar cyclosporine-prednisone immunosuppressive regimens, the frequency of CMV disease may vary greatly depending on the type of transplant [43]. Patients undergoing cardiac transplantation had more CMV disease than those who had kidney transplants. In this early phase, ALS was not used for routine immunosuppression after any of our organ transplantations, although it was used for rejection. The use of ATG for this purpose could not account for this difference [25].

More recently, ATG has been used more liberally in our transplant groups. A summary of CMV infections and morbidity is presented in Table 2 [26, 27, 43], which shows that the frequency of infection varies between 59% and 92% in different transplant groups. Whether this is a true difference or a reflection of differences in the serologic status of donors and recipients and other variables is not known.

Out of 131 renal transplant patients, only 10 (8%) had symptomatic CMV infection. By contrast, the other three transplant groups had significantly more symptomatic CMV disease. Whether there is a significant difference in CMV morbidity among liver, heart, and heart–lung recipients is not clear. What was significant is the finding that 32% of the heart–lung recipients had CMV pneumonia. This frequency approximates the frequency of symptomatic infections (39%) and suggests that the lung is particularly vulnerable to CMV disease after heart–lung transplantation. The question arises as to whether an allograft undergoing various degrees of allograft rejection is particularly vulnerable to CMV infection.

Table 2. Infection and morbidity of CMV infection in different transplant groups in Pittsburgh after 1981 (from [26, 27, 43])

Type of transplant	Total no. patients	Patients with infections		Symptomatic patients		Patients with CMV pneumonia	
		n	% of total	Infected (%)	Total (%)	Infected (%)	Total (%)
Kidney	131	79	60	13	8	4	2
Liver	93	55	59	49	29	5	3
Heart	48	44	92	27	25	9	8
Heart–lung	31	22	71	55	39	45	32

The situation is comparable to allogeneic marrow transplantation where CMV pneumonia has been a uniquely difficult problem. Meyers et al. [55] report an incidence of 16.7% in 545 marrow transplant recipients. In bone marrow transplantation, the lung is a target organ for GvH reaction. GvH reactions have consistently been found to be a significant risk factor.

The frequency of CMV hepatitis after liver transplantation also suggests that allografts are peculiarly vulnerable to CMV infection, perhaps as a consequence of or an accompaniment of an allograft reaction. While chemical hepatitis is a frequent accompaniment to the CMV "viral syndrome", severe life-threatening CMV hepatitis is a unique problem after liver transplantation.

From 1980 to 1985, 17 cases of CMV hepatitis were diagnosed in 429 patients who underwent liver transplantation at the University of Pittsburgh [9]. The most common presenting symptoms were prolonged fever, elevation in total serum bilirubin, and elevation in liver enzymes. Clinically, CMV hepatitis could not be distinguished from other causes of liver failure, especially rejection. Tissue diagnosis is essential [20]. Evidence of CMV in cells is always found, either in terms of inclusion bodies, viral antigens detected by polyclonal or monoclonal antibodies, or culture of CMV from the tissue specimen. Microabscesses were typical early reactions. Early diagnosis is lifesaving, since the treatment, reduction in immunosuppression, is opposite to treatment of rejection. Initially, cases were diagnosed at time of retransplantation; four out of five patients so diagnosed died. In contrast, only 4 of 12 patients diagnosed by percutaneous biopsy died. Biopsies were later more liberally taken.

In summary, it appears that besides immunosuppression, the type of transplant is a determinant of the type of severity of CMV disease. CMV disease preferentially attacks the lung in bone marrow and heart-lung recipients, and the liver in liver transplantation. Why the allograft becomes more vulnerable requires further study. The factors to be considered are a local allograft reaction and the possible local reactivation of the latently infected allograft.

The Spectrum of CMV Disease

There is a wide spectrum of CMV diseases. As in many infectious diseases, the most severe form was first recognized and was thought for some time to be the only disease. Congenital cytomegalic inclusion disease was recognized as early as 1881 by Ribbert [73]. The much milder form of disease, almost invariably benign in outcome, CMV mononucleosis in normal subjects, was not recognized until 1965 [46]. These two clinical syndromes may serve as extremes of the clinical manifestations of CMV disease in the immunosuppressed transplant patient.

The majority of symptomatic diseases even in transplant patients will be variants of the CMV mononucleosis syndrome. Prolonged fever is the most common manifestation. Leukopenia and chemical hepatitis are common, lymphadenopathy and hepatosplenomegaly are unusual, and arthralgia, arthritis, and skin rashes may occur. This syndrome is usually benign in outcome [44].

Many types of visceral involvement in CMV disease may occur. Peterson et al. [64] point to the frequency of gastrointestinal system. Esophageal, gastric, duodenal, small intestinal, or cecal involvement is common. Cohen et al. [18] note that gastroduodenal ulcers in transplant patients are frequently erroneously diagnosed as peptic or stress ulcers. Renal involvement is a common pathologic finding, but frank clinical involvement is rare. Richardson et al. [75] described a glomerulopathy in renal transplant recipients with CMV viremia associated with acute deterioration of the function of the allograft. Often, however, no local evidence of CMV infection is found, and some authors believe that the glomerulopathy represents an unusual form of rejection [41]. Tubulointerstitial involvement with CMV including typical giant cells is one of the best known pathologic lesions of CMV infection (reviewed in [44]), but renal dysfunction or failure due to CMV has been rarely described. Cameron et al. [10] did describe such a case of renal allograft. Shorr et al. [82] described a case of hemorrhagic cystitis in a bone marrow recipient who had CMV-associated tubulointerstitial nephritis. No evidence of vascular rejection was found.

Does the severity of particular types of CMV disease remain constant in different transplant groups? Two types of CMV disease are reported with sufficient frequency so that valid impressions may be formed. One is the "viral" mononucleosis syndrome, which appears to be a benign self-limited syndrome and as such has no definable mortality. However, the viral syndrome may precede more severe systemic form of CMV disease, such as pneumonitis or other forms of dissemination. For example, all eight cases of CMV pneumonia developing in 55 heart and heart–lung recipients had a preceding viral syndrome due to CMV [26]. The mortality of these patients was high (6/8 or 75%), and comparable to that of CMV pneumonia in bone marrow recipients (84%) [55].

Secondly, the morbidity of CMV pneumonia may vary in different transplant groups, although the evidence is incomplete. Peterson et al. [64] studied types of CMV diseases in renal recipients from Minnesota, and all 12 patients in his series who died of CMV disease had evidence of CMV pneumonia. Patients with CMV pneumonia had a 48% (12/25) mortality. While high, this is significantly lower than CMV interstitial pneumonia after marrow transplantation (84%) [55]. The clinical picture of CMV pneumonitis is worth commenting on. Most patients (96%) had bilateral interstitial or intra-alveolar infiltrates. Nodular infiltrates, often associated with other superinfectious pulmonary pathogens, pleural effusions, and discoid atelectasis were also seen. Most patients with CMV pneumonia (65%) were hypoxemic, and hypoxemia predated the onset of X-ray findings [44, 64]. Most who required respiratory assistance died.

Because of the lack of response of CMV interstitial pneumonia in marrow recipients to effective antiviral therapy (see below), it has been postulated that there must be an essential immunopathologic factor besides the presence of the virus [38]. According to this theory, pneumonia results from the development of a T cell cytotoxicity directed against viral antigens expressed on infected cells in the lung. There is as yet no direct evidence for this theory. Circumstantial evidence consists of reported efficacy of CMV immunoglobulin combined with ganciclovir in the treatment of CMV interstitial pneumonia in the marrow recipient (see below).

Two mouse models of CMV pneumonitis provide some insight. The virus alone usually does not produce pneumonia; it has to be administered to a preconditioned animal. In one case this animal is undergoing a GvH reaction [37]; in the other [79], the mouse has been immunosuppressed by one injection of cyclophosphamide. However, excess immunosuppression produced by repeated injections will obviate the development of pneumonitis, presumably because an essential immune reaction is suppressed.

Summarizing the above, it is quite possible that CMV pneumonitis is not a single disease, depending on whether an immunologic process is involved and what that process is. Four types of CMV pneumonia may be recognized. Firstly, there is an interstitial pneumonia associated with CMV mononucleosis [11, 47, 90], which appears to be self-limited and requires no treatment. Secondly, there is the type seen after solid organ transplantation, with the exception of lung transplantations. Morbidity may be lower in this type than in the next two groups. Thirdly, there is the type seen after lung or heart-lung transplantation where there may be an associated allograft reaction in the grafted lung. Fourthly, there is CMV pneumonia in the marrow recipient, which is often associated with GvH reaction. Whether the severity of CMV pneumonia in renal and other non-lung transplant recipients under different immunosuppressive regimes has different mortality rates is not clear. It is important to find out because treatment modalities may differ.

Chemotherapy and Chemoprophylaxis

Attempts to treat CMV disease with vidarabine, acyclovir, or interferon have not been successful. Alphainterferon, whether alone or in combination with vidarabine, was without effect on CMV pneumonia in marrow transplant recipients [80, 95].

Ganciclovir (or Dihydroxy-propoxy methyl-guanine, DHPG) is an analogue of acyclovir which has significantly more activity against CMV than acyclovir. Clinical trials in patients with AIDS and in bone marrow transplant recipients show promising results in the treatment of CMV retinitis [19, 31]. Vision improved, and in most cases there was virologic evidence of improvement. But ganciclovir did not have the effect of reducing mortality from CMV pneumonitis in bone marrow recipients [81]. Nine out of 10 treated patients died, and the tenth showed no clinical improvement.

Some recent data on the treatment of CMV pneumonia and other systemic disease due to CMV are somewhat more encouraging. Erice et al. [30] report that 17 (55%) of 31 immunosuppressed patients with various types of CMV disease who received 2.5 mg ganciclovir per kilogram body weight I.V. every 8 h improved clinically during therapy. Viremia ceased in 93% (14:15) of patients after 4.7 days of therapy. Unfortunately, in these anecdotal trials it is difficult to document efficacy because a control group is not available for comparison. Let us consider only the case of CMV pneumonia in marrow recipients, for which there is a great deal of historical data. In this study, 11 such patients were treated and 5 (45%) were said to improve with therapy, while 6 did not. However, three of the five eventually died, giving a mortality rate for the total group of 82% (9:11), which is the same as the mortality for untreated CMV pneumonia in marrow recipients (84%) [55]. As for the favorable responses in CMV disease in other types of transplant recipients, such as CMV pneumonitis in renal transplant recipients, or gastrointestinal disease or hepatitis, there is insufficient historical data to be sure that untreated patients would not have fared as well.

A possible significant advance has been the reduction of mortality from CMV pneumonia in marrow recipients to 48% and 30% if in addition to ganciclovir, immune globulin was added [29, 72]. Unfortunately, a rigorous placebo controlled trial may not be forthcoming, because many clinicians believe that ganciclovir therapy is effective in a potentially lethal disease, and it may not be possible to withhold ganciclovir.

Earlier attempts to prevent CMV infection along with herpes simplex virus (HSV) infections with oral acyclovir were either unconfirmed or unsuccessful [35, 96]. Meyers et al. [56] administered acyclovir at 500 mg/m^2 of body surface every 8 h to 86 CMV-seropositive bone marrow recipients from 5 days before transplantation to 30 days afterward. These patients were also seropositive for HSV. A group of 65 patients seropositive for CMV but not HSV served as controls. Cytomegalic disease, mostly interstitial pneumonia, developed in 19 (22%) acyclovir recipients and 25 (38%) controls ($p=0.008$). Survival in the first 100 days after transplantation was significantly increased in acyclovir recipients. CMV infection was also significantly decreased in acyclovir recipients from 87% to 70%.

The above study could be criticized because it was not randomized or blind. As a follow-up, Balfour et al. [4] conducted a randomized double blind controlled study of acyclovir administered orally, 800–3200 mg/day for 12 weeks, depending on the patient's renal function. During the first year after cadaveric kidney transplantation, 4 of 53 patients (7.5%) in the acyclovir groups had symptomatic disease compared with 15 of 51 (29%) in the placebo groups ($p=0.002$). The greatest prophylactic benefit was in the seronegative recipients who received a kidney from a seropositive donor. Only one out of six such patients in the treated group had CMV disease compared with seven out of seven in the placebo group. Acyclovir, unlike most immune globulins which do not affect infection rates, also reduced the CMV infection rate from 61% to 36% ($p=0.01$).

It is unclear why acyclovir was effective. The mean inhibitory dose (ID_{50}) for local isolates was 62.1 mM, while peak acyclovir levels in patients who received the drugs 1 week after transplantation was only 25 m*M*. It is possible that these measurements do not truly reflect intracellular triphosphate levels, which may have been higher.

Other drugs are being or will be tested in patients at high risk for CMV infection, including both parenterally and orally administered ganciclovir. Recently, Merigan et al. [52a] gave heart recipients intravenous ganciclovir for 4 weeks after transplantation. CMV disease was reduced in secondary infections (9%) compared to untreated controls (46%), but not in patients with primary CMV infection.

Passive Immune Prophylaxis

Six studies of hyperimmune plasma or globulin in bone marrow transplant recipients [48, 54, 59, 100, 102] and one study in kidney recipients [86] have demonstrated the efficacy of high-titered immune globulin in decreasing disease, although not in preventing infection, in CMV-seronegative transplant recipients.

Winston et al. [102], for example, studied 38 recipients who were given an equivalent of 1.0 g immune globulin per kilogram body weight once weekly until day 120 after marrow transplantation. There were 37 controls. CMV infection rates in the two groups (47% and 57%) were not significantly different, although symptomatic infection rates differed (21% vs 46%). Interstitial pneumonia due to CMV (16% vs 32%) and deaths due to interstitial pneumonia (6% vs 14%) were reduced. Most of the subjects in this study (63:75 or 84%) were negative for CMV antibodies prior to receiving transplants. If only primary infections were counted, these were also significantly reduced by immune globulin (25% vs 52%).

The antibody titer of the preparation used in this study was 1:6400 by enzyme-linked immunosorbent assay (ELISA) and 1:64 by neutralization. It should be pointed out that the best antibody test to titer immune serum is still unknown.

In the one negative study [8], immune globulin alone did not reduce primary infection in CMV-seronegative subjects (4/14 vs 4/11) or affect the number of symptomatic infections (2/14 vs 2/11). On the other hand, seronegative blood products significantly reduced CMV infection (1/32 vs 8/25). Perhaps the main problem with this study was that the number of symptomatic infections in the entire study was too small.

These results suggest that immune globulin may be effective in reducing but not eliminating CMV disease in seronegative transplant marrow recipients. Many centers are using immune globulin in the study of patients. Whether or not other types of transplant recipients should also be treated is not clear, particularly in view of the low morbidity due to CMV in some patient groups, the large amount of immune globulin required, and its high cost. Syndman et al. [86] showed, in an important study of 59 seronegative renal transplant recipients given 150 mg of a hyperimmune globulin per kilogram body weight within 72 h of transplantation and 50–100 mg/kg every 2 weeks up to 16 weeks after transplantation, that immune globulin did not reduce rate of CMV infection (71% vs 77%) but did reduce rates of symptomatic disease (21% and 60%). The rate of deaths ascribed to CMV were also reduced (1/17 vs 5/27). These results are provocative and suggest that immune prophylaxis should be considered for seronegative kidney allograft recipients. However, it should be noted that this group of renal transplant patients seemed to have unusually high rates of symptomatic CMV disease and deaths due to CMV, possibly due to the use of ATG. As pointed out, the risk of developing CMV disease in kidney recipients fluctuates with the type of immunosuppression. This risk must also be assessed for other types of transplant recipients.

Active Immunization

Though imperfect, active immunity develops after natural CMV infection and is an important part of man's acquired immunity. The beneficial role of acquired immunity is attested to by the fact that most problems with CMV occur when this immunity is absent in the host. Thus, congenital CMV disease follows primary infection in the mother when she has no acquired immunity; and in transplant patients, most severe symptomatic disease is also a consequence of primary infection in transplant patients. The efficacy of passive immunization in reducing CMV disease in seronegative transplant patients is further indirect proof of the importance of acquired humoral immunity. Hence, the development of acquired immunity by active immunization is justifiable. Two primary target populations may be considered for protective active immunization, the seronegative mother and the seronegative transplant recipient.

So far one live attenuated vaccine has been tested clinically in renal transplant recipients. There have been a number of objections to the concept of using live CMV vaccine. There are unanswered questions about strain variability of CMV isolates and, hence, possible lack of efficacy of a vaccine strain; and questions about the efficacy of humoral and cellular immunity developed by a vaccine. Live CMV vaccines may have troublesome long-term toxicity related to their persistence, latency, and potential transmissibility. CMV and other herpesviruses are also potentially oncogenic [60]. Tests of the Towne strain of cell-culture-attenuated vaccine developed by Plotkin et al. [34, 66, 67] seem to show that fears about its toxicity, persistence, and transmissibility are largely unfounded. Efficacy and cost-effectiveness in the immunosuppressed transplant patient, however, has not yet been conclusively proven.

The Towne attenuated vaccines produced an asymptomatic apparently self-limited infection which resulted in the production of detectable antibodies and the development of CMV-specific lymphocyte proliferative response in almost all healthy volunteers [88]. In a controlled clinical trial of 91 renal transplant recipients [67], 9 out of 37 (24%) CMV-seronegative patients who received the vaccine failed to produce antibodies. Five out of six also failed to develop a specific positive lymphocyte response while all eight normal controls responded. Primary infection developed in both vaccinated and unvaccinated seronegative recipients who received kidneys from seropositive donors. The frequency of such infection was similar in vaccinees and the placebo-treated subjects (15/16 or 94% vs 11/14 or 78%). Also, the proportion of those infected who were symptomatic was not significantly different (60% vs. 91%). However, the degree of morbidity in the vaccines measured according to a quantitative scoring system was significantly lower (2.7 vs. 5.7).

Vaccinated CMV-seronegative patients who received kidneys from seronegative donors and were not infected extraneously did not shed vaccine virus in the urine, throat, or blood, suggesting that the vaccine strain neither spread nor persisted in the host. Furthermore, CMV strains isolated from primary infections in vaccinees have been shown by restriction endonuclease fragment polymorphism to be unrelated to the vaccine strain [87].

The modest reduction in morbidity of CMV by the vaccine was not supported in a parallel study employing the same vaccine in Minnesota [3, 91]. A total of 117 received the vaccine (6.6×10^3 viral infectious plaques), and 119 received placebo. Of 63 CMV-seronegative subjects, 76% converted their antibody status after being immunized. Seropositive subjects also had a boost in their antibody titers.

Of the 236 subjects studied, 47 (20%) developed CMV disease. There was no difference in incidence or severity of CMV disease between vaccinees and the placebo group among seropositive subjects or seronegative subjects who received a kidney from a seropositive donor. There was suggestion of protection by the vaccine among seronegative subjects who were given a seropositive kidney. Two of eight vaccinees with CMV disease had severe or lethal disease, while five of six placebo subjects with CMV disease experienced severe or lethal illness. This suggests that CMV disease was ameliorated, although the frequency of CMV disease in the vaccinated and placebo groups (38% and 43%) was not changed.

In summary, the Towne vaccine may have at best a marginal effect in alleviating CMV disease due to primary infection. Future developments should aim at improving the immunogenicity of the vaccine in potential transplant recipients. Other classes of vaccines, such as subunits and recombinant vaccines, remain to be developed.

References

1. Allessiani M, Kusne S, Martin FM et al. (1990) Infections under FK506 immunosuppression: preliminary results with primary therapy. Transplant Proc 22:44–46
2. Andreone PA, Olivari MT, Elick B et al. (1986) Reduction of infectious complications following heart transplantation with triple-drug immunotherapy. J Heart Transplant 5:13–19
3. Balfour HH Jr, Welo PK, Sach GW (1985) Cytemegalovirus vaccine trial in 400 renal transplant candidates. Transplant Proc 17:81–83

4. Balfour HH, Chace BA, Stapleton JT et al. (1989) A randomized, placebo-controlled trial of oral acyclovir for the prevention of cytomegalovirus disease in recipients of renal allografts. N Engl J Med 320:1381–1387
5. Betts RF, Freeman RB, Douglas RG Jr et al. (1975) Transmission of cytomegalovirus infection with renal allograft. Kidney Int 8:387–394
6. Betts RF, Freeman RB, Douglas RG Jr, Talley TE (1977) Clinical manifestations of renal allograft derived primary cytomegalovirus infection. Am J Dis Child 131:759–763
7. Bia MJ, Andiman W, Gaudio K et al. (1985) Effect of treatment with cyclosporine versus azathioprine on incidence and severity of cytomegalovirus infection post-transplantation. Transplantation 40:610–614
8. Bowden RA, Sayers M, Flourney N et al. (1986) Cytomegalovirus immune globulin and seronegative blood products to prevent primary cytomegalovirus infection after marrow transplantation. N Engl J Med 314:1006–1010
9. Bronsther O, Makowaka L, Jaffe R (1988) Occurrence of cytomegalovirus hepatitis in liver transplant patients. J Med Virol 24:423–434
10. Cameron J, Rigby RJ, van Deth AG, Petrie JJB (1982) Severe tubulo-interstitial disease in a renal allograft due to cytomegalovirus infection. Clin Nephrol 18:321–325
11. Carlström G, Alden J, Belfrage S et al. (1968) Acquired cytomegalovirus infection. Br Med J 2:521–525
12. Carney WP, Rubin RH, Hoffman RA et al. (1981) Analysis of T lymphocyte subsets in cytomegalovirus mononucleosis. J Immunol 126:2114–2116
13. Chandler SH, Handsfield HH, McDougall JK (1987) Isolation of multiple strains of cytomegalovirus from women attending a clinic for sexually transmitted diseases. J Infect Dis 155:655–660
14. Chatterjee SN, Fiala M, Wiener J (1978) Primary cytomegalovirus and opportunistic infections. Incidence in renal transplant recipients. JAMA 240:2446–2449
15. Chou S (1986) Acquisition of donor strains of cytomegalovirus by renal-transplant recipients. N Engl J Med 314:1418–1423
16. Chou S (1987) Cytomegalovirus infection and reinfection transmitted by heart transplantation. J Infect Dis 155:1054–1056
17. Chou S (1989) Reactivation and recombination of multiple cytomegalovirus strains from individual organ donors. J Infect Dis 160:11–15
18. Cohen EB, Komorowski RA, Kauffman HM Jr, Adams M (1985) Unexpectedly high incidence of cytomegalovirus infection in apparent peptic ulcers in renal transplant recipients. Surgery 97:606–612
19. Collaborative DHPG Treatment Study Group (1986) Treatment of serious cytomegalovirus infections with 9-(1,3-Dihydroxy-2-Propoxymethyl) guanine in patients with AIDS and other immunodeficies. N Engl J Med 314:801–805
20. Demetrius AJ, Lasky S, van Thiel DH et al. (1985) Pathology of hepatic transplantation: a review of 62 adult allograft recipients immunosuppressed with a cyclosporine/steroid regimen. Am J Pathol 118:151–161
21. Donaldson PT, O'Grady J, Portmann B et al. (1987) Evidence for an immune response to HLA class I antigens in the vanishing-bile duct syndrome after liver transplantation. Lancet 1:945–948
22. Dowling JN, Saslow AR, Armstrong JA, Ho M (1976) Cytomegalovirus infection in patients receiving immunosuppressive therapy for rheumatologic disorders. J Infect Dis 133:399–408
23. Dowling JN, Wu BC, Armstrong JA, Ho M (1977) Enhancement of murine cytomegalovirus infection during graft versus host reaction. J Infect Dis 135:990
24. Dummer JS, Bahnson HT, Griffith BP, Ho M (1983) Infections in patients on cyclosporine and prednisone following cardiac transplantation. Transplant Proc 15:2779–2781
25. Dummer JS, Hardy A, Poorsattar A, Ho M (1983) Early infections in kidney, heart and liver transplant recipients on cyclosporine. Transplantation 36:259–267

26. Dummer JS, White LT, Ho M et al. (1985) The morbidity of cytomegalovirus infection in heart and hear–lung transplant recipients on cyclosporine. J Infect Dis 152:1182–1191
27. Dummer JS, Montero CG, Griffith BP et al. (1986) Infections in heart-lung transplant recipients. Transplantation 41:725–729
28. Einhorn L, Ost A (1984) Cytomegalovirus infection of human blood cells. J Infect Dis 149:207–214
29. Emanuel D, Cunningham I, Jules-Elysee K et al. (1988) Cytomegalovirus pneumonia after bone marrow transplantation successfully treated with the combination of ganciclovir and high-dose intravenous immune globulin. Ann Intern Med 109:777–782
30. Erice A, Jordan MC, Chace BA et al. (1987) Ganciclovir treatment of cytomegalovirus disease in transplant recipients and other immunocompromised hosts. JAMA 257:3082–3087
31. Felsenstein D, d'Amico DJ, Hirsch MS et al. (1985) Treatment of cytomegalovirus retinitis with 9-[2-hydroxy-1-(hydroxymethyl) ethoxymethyl] guanine. Ann Intern Med 103:377–380
32. Fiala M, Payne JE, Berne TV et al. (1975) Epidemiology of cytomegalovirus infection after transplantation and immunosuppression. J Infect Dis 132:421–433
33. Fox AS, Tolpin MD, Baker AL et al. (1988) Seropositivity in liver transplant recipients as a predictor of cytomegalovirus disease. J Infect Dis 157:383–385
34. Glazer JP, Friedman HM, Grossman RA (1979) Live cytomegalovirus vaccination of renal transplant candidates. A preliminary trial. Ann Intern Med 91:676–683
35. Gluckman E, Lotsberg J, Devergie A et al. (1983) Prophylaxis of herpes infections after bone-marrow transplantation by oral acyclovir. Lancet 2:706–708
36. Grattan M, Moreno-Cabral CE, Starnes VA et al. (1989) Cytomegalovirus infection is associated with cardiac allograft rejection and atherosclerosis. JAMA 261:3561–3566
37. Grundy JE, Shanley JD, Shearer GM (1985) Augmentation of graft-versus-host reaction by cytomegalovirus infection resulting in interstitial pneumonitis. Transplantation 39:548–553
38. Grundy JE, Shanley JD, Griffiths PD (1987) Is cytomegalovirus interstitial pneumonitis in transplant recipients an immunopathological condition? Lancet 2:996–999
39. Grundy JE, Super M, Lui S et al. (1987) The source of cytomegalovirus infection in seropositive renal allograft recipients is frequently the donor kidney. Transplant Proc 19:2126–2128
40. Grundy JE, Super M, Berry NJ et al. (1988) Symptomatic cytomegalovirus infection in seropositive kidney recipients: reinfection with donor virus rather than reactivation of recipient virus. Lancet 2:132–135
41. Herrera GA, Alexander RW, Cooley CF et al. (1986) Cytomegalovirus glomerulopathy: a controversial lesion. Kidney Int 29:725–733
42. Ho M (1977) Virus infections after transplantation in man. Arch Virol 55:1–24
43. Ho M (1987) Infection and organ transplantation. In Gelman S (ed) Anesthesia and organ transplantation. Saunders, Philadelphia, pp 49–60
44. Ho M (1991) Cytomegalovirus: biology and infection, 2nd ed. Plenum, New York
45. Ho M, Suwansirikul S, Dowling JN et al. (1975) The transplanted kidney as a source of cytomegalovirus infections. N Engl J Med 293:1109–1112
46. Klemola E, Kaariainen L (1965) Cytomegalovirus as a possible cause of a disease resembling infectious mononucleosis. Br Med J 2:1099–1102
47. Klemola E, Stenstrom R, von Essen R (1972) Pneumonia as a clinical manifestation of cytomegalovirus infection in previously healthy adults. Scand J Infect Dis 4:7–10
48. Kubanek B, Ernst P, Ostendorf P et al. (1985) Preliminary data of a controlled trial of intravenous hyperimmune globulin in the prevention of cytomegalovirus infection in bone marrow transplant recipients. Transplant Proc 17:468–469
49. Kusne S, Schwartz M, Ho M et al. (1991) Herpes simplex virus hepatitis after solid organ transplantation in adults. J Infect Dis 163:1001–1007
50. Lopez C, Simmons RL, Mauer SM et al. (1974) Association of renal allograft rejection with virus infections. Am J Med 56:280–289

51. Marker SC, Howard RJ, Simmons RL et al. (1981) Cytomegalovirus infection: a quantitative prospective study of 320 consecutive renal transplants. Surgery 89:660–671
52. Melnick JL, Petrie BL, Dreesman GR et al. (1983) Cytomegalovirus antigen within human arterial smooth muscle cells. Lancet 2:644–647
52a. Merigan TC, Renlund DG, Keay S et al. (1992) A controlled trial of ganciclovir to prevent cytomegalovirus disease after heart transplantation. N Engl J Med 326:1182–1186
53. Meyers JD, Flournoy N, Thomas ED (1980) Cytomegalovirus infection and specific cell-mediated immunity after marrow transplant. J Infect Dis 142:816–824
54. Meyers JD, Leszczynski J, Zaia JA et al. (1983) Prevention of cytomegalovirus infection by cytomegalovirus immune globulin after marrow transplantation. Ann Intern Med 98:442–446
55. Meyers JD, Flournoy N, Thomas ED (1986) Risk factors for cytomegalovirus infection after human marrow transplant. J Infect Dis 153:478–488
56. Meyers JD, Reed EC, Shepp DH et al. (1988) Acyclovir for the prevention of cytomegalovirus infection and disease after allogenic marrow transplantation. N Engl J Med 318:70–75
57. Najarian JS, Fryd DS, Strand M et al. (1985) A single institution, randomized, prospective trial of cyclosporine versus azathioprine-antilymphocyte globulin for immunosuppression in renal allograft recipients. Ann Surg 201:142–157
58. O'Grady JG, Sutherland S, Harvey F et al. (1988) Cytomegalovirus infection and donor/recipient HLA antigens: interdependent cofactors in pathogenesis of vanishing bileduct syndrome after liver transplantation. Lancet 2:302–305
59. O'Reilly RJ, Reich L, Gold J et al. (1983) A randomized trial of intravenous hyperimmune globulin for the prevention of cytomegalovirus infections following marrow transplantation: preliminary results. Transplant Proc 15:1405–1411
60. Osborn JE (1981) Cytomegalovirus: pathogenicity, immunology, and vaccine initiatives. J Infect Dis 143:618–630
61. Pass RF, Long WK, Whitley RJ et al. (1978) Productive infection with cytomegalovirus and herpes simplex virus in renal transplant recipients: role of source of kidney. J Infect Dis 137:556–563
62. Pass RF, Reynolds DW, Whelchel JD et al. (1981) Impaired lymphocyte transformation response to cytomegalovirus and phytohemagglutinin in recipients of renal transplants: association with antithymocyte globulin. J Infect Dis 143:259–265
63. Pecego R, Hill R, Appelbaum FR et al. (1986) Interstitial pneumonitis following autologous bone marrow transplantation. Transplantation 42:515–517
64. Peterson PK, Balfour HH Jr, Marker SC et al. (1980) Cytomegalovirus disease in renal allograft recipients: a prospective study of the clinical features, risk factors and impact on renal transplantation. Medicine (Baltimore) 59:283–300
65. Peterson PK, Balfour HH Jr, Fryd DS et al. (1983) Risk factors in the development of cytomegalovirus-related pneumonia in renal transplant recipients. J Infect Dis 148:1121
66. Plotkin SA, Farquhar J, Hornberger E (1976) Clinical trials of immunization with the Towne 125 strain of human cytomegalovirus. J Infect Dis 134:470–475
67. Plotkin SA, Smiley ML, Friedman HM et al. (1984) Towne-vaccine-induced prevention of cytomegalovirus disease after renal transplants. Lancet 1:528–530
68. Pollard RB, Rand KH, Arvin AM, Merigan TC (1978) Cell-mediated immunity to cytomegalovirus infection in normal subjects and cardiac transplant patients. J Infect Dis 137:541–549
69. Preiksaitis JK, Rosno S, Grumet C, Merigan TC (1983) Infections due to herpesviruses in cardiac transplant recipients: role of the donor heart and immunosuppressive therapy. J Infect Dis 147:974–981
70. Preiksaitis JK, Brown L, McKenzie M (1988) The risk of cytomegalovirus infection in seronegative transfusion recipients not receiving exogenous immunosuppression. J Infect Dis 157:523–529
71. Rand KH, Pollard RB, Merigan TC (1978) Increased pulmonary superinfections in cardiac transplant patients undergoing primary cytomegalovirus infection. N Engl J Med 298:951–953

72. Reed EC, Bowden RA, Dandliker PS, Lilleby KE, Meyers JD (1988) Treatment of cytomegalovirus pneumonia with ganciclovir and intravenous cytomegalovirus immunoglobulin in patients with bone marrow transplants. Ann Intern Med 109:783–788
73. Ribbert H (1904) Ueber proozoanartige Zellen in der Niere eines syphilitischen Neugeborenen und in der Parotis von Kindern. Zentralbl Allg Pathol 15:945–948
74. Rice GPA, Schrier RD, Oldstone MBA (1984) Cytomegalovirus infects human lymphocytes and monocytes: virus expression is restricted to immediate early antigen products. Proc Natl Acad Sci USA 81:6134–6138
75. Richardson WP, Colvin RB, Cheeseman SH et al. (1981) Glomerulopathy associated with cytomegalovirus viremia in renal allografts. N Engl J Med 305:57–63
76. Rinaldo CR Jr, Black PH, Hirsch MS (1977) Interactions of cytomegalovirus with leucocyte from patients with mononucleosis due to cytomegalovirus. J Infect Dis 136:667–678
77. Rubin RH, Tolkoff-Rubin NE, Oliver D et al. (1985) Multicenter seroepidemiologic study of the impact of cytomegalovirus infection on renal transplantation. Transplantation 40:243–429
78. Schrier KD, Nelson TA, Oldstone MBA (1985) Detection of human cytomegalovirus in peripheral blood lymphocytes in a natural infection. Science 230:1048–1051
79. Shanley JD, Pesanti EL, Nugent KM (1982) The pathogenesis of pneumonitis due to murine cytomegalovirus. J Infect Dis 156:388–396
80. Shepp DH, Newton BA, Meyers JD (1984) Intravenous lymphoblastoid interferon and acyclovir for treatment of cytomegaloviral pneumonia. J Infect Dis 150:776–777
81. Shepp DH, Dandliker PS, de Miranda P et al. (1985) Activity of 9-[2-hydroxy-1-(hydroxymethyl)ethoxymethyl] guanine in the treatment of cytomegalovirus pneumonia. Ann Intern Med 103:368–373
82. Shorr RI, Longo WL, Oberley TD et al. (1987) Cytomegalovirus-associated tubulointerstitial nephritis in an allogeneic bone marrow transplant recipient. Ann Intern Med 107:351–352
83. Simmons RL, Weil R, Tallent MB et al. (1970) Do mild infections trigger the rejection of renal allografts? Transplant Proc 2:419–423
84. Singh N, Dummer JS, Ho M et al. (1988) Infections with cytomegalovirus and other herpesvirus in 121 liver transplant recipients: transmission by donated organ and the effect of OKT3 antibodies. J Infect Dis 158:124–131
85. Smiley ML, Wlodaver CG, Grossman RA et al. (1985) The role of pretransplant immunity in protection from cytomegalovirus disease following renal transplantation. Transplantation 40:157–161
86. Snydman DR, Werner BG, Heinze-Lacey B et al. (1987) Use of cytomegalovirus immune globulin to prevent cytomegalovirus disease in renal-transplant recipients. N Engl J Med 317:1049–1054
87. Spector SA, Hirata KK, Neuman PR (1984) Identification of multiple cytomegalovirus strains in homosexual men with acquired immunodeficiency syndrome. J Infect Dis 150:953–956
88. Starr SE, Glazer JP, Friedman HM et al. (1981) Specific cellular and humoral immunity following immunization with live Towne strain of cytomegalovirus vaccine. J Infect Dis 143:585–589
89. Starzl TE, Klintmalm GBG, Porter KA et al. (1981) Liver transplantation with use of cyclosporin A and prednisone. N Engl J Med 305:266–269
90. Sterner G, Agell BO, Sahren B, Espmark A (1970) Acquired cytomegalovirus infection in older children and adults. Scand J Infect Dis 2:95–103
91. Taylor DL, Taylor-Robinson D, Jeffries DJ, Tyms AS (1988) Characterization of cytomegalovirus isolates from patients with AIDS by DNA-restriction analysis. Epidemiol Infect 101:483–493
92. Toorkey CB, Carrigan DR (1989) Immunohistochemical detection of an immediate early antigen of human cytomegalovirus in normal tissues. J Infect Dis 160:741–751
93. Via CS, Shanley JD, Weatherly BR et al. (1988) Altered threshold for the induction of graft-versus-host immunodeficiency following murine cytomegalovirus infection. Transplantation 30:298–302

94. Von Willebrand EV, Pettersson E, Ahonen J, Hayry P (1986) CMV infection, class II antigen expression, and human kidney allograft rejection. Transplantation 42:364–367
95. Wade JC, Hintz M, McGuffin RW, Springmeyer SC, Conner JD, Meyers JD (1982) Treatment of cytomegalovirus pneumonia with high-dose acyclovir. Am J Med 73:249–256
96. Wade JC, Newton B, Flournoy N, Meyers JD (1984) Oral acyclovir for prevention of herpes simplex virus reactivation after marrow transplant. Ann Intern Med 100:823–828
97. Weir MR, Irwin BC, Maters AW et al. (1987) Incidence of cytomegalovirus disease in cyclosporine-treated renal transplant recipients based on donor/recipient pretransplant immunity. Transplantation 43:187–193
98. Wilhelm JA, Matter L, Schopfer K (1986) The risk of transmitting cytomegalovirus to patients receiving blood transfusions. J Infect Dis 154:169–171
99. Wingard JR, Chen DY-H, Burns WH et al. (1988) Cytomegalovirus infection after autologous bone marrow transplantation with comparison to infection after allogenic bone marrow transplantation. Blood 71:1432–1437
100. Winston DJ, Pollard RB, Ho WG et al. (1982) Cytomegalovirus immune plasma in bone marrow transplant recipients. Ann Intern Med 97:11–18
101. Winston DJ, Huang ES, Miller MJ et al. (1985) Molecular epidemiology of cytomegalovirus infections associated with bone marrow transplantation. Ann Intern Med 102:16–20
102. Winston DJ, Ho WG, Lin CH et al. (1987) Intravenous immune globulin for prevention of cytomegalovirus infection and interstitial pneumonia after bone marrow transplantation. Ann Intern Med 106:12–18
103. Wu BC, Dowling JN, Ho M et al. (1975) Enhancement of mouse cytomegalovirus infection during host versus graft reaction. Science 190:56–58
104. Yamashiroya HM, Ghosh L, Yang R, Robertson AL (1988) Herpesviridae in the coronary arteries and aorta of young trauma victims. Am J Pathol 130:71–79

Chapter 11 Cytomegalovirus Infection in Bone Marrow Transplantation

Drew J. Winston

Summary

Cytomegalovirus (CMV) infection occurs in approximately 50% of all marrow transplant recipients, but is more common in CMV-seropositive patients than CMV-seronegative patients. Sources of infection include reactivation of latent endogenous virus, blood products from CMV-seropositive blood donors, and bone marrow from a CMV-seropositive donor. The most common and severe clinical syndrome associated with CMV infection is interstitial pneumonia, which occurs in about 15% of all allotransplants but is less frequent in syngeneic and autologous transplants. Risk factors for CMV pneumonia include CMV-seropositivity before transplant, older age, conditioning with total-body irradiation, and severe graft-versus-host disease (GVHD). The rapid diagnosis of CMV pneumonia has been facilitated by using CMV monoclonal antibodies in either immunochemical stains or centrifugation cell cultures of bronchoalveolar lavage fluid. Treatment of CMV pneumonia remains problematic, but therapy with a combination of intravenous immune globulin (IVIG) plus ganciclovir has resulted in the best survival rates. In CMV-seronegative patients, CMV infection and pneumonia can be prevented or modified by the use of CMV-seronegative blood products and IVIG. IVIG also reduces other infections and GVHD. For CMV-seropositive patients, effective prophylaxis for CMV reactivation and pneumonia has not yet been established, but trials of prophylactic ganciclovir are being conducted.

Introduction

Bone marrow transplantation is increasingly used in the treatment of aplastic anemia, hematologic malignancy, solid tumors, genetic diseases, metabolic deficiencies, and primary immunodeficiency conditions [6]. Over 4000 patients per year receive allogeneic bone marrow transplants from related or unrelated donors, while more than 1500 autologous transplants are being performed annually. There are more than 250 marrow transplant centers worldwide. Major complications of transplantation include toxicity of the conditioning regimen, graft rejection or failure, graft-versus-host disease (GVHD), relapse of under-

Division of Hematology/Oncology, University of California Medical Center, 10833 Le Conte Avenue, Los Angeles, CA90024-1678, USA lying disease, immunodeficiency, and infection [82]. Many of the risk factors and common infections associated with bone marrow transplantation are now well defined as a result of clinical and laboratory studies performed over the last two decades [36, 98, 103]. Among the viral pathogens producing disease in marrow transplant recipients, cytomegalovirus (CMV) causes the greatest morbidity and mortality [42, 106]. This review will focus on recent progress in defining the epidemiology and pathogenesis of CMV infection after marrow transplantation and current approaches for controlling the infection.

Epidemiology of Cytomegalovirus Infection and Disease

The incidences of cytomegalovirus (CMV) infection after allogeneic and autologous transplantation at different centers are shown in Tables 1 and 2. Approximately 50% of allogeneic transplant recipients develop CMV infection [38, 42, 45, 48, 51, 92, 94], which is similar to the 40%–45% incidence of infection after autologous transplantation [60, 91]. CMV infections are more common in patients who are seropositive before transplant (mean incidence of 65%, range 42%–87%) than in patients who are CMV-seronegative (mean incidence of 31%, range 13%–54%; Table 1).

The most consistent risk factors for CMV infection are CMV infection in the marrow recipient before transplant (usually defined as seropositivity for CMV antibody), frequent blood transfusions (especially granulocyte transfusions) from CMV-seropositive donors, and, in allogeneic transplants, a CMV-seropositive marrow donor for a CMV-seronegative recipient [42, 106]. Acute GVHD has also been correlated with an increased likelihood of CMV infection in some studies [42, 45, 51] but not others [92, 94, 106].

It is assumed that viral reactivation is responsible for most infections in CMV-seropositive patients. Indeed, studies of the molecular epidemiology of CMV infection after marrow transplantation show that CMV-seropositive patients can develop pneumonia after transplantation, caused by a CMV strain genetically identical to a CMV isolate present in the urine pretransplant [99]. Nonetheless, these observations do not preclude the possibility of exogeneous infection with a different CMV strain [37] as described in renal and cardiac transplants [14, 28]. The mechanism of viral reactivation is not completely understood but may be related to effects of immunosuppressive therapy [32, 34] or immunological events associated with graft-versus-host disease (GVHD) [18].

In CMV-seronegative marrow transplant recipients, primary CMV infection can be acquired from blood products or bone marrow from a CMV-seropositive donor. The risk of acquiring CMV from blood products is greatest in patients receiving granulocyte transfusions or other blood products from CMV-seropositive blood donors [9, 30, 95]. In contrast, CMV-seronegative patients transfused with blood products only from CMV-seronegative donors have a much lower incidence of CMV infection [8, 9]. Similarly, the use of a CMV-seronegative marrow donor instead of a CMV-seropositive donor de-

Table 1. Incidence of cytomegalovirus infection after allogeneic bone marrow transplantation (adapted from [106] with permission)

Pretransplant CMV serology	Seattle, 1977 Neiman et al. [48]	UCLA, 1979 Winston et al. [94]	Seattle, 1980 Meyers et al. [38]	Seattle, 1986 Meyers et al. [42]	Sweden, 1986 Paulin et al. [51]	Minnesota, 1986 Miller et al. [45]	Johns Hopkins, 1988 Wingard et al. [92]
Seronegative (*n*)	44	30	79	285	22	137	115
No. infected	10	12	43	103	8	26	15
Percentage infected	23	40	54	36	35	19	13
Seropositive (*n*)	36	10	79	258	45	44	232
No. infected	27	6	49	178	39	28	97
Percentage infected	75	60	62	69	87	64	42
Total patients (*n*)	80	40	158	543	67	181	347
Total infected (*n*)	37	18	92	281	47	54	112
Total infected (%)	46	45	58	52	70	30	32

Table 2. Incidence of cytomegalovirus infection and disease after autologous bone marrow transplantation (adapted from [105])

Reference	Patients			Patients			Other CMV disease
	Total	CMV infection		Total	CMV pneumonia		
	(*n*)	*n*	%	(*n*)	*n*	%	
Seattle, 1986, Pecego et al. [52]				70	3	4.0	
Johns Hopkins, 1988, Wingard et al. [91, 93]	143	65	45	143	3	2.0	Delay in platelet and neutrophil recovery
Institute Gustave-Roussy, 1988, Valteau et al. [84]				165	5	3.0	
UCLA, 1988, Winston et al. [105]				139	1	0.7	
Seattle, 1988, Reusser et al. [60]	159	63	40	159	12	8.0	
Total	302	128	42	676	24	3.5	

creases the risk of CMV infection in a CMV-negative recipient [42, 106]. On the other hand, when the transplant recipient is CMV seropositive before the transplant, the serologic status of the marrow donor has no effect.

Immunity to CMV

Evaluation of the immune response to CMV in marrow transplants is complex due to multiple factors affecting the immune response, including immunocompetent cells of donor origin, immunosuppressive agents, and GVHD. CMV infection itself also affects the host immune system [63].

It is generally believed that cell-mediated immunity is of primary importance in determining the severity and outcome of CMV infection in bone marrow transplant recipients. Whereas the activity of nonspecific cytotoxic cells correlates poorly with the outcome of CMV infection, T-cell activity against CMV-specific target cells appears to be an important determinant of the outcome of CMV infection. It has been shown that all marrow transplant recipients have depressed CMV-specific cytotoxic T-lymphocyte activity before the onset of CMV infection. However, CMV-specific T-cell cytotoxicity usually develops in survivors of infection and rarely in patients with fatal CMV infection [10, 54].

While it is clear that CMV-specific antibody does not necessarily protect against the development of CMV infection, current evidence suggests that humoral immunity can modify the severity of infection. Bone marrow transplant recipients can produce antibodies to a wide range of CMV proteins in a pattern similar to that shown by persons with natural infection [110]. Some studies describe a lower mortality from CMV pneumonia in marrow transplant recipients who develop an antibody response to the virus [48, 94], although other studies were not able to confirm this observation [38]. Passively acquired CMV antibody prevents viral replication and dissemination and protects against lethal infection in murine models of CMV infection [3, 64, 70, 71]. Administration of CMV immune globulin or plasma to CMV-seronegative recipients of bone marrow or a renal allograft reduces the incidence of CMV pneumonia and other CMV-related clinical syndromes [41, 49, 81, 97, 100].

The importance of donor immunity to CMV on the incidence and outcome of CMV infection after marrow transplantation is uncertain. Both cellular and humoral immunity are transferred by bone marrow transplantation, and donor lymphocytes of T and B cell type predominate after successful grafting [66, 89, 108]. Nonetheless, most studies have found no significant correlation between the donor's CMV immune status and the outcome of CMV infection in the marrow recipient [27, 39, 42, 61].

Clinical Manifestations of CMV Disease

CMV disease usually appears between 3 and 16 weeks after transplantation [2, 38, 42, 106]. Persistent unexplained fever and nonspecific constitutional symptoms in the presence of cultures negative for bacteria and fungi are frequently the initial manifestations. Patients may also develop leukopenia, thrombocytopenia, or hepatitis, but it is frequently difficult to distinguish GVHD or drug toxicity from CMV infection as the cause of these complications. A liver biopsy rarely shows intranuclear inclusion bodies and is frequently negative for CMV in culture. CMV is the most common infectious cause of esophagitis, and enigmatic nausea and vomiting after marrow transplantation, but endoscopy with biopsy, brushings, and culture is required for distinguishing CMV infection from herpes simplex infection or GVHD of the gastrointestinal (GI) tract [35, 76]. Interstitial pneumonia associated with CMV is the clinical syndrome of greatest significance in allogeneic marrow transplant recipients and is discussed below. Hemorrhagic cystitis, retinitis, and central nervous system (CNS) disease are rare manifestations of CMV infection in marrow transplant recipients. Delay in recovery of the neutrophil and platelet counts has been reported in autologous transplant recipients with CMV infection [91].

Confirmation of the diagnosis of CMV infection in marrow transplant recipients is best achieved by isolation of virus from a culture of body fluids or tissue. The oropharynx, buffy coat, urine, lung, and GI tract are the most frequent sites from which CMV is isolated [38, 42, 44, 48, 94]. However, isolation of CMV from a particular site is not conclusive proof that CMV is a pathogen and requires correlation with clinical symptoms and signs and the exclusion of other possible pathogens or noninfectious causes to determine its significance. Indeed, CMV has been isolated from the bronchoalveolar lavage fluid of bone marrow transplant recipients without pneumonia [65, 68, 96], while CMV may continue to be excreted in the urine or oropharynx for several months without any symptoms [38, 42, 44, 48, 94]. The detection of CMV in tissue culture has been recently enhanced by the rapid centrifugation culture technique [22, 23]. Serologic tests on blood for the rapid diagnosis of CMV infection (such as CMV IgM antibody) lack sensitivity in marrow transplant recipients [50]. Similarly, CMV intranuclear inclusions are rarely numerous in tissue specimens and cannot be relied upon for diagnosis [47]. On the other hand, more sensitive techniques for detection of CMV, such as DNA–DNA or DNA–RNA hybridization and the polymerase chain reaction, frequently lack specificity and may not be predictive of CMV disease [17, 31, 47, 75].

Interstitial Pneumonia Associated with CMV

Interstitial pneumonia occurs in 20%–40% of allogeneic marrow transplants (Table 3) [39, 86, 87, 92, 106]. CMV is associated with approximately one half of the cases; thus, the average incidence of CMV interstitial pneumonia among allogeneic transplants is 15%. In contrast, CMV interstitial pneumonia is uncommon after syngeneic (no cases reported in 100 identical-twin transplants

Table 3. Incidence of interstitial pneumonia after allogeneic bone marrow transplantation (adapted from [106] with permission)

Type of pneumonia	Seattle, 1969–1979, Meyers et al. [39]		UCLA, 1974–1987, Winston et al. [106]		Johns Hopkins, 1976–1985, Wingard et al. [92]		International marrow transplant registry, 1978–1983, Weiner et al. [87] [a]		International marrow transplant registry, 1978–1985, Weiner et al. [86] [b]	
	n	%	*n*	%	*n*	%	*n*	%	*n*	%
Cytomegalovirus	85	15	67	14	45	12	99	11	31	7
Idiopathic	63	12	34	7	57	15	134	14	32	7
Pneumocystis	34	6	7	2	6	2	11	1	} 16	4
Other viruses	16	3	4	1	5	1	11	1		
Clinically diagnosed	32	6	–		53	14	13	1		
Total [c]	215/525	41	112/469	24	166/386	43	268/932	29	79/439	18

[a] Only patients with leukemia
[b] Only patients with severe aplastic anemia
[c] Number of patients with pneumonia/total number patients in group

Table 4. Severity of cytomegalovirus infection in allogeneic bone marrow transplant recipients, shown by pretransplant cytomegalovirus serology (adapted from [106])

Reference	Pretransplant CMV serology	Patients	CMV infection		CMV pneumonia	
		n	*n*	%	*n*	%
Seattle, 1986, Meyers et al. [42]	Negative vs positive	285 258	103 178	36 vs 69	30 60	10 vs 23
Minnesota, 1986, Miller et al. [45]	Negative vs positive	137 44	26 28	19 vs 64	12 11	9 vs 25
Johns Hopkins, 1988, Wingard et al. [92]	Negative vs positive	115 232	15 97	13 vs 42	1 37	1 vs 16

from Seattle [1]) and autologous transplantation (3.5% incidence, Table 2) [52, 60, 84, 91, 93, 105]. CMV-seropositive patients have a higher incidence of CMV pneumonia (16%–25%) than CMV-seronegative patients (1%–10%; Table 4) [42, 45, 92, 106]. Patients with aplastic anemia not treated with radiation also experience fewer pneumonias than leukemia patients who usually receive radiation therapy [39, 40, 86, 87, 92]. Most of the other interstitial pneumonias are either idiopathic or less commonly caused by other viruses or *Pneumocystis carinii.* The idiopathic cases have been attributed to pulmonary toxicity of the pretransplant chemotherapy and radiotherapy used to prepare the patient for transplantation [40, 87]. The overall mortality from interstitial pneumonia is high (60%–80%) and is somewhat greater in patients with CMV pneumonia (80–90%) than in patients with idiopathic pneumonia (60–80%). Administration of prophylactic trimethoprim-sulfamethoxazole has greatly reduced the incidence and mortality of pneumonia due to *Pneumocystis carinii* [101].

Risk factors for the development of interstitial pneumonia are CMV-seropositivity before the transplant, older age, severe GVHD, pretransplant conditioning with total body irradiation, and the use of posttransplant methotrexate instead of cyclosporine for GVHD prophylaxis [39, 87, 92, 106]. Interestingly, UCLA and other transplant centers [92] have noted a decrease in interstitial pneumonia among allogeneic marrow transplant recipients since 1983. As shown in Fig. 1, the overall incidence of interstitial pneumonia at UCLA was 32% before 1984 but only 14% from 1984 to 1988. The decline in pneumonia was due more to a decrease in CMV pneumonia than to a change in the incidence of idiopathic pneumonia. The reasons for the lower incidence of CMV interstitial pneumonia are not entirely clear but may include better control of GVHD with cyclosporine or T-cell depletion of the donor marrow, the use of CMV-seronegative blood products and intravenous immune globulin in CMV-seronegative patients, and the use of prophylactic antiviral drugs in CMV-seropositive patients.

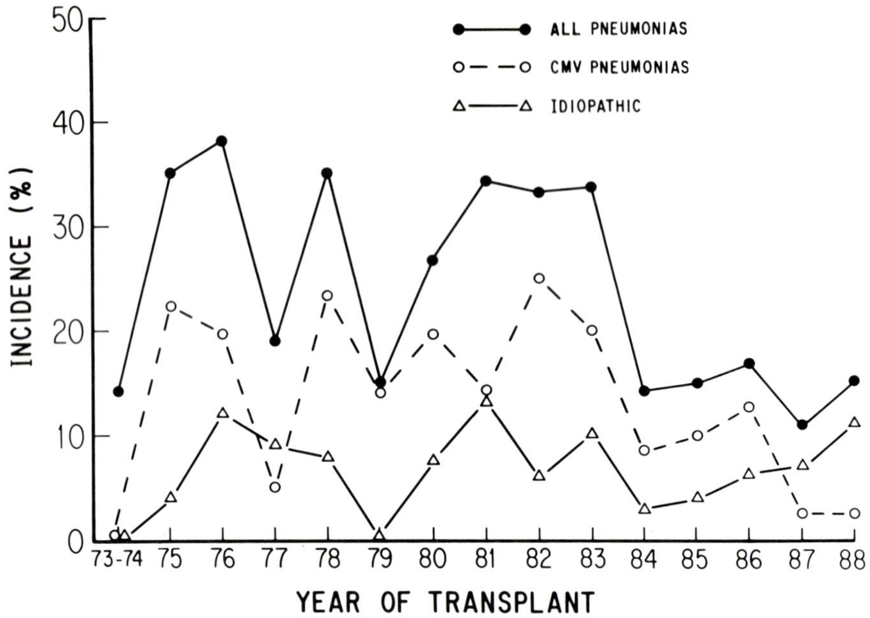

Fig. 1. Incidence of interstitial pneumonia, by year of transplantation, among recipients of allogeneic marrow transplants at the University of California, Los Angeles, between 1973 and 1988 (adapted from [106])

The pathogenesis of CMV interstitial pneumonia after bone marrow transplantation has been the subject of considerable speculation. The simplest explanation is that the immunosuppressive agents and radiation used before and after the transplant impair the patient's ability to control replication and dissemination of the virus and damage to the pulmonary tissues [10, 38, 54, 87, 96]. However, despite a similar incidence of CMV infection and the use of similar immunosuppressive agents among all types of marrow transplants, CMV pneumonia is rare in both syngeneic twin transplants and autologous transplants [1, 52, 60, 84, 91, 93, 105]. On the other hand, GVHD, which is not an expected complication of syngeneic or autologous transplantation, is commonly associated with CMV interstitial pneumonia in allogeneic transplants [39, 87, 92, 106]. These observations suggest that immunological events associated with GVHD may be involved in the development of CMV pneumonia [29]. Indeed, CMV pneumonia in both marrow transplant patients and animals is associated with an increased number of cytotoxic T cells in the lungs [11, 73], and the absence of these T cells in athymic/nude mice prevents CMV pneumonia despite viral replication in the lung tissue [69]. The blockage of a T-cell response by immunomodulating agents may explain the lower mortality of CMV pneumonia in transplant patients treated with intravenous immune globulin plus ganciclovir [20, 57] and in mice treated with continuous cyclophosphamide [72].

Interstitial pneumonia associated with CMV typically occurs between 3 and 12 weeks after transplant and has a median time to onset of 7 weeks [39, 87, 92, 106]. Interstitial pneumonias occurring earlier, before 3 weeks, or later, after 12 weeks, are usually idiopathic or caused by other organisms [39, 90, 106]. The onset may be rapid, with fulminant respiratory failure developing over 2–3 days in association with bilateral diffuse interstitial infiltrates [5]. Many other cases have a more insidious course characterized by prolonged fever for one or more weeks followed by the development of a nonproductive cough, dyspnea, and lower lobe interstitial infiltrates which progress to more diffuse infiltrates. Previous CMV viremia has been associated with an increased risk of subsequent CMV pneumonia in some studies [13, 44] but not in others [109]. Detection of CMV in routine bronchoalveolar lavage at day 35 after transplant may also be predictive of the later development of CMV pneumonia [68]. Open lung biopsy was once considered the procedure of choice for the diagnosis of CMV pneumonia [77]. However, the use of the centrifugation culture technique, direct immunochemical staining with CMV monoclonal antibodies, and DNA hybridization have greatly enhanced the sensitivity of bronchoalveolar lavage for the diagnosis of CMV pneumonia and obviated the need for open lung biopsy in many cases [15, 16, 19, 24]. Cytological methods are the least sensitive for diagnosis. Centrifugation culture is more sensitive than direct immunochemical staining which is more sensitive than DNA hybridization for finding CMV in bronchoalveolar lavage fluid.

Treatment of CMV Disease

Previously available antiviral agents were ineffective therapy for CMV pneumonia in marrow transplant recipients. Earlier studies used vidarabine (adenine arabinoside), human leukocyte interferon, acyclovir, recombinant leukocyte interferon, lymphoblastoid interferon, foscarnet (trisodium phosphonoformate), or combinations of these agents [101]. Responses were unfavorable in most cases and frequently associated with toxicity to the marrow, CNS, or kidneys.

More recently, ganciclovir has been used to treat CMV pneumonia in recipients of marrow transplants. Ganciclovir is approximately 50-fold more active in vitro than acyclovir against CMV isolates [83]. Nonetheless, despite the elimination of CMV from cultures of respiratory secretions and other body fluids, only 6 of 30 patients (20%) with CMV pneumonia treated with ganciclovir at the Seattle, Minnesota, and University of California in Los Angeles (UCLA) transplant centers survived [21, 74, 102, 104]. Combining the anti-inflammatory effect of high doses of corticosteroids with the antiviral effects of ganciclovir also did not improve the outcome (only 1 of 6 patients survived) [55]. The most frequent toxicity of ganciclovir is neutropenia, which usually occurs after one or more weeks of therapy and is reversible after the drug is discontinued.

The results of using CMV immune globulin alone for treatment of CMV pneumonia have been conflicting. Nine of 18 marrow transplants with CMV pneumonia treated with a CMV immune globulin by Griffiths et al. [26] in London survived. In contrast, only 3 of 14 patients treated with a CMV immune globulin by Reed et al. [57] in Seattle survived. However, improved survival has been observed in recent uncontrolled trials combining CMV immune globulin (400 mg/kg every other day) or a polyvalent intravenous immune globulin containing CMV antibody (500 mg/kg every other day) with ganciclovir (7.5–10 mg/kg per day in 2 or 3 divided doses; Table 5) [4, 12, 20, 57, 67, 85, 107]. Patients who improve after 14–21 days of induction therapy are given maintenance therapy with ganciclovir (5 mg/kg per day, 5–7 times each week) and intravenous immune globulin (500 mg/kg once weekly), for at least 4 weeks. As summarized in Table 5, the overall survival among patients treated at seven transplant centers is 54%. Survival appears to be influenced by the need for mechanical ventilation at the start of therapy. At the Wisconsin, Sloan-Kettering, Seattle, and City of Hope transplant centers, where pa-

Table 5. Results of treatment of cytomegalovirus pneumonia after bone marrow transplantation with intravenous immune globulin plus ganciclovir (adapted from [107])

Reference	Treatment	Response			Ventilator-dependent at start of therapy
		Survivors	Treated		
		n	*n*	%	
Wisconsin, 1987, Bratanow et al. [12]	Immune globulin (Gamimune) + ganciclovir	6	12	50	No data
Sloan-Kettering, 1988, Emanuel et al. [20]	Immune globulin (Gammagard) + ganciclovir	7	10	70	None
Seattle, 1988, Reed et al. [57]	CMV immune globulin (Cutter) + ganciclovir	13	24	52	None (ventilator pts excluded)
City of Hope, 1988, Schmidt [67]	Immune globulin (Gammagard) + ganciclovir	11	13	85	None
Innsbruck, 1988, Aulitzky et al. [4]	Immune globulin (Sandoglobulin) + ganciclovir	1	4	25	3 patients
Utrecht, 1989, Verdonck et al. [85]	CMV immune globulin (Cytotect) + ganciclovir	0	4	0	2 patients
UCLA, 1989, Winston et al. [107]	Immune globulin (Gammagard) + ganciclovir	3	8	38	5 patients
		41	76	54	

tients requiring mechanical ventilation were excluded from therapy, survival was 50%–85%. At the Innsbruck, Utrecht, and UCLA transplant centers, where patients requiring mechanical ventilation were not excluded, survival was 0%–38%. At UCLA, none of five patients on mechanical ventilation at the start of therapy with ganciclovir plus intravenous immune globulin for CMV pneumonia survived. On the other hand, three of three patients with interstitial infiltrates on chest X-ray due to CMV but minimal respiratory systems survived [107]. These data suggest that combination therapy with ganciclovir plus intravenous immune globulin is more likely to be effective when the diagnosis of CMV pneumonia is established earlier. The detection of CMV in routine bronchoalveolar lavage at day 35 after transplant may be a predictor for the later development of interstitial pneumonia and thus a basis for the early initiation of therapy [68]. The mechanism by which the combination of ganciclovir and intravenous immune globulin is effective is not clearly understood. It has been speculated that CMV pneumonia after marrow transplantation involves abnormal immune responses which are blocked by the intravenous immune globulin [29]. Ganciclovir plus CMV antiserum is also more effective for murine CMV infection than treatment with either agent alone [88].

There are no controlled studies supporting the efficacy of either intravenous immune globulin or ganciclovir given singly or in combination for treatment of other CMV diseases in marrow transplant recipients. Ganciclovir alone has been used to treat CMV GI infection, retinitis, and wasting syndrome [21, 102, 104]. However, in a randomized, double-blind, placebo-controlled trial, treatment of CMV gastroenteritis with two weeks of ganciclovir was not associated with clinical or endoscopic improvement compared to placebo and supportive care [59]. Whether the addition of intravenous immune globulin to ganciclovir would improve the effectiveness of therapy for CMV gastroenteritis or other CMV diseases is not known and requires additional controlled studies.

Prevention of CMV Infection and Disease

Due to the ineffectiveness of previous antiviral drugs for prevention or treatment of CMV infection and pneumonia, many of the earliest prophylactic trials in recipients of marrow transplants used passive immunization with immune plasma or globulin containing CMV antibodies. These trials were based upon clinical observations that CMV antibody snythesis is associated with less severe CMV infection [48, 94] and animal studies demonstrating that passive immunoprophylaxis modifies the severity of CMV infection (Table 6) [3, 64, 70, 71, 78].

Table 7 summarizes the results of six controlled trials of prophylactic CMV immune plasma, CMV hyperimmune globulin, or polyvalent intravenous immune globulin containing CMV antibodies [8, 33, 41, 49, 97, 100]. Most of the patients in these trials were seronegative for CMV antibody before transplan-

Table 6. Results of passive cytomegalovirus immunoprophylaxis in murine animal models (adapted from [104])

Reference	Results	Benefit
Starr and Allison [78[	CMV immune serum not effective when given in a single dose 24 h after infection	No
Araullo-Cruz et al. [3]	CMV immune serum protective from lethal infection when given 24 h before infection	Yes
Shanley et al. [71]	CMV immune serum prevents viral replication and reduces viral dissemination when given before infection	Yes
Shanley and Pesanti [70]	CMV immune serum reduces virus in lungs and severity of pneumonia when given after infection	Yes
Rubin et al. [64]	CMV immune serum protects against lethal infection when given as long as 24 h after infection	Yes

tation. Five of the six studies found a beneficial effect of passive immunoprophylaxis for modifying the severity of CMV infection and reducing the incidence of CMV pneumonia. In the one study showing no beneficial results, from Seattle [8], the incidence of CMV pneumonia in the control patients (5%) was much lower than the incidence of pneumonia in the controls in the other trials (20%–33%) and likely precluded any opportunity to demonstrate the alleviating effect of immune globulin on the severity of CMV infection observed in the other studies.

Another approach for prevention of CMV infection and pneumonia in CMV-seronegative transplants is the exclusive use of CMV-seronegative blood products [8, 46, 101]. The effectiveness of this approach and the significant expense of intravenous immune globulin has raised questions about the need and cost-effectiveness of intravenous immune globulin in CMV-seronegative marrow transplants. We have been conducting a controlled trial at UCLA of prophylactic intravenous immune globulin (1000 mg/kg once weekly from 7 days before to 120 days after transplant) in CMV-seronegative marrow transplants receiving only CMV-seronegative blood products [107]. Preliminary results are shown in Table 8. The overall incidence of CMV infection was very low in both groups. There were no cases of CMV-associated interstitial pneumonia. These results suggest that intravenous immune globulin is not necessary for the prevention or modification of CMV infection in CMV-seronegative patients receiving only CMV-seronegative blood products. On the other hand, the incidence of GVHD was lower in patients receiving intravenous immune globulin (7 of 17 or 41% vs 12 of 17 or 71%) and is similar to the reduction of GVHD reported in previous trials of intravenous immune globulin (Table 9) [79, 100]. In addition, intravenous immune globulin has been found to lower the number of bacterial, fungal, and other viral infections in marrow transplants [25, 53, 79]. Thus, in CMV-seronegative patients receiving CMV-seronegative blood products, intravenous immune

Table 7. Results of controlled trials of prophylactic immune plasma or globulin in allogeneic bone marrow transplants

Reference	Regimen	Patients						Benefit	Comments
			CMV infection			CMV pneumonia			
		n	*n*	%	*n*	*n*	%		
UCLA, 1982, Winston et al. [97]	CMV immune plasma vs *no* prophylaxis	24 24	12 15	50 vs 63	24 24	3 8	13 vs 33	Yes	Greater benefit with *no* WBC transfusions
Seattle, 1983, Meyers et al. [41]	CMV immune globulin vs *no* prophylaxis	30 32	10 14	33 vs 44	30 32	2 3	7 vs 9	Yes	Greater benefit with *no* WBC transfusions
Sloan-Kettering, 1983, O'Reilly et al. [49]	CMV immune globulin vs *no* prophylaxis	17 20	0 10	0 vs 50	17 20	0 6	0 vs 30	Yes	
Europe, 1985, Kubanek et al. [33]	CMV immune globulin vs normal immune globulin				26 23	1 6	4 vs 20	Yes	
Seattle, 1986, Bowden et al. [8]	CMV immune globulin vs *no* prophylaxis	21 20	5 8	24 vs 40	21 20	1 1	5 vs 5	No	Very low incidence of pneumonia in controls
UCLA, 1987, Winston et al. [100]	Gamimune vs *no* prophylaxis	38 37	18 21	48 vs 54	38 37	6 12	10 vs 32	Yes	
Total	Immune plasma/globulin vs controls	130 133	45 68	35 vs 51	156 156	13 36	8 vs 23		

Table 8. Results of University of California, Los Angeles, controlled trial of intravenous immune globulin in cytomegalovirus (CMV) seronegative allogeneic bone marrow transplant patients receiving CMV seronegative blood products (adapted from [107])

	CMV-seronegative blood	CMV-seronegative blood + IVIG [a]
No. of patients	17	17
CMV infection	2 (12%) [b]	0
CMV pneumonia	0	0
Idiopathic interstitial pneumonia	1	2
Acute graft-versus-host disease	12 (71%)	7 (41%)

IVIG, intravenous immune globulin
[a] 1000 mg/kg IVIG once weekly, days −7 to +120
[b] Both CMV infections asymptomatic

Table 9. Effects of intravenous immune globulin on acute graft-versus-host disease (adapted from [107] with permission)

Reference	IVIG regimen	Controls			IVIG			*p* value
			Acute GVHD			Acute GVHD		
		n	*n*	%	*n*	*n*	%	
UCLA, 1987, Winston et al. [100]	1000 mg/kg Gamimune, once weekly, days −7 to +120	37	24	65	38	13	34	0.01
Seattle, 1988, Sullivan et al. [79]	500 mg/kg Gamimune, once weekly, days −7 to +90; once monthly, days +120 to +360	185	107	58	183	79	43	0.02
UCLA, 1989, Winston et al. [107]	1000 mg/kg Sandoglobulin, once weekly, days −7 to +120	17	12	71	17	7	41	0.16
		239	143	60	238	89	37	

globulin appears to have a beneficial role in the modification of GVHD and in preventing infections other than CMV.

Trials of immune plasma or globulin in CMV-seropositive patients are summarized in Table 10 [62, 80, 97, 100]. The Nordic transplant group reported no apparent prevention of CMV pneumonia by CMV immune plasma, but the low incidence of pneumonia in the control patients likely prevented any possibility of detecting a difference. In contrast, earlier studies from UCLA

Table 10. Results of controlled trials of prophylactic immune plasma or globulin in cytomegalovirus (CMV)-seropositive allogeneic bone marrow transplants (adapted from [107] with permission)

Reference	Regimen	Patients						Benefit
			CMV infection			Interstitial pneumonia		
		n	*n*	%	*n*	*n*	%	
Nordic, 1987, Ringden et al. [62]	CMV immune plasma vs controls	27	21	78	27	3	11	No
			vs			vs		
		27	18	67	27	3	11	
UCLA, 1982, 1989, Winston et al. [97, 100]	CMV immune plasma or gamimune vs controls	11	3	27	11	0	0	Yes
			vs			vs		
		11	6	55	11	4	36	
Seattle, 1990, Sullivan et al. [80]	Gamimune vs controls				154	20	13 vs	Yes
					154	34	22	
	Immune plasma/globulin vs controls	38	24	63	192	23	12	
			vs			vs		
		38	24	63	192	41	21	

and a much larger study from Seattle found a reduction in interstitial pneumonia in CMV-seropositive patients receiving intravenous immune globulin. Multivariate analysis of the Seattle data indicated the reduction of interstitial pneumonia by intravenous immune globulin may be related to a modification of GVHD [80]. Thus, intravenous immune globulin may benefit CMV-seropositive patients by modifying GVHD, reducing the risk for interstitial pneumonia, and lowering the number of bacterial infections.

Antiviral drugs have also been used for prophylaxis of CMV reactivation and pneumonia in patients who are CMV-seropositive before transplantation. Previous trials of prophylactic vidarabine (adenine arabinoside), human leukocyte interferon, and low-dose acyclovir showed no benefit [101]. Recently, prophylactic high-dose intravenous acyclovir and ganciclovir have been evaluated in CMV-seropositive patients. In the acyclovir trial, patients seropositive for both CMV and herpes simplex viral antibodies were given high doses of prophylactic intravenous acyclovir (500 mg/m^2 every 8 h for 5 days before to 30 days after transplant) and compared with nonrandomized control patients who were seropositive for CMV but seronegative for herpes simplex [43]. The incidences of CMV infection and pneumonia were high in both groups but less in the recipients of high-dose acyclovir (Table 11). In a trial of prophylactic ganciclovir at UCLA, ganciclovir is given at a dosage of 2.5 mg/kg every 8 h for 1 week before transplantation and then stopped on the day of infusion of the donor marrow [102, 106]. After transplantation, when the granulocyte count reaches 1000 cells/mm^3, the ganciclovir is resumed at a

Table 11. Effects of intravenous high-dose acyclovir or ganciclovir on prevention of cytomegalovirus (CMV) reactivation and pneumonia in CMV-seropositive allogeneic bone marrow transplant recipients (adapted from [106] with permission)

Reference	Study groups	Patients						Comments
			CMV infection			CMV pneumonia		
		n	*n*	%	*n*	*n*	%	
Seattle and Minnesota [43]	Acyclovir vs controls	85 65	51 49	59 vs 75	86 65	16 20	19 vs 31	Nor randomized
UCLA [106]	Ganciclovir vs placebo, double blinded	68	22	32	68	6	9	Study code not broken; neutropenia in 28 of 68 (41%) patients

dosage of 6 mg/kg per day, Monday through Friday, until day 120 after transplantation. The trial is double-blinded and placebo-controlled; the study code has not been broken. Nonetheless, the overall incidences of CMV infection (32%) and pneumonia (9%) are approximately one half of the expected incidences of infection and pneumonia in CMV-seropositive patients and are much less than the incidences of infection and pneumonia in patients given prophylactic high-dose intravenous acyclovir. A similar double-blinded, placebo-controlled study of prophylactic ganciclovir is being conducted at the Seattle transplant center, expect that the ganciclovir or placebo is being administered only to patients who excrete CMV after transplant [7].

Acknowledgement. This work was supported by grant CA23175 from the National Cancer Institute.

References

1. Appelbaum FR, Meyers JD, Fefer A, Flournoy N, Cheever MA, Greenberg PD, Hackman R, Thomas ED (1982) Nonbacterial nonfungal pneumonia following marrow transplantation in 100 identical twins. Transplantation 33:265–268
2. Apperly JF, Goldman JM (1988) Cytomegalovirus: biology, clinical features and methods for diagnosis. Bone Marrow Transplant 2:253–264
3. Araullo-Cruz TP, Ho M, Armstrong JA (1978) Protective effect of early serum from mice after cytomegalovirus infection. Infect Immun 21:840–842
4. Aulitzky WE, Tilg H, Niederweiser D, Hack M, Meister B, Huber C (1988) Human monoclonal antibodies neutralizing cytomegalovirus (CMV) for prophylaxis of CMV disease: report of a phase 1 trial in bone marrow transplant recipients. J Infect Dis 158:488–489

5. Beschorner WE, Hutchins GM, Burns WH, Saral R, Tutschka P, Santos GW (1980) Cytomegalovirus pneumonia in bone marrow transplant recipients: miliary and diffuse patterns. Am Rev Respir Dis 122:107–114
6. Bortin MM, Rimm AA (1989) Increasing utilization of bone marrow transplantation. II. Results of the 1985–1987 survey. Transplantation 48:453–458
7. Bowden RA, Meyers JD (1990) Prophylaxis of cytomegalovirus infection. Semin Hematol 27 Suppl 1:17–21
8. Bowden RA, Sayers M, Flournoy N, Newton B, Banaji M, Thomas ED, Meyers JD (1986) Cytomegalovirus immune globulin and seronegative blood products to prevent primary cytomegalovirus infection after marrow transplantation. N Engl J Med 314:1006–1010
9. Bowden RA, Sayers M, Gleaves CA, Banaji B, Newton B, Meyers JD (1987) Cytomegalovirus-seronegative blood components for the prevention of primary cytomegalovirus infection after marrow transplantation. Considerations for blood banks. Transfusion 27:478–481
10. Bowden RA, Day LM, Amos DE, Meyers JD (1987) Natural cytotoxic activity against cytomegalovirus-infected target cells following marrow transplantation. Transplantation 44:504–507
11. Bowden RA, Dobbs S, Kopecky KJ, Crawford S, Meyers JD (1988) Increased cytotoxicity against cytomegalovirus-infected target cells by bronchoalveolar lavage cells from bone marrow transplant recipients with cytomegalovirus pneumonia. J Infect Dis 158:773–779
12. Bratanow NC, Ash RC, Turner PA, Smith R, Haasler G, Chitambar C, Hansen R, Casper J (1987) Successful treatment of serious cytomegalovirus (CMV) disease with 9(1,3-dihydroxy-2-propoxymethyl)guanine(ganciclovir, DHPG) and intravenious immunoglobulin (IVIG) in bone marrow transplant (BMT) patients (Abstract no 254). Exp Hematol 15:541
13. Bryson YJ, Jorgan MC, Winston DJ, Coloma L, Gale RP (1980) Prospective study of viral infections and interstitial pneumonia in bone marrow transplant recipients (Abstr). Clin Res 28:111 a
14. Chou S (1987) Cytomegalovirus infection and reinfection transmitted by heart transplantation. J Infect Dis 155:1054–1066
15. Cordonnier C, Escudier E, Nicolas JC, Fleury J, Deforges L, Ingrand D, Bircout F, Bernandin JF (1987) Evaluation of three assays on alveolar lavage fluid in the diagnosis of cytomegalovirus pneumonitis after bone marrow transplantation. J Infect Dis 155:495–500
16. Crawford SW, Bowde RA, Hackman RC, Gleaves CA, Meyers JD, Clark JG (1988) Rapid detection of cytomegalovirus pulmonary infection by bronchoalveolar lavage and centrifugation culture. Ann Intern Med 108:180–185
17. Dankner WM, McCutchan JA, Richman DD, Hirata K, Spector SA (1990) Localization of human cytomegalovirus in peripheral blood leukocytes by in situ hybridization. J Infect Dis 161:31–36
18. Dowling JN, Wu BC, Armstrong JA, Ho M (1977) Enhancement of murine cytomegalovirus infection during graft-versus-host reaction. J Infect Dis 135:990–994
19. Emanuel D, Peppard J, Stover D, Gold J, Armstrong D, Hammerling V (1986) Rapid immunodiagnosis of cytomegalovirus pneumonia by bronchoalveolar lavage using human and murine monoclonal antibodies. Ann Intern Med 104:476–481
20. Emanuel D, Cunningham I, Jules-Elysee K, Brochstein JA, Kerman NA, Laver J, Stover D, White DA, Fels A, Polsky B, Castro-Malaspina H, Peppard JR, Bartus P, Hammerling U, O'Reilly RJ (1988) Cytomegalovirus pneumonia after bone marrow transplantation successfully treated with the combination of ganciclovir and high-dose intravenous immune globulin. Ann Intern Med 109:777–782
21. Erice A, Jordan MC, Chace BA, Fletcher C, Chinnock BJ, Balfour HH (1987) Ganciclovir treatment of cytomegalovirus disease in transplant recipients and other immunocompromised hosts. JAMA 257:3082–3087

22. Gleaves CA, Smith TF, Shuster EA, Pearson GR (1985) Comparison of standard tube and shell vial cell culture techniques for the detection of cytomegalovirus in clinical specimens. J Clin Microbiol 21:217–221
23. Gleaves CA, Reed EC, Hackman RC, Meyers JD (1987) Rapid diagnosis of invasive cytomegalovirus infection by examination of tissue specimens in centrifugation culture. Am J Clin Pathol 88:354–358
24. Gleaves CA, Myerson D, Bowden RA, Hackman RC, Meyers JD (1988) Direct detection of cytomegalovirus from bronchoalveolar lavage using a rapid in situ DNA hybridization assay compared to centrifugation culture (abstr no 808). In: 28th Interscience Conference on Antimicrobial Agents and Chemotherapy. American Society for Microbiology, Washington, p 252
25. Graham-Pole J, Camitta B, Gross S, Herzig R, Koch P, Mahoney D, Casper J, Elfenbein G, Marcus R, Munoz L, Pick T, Spruce W, Steuber P, Weiner R (1988) Intravenous immunoglobulin may lessen all forms of injection in patients receiving allogeneic bone marrow transplantation for acute lymphoblastic leukemia: a Pediatric Oncology Group study. Bone Marrow Transplant 3:559–566
26. Griffiths PD, Stirk PR, Blacklock HA, Milburn HJ, DuBois RM, Prentice HG (1987) Rapid diagnosis and treatment of cytomegalovirus pneumonitis. In: Gale RP, Champlin RE (eds) Progress in bone marrow transplantation. Liss, New York, pp 583–587
27. Grob JP, Grundy JE, Prentice HG, Griffiths PD, Hoffbrand AV, Hughes MD, Tate T, Wimperis JZ, Brenner MK (1987) Immune donors can protect marrow-transplant recipients from severe cytomegalovirus infections. Lancet 1:774–776
28. Grundly JE, Super M, Griffiths PD (1986) Reinfection of seropositive allograft recipient by cytomegalovirus from donor kidney. Lancet 1:159–160
29. Grundy JE, Shanley JD, Griffiths PD (1987) Is cytomegalovirus interstitial pneumonitis in transplant recipients an immunopathological condition? Lancet 2:996–998
30. Hersman J, Meyers JD, Thomas ED, Buckner CD, Clift R (1982) The effect of granulocyte transfusions on the incidence of CMV infection after allogeneic marrow transplantation. Ann Intern Med 96:149–152
31. Hsia K, Spector DH, Lawrie J, Spector SA (1989) Enzymatic amplification of human cytomegalovirus sequences by polymerase chain reaction. J Clin Microbiol 27:1802–1809
32. Jordan MC, Shanley JD, Stevens JG (1977) Immunosuppression reactivates and disseminates latent murine cytomegalovirus. J Gen Virol 37:419–423
33. Kubanek B, Ernst P, Ostendorf P, Schaften U, Wolf PH (1985) Preliminary data of a controlled trial of intravenous hyperimmune globulin in the prevention of cytomegalovirus in bone marrow recipients. Transplant Proc 17:468–469
34. Mayo DR, Armstrong JA, Ho M (1977) Reactivation of murine cytomegalovirus by cyclophosphamide. Nature 267:721–723
35. McDonald GB, Sharma P, Hackman RC, Meyers JD, Thomas ED (1985) Esophageal infections in immunosuppressed patients after marrow transplantation. Gastroenterology 88:1111–1117
36. Meyers JD (1985) Infection in bone marrow transplantation. In: Remington JS, Swartz MN (eds) Current clinical topics in infectious diseases. McGraw-Hill, New York, pp 261–292
37. Meyers JD (1989) Prevention of cytomegalovirus infection after marrow transplantation. Rev Infect Dis 11[Suppl 7]:S1691–S1705
38. Meyers JD, Flournoy N, Thomas ED (1980) Cytomegalovirus infection and specific cell-mediated immunity after marrow transplant. J Infect Dis 142:816–824
39. Meyers JD, Flournoy N, Thomas ED (1982) Nonbacterial pneumonia after allogeneic marrow transplantation: a review of 10 years' experience. Rev Infect Dis 4:1119–1132
40. Meyers JD, Flournoy N, Wade JC, Hackman RC, McDougall JK, Neiman PE, Thomas ED (1983) Biology of interstitial pneumonia after marrow tranplantation. In: Gale RP, Champlin RE (eds) Progress in bone marrow transplantation. Liss, New York pp 405–423

41. Meyers JD, Leszcynski J, Zaia JA, Flournoy N, Newton B, Syndman DR, Wright GG, Levin MJ, Thomas ED (1983) Prevention of cytomegalovirus infection by cytomegalovirus immuneglobulin after marrow transplantation. Ann Intern Med 98:442–446
42. Meyers JD, Flournoy N, Thomas ED (1986) Risk factors for CMV infection after human marrow transplantation. J Infect Dis 153:478–488
43. Meyers JD, Reed EC, Shepp DH, Thornquist M, Dandliker PS, Vicary CA, Flournoy N, Kirk LE, Kersey JH, Thomas ED, Balfour HH (1988) Acyclovir for prevention of cytomegalovirus infection and disease after allogeneic marrow transplantation. N Engl J Med 318:70–75
44. Meyers JD, Ljungman P, Fisher LD (1990) Cytomegalovirus excretion as a predictor of cytomegalovirus disease after marrow transplantation: importance of cytomegalovirus viremia. J Infect Dis 162:373–380
45. Miller W, Flynn P, McCullough J, Balfour HH, Goldman A, Haake R, McGlave P, Ramsey N, Kersey J (1986) Cytomegalovirus infection after bone marrow transplantation: an association with acute graft-versus-host disease. Blood 67:1162–1167
46. Miller W, McCullough J, Balfour HH, Haake R, Ramsey NKC, Goldman A, Bowman R, Kersey J (1988) Prevention of CMV infection by blood products: a randomized trial. J Cell Biochem 12 [Suppl c]:93
47. Myerson D, Hackman RC, Nelson JA, Ward DC, McDougall JK (1984) Widespread presence of histologically occult cytomegalovirus. Hum Pathol 15:430–439
48. Neiman PE, Reeves W, Ray G, Flournoy N, Lerner KG, Sale GE, Thomas ED (1977) A prospective analysis of interstitial pneumonia and opportunistic viral infection among recipients of allogeneic bone marrow grafts. J Infect Dis 136:754–767
49. O'Reilly RJ, Reich L, Gold J, Kirkpatrick D, Dinsmore R, Kapoor N, Condie R (1983) A randomized trial of intravenous hyperimmune globulin for the prevention of cytomegalovirus (CMV) infections following marrow transplantation: preliminary results. Transplant Proc 15:1405–1411
50. Panjwani DD, Ball MG, Berry NJ, Wimperis JZ, Blacklock HA, Prentice HG, Hoffbrand AV, Griffiths PD (1985) Virological and serological diagnosis of cytomegalovirus infection in bone marrow allograft recipients. J Med Virology 16:357–365
51. Paulin T, Ringden O, Lönnqvist B, Wahren B, Nilsson B (1986) The importance of pre bone marrow transplantation serology in determining subsequent cytomegalovirus infection. An analysis of risk factors. Scand J Infect Dis 18:199–209
52. Pecego R, Hill R, Appelbaum FR, Amos D, Buckner CD, Fefer A, Thomas ED (1986) Interstitial pneumonitis following autologous bone marrow transplantation. Transplantation 42:515–517
53. Petersen FB, Bowden RA, Thornquist M, Meyers JD, Buckner CD, Counts GW, Nelson N, Newton BA, Sullivan KM, McIver J, Thomas E (1987) The effect of prophylactic intravenous immune globulin on the incidence of septicemia in marrow transplant recipients. Bone Marrow Transplant 2:141–148
54. Quinnan G, Kirmani N, Rook AH, Manischewitz JF, Jackson L, Moreschi G, Santos GW, Saral R, Burns WH (1982) Cytotoxic t cells in cytomegalovirus infection: HLA-restricted T-lymphocyte and non-T-lymphocyte cytotoxic responses correlate with recovery from cytomegalovirus infection in bone marrow transplant recipients. N Engl J Med 307:7–13
55. Reed EC, Dandliker PS, Meyers JD (1986) Treatment of cytomegalovirus pneumonia with 9-[2-hydroxy-1-(hydroxymethyl)ethoxymethyl]guanine and high-dose corticosteroids. Ann Intern Med 103:214–215
56. Reed EC, Bowden RA, Dandliker PS, Gleaves CA, Meyers JD (1987) Efficacy of cytomegalovirus immunoglobulin in marrow transplant recipients with cytomegalovirus pneumonia. J Infect Dis 156:641–645
57. Reed EC, Bowden RA, Dandliker PS, Lilleby KE, Meyers JD (1988) Treatment of cytomegalovirus pneumonia with ganciclovir and intravenous cytomegalovirus immunoglobulin in patients with bone marrow transplants. Ann Intern Med 109:783–788

58. Reed EC, Shepp DH, Dandliker PS, Meyers JD (1988) Ganciclovir treatment of CMV infection of the gastrointestinal tract after marrow transplantation. Bone Marrow Transplant 3:199–206
59. Reed EC, Wolford JL, Kopecky KL, Lilleby KE, Dandliker PS, Todaro JL, McDonald GB, Meyers JD (1990) Ganciclovir for the treatment of cytomegalovirus gastroenteritis in bone marrow transplant patients. A randomized, placebo-controlled trial. Ann Intern Med 112:505–510
60. Reusser P, Schoch HG, Fisher L, Thomas ED, Buckner CD, Meyers JD (1988) Cytomegalovirus (CMV) infection after autologous bone marrow transplantation (ABMT): occurrence of disease and impact on engraftment. Blood 72 Suppl 1:402a
61. Ringden O, Lönnqvist B, Sundberg B (1987) Cytomegalovirus immune bone marrow donors and interstitial pneumonitis. Lancet 2:105–106
62. Ringden O, Pihlstedt P, Volin L, Nikoskelainen J, Lönnqvist B, Ruutu P, Ruutu T, Tuivanen A, Wahren B (1987) Failure to prevent cytomegalovirus infection by cytomegalovirus hyperimmune plasma: a randomized trial by the Nordic BMT group. Bone Marrow Transplant 2:299–305
63. Rook AH (1988) Interactions of cytomegalovirus with the human immune system. Rev Infect Dis 10(Suppl 3):S460–S467
64. Rubin RH, Wilson EJ, Barrett LV, Medearis DN (1986) The protective effects of hyperimmune anti-murine cytomegalovirus antiserum against lethal viral challenge: the case for passive-active immunization. Clin Immunol Immunopathol 39:151–158
65. Ruutu P, Ruutu T, Volin L, Tukiainen P, Ukkonen P, Hovi T (1990) Cytomegalovirus is frequently isolated in bronchoalveolar lavage fluid of bone marrow transplant recipients without pneumonia. Ann Intern Med 112:913–916
66. Saxon A, Mitsuyasu R, Stevens R, Champlin RE, Kimata H, Gale RP (1986) Designed transfer of specific immune responses with bone marrow transplantation. J Clin Invest 78:959–967
67. Schmidt GM, Kovacs A, Zaia JA, Horak DA, Blume KG, Nademanee AP, O'Donnell MR, Synder DS, Forman SJ (1988) Ganciclovir/immunoglobulin combination therapy for the treatment of human cytomegalovirus-associated interstitial pneumonia in bone marrow allograft patients. Transplantation 46:905–907
68. Schmidt GM, Zaia J, Horak D, Kovacs A, Hawkins G, Nademanee A, O'Donnell MR, Synder DS, Stein AS, Paarker PM, Hill R, Blume KG, Forman SJ (1988) Human cytomegalovirus (HCMV) detection in routine bronchoalveolar lavage (BAL) specimen as a predictor for interstitial pneumonia (IP) in allogeneic bone marrow transplantation (BMT) recipients. Blood 72 Suppl 1:405a
69. Shanley JD (1987) Murine cytomegalovirus pneumonitis in T-cell deficient nude mice (Abstr). 12th Herpes Virus Workshop, Philadelphia
70. Shanley JD, Pesanti EL (1985) The relation of viral replication to interstitial pneumonitis in murine cytomegalovirus lung infection. J Infect Dis 151:454–458
71. Shanley JD, Jordan MC, Stevens JG (1981) Modification by adoptive humoral immunity of murine cytomegalovirus infection. J Infect Dis 143:231–237
72. Shanley JD, Pesanti EL, Nugent KM (1982) The pathogenesis of pneumonitis due to murine cytomegalovirus. J Infect Dis 146:388–396
73. Shanley JD, Via CS, Sharrow SO, Shearer GM (1987) Interstitial pneumonitis during murine cytomegalovirus infection and graft-versus-host reaction. Characterization of bronchoalveolar lavage cells. Transplantation 44:658–662
74. Shepp DH, Dandliker PS, DeMiranda P, Burnette TC, Cederberg DM, Kirk LE, Meyers JD (1986) Activity of 9-[2-Hydroxy-1(hydroxymethyl)ethoxymethyl]guanine in the treatment of cytomegalovirus pneumonia. Ann Intern Med 103:368–373
75. Spector SA, Rua JA, Spector DH, McMillan R (1984) Detection of human cytomegalovirus in clinical specimens by DNA–DNA hybridization. J Infect Dis 150:121–126
76. Spencer GD, Hackman RC, McDonald GB, Amos DE, Cunningham BA, Meyers JD, Thomas ED (1986) A prospective study of unexplained nausea and vomiting after marrow transplantation. Transplantation 42:602–607

77. Springmeyer SC, Silvestri RC, Sale GE, Peterson DC, Weems CE, Huseby JS, Hudson LD, Thomas ED (1982) The role of transbronchial biopsy for the diagnosis of diffuse pneumonias in immunocompromised marrow transplant recipients. Am Rev Respir Dis 126:763–765
78. Starr SE, Allison AC (1977) Role of T lymphocytes in recovery from murine cytomegalovirus infection. Infect Immun 17:458–462
79. Sullivan KM, Kopecky K, Jocom J, Buckner CD, Counts G, Meyers JD, Witherspoon RP, Storb R, Thomas ED (1988) Antimicrobial and immunomodulatory effects of intravenous immunoglobulin in bone marrow transplantation. In: 28th Interscience Conference on Antimicrobial Agents and Chemotherapy. American Society for Microbiology. Washington, p 216
80. Sullivan KM, Kopecky K, Meyers J, Buckner CD (1990) Immunoglobulin prophylaxis in marrow transplantation. 6th International Symposium on Infections in the Immunocompromised Host, Peebles
81. Syndman DR, Werner BG, Heinze-Lacey B, Berandi VP, Tilney NL, Kirkman RL, Milford EL, Cho SI, Bush HL, Levey AS, Strom TB (1987) Use of cytomegalovirus immune globulin to prevent cytomegalovirus disease in renal transplant recipients. N Engl J Med 317:1049–1054
82. Thomas ED, Storb R, Clift A, Fefer A, Johnson FL, Lerner KG, Glucksberg H, Buckner CD (1975) Bone marrow transplantation. N Engl J Med 292:832–843, 895–902
83. Tyms AS, Davis JM, Jeffries DJ, Meyers JD (1984) BWB759U, an analogue of acyclovir, inhibits human cytomegalovirus in vitro. Lancet 2:924–925
84. Valteau P, Hartmann O, Benhamon E, Callaud JM, Brugieres L, Beaujeau F, Patte C, Flamant P, Lemerle J (1988) Nonbacterial nonfungal interstitial pneumonitis following autologous bone marrow transplantation in children treated with high-dose chemotherapy without total body radiation. Transplantation 45:737–740
85. Verdonck LF, DeGast GC, Dekker AW, DeWeger RA, Schuurman HJ, Rozenberg-Arska M (1989) Treatment of cytomegalovirus pneumonia after bone marrow transplantation with cytomegalovirus immunoglobulin combined with ganciclovir. Bone Marrow Transplant 4:187–189
86. Weiner RS (1987) Interstitial pneumonia following bone marrow transplantation. In: Gale RP, Champlin RE (eds) Progress in bone marrow transplantation. Liss, New York, pp 507–523
87. Weiner RS, Bortin MM, Gale RP, Gluckman E, Kay HEM, Kolb HJ, Hartz AJ, Rimm AA (1986) Interstitial pneumonitis after bone marrow transplantation. Ann Intern Med 104:168–175
88. Wilson EJ, Medearis DN, Hansen LA, Rubin RH (1987) 9-(1-3-Dihydroxy-2-propoxymethyl)guanine prevents death but not immunity in cytomegalovirus-infected normal and immunosuppressed BALB/c mice. Antimicrob Agents Chemother 31:1017–1020
89. Wimperis JZ, Brenner MK, Prentice HG, Reittie JE, Karayiannis P, Griffiths PD, Hoffbrand AV (1986) Transfer of a functioning humoral immune system in transplantation of T-lymphocyte-depleted bone marrow. Lancet 1:339–343
90. Wingard JR, Santos GW, Saral R (1985) Late-onset interstitial pneumonia following allogeneic bone marrow transplantation. Transplantation 39:21–23
91. Wingard JR, Chen DVH, Burns WH, Fuller DJ, Braine HG, Yeager AM, Kaiser H, Burke PJ, Graham ML, Santos GW, Saral R (1988) Cytomegalovirus infection after autologous bone marrow transplantation with comparison to infection after allogeneic bone marrow transplantation. Blood 71:1432–1437
92. Wingard JR, Mellits ED, Sostrin MB, Chen DVH, Burns WH, Santos GH, Vriesendorp HM, Beschorner WE, Saral R (1988) Interstitial pneumonitis after allogeneic bone marrow transplantation. Nine-year experience at a single institution. Medicine (Baltimore) 67:175–186
93. Wingard JR, Sostrin MB, Vriesendorp HM, Mellits ED, Santos GW, Fuller DJ, Braine HG, Yeager AM, Burns WH, Saral R (1988) Interstitial pneumonitis following autologous bone marrow transplantation. Transplantation 46:61–65

94. Winston DJ, Gale RP, Meyers DV, Young LS, UCLA Bone Marrow Transplant Group (1979) Infectious complications of human bone marrow transplantation. Medicine (Baltimore) 58:1–31
95. Winston DJ, Ho WG, Howell CL, Miller MJ, Mickey R, Martin WJ, Lin CH, Gale RP (1980) Cytomegalovirus infections associated with leukocyte transfusions. Ann Intern Med 93:671–678
96. Winston DJ, Territo MC, Ho WG, Miller MJ, Gale RP, Golde DW (1982) Alveolar macrophage dysfunction in human bone marrow transplant recipients. Am J Med 73:859–866
97. Winston DJ, Pollard RB, Ho WG, Gallagher JG, Rasmussen LE, Huang SH, Lin CH, Gosset TG, Merigan TC, Gale RP (1982) Cytomegalovirus immune plasma in bone marrow transplant recipients. Ann Intern Med 97:11–18
98. Winston DJ, Ho WG, Champlin RE, Gale RP (1984) Infectious complications of bone marrow transplantation. Exp Hematol 12:205–215
99. Winston DJ, Huang ES, Miller MJ, Lin CH, Ho WG, Gale RP, Champlin RE (1985) Molecular epidemiology of cytomegalovirus infections associated with bone marrow transplantation. Ann Intern Med 102:16–20
100. Winston DJ, Ho WG, Lin CH, Bartoni K, Budinger MD, Gale RP, Champlin RE (1987) Intravenous immune globulin for prevention of cytomegalovirus infection and interstitial pneumonia after bone marrow transplantation. Ann Intern Med 106:12–18
101. Winston PJ, Ho WG, Gale RP, Champlin RE (1987) Treatment and prevention of interstitial pneumonia after bone marrow transplantation. In: Gale RP, Champlin RE (eds) Progress in bone marrow transplantation. Liss, New York, pp 525–544
102. Winston DJ, Ho WG, Bartoni K, Holland GN, Mitsuyasu RT, Gale RP, Busuttil RW, Champlin RE (1988) Ganciclovir therapy for cytomegalovirus infection in recipients of bone marrow transplants and other immunosuppressed patients. Rev Infect Dis 10 Suppl 3:S540–S553
103. Winston DJ, Ho WG, Champlin RE (1989) Current approaches to management of infections in bone marrow transplants. Eur J Clin Oncol 25 Suppl 2:S25–S35
104. Winston DJ, Ho WG, Champlin RE (1989) Use of DHPG (ganciclovir) and intravenous immune globulin in bone marrow transplantation. In: Gale RP, Champlin RE (eds) Bone marrow transplantation: current controversies. Liss, New York, pp 553–561
105. Winston DJ, Ho WG, Champlin RE (1990) Cytomegaovirus infection and interstitial pneumonia after bone marrow transplantation. In: Champlin RE (ed) Bone marrow transplantation. Kluwer, Norwell, pp 113–128
106. Winston DJ, Ho WG, Champlin RE (1990) Cytomegalovirus infections after allogeneic bone marrow transplantation. Rev Infect Dis 12 Suppl 7:S776–S792
107. Winston DJ, Ho WG, Champlin RE (1991) Ganciclovir and intravenous immunoglobulin in bone marrow transplants. In: Gale RP, Champlin RE (eds) New strategies in bone marrow transplantation. Wiley-Liss, New York, pp 337–348
108. Witherspoon RP, Lum LG, Storb R (1984) Immunologic reconstitution after human marrow grafting. Semin Hematol 21:2–10
109. Zaia JA, Forman SJ, Gallagher MT, Vanderwal-Urbina E, Blume KG (1984) Prolonged human cytomegalovirus viremia following bone marrow transplantation. Transplantation 37:315–317
110. Zaia JA, Forman SJ, Ting YP, Vanderwal-Urbina E, Blume KG (1986) Polypeptide-specific antibody response to human cytomegalovirus after infection in bone marrow transplant recipients. J Infect Dis 153:780–787

Chapter 12 The Management of Cytomegalovirus Infection in Heart-Lung Transplant Recipients

R. L. Smyth [1,2], T. W. Higenbottam [1], J. P. Scott [1] and J. Wallwork [1]

Summary

In the 1980s heart-lung transplantation (HLT) [1, 2], evolved from an experimental and innovative stage to a clinical treatment. Despite improvements in survival and understanding of pathogenesis of the lung disease in HLT recipients, cytomegalovirus (CMV) infection remains an important cause of death and morbidity. Donor-acquired primary CMV disease may be effectively prevented by prospective donor and recipient matching. Considerable progress has been made in the diagnosis of CMV pneumonia by the use of transbronchial lung biopsy (TBB), and the antiviral drug ganciclovir provides effective treatment of reactivation or reinfection. However, the mechanisms and immunological response to CMV infection in this patient population remain poorly understood.

Introduction

Cytomegalovirus (CMV) infection, identified as early as 1964 as a cause of death in renal transplant recipients [3], is now acknowledged to be one of the major complications of solid organ and bone marrow transplantation [4–7]. Clinical studies have reported an incidence of CMV infection approaching 100% in seropositive recipients of renal, liver and heart allografts [4, 8, 9]. The clinical manifestations and severity of CMV infection vary with the type of allograft received [10], the primary cause of death being CMV pneumonia [4, 7, 11]. When compared with heart transplant recipients, heart-lung transplantation (HLT) recipients experience a more severe CMV pneumonia [9, 12]. This review will attempt to summarise the epidemiology, clinical presentations and diagnosis of CMV infection in HLT patients and address issues of prevention and treatment. For the purposes of this discussion, CMV infection refers to laboratory evidence (either serological, histological or by virus isolation) of

[1] Heart-Lung Transplant Research Unit, Papworth Hospital, Cambridge CB3 8RE, UK
[2] Oncology Unit, Ward C3, Royal Liverpool Children's Hospital, Alder Hey, Liverpool, L12 2AP, UK

primary or recurrent CMV infection. CMV disease is defined as clinical evidence of CMV infection in one or more organs together with laboratory evidence of CMV infection of that organ.

Mechanisms of Disease

The CMV-Seronegative Recipient

In the normal population CMV infections are common and largely undiagnosed [13]. The risk of an individual having acquired CMV varies with age, sex, socioeconomic status and geographic location. Reflecting these demographic differences, 45% of our HLT recipients were reported to be CMV-seropositive [14] compared with 60% in the United States [9]. A further problem is in defining seropositivity, which may depend on the sensitivity of the method used to measure antibody [15]. The seronegative transplant recipient may acquire CMV infection from the donor organ, cellular blood products or by nosocomial transmission.

Allograft transmission of CMV was first established in the kidney [16] and later demonstrated for bone marrow [7], liver [8], heart [6, 17–19] and heart–lung [6, 14, 17] transplants. The most severe form of infection is primary organ-transmitted disease [6, 14, 20]. The site in the donor organ where CMV remains dormant is uncertain, and even using the sensitive in situ hybridization technique Gnann et al. [21] were unable to demonstrate the CMV nucleic acids in kidneys prior to transplantation. A recent study by Chou and Norman [22] in heart and kidney recipients suggested that not all seropositive donors are equally capable of transmitting CMV infection. They studied nine pairs of seronegative recipients, each pair of whom received organs from the same seropositive donor. In four pairs, both recipients developed CMV infection, defined by seroconversion, whereas in the remaining five pairs, neither recipient did so. These observations suggest that additional factors other than serological status determine the CMV infectivity of donor organs. We have reported primary CMV disease in seven of ten HLT-seronegative recipients who received organs from seropositive donors. Four died [23], and the three survivors remained seriously ill, requiring hospitalisation and treatment for many months.

Prospective matching of CMV-negative recipients with CMV-negative donors effectively prevents donor transmission of CMV (Table 1) [14, 23]. Because of the short ischaemic times required for HLT, matching was only possible when a rapid test for CMV antibody status became available [24] and has been our policy since 1986.

The seronegative patient may also develop primary CMV infection from blood or cellular blood products. Although a significant route of infection in bone marrow recipients [7], this form of primary infection in heart transplant and HLT patients causes less morbidity than organ-transmitted disease [6, 14].

Table 1. Incidence of primary CMV disease before and after matching in Papworth Hospital

	Before matching	After matching
Number of patients	17	49
$R^- D^+$	8	3
Primary CMV disease	5	1
Deaths associated with primary CMV disease	3	1

R^-, CMV-seronegative recipient; D^+, CMV-seropositive donors

Table 2. CMV infection in the 56 HLT recipients in the Papworth series who were not at risk of organ-transmitted primary CMV infection

	$D^+ R^+$		$D^- R^+$		$D^- R^-$
	n	%	*n*	%	
Number of patients	18		15		24
CMV infection	13	72	11	80	1
CMV pneumonia	10	56	7	53	1

D^+, CMV-seropositive donor; R^+, CMV-seropositive recipient; D^-, CMV-seronegative donor; R^-, CMV-seronegative recipient

Of our 24 seronegative recipients who received organs from seronegative donors only one developed CMV pneumonia, presumed to be blood-borne (Table 2). This resulted in pneumonia which was not life-threatening. The early use of transbronchial lung biopsy (TBB) to investigate all patients with clinical or radiological evidence of lung disease contributes to the success of antiviral therapy. It also provides accurate estimates of prevalence of disease in our population.

The CMV-Seropositive Recipient

The source of infection in the CMV-seropositive recipient is more difficult to assess. While in seropositive patients exposed only to seronegative organs and blood products CMV infection is presumed to be the result of reactivation of endogenous virus [19].

The relative roles of reactivation or reinfection in seropositive recipients who receive seropositive organs remain unknown. Grundy et al. [25], in renal allograft recipient pairs who received organs from the same donor, have performed restriction enzyme typing of virus isolates and suggest that a high proportion of such infections are donor acquired. The authors do not state where the virus strains studied were excreted or if isolates from multiple sites in the same individual were compared. However, these results imply that previous exposure to CMV does not protect a recipient from significant CMV infection of donor origin. They also conclude [25] that CMV infection in seropositive recipients who have received seropositive organs is both more frequent and severe than in those patients who have received seronegative organs. Not all studies, including our own [23] (Table 2), concur with these findings [8, 19]. We, studying HLT patients, showed no increased CMV disease in seropositive recipients with seropositive donors.

A further confounding factor is introduced by the study from Chou [26] who suggested that individual organ donors can transmit more than one strain of CMV to their recipients. Conceivably each recipient of such an organ would be latently infected with many different CMV strains. This study also demonstrated that in vitro new viral strains can arise readily through recombination of existing strains. By implication, the development of CMV disease in a recipient when presented with such a heterogeneity of viral strains is not dependent on the source of virus, but more the immunological responses by the recipient.

Immunosuppressive Therapy

Immunosuppressive therapy is known to influence the development of CMV disease. Drugs which profoundly depress the number of circulating T lymphocytes, such as antithymocytic globulin and Orthoclone OKT3, have been associated with increased incidence of infection [8, 19]. These observations are consistent with the proposed central role of CMV-specific cytotoxic T lymphocytes (CTLs) in providing protective immunity to infection. Absence of such CMV-specific CTLs has been correlated with poor outcome of CMV reactivation in bone marrow transplant patients [27].

It has been shown in normal individuals that the 72-kDa immediate early (IE) protein, which is known to be produced within the first few hours of CMV replication, is an important determinant for CMV-specific cytotoxic T cells [28]. The significance of this observation is that IE-specific cytotoxic T cells may recognise and lyse infected cells before viral replication, thereby eliminating foci of reactivation. Loss or severe depression of such an immunosurveillance mechanism as a result of immunosuppressive therapy could be responsible for reactivation of CMV.

It has been suggested that CMV pneumonia is predominantly a cell-mediated immunological process [29] and is related to the development of host T cell response which causes lung injury rather than virus replication. Clinical evidence cited in support of this hypothesis is that in patients with the acquired immunodeficiency syndrome (who have an impaired ability to mount a T cell response and a high incidence of CMV pneumonia) deaths from this complication are rare and response to antiviral agents generally satisfactory. This may be true and in bone marrow transplant recipients, graft-versus-host disease is often associated with the development of CMV pneumonia, and antiviral agents, while reducing the titre of CMV in the lung, do not prevent death. Our experience in HLT patients is that CMV pneumonia in the seropositive HLT patient is a mild disease which responds readily to antiviral treatment. The uniqueness of this model is that CMV pneumonia occurs in the allograft itself, in the presence of alloreactive cytotoxic T cells, and may indeed be concomitant with lung rejection [30]. These clinical observations suggest that, at least in the seropositive HLT recipient, CMV pneumonia may run a mild clinical course despite the ability to mount a pathogenic T cell response in the lung. We suspect, in part, the problem of pulmonary complications after bone marrow transplantation is failure to diagnose the cause of pulmonary shadows on chest radiographs in over 40% of patients [31]. Imprecise diagnosis is unhelpful in organizing rational theories on pathogens.

Clinical CMV Disease

Clinical Manifestations

Pulmonary infections, including CMV pneumonia, are common in HLT recipients [32, 33]. Unfortunately, one infection is not distinguishable from another and, in the case of the HLT patients, not distinguishable from acute rejection (Fig. 1). CMV disease occurs most commonly in the transplanted organ; HLT patients have a much higher incidence of CMV pneumonia than do heart transplant patients [12], whereas after liver transplantation the most common manifestation is CMV hepatitis [34]. Compared with CMV pneumonia, which occurred in 47% of seropositive patients [23], CMV involvement of the liver, eyes, gastrointestinal tract and pancreas is unusual in our series.

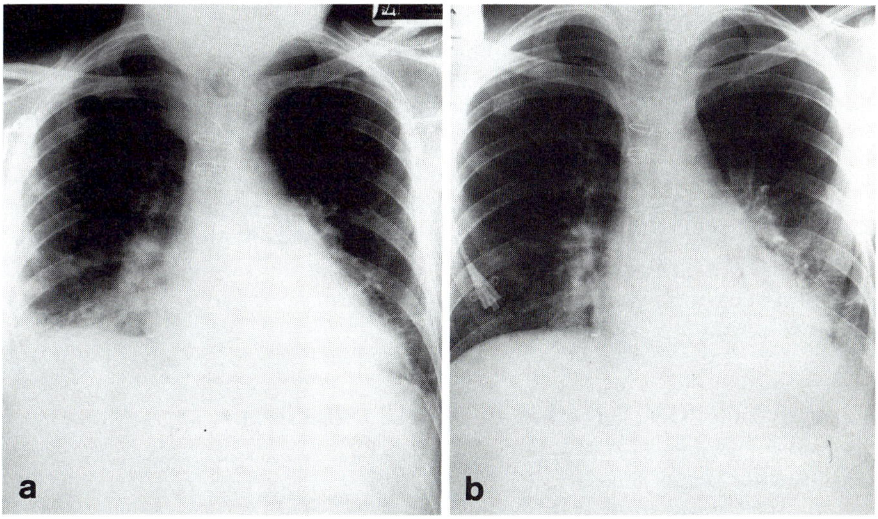

Fig. 1 a, b. Chest radiographs from a heart-lung transplant patient during episodes of rejection (**a**) and cytomegalovirus pneumonia (**b**), showing similarities in appearance

CMV not only causes clinical disease directly, but may facilitate additional infections by exerting immunosuppressive effects [35]. Rinaldo et al. [36] demonstrated in vitro that during acute CMV mononucleosis, mononuclear leukocytes displayed diminished responsiveness to certain mitogens, which they suggested was mediated by suppressor cells. Clinically, CMV pneumonia is associated with viral, bacterial and fungal superinfections [23, 37, 38], although it is often impossible to distinguish the effects of CMV infection from immunosuppression which predisposes to CMV and other infections. We have noted a close association between CMV and herpes simplex virus (HSV) pneumonia [38]. All episodes of HSV pneumonia in CMV-positive patients have occurred within 3 months of CMV pneumonia. Indeed, experimentally, in vivo CMV has been shown to stimulate reactivation of HSV from the latent state [39]. Invasive pulmonary aspergillosis, which has a grave prognosis, almost invariably (in six out of seven patients in our series) occurs in HLT patients who have suffered previous lung injury from CMV [1, 23].

Relationship to Lung Rejection

The relationship of CMV infection to allograft rejection has been suggested for kidney transplant recipients, but not yet demonstrated for HLT recipients [40]. Support for this association has come from the observation that CMV infection is associated with enhanced expression of MHC class II antigens in the graft [41]. More recently, it has been deomonstrated in vitro that endothelial cells exhibit an increase in MHC class I but not class II antigens after CMV infection [42]. Experimentally, if gamma interferon was added to the culture medium it also produced an increase in class II expression, suggesting that the earlier observation was due to gammainterferon or interleukin-2 released by virus-activated T cells in response to virus infection or concomitant rejection. In this context it is interesting to note that the CMV genome encodes a protein with homology to class 1 antigens, although its function in the virus is unknown [43]. In HLT patients, as lung rejection can be reliably distinguished from pulmonary infection [44] by means of transbronchial biopsy (vide infra), we have been able to consider risk factors for both infection and lung rejection. At present all we can conclude is that repeated courses of enhanced immunosuppression for the treatment of rejection are associated with subsequent reactivation of CMV in seropositive recipients. In view of these observations and the immunosuppressive effects of CMV disease it seems unlikely that CMV induces rejection.

Diagnosis of CMV Infection in the HLT Recipient

Transbronchial Lung Biopsy

In this patient population pulmonary infections cannot be distinguished from lung rejection by either clinical [44] or radiological [45] criteria (Fig. 1). This observation underlined the need to develop an accurate histological diagnosis of lung disease. TBB performed through a fibreoptic bronchoscope (and rigid bronchoscope in small children) has been used successfully in HLT patients to accurately diagnose lung infection and rejection [44]. We have established histological classification of acute lung rejection which has been shown to correlate with prognosis [46] and to identify patients at high risk of developing disabling obliterative bronchiolitis [47]. The sensitivity of this technique is further enhanced by sampling all three lobes of one lung (lingula being regarded as a separate lobe) and taking at least three biopsies from each lobe [30]. This approach leads to safe, accurate diagnosis even in the critically ill patient in whom more than one opportunistic infection is frequently found [48].

Indeed, rejection and infection have been shown to occur concomitantly in over a quarter of our cases [30]. The characteristic findings in CMV pneumonia as shown in Fig. 2 are of enlarged (cytomegalic) cells containing large basophilic intranuclear inclusions (referred to as "owls eye" inclusions because they are separated from the nuclear membrane by a halo). These appearances are quite distinct from those of acute lung rejection (Fig. 3). CMV inclusions may occasionally be seen in the absence of changes of viral alveolitis, and in this situation a diagnosis of active CMV pneumonia cannot be made [49].

Bronchoalveolar Lavage

At the time of fibreoptic bronchoscopy we also perform bronchoalveolar lavage (BAL), which has enabled us to compare BAL with TBB (Table 3). We have studied the lymphocyte counts obtained from BAL during rejection and infection [50]. Although there were differences in lymphocyte counts between acute lung rejection and normal or infected lung, the sensitivity of this method in the diagnosis of lung rejection was low (approximately 21%). In the diagnosis of CMV pneumonia cytological examination of BAL cells may reveal characteristic viral inclusions [51]. Use of other diagnostic methods including viral culture and immunocytochemistry of BAL are discussed below.

Table 3. Bronchoalveolar lavage cell counts in HLT patients with normal lung histology compared with those during acute rejection and acute infection. Shown as mean ± standard deviation

	Histology of TBB		
	Normal	Rejection	CMV
Number of samples	10	57	9
Total cell count ($\times 10^6$/l)	0.13 ± 0.07	0.25 ± 0.33	0.32 ± 0.24
Lymphocytes (%)	11 ± 6	14 ± 12	10 ± 7
Neutrophils (%)	3 ± 3	15 ± 20	24 ± 30

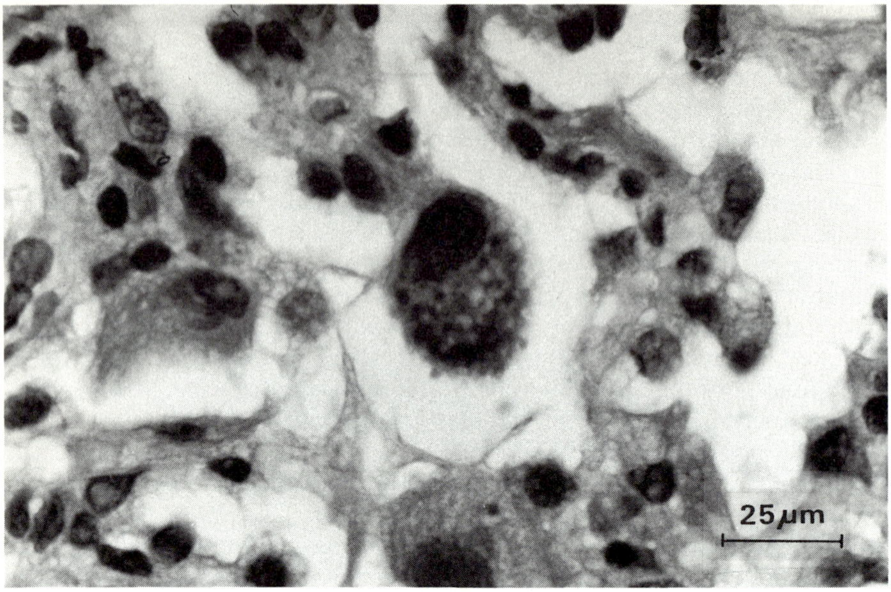

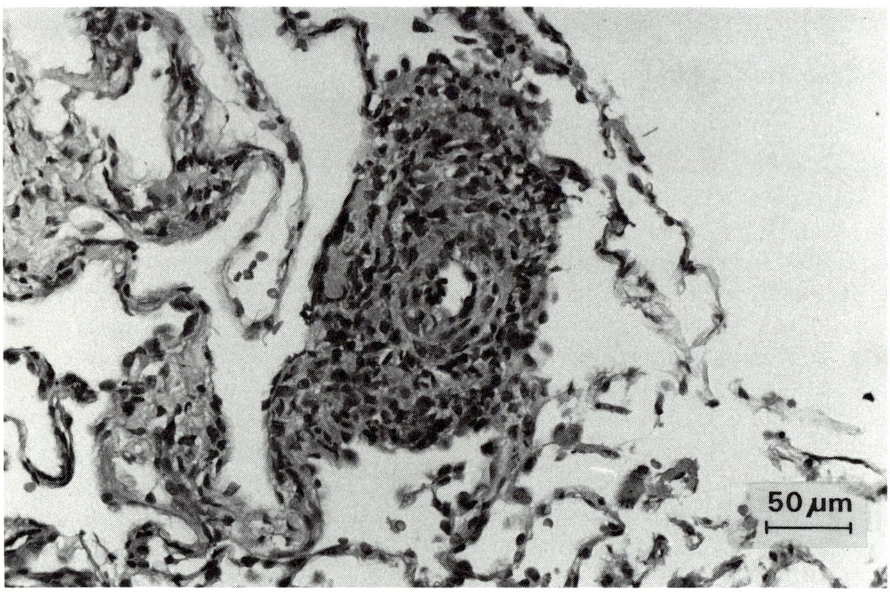

Fig. 2 (*above*). Transbronchial lung biopsy, showing the characteristic "owls eye" inclusion of cytomegalovirus pneumonia

Fig. 3 (*below*). Transbronchial lung biopsy from a patient with acute lung rejection, showing a perivascular, mononuclear cell infiltrate

Serology

Serology has a limited role as a diagnostic tool in the HLT recipient. Seroconversion (the development of CMV antibody in a previously seronegative individual) is a useful marker for the occurrence of primary infection. A fourfold rise in IgG titre or the appearance of CMV-specific IgM is frequently taken to indicate recurrent infection. However, in normal individuals levels of IgG antibody are known to fluctuate considerably [15] and in the immunocompromised individual the ability to mount normal IgG or IgM antibody responses may be severely depressed, making interpretation even more difficult [52].

Techniques of Viral Detection

A major drawback of viral culture is that it can take many days or weeks to obtain a positive result, which may not allow a diagnosis in life [53]. The use of fluoresceinated monoclonal antibodies against IE or early proteins [54] (sometimes referred to as detection of early antigen fluorescent foci, DEAFF, test) may allow CMV to be detected in tissue culture within 24–48 h prior to development of the characteristic cytopathogenic effect.

The direct detection of CMV antigen in lung biopsy and BAL specimens is possible using monoclonal antibodies to CMV proteins, and this has now been evaluated in a number of studies [53, 55]. Because of the huge variability of clinical isolates of CMV, optimal detection will probably only be obtained when a pool of monoclonal antibodies is used.

Another technique allowing rapid identification of CMV in the lung is the use of DNA probes [55–57]. Again, selection of the right probes is important, particularly as some regions of the CMV genome show homology to cellular DNA. This may explain some of the puzzling results, although it simply may be over-sensitive. For example, the study by Myerson et al. showed the presence of CMV in many apparently normal as well as cytomegalic cells [56].

The polymerase chain reaction (PCR), an in vitro DNA amplification technique, has been applied to the rapid detection of CMV DNA in peripheral blood leucocytes of viraemic transplant recipients [58]. When compared with the DEAFF test PCR was more sensitive and produced earlier results (within 6–8 h). Use of PCR to detect CMV DNA in lung tissues has yet to be evaluated.

A major shortcoming of viral culture and direct detection of CMV by monoclonal antibodies and DNA probes is in determining whether the CMV identified is responsible for active pneumonia or is merely an "innocent bystander". This difficulty has been acknowledged by many authors [15, 53, 59]. Patients may excrete virus in urine, semen or cervical secretions for years following its acquisition. We have shown that positive viral culture from lung or BAL may occur in the absence of clinical disease and in histologically normal lung from samples of all three lobes of one lung. These patients remained well without treatment [49, 60].

Approach to Clinical Diagnosis

Several authors have criticised the use of TBB in the diagnosis of CMV pneumonia on the grounds that it is not sufficiently sensitive [15, 55, 57, 61]. We have demonstrated that by sampling all the lobes of one lung the sensitivity of this method may be considerably increased [30]. In addition, rejection may also be effectively diagnosed or excluded. In contrast, methods that rely solely on BAL provide no means of directly assessing lung pathology. Paradis et al. [51] evaluated viral culture, immunocytochemistry and cytology of BAL cells in the diagnosis of CMV pneumonia. They used as their "gold standard" histology or culture of lung tissue. Not surprisingly, viral culture had a sensitivity of 100% but a specificity of 70%, compared with sensitivities of 21% and 82% for cytology and immunocytochemistry respectively. What was disappointing was that in none of the five patients who died from CMV pneumonia was this diagnosis made in life. In our series, all patients with evidence of CMV pneumonia at autopsy had been diagnosed by TBB antemortem. In certain cases accurate histological diagnosis may be difficult. Early in the course of infection the biopsies may show a nonspecific viral alveolitis before the inclusions are visible to light microscopy. This may be distinguished from rejection by perivascular oedema, polymorphonuclear microabscesses and lack of perivascular mononuclear cell infiltrates [38]. Following treatment with antiviral agents the inclusions may become degenerate and lack specific morphological features [49]. In these situations highly sensitive techniques such as immunohistochemistry and DNA probes [55] may also have a role, but their use in treated CMV pneumonia has yet to be evaluated. We perform viral culture of lung tissue and BAL fluid [38] in all cases of suspected viral pneumonias and use the DEAFF test [54] to provide an early result in the diagnosis of CMV pneumonia.

We therefore caution the clinicians against diagnosing CMV pneumonia without histological evidence of alveolar disease. Less invasive tests will probably result in detection of viral colonisation rather than pathogenic infection.

Prevention

As has already been described, we perform prospective matching of CMV-seronegative recipients with seronegative donors. In all but two inadvertently mismatched patients this has eliminated the risk of primary organ-transmitted disease [23]. We do not use CMV-seronegative blood products for seronegative recipients as primary CMV infection from this source is unusual and uncomplicated [6, 19, 23].

The logical approach to preventing primary CMV disease is to develop a vaccine which could be administered to seronegative individuals before transplant. Trials using live attenuated viral strains in seronegative transplant recipients have been performed and whilst the vaccine may reduce the severity of primary CMV disease, it does not prevent superinfection with other viral strains [62]. Therefore, additional theoretical problems are encountered with the use of a live virus vaccine, which include malignant transformation, immune impairment, reactivation and reversion to a more virulent phenotype. Other approaches include the development of an effective subunit vaccine and these are currently under study.

Modification or prevention of CMV infection in HLT patients may be possible by the administration of passive antibody in the form of CMV hyperimmune globulin. Its use in seronegative renal allograft recipients with seropositive donors was associated with a reduction in severity of CMV disease, viral and fungal superinfections when evaluated in a controlled clinical trial [63]. The mechanism of action of CMV hyperimmune globulin is poorly understood. The major drawback to the use of CMV hyperimmune globulin is its cost and because of this we reserve its use in those now rare situations of inadvertant transplant to a seronegative recipient from a seropositive donor. We administer it weekly from the time the mismatch has been identified for the first 3 months or until resolution of any CMV disease which may have developed [1].

Acyclovir was initially the only anti-CMV drug available and was used as treatment in the first three patients in our series, with disappointing results [14]. However, there have been two recent studies suggesting that acyclovir may reduce the incidence of CMV disease when used preventatively in bone marrow and renal transplant recipients [64, 65]. In the first study [64], which was neither randomised nor double-blind, high-dose intravenous acyclovir was being used for prevention of herpes simplex virus infections in bone marrow recipients. The incidence and severity of CMV infections was found to be slightly lower in the acyclovir-treated group. The second [65], a randomised, double-blind, placebo-controlled trial evaluated high-dose prophylactic oral acyclovir for 3 months after surgery in renal transplant recipients. They found that the acyclovir-treated group had less symptomatic and subclinical CMV disease, the effect being greatest in seronegative recipients of seropositive organs. The mechanism of action of acyclovir is unclear. CMV does not possess its own thymidine kinase and cannot phosphorylate acyclovir. However, Balfour et al. [65] suggest that, as acyclovir triphosphate is a competitive inhibitor of CMV DNA polymerase, concentrations of acyclovir may be sufficient inside the cell to inhibit the replication of CMV. Acyclovir in the doses used in these studies may be associated with renal impairment which together with cyclosporine-induced nephrotoxicity in the early postoperative period may precipitate renal failure. We routinely use low-dose orally administered acyclovir as a preventative agent in HSV-positive recipients in the first 3 months after transplant [38] and are currently evaluating a similar regime for prophylaxis in patients who have had one or more episodes of CMV pneumonia.

Treatment

Experience of the use of CMV hyperimmune globulin as a therapeutic agent has been disappointing. As a single agent in the treatment of CMV pneumonia it has not shown benefit [66]. The combination of CMV hyperimmune globulin with the antiviral agent ganciclovir to treat CMV pneumonia in bone marrow transplant recipients has shown more encouraging results [67, 68].

In the last 5 years the management of CMV disease has been transformed by the introduction of new antiviral drugs. The antiviral agent foscarnet is a competitive inhibitor of viral DNA polymerase and has been shown to inhibit CMV replication in vitro. Its use has not been evaluated by controlled clinical trials, although there are limited reports suggesting benefit in transplant recipients [69, 70]. It was used in one of our patients in an earlier study [14] but has since been superceded by ganciclovir.

Ganciclovir, which effectively inhibits CMV replication in vitro, has been used with encouraging results in numerous studies with solid organ transplant recipients [12, 71]. By contrast, studies of ganciclovir therapy in bone marrow recipients with CMV pneumonia demonstrated cessation of viral excretion but little impact on patient survival [11, 72]. The reason for these disappointing results may be that treatment was started too late, as diagnosis relied in the majority of cases on open lung biopsy. Although, for ethical reasons, none of these trials were controlled, in six HLT patients, all of whom had CMV pneumonia, treatment with ganciclovir resulted in recovery in every case [12]. These results are supported by our own experience. We reported 19 episodes of CMV pneumonia occurring in 15 previously seropositive HLT recipients which all responded to ganciclovir [23]. Three of these patients subsequently died and were found to have CMV inclusions in their lungs at autopsy. In only one was the primary cause of death considered to be CMV infection. Shortly before death this patient had received a 2-week course of treatment with ganciclovir for CMV pneumonia, but 3 days after discontinuation of this treatment was admitted to hospital in a moribund state. TBB showed severe CMV pneumonia, but despite treatment with ganciclovir the patient died 3 days later. This case illustrates one of the difficulties with ganciclovir, which is in knowing when an adequate course of treatment has been given. We suspect that until a reliable measure of return of CMV-specific cell-mediated immunity in the lung is available the duration of treatment will be empirical. Our results of treatment for primary organ-transmitted CMV infection with ganciclovir are more varied. Two of our three survivors from this form of disease and two of the four patients who died received ganciclovir, reflecting perhaps the more severe disease in this context. Because ganciclovir is only active if given intravenously its use as a prophylactic agent will be limited until an oral form becomes available. It is known to cause neutropenia in up to 40% of individuals treated [12], but this has been the only significant adverse effect observed in our series. The more widespread use of ganciclovir will inevitably result in the emergence of resistant strains. This phenomenon, which is well recognised for acyclovir [73], has recently also been reported for ganciclovir

[74]. Although this has not become a widespread clinical problem it underlines the need to restrict the use of this drug to symptomatic patients and to continue to search for more effective strategies of prevention.

Conclusion

There is still much to be learnt about the mechanisms and treatment of CMV pneumonia in HLT patients. However, with a clearly effective diagnostic technique in the form of TBB, management of patients can become more rational and less empirical. Lessons from the HLT patients can be applied to other transplant patient groups. Preventative therapy is urgently required as the policy of matching donor and recipient in CMV serology is not without error and contributes significantly to the shortage of suitable donors.

References

1. Smyth RL, Higenbottam TW, Scott JP, Wallwork J (1989) Transplantation of the lungs. Respir Med 83:459–466
2. Reitz BA, Wallwork JL, Hunt SA, Pennock JL, Billingham ME, Oyer PE, Stinson EB, Shumway NE (1982) Heart-lung transplantation: successful therapy for patients with pulmonary vascular disease. N Engl J Med 306:557–564
3. Hill RB, Rowlands DT, Rifkind D (1984) Infectious pulmonary disease in patients receiving immunosuppressive therapy for organ transplantation. N Engl J Med 271:1021–1027
4. Peterson PK, Balfour HH, Marker SC, Fryd DS, Howard RJ, Simmons RL (1980) Cytomegalovirus in renal allograft recipients: a prospective study of the clinical features, risk factors and impact on renal transplantation. Medicine (Baltimore) 59:283–300
5. Wreghitt T, Hughes M, Calne R (1987) A retrospective study of viral and Toxoplasma gondii infections in 54 liver transplant recipients in Cambridge. Serodiagn Immunother 1:219–239
6. Wreghitt TG, Hakim M, Gray JJ, Kucia S, Wallwork J, English TAH (1988) Cytomegalovirus infections in heart and heart and lung transplant recipients. J Clin Pathol 41:660–667
7. Meyers JD, Flournoy N, Thomas ED (1986) Risk factors for cytomegalovirus infection after human marrow transplantation. J Infect Dis 153:478–488
8. Singh N, Dummer S, Kisne S et al. (1988) Infections with cytomegalovirus another herpesviruses in 121 liver transplant recipients: transmission by donated organ and effect of OKT3 antibodies. J Infect Dis 158:124–131
9. Dummer JS, White LT, Ho M, Griffith BP, Hardesty RL, Bahnson HT (1985) Morbidity of cytomegalovirus infection in recipients of heart or heart–lung transplants who received cyclosporine. J Infect Dis 152:1182–1191
10. Preiksaitis JK (1989) Cytomegalovirus infection in transplant recipients. Immunol Allergy Clin North Am 9:137–151
11. Crumpacker C, Marlowe S, Zhang JL, Abrams S, Watkins P (1988) Treatment of cytomegalovirus pneumonia. Rev Infect Dis 10 Suppl:S538–S546
12. Keay S, Peterson E, Icenogle T, Zeluff BJ, Samo T, Busch D, Newman CL, Buhles WC, Merigan TC (1988) Ganciclovir treatment of serious cytomegalovirus infection in heart and heart–lung transplant recipients. Rev Infect Dis 10:S563–S572

13. Weller TH (1971) The cytomegaloviruses: ubiquitous agents with protean clinical manifestations. I. N Engl J Med 285:203–214
14. Hutter JA, Scott J, Wreghitt T, Higenbottam T, Wallwork J (1989) The importance of cytomegalovirus in heart–lung transplant recipients. Chest 95:627–631
15. Drew WL (1988) Diagnosis of cytomegalovirus infection. Rev Infect Dis 10 Suppl:S468–S476
16. Ho M, Suwansirikul S, Dowling JN, Youngblood LA, Armstrong JA (1975) The transplanted kidney as a source of cytomegalovirus infection. N Engl J Med 293:1109–1112
17. Hakim M, Wreghitt TG, English TAH, Stovin PGI, Cory-Pearce R, Wallwork J (1985) Significance of donor transmitted disease in cardiac transplantation. Heart Transplant 4:302–305
18. Chou S (1987) Cytomegalovirus infection and reinfection transmitted by heart transplantation. J Infect Dis 155:1054–1056
19. Preiksaitis JK, Rosno S, Grumet C, Merigan TC (1983) Infections due to herpesviruses in cardiac transplant recipients: role of the donor heart and immunosuppressive therapy. J Infect Dis 147:974–981
20. Smiley ML, Wlodaver CG, Grossman RA, Barker CF, Perloff LJ, Tustin NB, Starr SE, Plotkin SA, Friedman HM (1985) The role of pretransplant immunity in protection from cytomegalovirus disease following renal transplantation. Transplantation 40:157–161
21. Gnann JW, Ahlmen J, Svalander C, Olding L, Oldstone MBA, Nelson JA (1988) Inflammatory cells in transplanted kidneys are infected by cytomegalovirus. Am J Pathol 132:239–248
22. Chou S, Norman DJ (1988) The influence of donor factors other than serologic status on transmission of cytomegalovirus to transplant recipients. Transplantation 46:89–93
23. Smyth RL, Scott JP, Higenbottam TW, Wreghitt TG, Stewart S, Fradet G, Clelland CA, Wallwork J (1990) Experience of cytomegalovirus infection in heart–lung transplant recipients. Transplant Proc 22:1822–1823
24. Gray JJ, Alvey B, Smith DJ, Wreghitt TG (1987) Evaluation of a commercial latex agglutination test for detecting antibodies to cytomegalovirus in organ donors and transplant recipients. J Virol Methods 16:13–19
25. Grundy JE, Lui SF, Super M, Berry NJ, Sweny P, Fernando ON, Moorhead J, Griffiths PD (1988) Symptomatic cytomegalovirus infection in seropositive recipients: reinfection with donor virus rather than reactivation of recipient virus. Lancet 2:132–135
26. Chou S (1989) Reactivation and recombination of multiple cytomegalovirus strains from individual organ donors. J Infect Dis 160:11–15
27. Quinnan GV, Burns WH, Kirmani N, Rook AH, Manischewitz J, Jackson L, Santos GW, Saral R (1984) HLA-restricted cytoxic T lymphocytes are an early immune response and important defence mechanism in cytomegalovirus infection. Rev Infect Dis 6:156–163
28. Borysiewicz LK, Hickling JK, Graham S, Sinclair J, Cranage MP, Sissons JGP (1988) Human cytomegalovirus-specific cytotoxic T cells – relative frequency of stage-specific CTL recognizing the 72-kD immediate early protein and glycoprotein B expressed by recombinant vaccinia viruses. J Exp Med 168:919–931
29. Grundy JE, Shanley JD, Griffiths PD (1987) Is cytomegalovirus interstitial pneumonitis in transplant recipients and immunopathological condition? Lancet 2:996–998
30. Smyth RL, Scott JP, Igboaka G, Clelland C, Higenbottam TW, Wallwork J (1989) Distribution of rejection within the transplanted lung (Abstr). Thorax 44:321P
31. Anonymous (1989) Lung disease following allogeneic marrow transplantation. Lancet 2:1368–1369
32. Dummer JS, Montero CG, Griffith BP, Hardesty RL, Paridis IL, Ho M (1986) Infections in heart–lung transplant recipients. Transplantation 41:725–729
33. Brooks RG, Hofflin JM, Jamieson SW, Stinson EB, Remington JS (1985) Infectious complications in heart–lung transplant recipients. Am J Med 79:412–422
34. Paya CV, Hermans PE, Wiesner RH, Ludwig J, Smith TF, Rakela J, Krom RAF (1989) Cytomegalovirus hepatitis in liver transplantation: prospective analysis of 93 consecutive orthotopic liver transplantations. J Infect Dis 160:752–758

35. Rook AH (1988) Interactions of cytomegalovirus with the human immune system. Rev Infect Dis 10:S460–S467
36. Rinaldo CR, Carney WP, Richter BS, Black PH, Hirsch MS (1980) Mechanisms of immunosuppression in cytomegaloviral mononucleosis. J Infect Dis 141:488–495
37. Rand KH, Pollard RB, Merigan TC (1978) Increased pulmonary superinfections in cardiac-transplant patients undergoing primary cytomegalovirus infection. N Engl J Med 298:951–953
38. Smyth RL, Higenbottam TW, Scott JP, Wreghitt TG, Stewart S, Clelland CA, McGoldrick J, Wallwork J (1990) Herpes simplex virus infection in heart–lung transplant recipients. Transplantation 49:735–739
39. Colberg-Poley AM, Isom HC, Rapp F (1979) Reactivation of herpes simplex virus type 2 from a quiescent state by human cytomegalovirus. Proc Natl Acad Sci USA 76:5948–5951
40. Glenn J (1981) Cytomegalovirus infections following renal transplantation. Rev Infect Dis 3:1151–1177
41. Von Willebrand E, Pettersson E, Ahonen J, Hayry P (1986) CMV infection, class II antigen expression and human kidney allograft rejection. Transplantation 42:364–367
42. Van Dorp WT, Jonges E, Bruggeman CA, Daha MR, van Es LA, van der Woude FJ (1989) Direct induction of MHC class I, but not class II expression on endothelial cells by cytomegalovirus infection. Transplantation 48:469–472
43. Beck S, Barrell BG (1988) Human cytomegalovirus encodes a glycoprotein homologous to MHC class-I antigens. Nature 331:269–272
44. Higenbottam T, Stewart S, Penketh A, Wallwork J (1988) Transbronchial biopsy for the diagnosis of rejection in heart–lung transplant patients. Transplantation 46:532–539
45. Millet B, Higenbottam TW, Flower CDR, Stewart S, Wallwork J (1989) The radiographic appearances of infection and acute rejection of the lung after heart–lung transplantation. Am Rev Respir Dis 140:62–67
46. Clelland CA, Higenbottam TW, Otulana BA, Stewart S, Scott J, McGoldrick J, Wallwork J (1989) A histological classification of acute lung rejection in heart–lung transplantation (Abstr). J Heart Transplant 8:98
47. Scott JP, Higenbottam TW, Clelland CA, Stewart S, Smyth RL, McGoldrick JP, Otulana BA, Wallwork J (1990) The natural history of chronic rejection in heart–lung transplant recipients. J Heart Transplant 9:510–515
48. Smyth RL, Scott JP, McGoldrick J, Wallwork J, Higenbottam T (1989) Successful use of repeated transbronchial lung biopsies in a patient with multiple opportunistic infections. Respir Med 83:505–507
49. Wreghitt TG, Smyth RL, Scott JP, Higenbottam TW, Gray JJ, Stewart S, Wallwork J (1990) Value of culture of biopsy material in diagnosis of viral infections in heart–lung transplant recipients. Transplant Proc 22:1809–1810
50. Clelland C, Higenbottam TW, Smyth RL, Scott JP, Stewart S, Wallwork J (1989) Lymphocyte counts in broncho-alveolar lavage (BAL) during acute lung rejection and infection in heart-lung transplantation (HLTx). Am Rev Respir Dis 139:A242
51. Paradis I, Grgurich WF, Dummer JS, Dekker A, Douber JH (1988) Rapid detection of cytomegalovirus pneumonia from lung lavage cells. Am Rev Respir Dis 138:697–702
52. Sissons JGP, Borysiewicz LK (1989) Human cytomegalovirus infection. Thorax 44:241–246
53. Emanuel D, Peppard J, Stover D, Gold J, Armstrong D, Hammerling U (1986) Rapid immunodiagnosis of cytomegalovirus pneumonia by bronchoalveolar lavage using human and murine monoclonal antibodies. Ann Intern Med 104:476–481
54. Griffiths PD, Panjwani DD, Stirk PR, Ball MG, Ganczakowski M, Blacklock HA, Prentice HG (1984) Rapid diagnosis of CMV infection in immunocompromised patients by detection of early antigen fluorescent foci. Lancet 2:1242–1245
55. Niedobitek G, Finn T, Herbst H, Gerdes J, Grillner L, Landqvist M, Wirgart BZ, Stein H (1988) Detection of cytomegalovirus by in situ hybridisation and immunohistochemistry using new monoclonal antibody CCH2: a comparison of methods. J Clin Pathol 41:1005–1009

56. Myerson D, Hackman RC, Nelson JA, Ward DC, Mcdougall JK (1984) Widespread presence of histologically occult cytomegalovirus. Hum Pathol 15:430–439
57. Churchill MA, Zaia JA, Froman SJ, Sheibani K, Azumi N, Blume KG (1987) Quantitation of human cytomegalovirus DNA in lungs from bone marrow transplant recipients with interstitial pneumonia. J Infect Dis 155:501–509
58. Jiwa NM, van Gemert GW, Raap AK, van de Rijke FM, Mulder A, Lens PF, Salimans MMM, Zwaan FE, van Dorp W, van der Ploeg M (1989) Rapid detection of human cytomegalovirus DNA in peripheral blood leukocytes of viremic transplant recipients by the polymerase chain reaction. Transplantation 48:72–76
59. Broaddus C, Dake MD, Stulbarg MS, Blumenfeld W, Hadley K, Golden JA, Hopewell PC (1985) Bronchoalveolar lavage and transbronchial biopsy for the diagnosis of pulmonary infections in the acquired immunodeficiency syndrome. Ann Intern Med 102:747–752
60. Scott JP, Higenbottam TW, Smyth RL, Wreghitt T, Clelland C, Solis E, Wallwork J (1990) The presence of cytomegalovirus (CMV) or herpes simplex virus (HSV) on culture of bronchial lavage (BAL) or transbronchial biopsy (TBB) does not diagnose viral pneumonitis in heart-lung transplant (HLT) recipients. Am Rev Respir Dis 141:A684
61. Crawford SW, Bowden RA, Hackman RC, Gleaves CA, Meyers JD, Clark JG (1988) Rapid detection of cytomegalovirus pulmonary infection by bronchoalveolar lavage and centrifugation culture. Ann Intern Med 108:180–185
62. Farrar GH, Bull JR, Greenaway PJ (1986) Prospects for the clinical management of human cytomegalovirus infections. Vaccine 4:217–224
63. Snydman DR, Werner BG, Heinze-Lacey B, Berardi VP, Tilney NL, Kirkman RL, Milford EL, Cho SI, Bush HL, Levey AS, Strom TB, Carpenter CB, Levey RH, Harmon WE, Zimmerman CE, Shapiro ME, Steinman T, LoGerfo F, Idelson B, Schroter GPJ, Levin MJ, McIver J, Lezczynski J, Grady GF (1987) Use of cytomegalovirus immune globulin to prevent cytomegalovirus disease in renal transplant recipients. N Engl J Med 317:1049–1054
64. Meyers JD, Reed EC, Shepp DH, Thornquist M, Dandliker PS, Vicary CA, Flournoy N, Kirk LE, Kersey JH, Thomas ED, Balfour HH (1988) Acyclovir for prevention of cytomegalovirus infection and disease after allogeneic marrow transplantation. N Engl J Med 318:70–75
65. Balfour HH, Chace BA, Stapleton JT, Simmons RL, Fryd DS (1989) A randomized, placebo-controlled trial of oral acyclovir for the prevention of cytomegalovirus disease in recipients of renal allografts. N Engl J Med 320:1381–1387
66. Reed EC, Bowden RA, Dandliker PS, Gleaves CA, Meyers JD (1987) Efficacy of cytomegalovirus immunoglobulin in marrow transplant recipients with cytomegalovirus pneumonia. J Infect Dis 156:641–645
67. Emanuel D, Cunningham I, Jules-Elysee K, Brochstein JA, Kernan NA, Laver J, Stover D, White DA, Fels A, Polsky B, Castro-Malaspina H, Peppard JR, Bartus P, Hammerling U, O-Reilly RJ (1988) Cytomegalovirus pneumonia after bone marrow transplantation successfully treated with the combination of ganciclovir and high-dose intravenous immune globulin. Ann Intern Med 109:777–782
68. Schmidt GM, Kovacs A, Zaia JA, Horak DA, Blume KG, Nademanee AP, O'Donnell MR, Snyder DS, Forman SJ (1988) Ganciclovir/immunoglobulin combination therapy for the treatment of human cytomegalovirus-associated interstitial pneumonia in bone marrow allograft recipients. Transplantation 46:905–907
69. Klintmalm G, Lonnqvist B, Oberg B, Gahrton G, Lernestedt J-O, Lundgren G, Ringden O, Roberg K-H, Wahren B, Groth C-G (1985) Intravenous foscarnet for the treatment of severe cytomegalovirus infection in allograft recipients. Scand J Infect Dis 17:157–163
70. Locke TJ, Odom NJ, Tapson JS, Freeman R, McGregor CGA (1987) Successful treatment with trisodium phosphonoformate for primary cytomegalovirus infection after heart transplantation. J Heart Transplant 6:120–122

71. Harbison MA, de Girolami PC, Jenkins RL, Hammer SM (1988) Ganciclovir therapy of severe cytomegalovirus infections in solid-organ transplant recipients. Transplantation 46:82–88
72. Shepp DH, Dandliker PS, de Miranda P, Burnett TC, Cederberg DM, Kirk LE, Meyers JD (1985) Activity of 9-[2-hydroxy-1-(hydroxymethyl)ethoxymethyl] guanine in the treatment of cytomegalovirus pneumonia. Ann Intern Med 103:368–373
73. Burns WH, Santos GW, Saral R, Laskin OL, Lietman PS (1982) Isolation and characterisation of resistant herpes simplex virus after acyclovir therapy. Lancet 1:421–424
74. Erice A, Chou S, Biron DD, Stanat SC, Balfour HH, Jordan MC (1989) Progressive disease due to ganciclovir-resistant cytomegalovirus in immunocompromised patients. N Engl J Med 320:289–293

Section III Diagnosis, Treatment and Prevention of Human Cytomegalovirus and Human Diseases

Chapter 13 Diagnosis of Human Cytomegalovirus Infection: Laboratory Approaches

Eng-Shang Huang and Timothy F. Kowalik

Summary

The association of cytomegalovirus (CMV) with a plethora of diseases and the recent development of potent anti-CMV compounds warrants the need for accurate verification of prior exposure to CMV as well as the identification of infectious virus in clinical specimens. This chapter initially reviews many of the traditional procedures used to detect CMV infections, including direct virus isolation and indirect immunological assays, for evidence of CMV infection. In so doing, procedures are outlined and the advantages and disadvantages of each method are discussed. Later, more detailed presentations of newer and, often, more sensitive procedures for CMV identification are given. Several of these approaches are designed to identify the presence of viral nucleic acid sequences in specimens by hybridization of probes to purified nucleic acids (Southern blotting) or directly to nucleic acids embedded in tissue sections (in situ hybridization). Also included here are significant discussion and instruction in the use of the polymerase chain reaction (PCR) and its application in identifying HCMV nucleic acid sequences in fresh and fixed specimens. Analysis of many of the advantages and disadvantages of using various reagents and samples is included. Finally, a brief description of virally associated cytomegalic cells in exfoliated and histological specimens is included in the hope that clinicians and laboratory scientists will be aware of a potential role for CMV in their diagnosis and prognosis of individual patients.

Introduction

Problems induced by human cytomegalovirus (CMV) infection have been overlooked for decades by clinicians and biomedical scientists because of the virus' ubiquitous, mostly asymptomatic infection and the lack of antiviral remedies. This situation has changed recently due to the discovery of potent

Lineberger Comprehensive Cancer Center, Departments of Medicine, Microbiology and Immunology and Curriculum of Genetics, University of North Carolina at Chapel Hill, School of Medicine, CB #7295, Rm. 117, Lineberger Building, Chapel Hill, NC, 27599-7295 anti-CMV compounds and an increase in the number of severe CMV infections in organ transplantation recipients and in patients with AIDS. Severe clinical complications associated with CMV, such as CMV-induced graft rejection, CMV retinitis, CMV pneumonitis, and CMV gastroenteritis, are frequently encountered in patients receiving organ transplants or infected with human immunodeficiency virus (HIV); such complications are the major causes of mortality and morbidity among these subjects. Therefore, accurate and rapid diagnostic method applying all possible approaches are needed both at the prevention and treatment levels.

The laboratory diagnosis of CMV infection can be achieved by the following approaches: (a) virus isolation, (b) serologic testing and viral antigen detection (by ELISA, immunofluorescence, and western blot), (c) nucleic acid hybridization (dot blot, Southern and northern, and in situ nucleic acid hybridization), (d) polymerase chain reaction (PCR), and (e) the search for cytomegalic inclusions in histological sections. The ideal method used for laboratory diagnosis of CMV infection is often dependent on clinical manifestations and the type of specimen collected. Specimens include blood, semen, urine, saliva, milk, stool, cervical discharge, paired sera for serological tests, and biopsied or even autopsied tissues.

Traditional approaches include virus isolation, antigen detection by immunofluorescence (FA) or immunoperoxidase (IP) test, and serological assays using neutralization, ELISA, and complement fixation (CF) tests. Virus isolation is limited by the slow development of CMV-induced cytopathic effect (CPE). Furthermore, final confirmation by immunocytochemistry or nucleic acid hybridization is needed. Immunocytochemical and serological methods offer faster results, but sensitivity is always a concern. The newer approaches include the use of various nucleic acid hybridization techniques and the polymerase chain reaction. In these options, specific radioactive labeled or biotinylated DNA probes and oligonucleotide-primers are needed. Because of the requirements for special reagents, instrumentation and radiosafety environments, these tests are not popularly used in the clinic to detect CMV infection at the present moment. In this chapter, we shall briefly describe classic methods which are well established and have been described in detail before [23, 39] and devote more effort to the newer approaches.

Detection of Infectious CMV

Virus Isolation and Rapid FA Test

Human CMV has been isolated from various body fluids (including urine, blood, semen, milk, stool, saliva, and cervical discharges) and from biopsied or autopsied tissue specimens. This virus has a very strong species specificity; it does not grow in cells other than those of human origin. Although CMV can be detected in many types of tissues and organs, it only replicates in human fibroblasts in cell culture. Human foreskin or embryonic fibroblast cells are commonly used for virus isolation. Susceptible fibroblast cell lines such as WI-38, HEL, and MRC-5 are available from ATCC (Rockville, Maryland).

Because viruria is frequently associated with most symptomatic CMV infections, urine is the most common specimen used for the diagnosis of CMV infection. Viruria at birth is the main indicator in the diagnosis of congenital CMV infection. Urine specimens should be neutralized with 0.1 N NaOH or HCl before inoculation. Infectious CMV is also frequently detected in the semen of asymptomatic homosexual men, approximating 30% of this population. Semen samples have to be diluted at least tenfold with MEM medium to avoid toxicity and proteolytic enzyme activity associated with this specimen. In biopsied or autopsied tissues, 10% of the tissue homogenate is prepared in MEM medium by homogenizing the tissue block in a sterile homogenizer. Supernatant fluid obtained by low speed centrifugation is then used for inoculation. Cervical and throat swabs are collected and suspended in MEM medium with 10% fetal calf serum. High concentrations of antibiotics and fungicides (200 units/ml penicillin, 200 μg/ml streptomycin, and 100 μg/ml of mycostatin or 50 μg/ml of amphitericin) are added to the samples or collection medium (MEM with 10% fetal calf serum) to prevent contaminating cell cultures during virus isolation. The inoculation volume is 0.1–0.2 ml per culture tube of late log phase fibroblasts. An absorption time of 1 h is needed and 2 h is recommended. For cervical, throat, urine, and semen specimens, the rinsing of the inoculated cultures with MEM medium containing antibiotics a couple of times after absorption is essential to cut down toxicity and contamination. The maintenance medium used after absorption is MEM with 6% fetal calf serum. The medium is changed 24 h after inoculation, then twice weekly, and the cultures are checked regularly for the appearance of CMV cytopathic effect (CPE). The inoculated cultures should be examined for 4 weeks before discarding or subculture.

For highly efficient recovery and rapid detection of CMV from blood or other exfoliative cells, the shell culture method (Viromed. Lab. Inc., Minnetonka, MN; Shell Vial Rapid FA Techniques) [17] with cells grown on coverslips has been used to isolate and identify CMV. In this method, human fibroblast cells are grown on a small round coverslip placed inside a glass vial, which resembles those used in scintillation counting. Absorption is carried out at room temperature or 37 °C for 1 h by centrifugation at 2000 rpm in a table top centrifuge to enhance the infection frequency. Duplicate or quarternary sets of vials are used for CMV isolation. One can be harvested 24 h after infection for rapid detection of CMV infection by identifying CMV immediate-early (IE) gene expression via indirect immunofluorescence or immunoperoxidase assays (see below). Another vial is used for continued observation. Monoclonal antibodies against HCMV IE and late nuclear antigens are available from Du Pont Specialty Diagnostics (Product 9221 and 9220, respectively). In all cases, the use of preconfluent log phase fibroblast cultures for inoculation and frequent changing of the maintenance medium results in a better isolation frequency.

An alternative way to isolate CMV from a blood sample is to use the buffy coat as an inoculant. This method is often used when CMV viremia is suspected, particularly in immunosuppressed patients after organ transplantation and patients suspected to have CMV mononucleosis. In these cases, 5–7 ml of blood is collected in a tube containing citrate anticoagulant (heparin cannot be used because of its anti-CMV effect by interfering with virus absorption). The blood sample is subjected to centrifugation in a tabletop centrifuge at 1500–2000 rpm (around 400 *g*) for 20 min. The leukocyte-rich buffy coat is then collected and inoculated into the shell vials or culture tubes (0.1 ml each). MEM medium with 6% fetal calf serum is added after absorption. The inoculant is not removed until 48 h later to enhance the recovery of latent CMV residing within white blood cells.

The morphology of CMV CPE in human fibroblast is quite distinguishable from that of other herpes group viruses, consisting of enlarged, ovary-shaped, refractile cells with intranuclear inclusions. This virus has the unusual characteristic of strong cell association. In clinical isolates it is rare to find extracellular infectious virus released at early stages of infection. Figure 1 a–f shows typical CMV-induced CPE in cultured cells at 72 h after inoculation. Cells with CPE frequently form longitudinal spindle clusters which result from contact infections of cells neighboring the initially infected cell. Degeneration and cytolysis of CMV-infected cells occur slowly and infected cells can remain attached to culture vessels for weeks.

In fixed and stained (with May-Greenwald-Giemsa or HE stain) tissue culture preparations, CMV-infected cells always contain typical intranuclear inclusion bodies surrounded by a halo zone on the inside of the enlarged nuclei after 48–72 h of infection. The nuclear inclusions are dense and oval or kidney shaped.

Serologic and Immunologic Tests for CMV Infections

The diagnosis of CMV infection can be achieved by measuring seroconversion and detecting viral antigen by immunocytochemistry. Complement fixation (CF) test, viral neutralization (NT) test, and immunofluorescence (FA) were used commonly a couple of decades ago to measure serum anti-CMV titer. More recently ELISA and western blot have become popular tests for both quantitation and characterization of CMV antigens and antibodies. Detection of CMV-specific antibodies in serum can be achieved by the following approaches.

Complement Fixation Test

The CF test uses hemolysin (anti-sheep RBC) sensitized sheep red blood cells (RBC) to measure the amount of complement bound by specific antigen-anti-

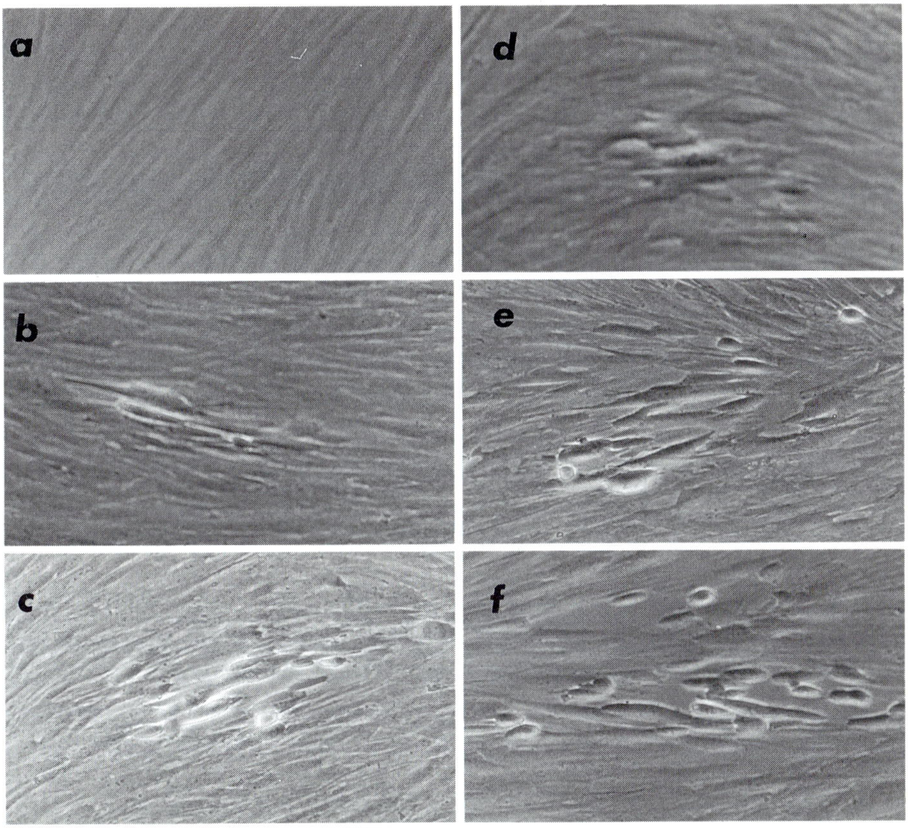

Fig. 1a–f. Cytopathic effect of human cytomegalovirus in human embryonic lung fibroblasts. Clustered cells with typical cytomegalovirus-CPE appeared 3 days after infection with urine samples (**b–f**) in this case. **a** HEL cells. ×400

body complexes in a defined assay condition. If a specific antigen-antibody reaction occurs, then the complement will be bound to the complex and no longer available to lyse the sensitized RBCs. On the other hand, the sensitized RBC will be lysed by the available complement if there is no specific antigen-antibody reaction occurring within the test. This method can be used to measure antibody titers using defined CMV antigen, or to detect the existence of CMV antigen using CMV antibodies.

There are at least two ways to prepare CMV CF antigen: the first method is to prepare CF antigen in veronal-buffer saline solution (VBS, pH 7.8). CMV-infected cells, 2 days after displaying 100% CPE, are harvested, washed three times with VBS, suspended in VBS, and then subjected to ultrasonification with a Branson sonifier (Branson Sonic Power Co., Connecticut). Cell debris is removed by centrifugation at 6000 rpm for 10 min at 4 °C in a Sorval HB-4 or SS34 rotor. The supernatant is used as the CF antigen. The second method uses 0.15 *M* glycine (pH 8.5–9.0) buffer to extract CMV antigen from virus-infected cells [2, 11]. The procedure is identical to that used above. Uninfected cells prepared in the same manner are used for control material. Microtiter U-shaped wells containing two units of complement, 2% sheep RBC sensitized with 2 units of hemolysin, and overnight incubation of antibody, CMV antigen and complement are employed [29]. The veronal-buffer saline, pH 7.8, is used for preparation of ingredients used in this assay.

Because of the heterogeneity of HCMV CF antigens among various CMV strains and because some strains have no crossover of CF antigens [29], it is important to have multivalent antisera or antigens to cover a broad spectrum of CMV strains for clinical diagnostic purposes. Anticomplement activity is frequently encountered in serum or antigen preparation. It can be preabsorbed out by pretreating serum or antigen with undiluted complement at 4 °C overnight and then heat-inactivating at 56 °C for 30 min to remove the excess complement. The technical details of CF test and the nature of CMV CF antigen and antibody have been carefully described elsewhere [23, 39].

Neutralization and Plaque Reduction Tests

Because of the antigenic heterogeneity and the lack of information on CMV serotyping by neutralization, the usefulness of neutralization and plaque reduction test in CMV diagnosis is limited. These tests are rarely used in the clinical laboratory today because of recent advances in rapid diagnosis of CMV by nucleic acid hybridization, PCR, and various immunocytochemical methods.

CMV is strongly cell-associated, so it is very important to have a cell-free virus for these tests. Clarifying the CMV-infected cell lysate at 8000 rpm for 15 min in a Sorvall HB-4 or SS-34 rotor will remove aggregation and cell debris, which might protect the virus from neutralization. Approximately 100 $TCID_{50}$ of virus in 0.1 ml and an equal volume of properly diluted serum are mixed for 1 h at room temperature, and then inoculated into culture tubes with WI-38 or HEL cells. At least four culture tubes are required for $TCID_{50}$ calculations. After 2 h of absorption, MEM maintenance media are added. Culture media are changed twice a week and the cells are microscopically examined for at least 3 weeks.

For plaque reduction tests, a virus dose of 100–300 PFU per petri dish (Falcon 3006) with duplicate samples are employed. Neutralization and absorption procedures are the same as in the tube neutralization test. After absorption, 7 ml of 1X high glucose MEM medium containing 2% methylcellulose (or 0.8% low melting point agarose, BRL), 6% fetal calf serum, penicillin, and streptomycin (100 units and 100 µg per ml, respectively), and mycostatin (50 µg/ml) is added. Culture plates are overlayed with the same medium on the 7th and 14th days after infection. By the end of third week, opaque plaques with a size of around 1 mm^2 should be observed by the eye without staining. The monolayers can then be stained with Giemsa stain or 0.03% methylene blue after the removal of agarose or methylcellulose.

Enzyme-Linked Immunosorbent Assay

Enzyme-linked immunosorbent assay (ELISA) can be used for detecting human CMV-specific IgG and IgM antibodies in serum or CMV-specific soluble antigens in body fluids or tissue extracts, depending upon whether viral antigen or virus-specific antibody is coated on the well surface of microtiter plates. Measuring CMV-specific IgG and IgM titers can provide useful reference to diagnose the prior history of human CMV infection as well as to distinguish primary infection from reactivation, or secondary infection, in pregnant women and neonates (see [23] for details).

For measuring human CMV-specific IgG or IgM titers in serum samples, infected cell extracts are first diluted with coating buffer to the concentration of 100 μg/ml and then absorbed on the well surface, 100 μl per well, at 4 °C overnight. The coating buffer is 0.1 *M* carbonate buffer, pH 9.6. Dynatech (Alexandria, Virginia) polystyrene 96-well plates (Immulon) as well as 12-well individual strips (Immulon 2) are used in our laboratory. After absorption, 300 μl/well of blocking solution containing 0.01 *M* Tris-HCl (pH 8.0), 2.5% ultra-pure sucrose, 2% protease free BSA (Boehringer Mannheim, FRG) and 0.1% thimersol is added to the well and set for 1 h at room temperature with frequent agitation. The blocking solution is then removed and the coated well is air dried or lyophilized. For long term storage the wells can be sealed with scotch tape and kept at 4 °C. Control cellular antigen is prepared and coated in the same way for background comparison.

A diluted serum sample of 100 μl (with PBS to 1:10 or to a desirable concentration) is added to the antigen coated wells and allowed to react at 37 °C for 1 h or at 4 °C overnight. After washing with PBS containing 0.05% Tween 20 three times, 100 μl of peroxidase- or alkaline phosphate-conjugated anti-human IgG or IgM secondary antibody in conjugate buffer (1% protease free BSA, 0.15 *M* Tris-HCl, pH 8.0, 0.2% PEG [Sigma, 4000 mol. wt.] and 0.1% thimersol) is added to the testing well and incubated at 37 °C for 1 h. After washing at least three time with PBS to remove unbound enzyme-antibody conjugates, the wells are then subjected to chromagenic reactions. There are numerous formulas available for preparing chromogenic reaction mixtures for either alkaline phosphotase- or peroxidase-conjugated antibodies. The most common one used in our laboratory for peroxidase-conjugated antibody is as follows:

Solution A (urea hydrogen peroxide solution)
0.1 *M* sodium citrate, adjusted to pH 5 with H_3PO_4
0.054 gm urea hydrogen peroxide per 100 ml of dH_2O
Solution B (substrate, chromogen)
i) dissolve 30 mg 3,3′,5,5′ tetramethyl benzidine (TMB) in the smallest volume of DMSO (probable concentration, 30 mg/ml)
ii) prepare solution B (kept away from light) using the following formula: 10% glycerol, 30% methanol, 59% distilled H_2O and concentrated TMB stock to a final concentration of 0.3 mg/ml.

To each testing well, 100 µl of solution A and 100 µl of solution B are added, gently mixed with a shaker or vibrator and incubated at 37 °C for 10 min. A positive blue color reaction should appear in positive wells. Other chromatogenic reactions are described in the next section.

The detection of specific IgM antibodies against human CMV is extremely important for diagnosis of primary and active infections in pregnant women as well as in neonates, but not in immunosuppressed patients. Unfortunately, false-positive tests and nonspecific IgM activities are frequently encountered due to the presence of rheumatoid factors and antinuclear antibodies in the sera when virus-infected cell extracts are used as antigen source [11, 23, 42]. In addition, nonspecific IgM titer against CMV has been found during Epstein-Barr virus (EBV) and varicella-zoster virus (VZV) infections. Hanshaw et al. [19] observed that out of 43 heterophil-positive sera, 42 were positive for anti-CMV macroglobulin. But after absorption of heterophil agglutinins, only seven of the 43 had CF antibodies against human CMV. Horwitz et al. [24] also reported that 21 out of 55 heterophil-positive sera had anti-CMV IgM titers at a level higher than 1:16. CMV-reactive macroglobulin was also found in six out of ten sera from patients with moderate to severe VZV infection. These data suggest that anti-CMV IgM antibodies can cross-react with antigens developed during EBV and VZV infections [23]. Therefore, the detection of viral antigen and the application of virus isolation in tissue culture become important approaches in the diagnosis of active CMV infections.

Several approaches have been used to eliminate nonspecific IgM activity and to improve the sensitivity of detection of specific anti-CMV IgM antibodies [9, 10, 34, 56]. These methods mainly target the removal of rheumatoid factor and the IgM class of anti-IgG antibodies. Approaches include the removal of IgG by staphylococcal protein-A (or Pansorbin, Calbiochem) or by high titer antihuman IgG serum from sheep, absorption of rheumatoid factor with IgG-coated latex beads, and fractionation of serum samples by column chromatography. These approaches have been found somewhat satisfactory in eliminating nonspecific activity and preserving the specific reaction in detecting IgM antibodies in pregnant mothers, neonates, and other patients with primary CMV infections. One more alternative method to improve the specificity of CMV IgM antibody detection is the application of anti-human IgM monoclonal or polyclonal antibody on the well to capture the human IgM antibody, then CMV antigen extract is added to react with the viral specific-IgM antibodies. The amount of CMV antigen captured by IgM antibody is subsequently quantitated or monitored by enzyme- or radioactive-labeled CMV-specific monoclonal or polyclonal antibodies. CMV-specific IgM antibody is, in this application, indirectly quantitated. CMV-specific IgA and IgE immunoglobulins can be detected using similar approaches.

CMV-specific antigens can be detected by ELISA using a pair of CMV-specific monoclonal antibodies which recognize different epitopes of viral antigens. In this case, the primary antibody (1 µg of antibody in 0.1 ml of 0.05 *M* Tris-HCl, pH 8.0, per well) is coated on the testing well overnight at 4 °C. The residual antibody is then decanted and the well is blocked with blocking solution (0.3 ml) for 1 h with frequent tapping or agitation. The subsequent procedures are identical to that described above for the detection of virus specific antibody in body fluids. Secondary antibody can be labeled either with enzymes or isotope.

Immunofluorescence and Immunoperoxidase Techniques

Immunofluorescence (FA) and immunoperoxidase (IP) tests have been successfully used in detecting virus-specific antigens or antibodies in the CMV system. The principles of these techniques are identical except the application of different labeling materials for fluorescent tag or enzymatic tag on the 1° or 2° antibody to trace the specific reactions. FA and IP tests can be categorized into direct and indirect methods based upon whether the first or the second antibody is being labeled. The common fluorescent conjugates are fluorescein isothiocyanate (FITC), tetramethylrhodamine isothiocyanate (TRITC), and R-phycoerythrin (PE) [18, 21, 38]. The enzymatic reaction employs horseradish peroxidase or alkaline phosphate and chromogenic substracts.

Immunofluorescence Assay. Frozen tissue sections with 5 μm thickness, exfoliated cells or infected cell cultures on chamber slides are first fixed with ice-chilled acetone for 15 min and rinsed with PBS (phosphate buffer saline) twice and then treated with 2% bovine serum albumin (blocking reagent, in PBS) before applying the properly diluted primary antibody. Freshly prepared paraformaldehyde (0.4%) in PBS can be used to replace acetone to fix the cells if preservation of the detailed cellular structures is needed. The reaction times for both primary and secondary antibodies are 1 h each at either 37 °C or room temperature. Extensive washing with PBS (three times, 5 min each) is needed after each antibody reaction. Slides are then mounted with coverslides and 50% glycerol in PBS.

In both direct or indirect immunofluorescent tests, a background reaction due to the presence of Fc receptors on the cell surface has to be taken into consideration. These Fc receptors can react nonspecifically with FITC- or enzyme-conjugated primary or secondary antibodies. Therefore, to minimize this nonspecific reaction the conjugated antibody should be diluted with buffer containing normal serum of the same animal species from which the specific antibody is derived. Monoclonal antibodies against CMV-specific proteins are available from various commercial sources such as DuPont. In addition, monoclonal antibodies against CMV-specific glycoproteins, structural and nonstructural proteins have been developed and are available for immunocytochemical studies (see Chap. 21, Pereira et al. for details).

Immunoperoxidase Assays. In immunoperoxidase assays, the antibody is labeled with horseradish peroxidase (HRPO) using either the periodate conjugation method [65] or the glutaraldehyde method [1]. In the periodate method, the alpha- and epsilon-amino groups and the hydroxy group of horseradish peroxidase (HRPO) are first completely blocked with fluorodinitrobenzene (FDNB), and then the carbohydrate portions of HRPO are oxidized by sodium m-periodate ($NaIO_4$) to form HRPO-aldehydes. The HRPO-aldehyde will form Schiff bases with antibodies having available alpha- or epsilon-amino groups at high efficiency. Using FDNB prior to the oxidation with $NaIO_4$ can prevent the self-coupling of HRPO-aldehyde. In the glutaraldehyde method, highly purified horseradish peroxidase is coupled to gamma-globulin by glutaraldehyde, and the excess conjugate blocked by L-lysine after coupling. The peroxidase-antibody conjugate is then purified by Sephadex G-150 or G-200 chromatography.

The degree of specificity of these techniques and the level of background depend strongly on the purity and specificity of the antibody. Fractionation and removal of nonspecific components from antisera by column chromatography, such DEAE cellulose column or DEAE-affigel blue (BioRad), is recommended. Peroxidase-labeled secondary antibodies are available from many commercial sources. The peroxidase activity of antigen-antibody complexes can be demonstrated intracellularly or extracellularly using various chromogens (e.g., diaminobenzidine, 4-chloronaphthol, and 3-amino-9-etyl-carbazole) [48, 60] in the presence of hydrogen peroxide.

The procedures for immunoperoxidase tests are identical to that of immunofluorescent assays except the final step of chromogenic reaction for immunoperoxidase test. The most common reagent used as a peroxidase substrate is 3,3′-diaminobenzidine tetrahydrochloride dihydrate (DAB). Freshly prepared 0.05% DAB (5 mg DAB in 10 ml of PBS) is mixed together with 10 μl of 10% hydrogen peroxide and applied to slides of fixed specimens. Cleavage of the DAB substrate by HRPO yields a brownish precipitate that is insoluble in alcohol, xylene, and water. The reaction can be stopped in 5 min with 0.05 *M* EDTA in PBS. DAB is a potential carcinogen and should be handled with great care.

In addition to FITC and HRP, secondary antibodies can be conjugated with alkaline phosphatase, biotin or different biochemical polymers. Streptavidin-peroxidase or streptavidin-peroxidase complexes can be used to detect biotinylated antibodies which in turn are chromagenized by DAB or nitroblue tetrazolium chloride (NBT). All of these chromagens are available from sources such as BRL (Gaithersburg, MD).

Anti-Complement (C′3) Immunofluorescence Assay. Besides the direct and indirect immunofluorescence assays, the anti-complement (C′3) immunofluorescence assay (ACIF) has been used to detect CMV in infected tissues [29]. The ACIF test is based on the ability of specific antigen and antibody reactions to fix C′3 complement. With FITC-conjugated anti-C′3 complement serum, the location of viral antigen can be indirectly demonstrated. This test has proven to be more sensitive than the direct and indirect FA tests [22] because it detects both IgM and IgG classes of antigen-antibody reactions that fix complement. Antiviral hyperimmune sera prepared from cattle and several species of birds cannot be used in this test because these sera are inactive in fixing complement.

The common complement sources we have used in this test are normal human sera without CMV, EBV, HSV, VZV and anti-nuclear antibodies. Complement sera and anti-human C′3 antibodies are available from Sigma (St. Louis, MO) or ICN Biomedicals (Costa Mesa, CA) FITC- or HRPO-conjugated anti-human C′3 complement polyclonal as well as monoclonal antibodies are available from Dako (Carpinteria, CA).

In this assay, virus-infected cells, frozen sections, or exfoliated cells are applied to precleaned microscope slides (Fisher Superfrost Plus, catalog No. 12-550-15) and fixed with ice-chilled acetone for 15 min. Anti-CMV monoclonal or polyclonal antibodies are mixed with complement, applied to the samples and placed in a moist CO_2 incubator for 1 hour. After extensive washing, the FITC-conjugated anti-human C′3 antibody with a rhodamine counterstain (final dilution of 1:200; BRL, Maryland) are applied to the samples and incubated for 1 h. Extensive washing with PBS is needed after incubation. A control to which CMV antiserum is not applied is essential. This control detects the presence of any cells which possess complement receptor sites that are able to fix complement and give a false positive result, such as human B lymphocytes. Figure 2 shows the detection of CMV-infected cells by ACIF test. The specimen is a frozen kidney section from a congenitally CMV-infected infant. The location of human CMV antigens is demonstrated primarily in cuboidal-epithelial cells of the collecting tubules. The FITC-conjugated anti-human C′3 antibody can be replaced with horseradish peroxidase (HRP)-conjugated anti-human C′3 antibody and by using a chromogenic reagent to localize the specific antigen-antibody reaction.

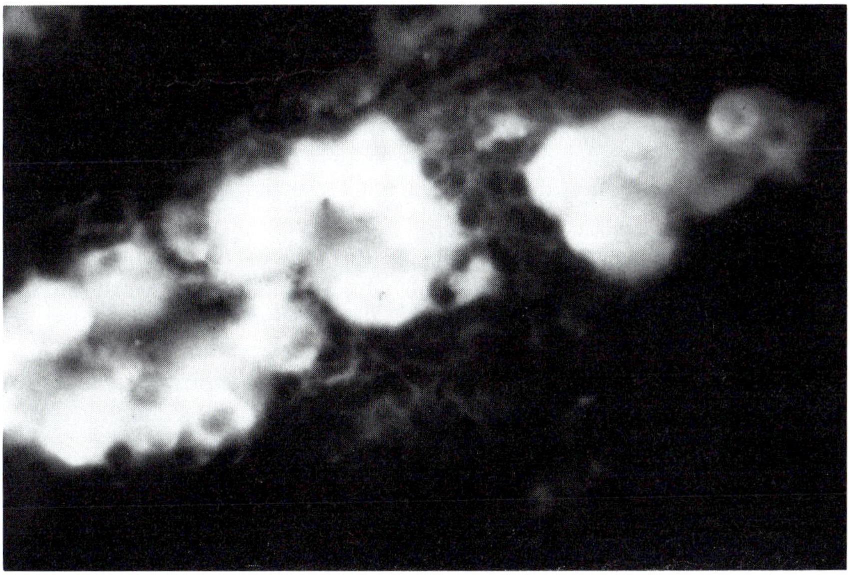

Fig. 2. Detection of human CMV in a frozen kidney section by anti-complement immunofluorescence test. The location of CMV antigen is mainly in cuboidal epithelial cells of the collection tubules. Magnification is about ×800

Detection of Human CMV-Specific DNA and RNA by Nucleic Acid Hybridization

Nucleic acid hybridization techniques have become powerful tools in virus diagnosis. Quantitation of CMV DNA, or mRNA, as well as the location of virus specific nucleic acid can be achieved by using various nucleic acid hybridization techniques [26, 27]. Classic DNA–DNA reassociation kinetic analyses can detect virus-specific nucleic acid and the percentage of homology between two viral strains at the subgenomic level. But this method requires extensive effort in analyzing the rates of DNA reassociation from several sets (or time courses) of reactions. This method is not practical for routine viral diagnosis. Therefore, no effort will be made here to reiterate this approach. The information and procedures related to the use of DNA–DNA reassociation kinetic analysis for diagnosis of CMV infections have been described before [26, 27]. Uses for nucleic acid hybridizations with nitrocellulose membrane as solid supports including classical DNA–DNA (or RNA) membrane hybridization (Southern), dot hybrdization, and northern blot hybridizations are very popular for the detection of CMV in various clinical specimens. In addition, recent advances in the development of nonradioactive DNA or RNA probes make these techniques very powerful tools in clinical virology.

Denatured single-stranded DNAs or RNAs are able to absorb onto solid nitrocellulose membrane filters in the presence of salt (6XSSC for DNA and 10XSCC for RNA). After baking, the single-strand DNAs orRNAs immobilized on the filters are then available to hybridize with radioactive or nonradioactive labeled nucleic acids probes that share sequences complementary to them. The Southern blot hybridization technique uses electrophoresis to separate restriction enzyme-fragmentated DNAs in agarose gels. The DNA fragments are then denatured in situ and transferred to nitrocellulose or nylon membranes for hybridization [49, 54, 64]. In this case the sample on the membrane is single-stranded DNA. Northern blot hybridizations use RNAs isolated from tissues or virus-infected cells. The RNAs are first separated by electrophoresis through agarose gels in the presence of formaldehyde or other denaturing agent, such as glyoxal. The RNAs are then blotted onto nitrocellulose or nylon membranes in the presence of 10XSSC and readied for hybridization [50, 59]. Dot hybridization can also be used to study virus-related sequences in the form of either DNA or RNA. In this assay, denatured DNA or single stranded RNA is immobilized on nitrocellulose membrane using a dot blot device, such as a Minifold apparatus (Schleicher and Schuell, Keene, N.H.).

DNA Extraction and RNA Purification

Total DNA and RNA can be extracted from cells or tissues by either of two approaches. When both total DNA and intact RNA are wanted, the guanidinium isothiocyanate-CsCl equilibrium centrifugation method should be applied [37, 61]. In this case, cells or cold powdered tissues are dissolved in a 6 *M* guanidinium isothiocyanate solution. The viscous lysate is passed through a 20-G needle six times to decrease the viscosity and then layered on top of a 5.7 *M* CsCl solution in a polyallomer ultracentrifuge tube. The sample is centrifuged at 35 000 rpm in a Beckman SW40 rotor overnight at 20 °C. The RNA should form a pellet and the DNA should be banded at a density of around 1.70 g/ml. In the second method, cells are lysed with a buffer containing 0.05 *M* Tris-HCl, pH 8.0, 0.01 *M* EDTA, 1% SDS, 0.001 *M* CaCl and 40–100 μg/ml of proteinase K. After incubation at 37° to hydrolyze proteins, the cell lysate is subjected to phenol extraction and alcohol precipitation following standard protocols. RNA can be removed by pancreatic RNase digestion followed by phenol extraction and alcohol precipitation to remove residual RNase.

Preparation of Radioactive or Nonradioactive Nucleic Acid Probes

There are many ways to prepare either radioactive or nonradioactive CMV-specific DNA or RNA probes. Table 1 is a brief outline of methods that are commonly used in our laboratory.

A wide variety of nucleic acid labeling kits are available commercially, such as those from BRL, Promega, Boehringer Mannheim Biochemicals, etc. The basic approaches used by various firms to label nucleic acids are almost identical for nick-translation, random priming, direct labeling using ^{125}I or photobiotin and the use of SP6 or T7 polymerases to synthesize riboprobes. The use of *E. coli* transcriptase (DNA-dependent RNA polymerase) to synthesize ^{3}H-labeled CMV cRNA for membrane hybridization and in situ cytohybridization has been described previously [26–28, 41]. The details for other approaches using commercial kits are provided by the manufacturers. Blot hybridization with radioactive probes are visualized by enhanced autoradiography, whereas hybridizations using nonradioactive probes are identified by colormetric reactions. Radioactive probes have the advantage of greater sensitivity, whereas nonradioactive probes require no special handling or disposal considerations.

It is extremely important to select appropriate CMV DNA fragments or gene sequences for use as probes because some regions of the CMV genome share homology with human DNA [44, 51]. In addition, the high GC content of some regions of the CMV genome frequently results in high background hybridization against cellular DNA. Via extensive study, we have found that a CMV IE2 cDNA (or a BamH1 fragment of CMV genome, recovered from plasmid pHD101SV1, which encodes the IE2 gene) [12] provides low background and an extremely specific hybridization signal for CMV. This DNA fragment has been inserted into pGEM2 at the *Eco*R1 site (pHDIE2) for synthesizing riboprobes for clinical diagnosis of CMV infections.

DNA or RNA probes can be purified by Sephadex G-25 or 50 column chromatography or through various spin columns available commercially,

Table 1. An outline of methods used to label nucleic acid probes for CMV detection

Probes	Label	Labeling method
Radioactive		
Radioactive CMV-DNA	^{32}P α-dXTP, or ^{3}H α-dXTP, or ^{32}S α-dATP, or (NEG-034N, NEN) ^{125}I dCTP	a. Nick-translation using Kornberg's enzyme (Nick translation system from Promega, product U1001, or BRL, product 8160SB) b. Random primer DNA labeling system using Klenow enzyme (BRL, product 8187SA)
Radioactive CMV-specific oligo DNA	^{32}P γ-ATP	a. 5′ end labeling with polynucleotide kinase (5′ DNA terminus labeling system from BRL, product 8060SA, or Promega, product U2010)
Radioactive CMV-cRNA, riboprobe	^{32}P α-XTP, or ^{3}H α-XTP, or ^{35}S α-ATP	a. In vitro transcription using *E. coli* transcriptase b. CMV DNA fragment is inserted into the multiple cloning sites of plasmid pGEX2. Riboprobe are synthesized using SP6 or T7 phage RNA polymerase after linearization of plasmid by the appropriate restriction enzyme (Promega, p2101)
Nonradioactive		
Biotin-labeled CMV-DNA	Biotin-14-dATP (BRL 9524SA)	a. Nick-translation using BioNick kit (BRL 8247SA) b. Random primed labeling system
	photobiotin acetate	a. Photobiotin labeling system (BRL, product 8186SA) [15]
DIG-labeled CMV-DNA	digoxigenin-11-dUTP	a. Nick-translation or, b. Random primed labeling system using digoxigenin -dUTP (DIG-UTP, Boehringer Mannheim Biochemicals, product 1175033)
Biotin or DIG-labeled CMV-cRNA (riboprobe)	Biotin-UTP DIG-11-UTP	a. In vitro transcription using *E. coli* transcriptase b. CMV DNA fragment to be transcribed is cloned into the multiple cloning sites of vectors containing promoters for SP6 or T7 polymerase adjacent to the insertion sites, such as pGEX2 (Promega). CMV cRNA is synthesized using SP6 or T7 after linearizing the plasmid at an appropriate site

such as Quick Spin Column G-25 and G-50 from Boehringer Mannheim Biochemicals (product 100420 and 100408, respectively), to remove free triphosphates and salt. Radioactive-labeled DNA and RNA can be further purified by phenol extraction and alcohol precipitation, but not the biotinylated or digoxiginin-labeled nonradioactive probes; these nonradioactive probes will be trapped at the aqueous and organic interphase.

Dot Blot Hybridization

Dot blot hybridization has been used to detect CMV in urine and leukocytes [8, 47, 55] (our unpublished data). Although this method is relatively simple, sensitivity is always a problem with this assay. Specimens containing low amounts of virus frequently have signals close to that of normal control DNA, particularly for DNA samples extracted from leukocytes or tissues.

Figure 3 shows the detection of CMV-specific DNA sequences in DNA extracted from the buffy coats of organ transplantation patients. DNA (5 μg) from buffy coats were denatured with 0.5 N NaOH for 3 min and neutralized with 1.1 N HCl in 0.2 *M* Tris. The DNA solution was then adjusted to 6X SSC (0.9 *M* CaCl, 0.09 *M* sodium citrate) and immobilized on nitrocellulose membrane via a BRL dot apparatus. After baking for 2 h at 80°C in vacuum oven, the filter was prehybridized for 1 h and then hybridized with CMV-specific ^{32}P cRNA (hybridization solution contained ^{32}P cRNA at 1×10^5 cpm/ml, specific activity of 1×10^7 cpm/μg, 6XSSC, 1 mg/ml yeast RNA, 100 μg/ml sonicated calf thymus DNA, 0.1% SDS). Hybridization was carried out overnight at 65 °C with agitation. Recently, we added formamide to the hybridization solution (final concentration 50%) to lower the hybridization temperature to 40 °C and Denhardt's solution (final 5X) to decrease hybridization background. Denhardt's solution contains 0.02% Ficoll, 0.02% polyvinylpyrrolidone and 0.02% BSA (Pentax fraction V) in dH_2O. After hybridization, the filter was washed with 2X SSC three times. Any remaining unhybridized

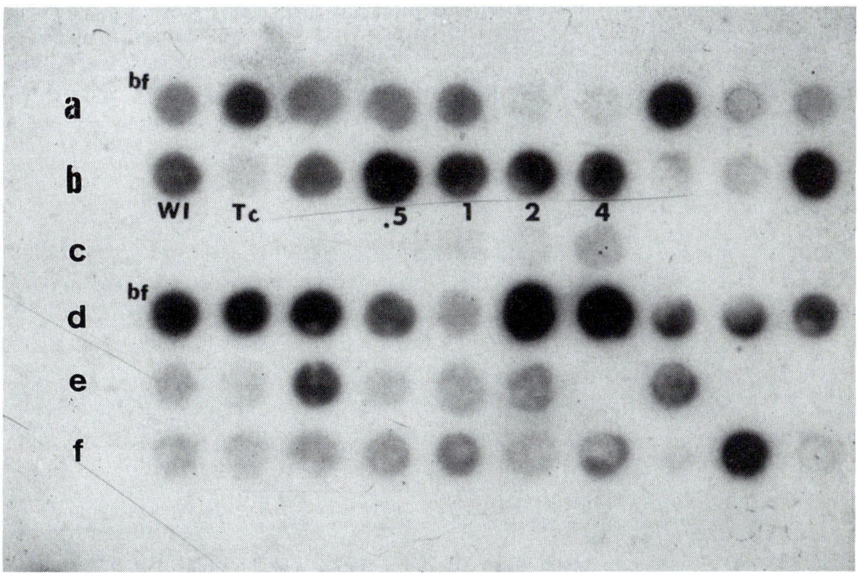

Fig. 3. Detection of CMV DNA in buffy coats from organ transplantation patients by RNA-DNA dot hybridization. 5 μg of DNA extracted from buffy coats was used in each case. CMV-specific ^{32}P-cRNA with a specific activity of 1×10^7 cpm/μg was used in this experiment. *Line c* shows the hybridization intensity for WI-38 cell (*WI*), calf thymus DNA (T_c), and positive CMV control at levels of 0.5, 1, 2 and 4 viral genomes per cell. The remaining samples on *lines a, b, d, e,* and *f* are various buffy coats obtained from bone marrow transplantation patients. Overnight exposure

cRNA was removed by RNase digestion (40 µg/ml, in 2X SSC for 30 min). The filter was washed again three times with 2X SSC, dried and subjected to autoradiography. Figure 3 (line C) shows the hybridization intensity for WI-38 cell (WI), calf thymus DNA (Tc) and positive CMV controls at levels of 0.5, 1, 2 and 4 viral genomes per cell. The remaining lines (A, B, D, E, and F) are various buffy coat samples obtained from bone marrow transplantation patients from the Bone Marrow Transplantation Center at the University of Washington at Seattle. This experiment was performed in 1974.

Nonradioactive DNA or riboprobes can also be used in dot blot hybridization; when DNA probes are used for hybridization, the RNase digestion step is not needed. Nonspecific hybridization can be partially reduced by raising the washing temperature to 60 °C in 2X SSC for 10 min for one cycle. Other stringent washing conditions, such as higher temperatures and lower ionic strengths, can be applied if the hybridization background is still too high. Biotinylated probes were used by Buffone et al. [4] to detect CMV in clinical urine specimens. In this study, the biotin-labeled CMV DNA probes, hybridized to DNA bound to nitrocellulose membranes, were bound by streptavidin-alkaline phosphatase complexes and detected by a chromogenic reaction using 5-bromo-4-chloro-3-indolyl phosphate (BCIP) and nitro blue tetrazolium. The authors claimed that they could detect CMV DNA in as little as 10 pg. Using ^{32}P-labeled radioactive probe, Spector et al. [55] could detect CMV DNA to the same level. For alkaline phosphatase-labeled complexes, the chemiluminescent formulation of Boehringer Mannheim Biochemical (Lumi-Phos 530, Cat. No. 1275 470) offers a rapid and sensitive way to detect the signal and location of specific hybridization. It can be used in dot blot as well as Southern blot hybridizations.

Southern Blot Hybridization

Southern blot hybridization applies restriction enzymes and agarose gel electrophoresis to fragment and separate DNAs which in turn are denatured in situ and transferred onto nitrocellulose by blotting. Detailed procedures have been provided previously [49, 54, 64]. Restriction enzymes commonly used in CMV study are *Eco*R1, *Bam*H1 and *Hin*dIII [30, 31, 36]. Because many of the generated CMV DNA fragments have sizes larger than 5 kb, highly efficient fragment transfer is necessary. Treatment of the DNA fragments in agarose gels with 1.5 N HCl before denaturation will facilitate transfer [64]. The acid treatment partially depurinates the DNA which will then be further fragmented by subsequent alkaline treatment. The nitrocellulose membrane bound DNA will then be subjected to hybridization following the protocol used for dot blot hybridization.

Southern blot hybridization offers more specific and detailed information for clinical CMV diagnosis. The resulting hybridization pattern can not only make positive CMV DNA detection, but can also provide information regarding viral strain relatedness. Due to the complicated nature of this procedure, Southern blot hybridization is not commonly used in clinical CMV detection.

In Situ Nucleic Acid Hybridization

In situ hybridization is derived from classic cRNA–DNA membrane hybridization. However, in this method the cellular DNA or RNA is not extracted, rather the hybridization of radioactive or nonradioactive labeled DNA or RNA probe to the complementary sample is carried out directly on slides of fixed cells or specimens. The site at which the specific hybridization occurs can be localized and detected by autoradiography or in situ chromogenic reactions. These methods are adapted from that of Gall and Pardue [16] and have been successfully used for the human CMV system [26–29]. The in situ hybridization method can be used to detect both viral DNA or RNA in either frozen sections or formalin fixed paraffin embedded samples. The sensitivity in formalin fixed specimens is far less than in frozen sections fixed with glacial acetate-alcohol (1:3) fixative. This is apparently due to the degree of covalent crosslinking between protein–protein and protein–nucleic acids caused by formalin fixation. Nucleic acid probes can be either radioactive or nonradioactive DNA or RNA, depending on the nature of the specimen to be studied.

Preparation of Slides. It is essential to have very clean slides for mounting frozen sections or exfoliated cells for in situ hybridization. Slides should be precleaned with Extran alkali-detergent (1:100, Merck cat. no. 7555) or chromic cleaning solution (Chromatic-sulfuric acid cleaning solution, Fisher cat. no. c57712) overnight, washed extensively with dH_2O, then coated with polylysine (use poly-L-lysine hydrobromide, MW > 30 kDa, Sigma P1274, P1300, P1524 or P2636, 0.1% W/V in 0.01 M Tris-HCl, pH 8.0) at 37 °C for 1 h or 4 °C overnight. After coating, the polylysine solution is removed and the slides are air dried and stored in a dust free desiccator. Alternatively, Superfrost/Plus precleaned microscope slides from Fisher Scientific (catalog no. 12-550-15) can be used directly to mount specimens without further cleaning and precoating processes.

Preparation of Tissues and Pretreatment of Sections. Biopsied or autopsied fresh tissues are frozen immediately after sampling by immersing specimens in liquid nitrogen or keeping in a −70 °C freezer. The frozen tissues are then immersed in O.T.C. compound (Lab-tech products, Naperville, IL) in an embedding mold on dry ice or at −70 °C for sectioning. Tissue sections with a 5–6 µm thickness are prepared using a cryostat at −20 °C, mounted onto slides at multiple locations and air dried. Sections can then be fixed using one of the following fixatives: (i) 4% paraformaldehyde in PBS, pH 7.2, for 15 min at 4 °C; (ii) 0.1% glutaraldehyde in PBS for 30 min at 4 °C; (iii) ice chilled Clark's fixative (glacial acetic acid : alcohol = 1:3 for 10 min); or (iv) Carnoy's fluid (ethanol : glacial acetic acid : chloroform = 6:3:1) at room temperature for 10 min. After fixation, the slides are washed with ethanol, air dried and stored at −20 °C.

Routinely processed, formalin fixed paraffin embedded autopsied or biopsied tissues can also be used for this assay [3, 5, 62]. Paraffin sections (5 µm) are cut, mounted on slides, dried at 37 °C for an hour, and baked at 60 °C for overnight to 24 h. Sections are dewaxed by three changes of xylene (10 min each) and incubated for two 10 min periods in absolute alcohol and then air dried. If the testing involves a peroxidase enzyme assay, endogenous peroxidase activity can be inactivated by treatment of slide-mounted samples with absolute methanol containing 1% H_2O_2 for 3 min, then rehydrated in a stepwise manner for hybridization.

Both frozen and paraffin sectioned samples should be pretreated with pronase or proteinase K, before hybridization, in order to increase the hybridization efficiency. Exfoliated cells which have been fixed on slides also need to be treated with pronase to open cell membranes allowing nucleic acid probes to enter into the cells. Slides are first treated with 0.01% Triton-X-100 in PBS for 1 min, washed three times in PBS for 3 min each, then digested with pronase solution (CalBiochem, 0.1–0.3 mg/ml in 0.05 *M* Tris-HCl, pH 7.4 and 5 m*M* EDTA) for 10 min at room temperature. Proteinase K can be used at a concentration of 10 µg/ml in 0.05 *M* Tris-HCl, pH 7.4 and 1 m*M* $CaCl_2$ place of pronase. The proteinase K reaction is at room temperature for 3 min. After proteolytic digestion, excess enzyme should be removed and the reaction stopped by washing the samples three times with TBS (0.05 *M* Tris-HCl, pH 7.4, 0.15 *M* NaCl) containing 2 mg/ml of glycine.

Hybridization. Radioactive- or nonradioactive-labeled DNA or RNA probe can be used for in situ hybridization. For CMV DNA detection, DNA and RNA probes derived from either strand are appropriate for use in this assay. For detection of mRNA transcripts (sense strand) in situ, an anti-sense strand probe should be used.

The hybridization mixture used in all experiments contains 50% ultrapure deionized formamide (Boehringer Mannheim Biochemicals, Cat. No. 100144), 6X SSC, 1X Denhardt's solution, 100 µg/ml of sonicated denatured salmon sperm DNA, 100 µg/ml of yeast RNA and $3-5 \times 10^6$ cpm/ml of radioactive DNA or RNA probe, or 2 µg/ml of biotinylated nucleic acid probe. Plastic electric tape is used to create a well around the tissue section. This is overlaid with hybridization mixture and covered with a coverslip, preventing the generation of air bubbles. The tissue and probe are then subjected to heat denaturation for 10 min by heating the slides on a sponge floating in the boiling water. The slides are then incubated in a 37 °C, humidified incubator for 16–24 h. After hybridization, the coverslips are carefully removed by dipping the slides into 2X SSC with 0.1X SDS. The slides are then subjected to three 5-min washes with 2X SSC-0.1% SDS at room temperature, one 3-min wash with 50% formamide in 2X SSC-0.1% SDS at 35 °C, and two 1-min washes in 2X SSC-0.1% SDS at room temperature. For samples with radioactive probes, the slides are dehydrated with alcohol and overlayed with Kodak NTB-2 immulsion for autoradiography. When ^3H-labeled probe is used, a 3–4 week exposure time is required if no ^3H enhancer is used. Exposure time can be shortened by dipping the emulsion coated slide in ^3H enhancer or 1% PPO and 0.2% POPOP (in dioxane) in the dark. For ^{32}P probe, 3–5 day exposures are required. After exposure, slides are developed in Kodak D-19 developer for 3 min, gently rinsed with water for 3 min and fixed in Kodak rapid fixer for 3 min.

For nonradioactive probes, the samples are blocked with 3% BSA in TBS and subjected to chromogenic reactions as described in the membrane hybridization section. Biotinylated DNA can be detected by (i) indirect immunofluorescence or peroxidase assay using a primary antibody against biotin, and secondary antibody labeled with FITC or peroxidase, or (ii) streptavidin horseradish peroxidase complex (from EnZo-Biochem), streptavidin-alkaline phosphatase or streptavidin-peroxidase from Promega, BRL, and Boehringer Mannheim Biochemicals.

When digoxigenin-labeled DNA is used, the hybridized probe can be detected by anti-DIG alkaline phosphate (AP) or peroxidase conjugated antibody. The color reaction for anti-DIG AP is developed in alkaline pH using X-phosphate and NTB (Boehringer Mannheim Biochemical, cat. no. 1175041) or BICP and NTB (Promega). A blue precipitate develops at the sites of positive hybridization.

Figure 4 shows the application of in situ nucleic acid hybridization to detect CMV genomes using radioactive and nonradioactive probes. In Fig. 4a and 4b, CMV-specific ^{3}H cRNA was used to detect human CMV-infected syncytial trophoblasts in placenta and in buffy coat white blood cells, respectively. Note the heavy silver granules clustered within CMV-infected cells. In Fig. 4c biotinylated DNA probe was used to detect CMV-infected cells within the lymph node of a patient with AIDS.

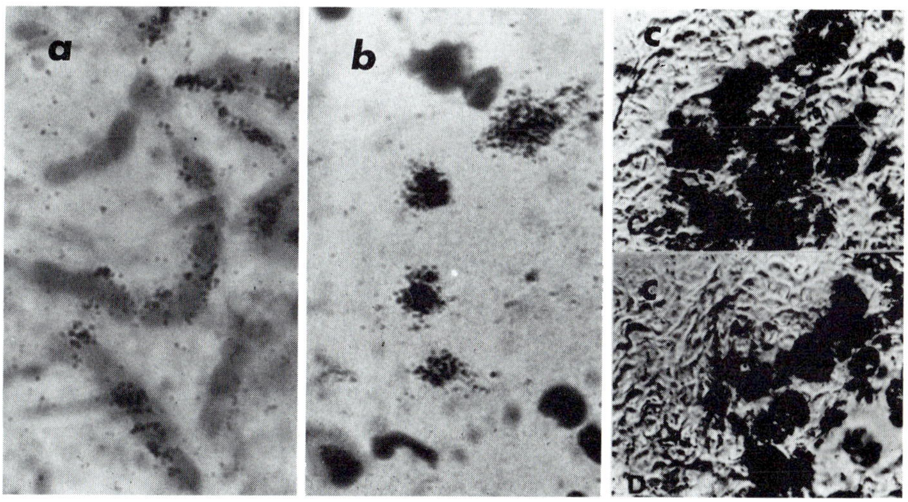

Fig. 4a–d. In situ nucleic acid hybridization with CMV-specific radioactive (**a** and **b**) and nonradioactive (**c**) probes. Panels **a** and **b** used ^{3}H labeled CMV cRNA to detect CMV-infected syncytial trophoblasts in the placenta and white blood cells (in buffy coats), respectively. In panel **c** biotinylated DNA probe was used to detect virus-infected cells within the lymph node of a patient with AIDS

Detection of CMV Infection by the Polymerase Chain Reaction

The polymerase chain reaction (PCR) offers the many advantages of sensitivity, speed, simplicity and effectiveness over other detection methods used in CMV diagnosis. In this assay, a specific segment of viral DNA is amplified by a thermal stable DNA-dependent DNA polymerase purified from thermophilic bacteria, such as Taq polymerase (Cetus) from *Thermus aquaticus* YT1(ATCC 25104). The procedure uses two oligonucleotide primers that hybridize with complementary DNA strands and flank the specific viral DNA fragment of interest. The DNA amplification occurs via a repetitive series of cycles involving template denaturation at 94 °C, primer annealing at 40° – 60°C and the extension of annealed primers at 72°C. After 20 – 30 cycles of PCR, the specific DNA fragment can be amplified up to one million-fold. The amplified DNA can be identified by dot blot hybridization, or by agarose gel electrophoresis and Southern blot hybridization. A restriction enzyme site can also be created during primer selection for verifying the fidelity of DNA amplification by restriction enzyme digestion.

The PCR technique has been successfully used to detect CMV in urine from newborns [13], in blood of patients with AIDS [40, 53], in patients undergoing organ transplantation [6, 14, 32, 43], in Kaposi's sarcoma specimens [63], in lung tissue of patients with interstitial pneumonitis [33], in the arterial walls of patients suffering from atherosclerosis [20], and in cervicovaginal cells [67]. The sensitivity of this assay was estimated to be at the level of one viral genome per 40,000 cells [6] or 0.01 pg of AD169 fragment D DNA [25]. In one study, this assay diagnosed viremia and viruria in 83% of seropositive patients (24 cases) after bone marrow transplantation, while virus isolation by cell culture showed 67% of these patients to be viruric and 37% to be viremic. Slot blot hybridization showed 50% positivity for both viruria and viremia in these subjects [14]. In this same study, positive PCR was demonstrated in five patients even before the onset of clinical symptoms of acute graft-versus-horst rejection. In addition to freshly collected specimens, sample DNA can be purified from paraffin-embedded tissues or by directly boiling deparaffinized sections for CMV PCR assay [7]. The superb sensitivity and specificity of PCR makes it one of the best methods in the clinical laboratory to detect CMV in a great variety of clinical samples.

Preparation of Samples for PCR

The PCR technique can be used to detect both virus-specific DNA or mRNA. For viral RNA detection, an additional reverse transcription step is needed to generate either single-stranded or double-stranded DNA for template. This involves the addition of oligo(dT) and reverse transcriptase to synthesize complementary DNA for subsequent amplification.

Total DNA for PCR assays can be purified from biopsied or autopsied tissues, peripheral blood cells, exfoliated cells, and body fluids by phenol extraction, as decribed above. Although positive reactions can be obtained by using proteinase K-digested crude cell lysates, the results are not consistent if only low levels of viral DNA are present in the specimens. Therefore, we recommended the use of purified DNA samples for critical experiments.

Beside peripheral blood cells, urine samples are the most common clinical samples encountered for CMV detection. Urine samples can be used either directly for PCR or after phenol extraction of DNA. Demmler et al. [13] successfully detected CMV in urine samples obtained from congenitally infected infants using urine directly without any further purification. The positive detection rate for PCR analysis of urine samples is more than 93% as compared to that of culture isolation. This approach is simple and specific, but the concentration of urea in the reaction mixture is a major concern. We have found, as has Khan et al. [35], that urea was the major component in urine that inhibited PCR reactions if concentrations reach 50 m*M*. Khan et al. [35] also discovered that urine samples from older children were more inhibitory than those from neonates. To increase the sensitivity and to avoid inhibitory effects from other components residing within urine samples, we first precipitate macromolecules with polyethylene glycol (final concentration 10%) and extract DNA from the resulting precipitate with phenol before PCR analysis.

The procedures for preparing urine samples are as follows:

a. 0.25 ml of a sterile 50% polyethylene glycol 6000 (PEG, Fisher Scientific, in dH_2O with 0.15 N NaCl) solution is added into 1 ml of a urine sample dispensed into a 1.5 ml microfuge tube. After mixing and incubating in the cold (4 °C) for 2 h, the precipitate is collected by centrifugation in a microfuge for 20 min at 12 000 rpm in cold room.
b. The supernant is removed and discarded (as complete as possible to decrease the amount of residual PEG), and the pellet dissolved in 0.25 ml of TE buffer (0.05 *M* Tris-HCl, pH 7.9, and 0.001 *M* EDTA) containing 1% SDS, 1 m*M* $CaCl_2$ and 40 µg/ml of proteinase K.
c. After 1 h incubation at 37 °C, the sample is then subjected to one phenol and one chloroform extraction. Thirty µl of 7 *M* NH_4Cl is added to the solution and the sample DNA as well as RNA are precipitated with 2.5 volumes of alcohol (approximately 1 ml) at −20 °C.
d. DNA and RNA precipitates are collected by centrifugation in a microfuge for 20 min, washed with 75% alcohol once, dried in a speed vac and dissolved in 30 µl of sterile dH_2O. For each PCR assay, 5 µl of dissolved specimen is used.
e. For PCR assays using urine directly without purification, the amount of urine used should be less than 5 µl per reaction to avoid any inhibitory effects [35].

The reagents and procedures used in our laboratory for PCR essentially followed that described in the Cetus protocol guide (GeneAmp DNA amplification reagent kit part. no. N801-0043) and in Saiki [46] with minor modification.

Reagents

a. 10X reaction buffer

0.1 *M*	Tris-HCl, pH 8.3
0.5 *M*	KCl
0.02 *M*	$MgCl_2$
0.1% (w/v)	gelatin (Sigma Cat. No. G2500)

This solution should be filtered and autoclaved before use. The optimal $MgCl_2$ concentration should be empirically determined if template DNA is in a solution containing EDTA or other chelating agent. The final concentration of nonchelated Mg^{2+} should be kept under 2 m*M* to avoid nonspecific amplification, a concentration of 1.5 m*M* is optimal. Insufficient Mg^{2+} will reduce the yield.

b. 10X dNTP solution (2.5 mM each of dNTP). The deoxyribonucleotide triphosphates (dXTP) are prepared in sterile dH_2O and the pH of solution titrated to 7.4. Aliquots are stored at −20 °C.

Primers and Probe

In our laboratory in early 1988, five pairs of oligonucleotide primers derived from five regions of the Towne strain human CMV genome, including IE2, DNA polymerase, pp67, pp71, and US18 gene (multiple hydrophobic membrane protein), were used to test their specificity and sensitivity against 49 CMV clinical isolates and six other kinds of herpes group viruses, including HSV type 1 (KOS), HSV-2 (333), EBV (P3HR1K), simian CMV (GR2757), herpes virus saimiri, and mouse CMV. Results indicated that only the CMV IE2 and US18 pairs of primers were suitable for use in our molecular epidemiology study. The IE2 pair reacted with all 49 clinical CMV isolates while the US18 pair only reacted with 46 out of 49 CMV strains. Both IE2 and US18 primers showed negative response to the other herpes viruses. The polymerase and pp71 pairs of primers showed a lesser degree of specificity and had strong cross reactivity with all seven herpes group viruses in PCR. High specificity was found when pp67 were used but its sensitivity was relatively low as compared to that of the others; only 70% of the CMV isolates showed positive PCR (Huang et al. in preparation). Based on these results, the IE2 pair of primers were then selected for further comparison with clinical virus isolation data. In one study, 19 urine samples from infants with congenital CMV infection or suspicious HCMV-induced hepatitis were subjected to virus isolation and PCR testing using the IE2 primers. CMV was isolated from 15 out of 19 specimens while 16 out of 19 were PCR positive. In this case, the PCR test picked up all positive samples identified by virus isolation. The second study involved the use of liver biopsied tissues from children with clinical symptoms of possible CMV hepatitis (see Chap. 3 by Chang and Lee, this volume). CMV was isolated from 14 out of 35 samples while positive PCR was demonstrated in 24 out of 35 liver specimens. Eleven samples were positive for both virus

Table 2. Sequences of oligonucleotide primers and probes used in our laboratory as well as others and their locations within the CMV genome

Primer or probe	Sequences (5′ to 3′)	Length of product	Location of primer or probe
a. *Our primers*			
Primer IE2a	TCCTCCTGCAGTTCGGCTTC	240	531– 550
Primer IE2b	TTTCATGATATTGCGCACCT		770– 751
Probe IE2	TGCTGAGCTGCGGCCATCAGA		661– 680
Primer US18a	CGCGTCATCGGTCTGTCGTT	209	397– 476
Primer US18b	GTCACCACCAGGACGTAGAG		605– 586
Probe US18	TACGGCTGGTCCGTCATCGT		508– 527
b. *Demmler et al. (1988)*			
Primer MIE-4	CCAAGCGGCCTCTGATAACCAAGCC	435	731– 755
Primer MIE-5	CAGCACCATCCTCCTCTTCCTCTGG		1165–1150
Probe MIE	GAGGCTATTGTAGCCTACACTTTGG		900– 925
Primer LA-1	CACCTGTCACCGCTGCTATATTTGC	400	2101–2125
Primer LA-6	CACCACGCAGCGGCCCTTGATGTTT		2500–2476
Probe LA	GTCGCCTGCACTGCCAGGTGCTTCG		2301–2325
c. *Shibata et al. (1988)*			
Primer IE1	CCACCCGTGGTGCCAGCTCC	162	1307–1326
Primer IE2	CCCGCTCCTCCTGAGCACCC		1468–1449
Primer IE3	CTGGTGTCACCCCCAGAGTC-CCCTGTACCCGCGACTATCC		1336–1375
Primer LA-1	CCGCAACCTGGTGCCCATGG	139	1818–1837
Primer LA-2	CGTTTGGGTTGCGCAGCGGG		1956–1937
Probe LA-3	TTCTTCTGGGACGCCAACGA-CATCTACCGCATCTTCGCCG		1877–1916

IE, immediate-early gene region of CMV; MIE, major immediate-early gene region of CMV; LA, late antigen region of CMV; US18, reading frame 18 of unique region S of CMV. The location is expressed as the nucleotide number, numbered sequentially within each gene as published or as cited in the sequences contained in Gene Bank. Sequences for primers IE2a, b and probe IE2 are derived from CMV IE2 gene (exon 5) region of Stenberg et al. [58]; sequences for US20a, b and Probe US18 are derived from our US18 sequences (Gao et al., in preparation); primer IE1, IE2 and probe IE3 for Shibata et al. [53] are derived from exon 4 of IE1 [57]; and primer LA-1, La-2 and probe LA-3 of Shibata et al. are derived from sequences published by Ruger et al. [45]

isolation and PCR. In our experience, the efficiency of isolating CMV from biopsied tissues or blood samples is far less than that from urine or cervical specimens. It is, therefore, concluded that the use of the IE2 primers we designed to detect CMV from urine, cervical swab or biopsied specimen is specific.

The sequences of the primers used in our laboratory and that of others are listed in Table 2.

Reaction and Amplification in a DNA Thermal Cycler

The typical PCR assay is done in a 50- to 100 µl volume. The reaction mixture used in our laboratory is assembled as follows:

Template or sample DNA (for urine samples, 5 µl)	1–3 µg
Primer A and primer B (100 µg each/ml)	2 µl
10X reaction buffer	10 µl
10X (2.5 mM each) dNTP	10 µl
5% Triton-X-100	2 µl
Steriled double-distilled dH_2O made up to a total volume	95 µl

All ingredients are mixed well and centrifuged in a microfuge to settle the mixture on the bottom of the tube (0.45 ml thin walled microfuge tubes). A couple of drops (100 µl) of autoclaved light grade liquid mineral oil is laid over the mixture. The mixture is then denatured by boiling in 100 °C water bath for 5 min and then 2 units of Taq polymerase (AmpliTaq, Cetus) is added to the reaction mixture for subsequent amplification.

Amplification is performed in a Perkin-Elmer Cetus DNA Thermal Cycler using the "Step Cycle" program to set denaturation, annealing and extension cycles as follows:

a. Two cycles of initial amplification with
   denaturation at 94 °C for 2 min
   annealing at 50 °C for 2 min
   extension at 72 °C for 2 min
b. Thirty cycles of subsequent amplification with
   denaturation at 94 °C for 1 min,
   annealing at 50 °C for 1 min,
   extension at 72 °C for 1 min.
c. Two cycles of completing reaction with
   denaturation at 94 °C for 1 min,
   annealing at 50°C for 2 min
   extension at 72 °C for 5 min
d. Soaking cycle is set at 4 °C.

Confirmation by Electrophoresis and Hybridization

The amplification products are subjected to 3% agarose gel electrophoresis in TBE buffer [66]. The best DNA molecular weight markers are *Hin*fI digested pBR322 DNA fragments, with sizes of 1631, 517, 506, 396, 344, 298, 221, 220, 154 and 75 bp. Ethidium bromide at concentration of 5 µg/ml in TBE buffer can be used to stain DNA fragments in the gel. The amplified PCR products can be verified by dot blot or Southern blot hybridization for its specificity using corresponding oligonucleotide probe, labelled with gamma ^{32}P ATP using polynucleotide kinase, or riboprobe synthesized from the DNA

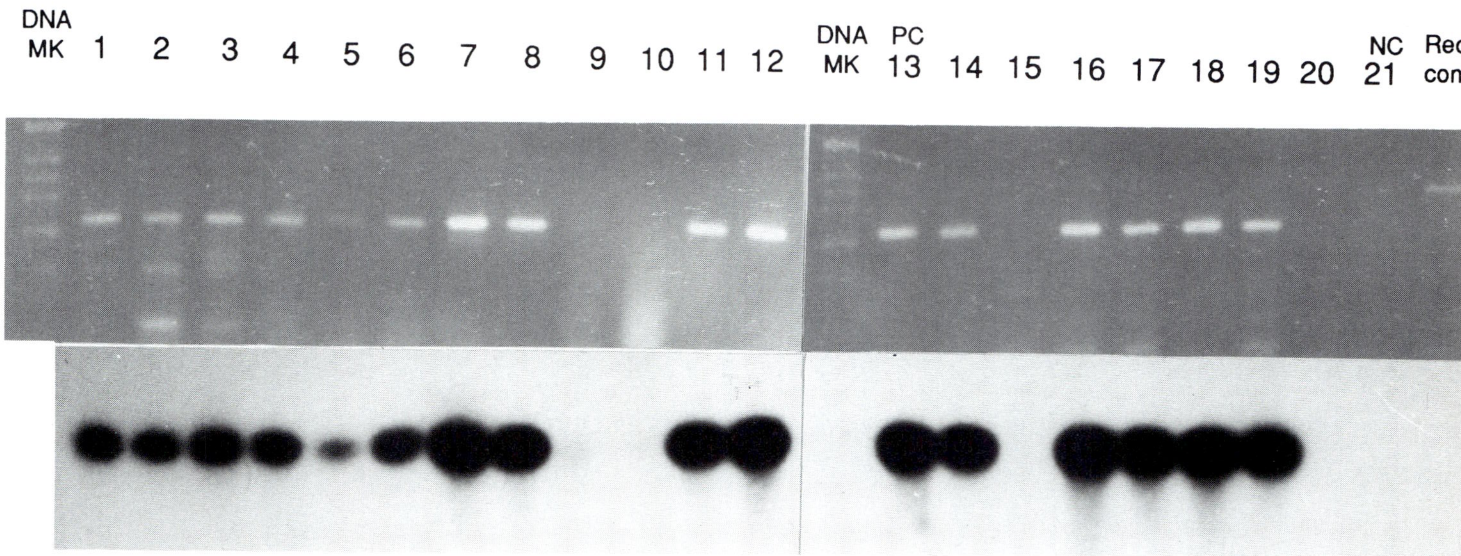

Fig. 5. PCR analysis of CMV DNA in urine samples of neonates suffering from infant hepatitis. The IE2a and IE2b pair of primers were used in this experiment. The *Hin*f1 digested pBR322 markers (DNA MK) are on the *left* of each gel. The lane marked with *PC 13* is the positive control using CMV IE2 recombinant plasmid pGEMIE2 as a control (1 ng). *NC 21* indicates negative cell control. The confirming hybridization results are shown immediately underneath the PCR figures

fragment from which the primers are derived from. Figure 5 shows the result of the detection of CMV in urine specimens of neonates suffering from infant hepatitis. CMV IE2a and b primers were used for amplification. The resulting products were subjected to 3% agarose gel electrophoresis and Southern blot hybridization using ^{32}P labeled CMV IE2 probe.

Paraffin Embedded Samples for CMV PCR

Shibata et al. [52] have successfully used paraffin embedded histological sections to detect papilloma virus DNA by PCR. The same approach can be used for CMV DNA detection. In this approach, paraffin sections are first deparaffinized in 500 μl of xylene. The tissue sections are washed with xylene and then 95% alcohol in a 1.5 ml centrifuge tube separated by short centrifugations in a microfuge. After washing one more time with 75% alcohol, the tissue sections are then dissolved in 100 μl of digestion solution containing 2.5 m*M* $MgCl_2$, 0.5% Tween-20, 0.5% NP-40, 50 m*M* KCl, 100 m*M* Tris-HCl, pH 8.3, 0.01% gelatin and 100 μg/ml of proteinase K. After overnight digestion in a 37 °C incubator, the specimens can then be subjected to phenol extraction to obtain purified DNA for PCR or directly subjected to the PCR reaction by adding dXTP (to 0.8 m*M*) and 5 units of Taq polymerase to the mixture [52].

Direct Microscopic Examination of Clinical Samples

Exfoliated Cells

CMV-infected cells are frequently demonstrated in exfoliated cells of urine sediment and bronchial lavage obtained from CMV viruria or CMV pneumonitis patients. With H and E or Giemsa stain, cytomegalic intranuclear inclusion-bearing cells are easily distinguished from normal cells under the light microscope. These cells are large, and each has a large intranuclear inclusion body which is separated from the peripheral chromatin by a distinct halo zone. These inclusion body-bearing cells also can be found in saliva, vaginal discharge, milk, and other body fluids of CMV-infected individuals. The morphological similarity of CMV inclusion-bearing cells to those of other herpes group viruses makes it important to examine specimens in parallel with other methods, such as virus-isolation, immunocytochemistry, nucleic acid hybridization, and/or PCR.

Histopathology Sections

As for exfoliated cells, routine histopathological techniques are sufficient to detect typical cytomegalic cells in sections of specimens obtained by biopsy or

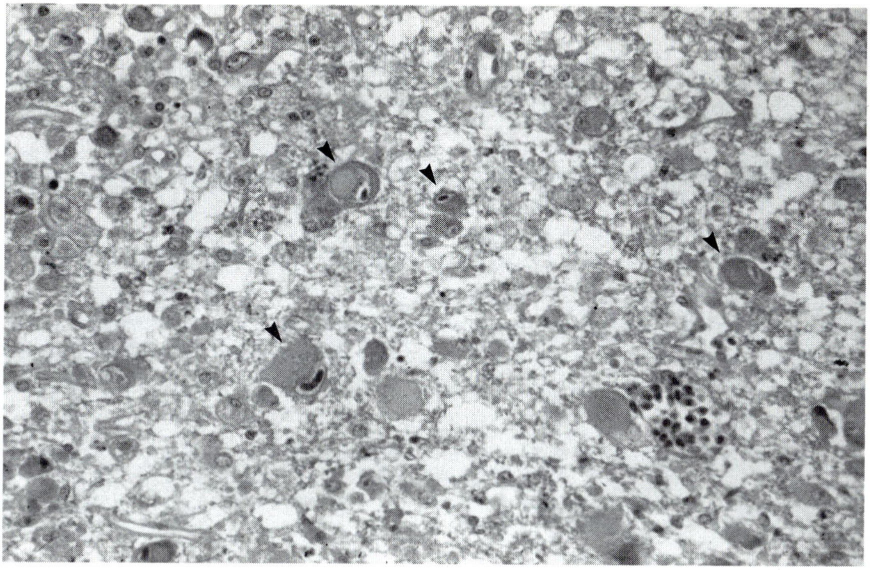

Fig. 6. Typical CMV cytomegalic inclusion-bearing cells in autopsied brain tissue from an AIDS patient with disseminated CMV infection. The *arrows* show cells bearing typical CMV-inclusion bodies

autopsy. However, confirmation by virus isolation, immunocytochemistry, and nucleic acid hybridization is needed. Figure 6 shows typical CMV cytomegalic inclusion-bearing cells in autopsied brain tissue from AIDS patient with disseminated CMV infection.

Conclusion

There are numerous methods and approaches to diagnose CMV infection in patients and normal individuals. Each has its own advantages and disadvantages. The optimal and appropriate method to be used frequently depends on the nature of the clinical samples collected and the clinical manifestation at the time a specimen is collected. In general, immunocytochemistry, either using fluorescent labeled or HRPO- (or AP-) labeled antibody is the best choice for rapid diagnosis of CMV infection in biopsied and autopsied specimens, just as for exfoliated cells with suspict CMV infection. ELISA offers rapid and accurate information of prior and currently active CMV infections, but it does not provide any accurate information when a patient or an individual has developed immunotolerance to human CMV. In a recent epidemiology survey carried out in Taiwan, we discovered children with persistent CMV infection without obvious CMV IgG and IgM responses (our unpublished data). Therefore, other measurements such as detecting CMV in urine by PCR or culture isolation is justified. In situ hybridization using a nonradioactive probe is a sophisticated and unique approach, but poor sensitivity and high background frequently create problems with this approach. This technique also requires a high viral genome number centralized within a cell for generating a positive signal.

Dot blot hybridization is simple but only good for detecting samples with a high number of active CMV-infected cells. It is extremely difficult to make any conclusion when a limited amount of CMV is present in a specimen. Southern hybridization is extremely useful for basic research and for identifying virus strain relatedness. It is not an ideal approach for routine viral diagnosis. Finally, the PCR assay is an innovative and revolutionary technique for current CMV detection. Its sensitivity and specificity are superb, better than any of the other presently available techniques for CMV detection, but precautions to avoid sample or droplet cross contaminations in laboratories should be carefully addressed.

References

1. Avrameas S, Ternync T, Guesdon JL (1978) Coupling of enzymes to antibodies and antigens. Scand J Immunol 8 Suppl 7(7)
2. Bernstein MT, Stewart JA (1971) Indirect hemagglutination test for detection of antibodies to cytomegalovirus. Appl Microbiol 21:84–89
3. Brigati DJ, Myerson D, Leary JJ, Spalholz B, Travis SZ, Fong CKY, Hsiung GD, Ward DC (1983) Detection of viral genomes in cultured and paraffin-embedded tissue sections using biotin-labeled hybridization probes. Virology 126:32–50
4. Buffone GJ, Schimbor CM, Demmler GJ, Wilson DR, Darington GJ (1986) Detection of cytomegalovirus in urine by nonisotopic DNA hybridization. J Infect Dis 154:163–166
5. Burns J, Redfern DRM, Esiri MM, McGee, J'OD (1986) Human and viral gene detection in routine paraffine embedded tissue by in situ hybridization with biotinylated probes: viral localization in herpes encephalitis. J Clin Pathol 39:1066–1073
6. Cassol SA, Poon MC, Pal R, Naylor MJ, Culver-James J, Bowen TJ, Russell JA, Krawetz SA, Pon RT, Hoar DI (1989) Primer-mediated enzymatic amplification of cytomegalovirus (CMV) DNA. Application to early diagnosis of CMV infection in marrow transplant recipients. J Clin Invest 83:1109–1115
7. Chehab FF, Xiao C, Kan YW, Yen TS (1989) Detection of cytomegalovirus infection in paraffin-embedded tissue specimens with the polymerase chain reaction. Mod Pathol 2:75–78
8. Chou S, Merigan TC (1983) Rapid detection and quantitation of human cytomegalovirus in urine through DNA hybridization. N Engl J Med 308:921–925
9. Chou S, Scott KM (1988) Latex agglutination and enzyme-linked immunosorbent assays to cytomegalovirus serologic screening of transplant donors and recipients. J Clin Microbiol 26:2116–2119
10. Chou S, Kim D, Scoot KM, Sewell DL (1987) Immunoglobulin M to cytomegalovirus in primary and reactivations in renal transplant recipients. J Clin Microbiol 25:52–55
11. Cremer NE, Schmidt NJ, Jensen F, Hoffman M, Osiro LS, Lennette EH (1975) Complement-fixing antibody in human sera reactive with viral and soluble antigens of cytomegalovirus. J Clin Microbiol 1:262–267
12. Davis MG, Kenney SC, Kamine J, Pagano JS, Huang ES (1987) Immediate-early gene region of human cytomegalovirus trans-activates the promoter of human immunodeficiency virus. Proc Natl Acad Sci USA 84:8642–8646

13. Demmler GJ, Buffone GJ, Schimbor CM, May RA (1988) Detection of cytomegalovirus in urine from newborns by using polymerase chain reaction DNA amplification. J Infect Dis 158:1177–1184
14. Einsele H, Steidle M, Vallbracht A, Sall JG, Ehninger G, Muller CA (1991) Early occurrence of human cytomegalovirus infection after bone marrow transplantation as demonstrated by the polymerase chain reaction technique. Blood 77:1104–1110
15. Forster AC, McInnes JL, Skingle DC, Symons RH (1985) Non-radioactive hybridization probes prepared by the chemical labeling of DNA and RNA with a novel reagent, photobiotin. Nucleic Acids Res 13:745–761
16. Gall JG, Pardue ML (1971) Nucleic acid hybridization in cytological preparation. Methods Enzymology 21D:470–480
17. Gleaves CA, Smith TF, Shuster EA, Pearson GR (1984) Rapid detection of CMV in MRC-5 cells inoculated with urine specimens by using low-speed centrifugation and monoclonal antibody to an early antigen. J Clin Microbiol 19:917–919
18. Goding JM (1976) Conjugation of antibodies with fluorochromes: modifications to the standard methods. J Immunol Methods 13:215–226
19. Hanshaw JB, Niederman JC, Chessin LN (1972) Cytomegalovirus macroglobulin in cell-associated herpesvirus infection. J Infect Dis 125:304–306
20. Hendrix MG, Salimans MM, van Boven CP, Bruggeman CA (1990) High prevalence of latently present cytomegalovirus in arterial walls of patients suffering from grade III atherosclerosis. Am J Pathol 136:23–38
21. Hijmans W, Schuit HRE, Klein F (1969) An immunofluorescence procedure for the detection of intracellular immunoglobulins. Clin Exp Immunol 4:457–472
22. Himuna Y, Ohta R, Miyamoto T, Ishida N (1962) Evaluation of the complement method of fluorescent antibody technique with myxoviruses. J Immunol 89:19–26
23. Ho M (1991) Human cytomegalovirus: biology and infection, 2nd ed. Plenum, New York, pp 101–126
24. Horwitz CA, Henle W, Henle G, Polesky H, Balfour HH, Siem RA, Borken S, Ward PCJ (1977) Heterophile-negative infectious mononucleosis and mononucleosis-like illnesses: laboratory confirmation of 43 cases. Am J Med 63:947–957
25. Hsia K, Spector DH, Lawrie J, Spector SA (1989) Enzymatic amplification of human cytomegalovirus sequences by polymerase chain reaction. J Clin Microbiol 27:1802–1809
26. Huang ES, Pagano JS (1977) Comparative diagnosis of cytomegalovirus: new approach. In: Kurstak E, Kurstak C (eds) Human and related virus, part A. Academic, New York, pp 241–285 (Comparative diagnosis of viral diseases, vol 1)
27. Huang ES, Pagano JS (1977) Nucleic acid hybridization technology and detection of proviral genomes. Methods Virol 6:457–497
28. Huang ES, Chen ST, Pagano JS (1973) Human cytomegalovirus. I. Purification and characterization of viral deoxyribonucleic acid. J Virol 12:1473–1481
29. Huang ES, Kilpatrick BA, Huang YT, Pagano JS (1976) Detection of human cytomegalovirus and analysis of strain variation. Yale J Biol Med 49:29–43
30. Huang ES, Alford C, Reynolds DW, Stagno S, Pass RF (1980) Molecular epidemiology of cytomegalovirus infections in women and their infants. N Engl J Med 303:958–962
31. Huang ES, Huong SM, Tegmeier P, Alford C (1980) Cytomegalovirus: genetic variation of viral genome. Ann NY Acad Sci 354:332–346
32. Jiwa NM, van Gemert GW, Raap AK, van de Rijke FM, Mulder A, Lens PF, Salimans MM, Zwaab FE, van Drop W, van der Ploeg M (1989) Rapid detection of human cytomegalovirus DNA in peripheral blood leukocytes of viremic transplant recipients by the polymerase chain reaction. Transplantation 48:72–76
33. Jiwa NM, Steenbergen RD, Zwaan FE, Kluin PM, Raap AK, van der Ploeg M (1990) Three sensitive methods for the detection of cytomegalovirus in lung tissue of patients with interstitial pneumonitis. Am J Clin Pathol 93:491–494
34. Joassin L, Reginster M (1986) Elimination of nonspecific cytomegalovirus immunoglobulin M activities in the enzyme-linked immunosorbent assay by using anti-human immunoglobulin G. J Clin Microbiol 23:576–581

35. Khan G, Kangro HO, Coates PJ, Heath RB (1991) Inhibitory effect of urine on the polymerase chain reaction of CMV DNA. J Clin Pathol 44:360–365
36. Kilpatrick BA, Huang ES, Pagano JS (1976) Analysis of cytomegalovirus genomes with restriction endonuclease *Hin*dIII and *Eco*RI. J Virol 18:1095–1105
37. Kingston RE (1987) Guanidinium method for total RNA preparation. In: Ausubel FM, Bret R, Kingston RE et al. (eds) Current protocols in molecular biology. Wiley, New York, pp 4.2.1–4.2.5
38. Kronick MN (1986) The use of phycobiliproteins as fluorescent labels in immunoassay. J Immunol Methods 92:1–13
39. Lennette EH, Schmidt NJ (1979) Diagnostic procedures for viral and rickettsial infection, 5th edn. American Public Health Association, New York, pp 399–439
40. Olive DM, al-Mufti S, Simsek M, Fayez H, al-Nakid W (1989) Direct detection of human cytomegalovirus in urine specimens from renal transplant patients following polymerase chain reaction amplification. J Med Virol 29:232–237
41. Pagano JS, Huang ES (1974) Application of RNA–DNA cytohybridization to viral diagnosis. In: Kurstak E, Morrisset R (eds) Comparative immunodiagnosis of viral infection. Academic, New York, pp 279–299
42. Reimer CB, Black CM, Philips DJ, Logan LC, Hunter EF, Pender BJ, McGrew BF (1975) The specificity of fetal IgM: antibody or antiantibody? Ann NY Acad Sci 254: 77–93
43. Rowley AH, Wolinsky SM, Sambol SP, Barkhol L, Ehrnst A, Andersson JP (1991) Rapid detection of cytomegalovirus DNA and RNA in blood of renal transplant patients by in vitro enzymatic amplification. Transplantation 51:1028–1033
44. Ruger R, Bornkamm GW, Fleckenstein B (1985) Human cytomegalovirus DNA sequences with homologies to the cellular genome. J Gen Virol 65:1351–1364
45. Ruger B, Klages S, Walla B, Albrecht J, Fleckenstein B, Tomlinson P, Barrell B (1987) Primary structure and transcription of the genes coding for the two virion phosphoproteins pp65 and pp71 of human cytomegalovirus. J Virol 61:446–453
46. Saiki RK (1989) The design and optimization of the PCR. In: Erlich HA (Ed) PCR technology: principles and applications for DNA amplification. Stockton, London, pp 7–16
47. Schuster V, Matz B, Wiegand H, Traub B, Kampa D, Neumann-Haefelin D (1986) Detection of human cytomegalovirus in urine by DNA–DNA and RNA–DNA hybridization. J Infect Dis 154:309–314
48. Scopsi L, Larsson LI (1987) Increased sensitivity in peroxidase immunocytochemistry. A comparative study of a number of peroxidase visualization methods employing a model system. Histochemistry 84:221–230
49. Selden RF (1987) Southern blotting and hybridization. In: Ausubel FM, Brent R, Kingston RE et al. (eds) Current protocols in molecular biology. Wiley, New York, pp 2.9.1.–2.9.10.
50. Selden RF (1987) Analysis of RNA by Northern hybridization. In: Ausubel FM, Brent R, Kingston RE et al. (eds) Current protocols in molecular biology. Wiley, New York, pp 4.9.1.–4.9.4.
51. Shaw SB, Rasmussen RD, McDonough SH, Staprans SI, Vacquier JP, Spector DH (1985) Cell-related sequences in the DNA genome of human cytomegalovirus AD169. J Virol 55:843–848
52. Shibata D, Anheim N, Martin WJ (1988) Detection of human papilloma virus in paraffin-embedded tissue using the polymerase chain reaction. J Exp Med 167:225–230
53. Shibata D, Martin WJ, Appleman MD, Causey DM, Leedon JM, Arnheim N (1988) Detection of cytomegalovirus in peripheral blood in patients infected with human immunodeficiency virus. J Infect Dis 158:1185–1192
54. Southern EM (1975) Detection of specific sequences among DNA fragments separated by gel electrophoresis. J Mol Biol 98:503–517
55. Spector SA, Rua JA, Spector DH, McMillan R (1984) Detection of human cytomegalovirus in clinical specimens by DNA–DNA hybridization. J Infect Dis 150:121–126

56. Stagno S, Tinker MK, Elrod C, Fuccillo DA, Cloud G, O'Beirne AJ (1985) Immunoglobulin M antibodies detected by enzyme-linked immunosorbent assay and radioimmunoassay in the diagnosis of cytomegalovirus infections in pregnant women and newborn infants. J Clin Microbiol 21:930–935
57. Stenberg RM, Thomsem DR, Stinski MF (1984) Structural analysis of the major immediate early gene of human cytomegalovirus. J Virol 49:190–199
58. Stenberg RM, Witte PR, Stinski MF (1985) Multiple spliced and unspliced transcripts from human cytomegalovirus immediate-early region 2 and evidence for a common initiation site within immediate-early region 1. J Virol 56:665–675
59. Thomas PS (1980) Hybridization of denatured RNA and small DNA fragments transferred to nitrocellulose. Proc Natl Acad Sci USA 77:5201–5205
60. Trojanowski JQ, Obrocka MA, Lee VMY (1983) A comparison of eight different chromogen protocols for the demonstration of immunoreactive neurofilaments or glial filaments in rat cerebellum using the peroxidase-antiperoxidase method and monoclonal antibodies. J Histochem Cytochem 31:1217–1223
61. Ullrich A, Shine J, Chirgwin J, Pictet R, Tischer E, Rutter WJ, Goodman HM (1977) Rat insulin genes: construction of plasmids containing the coding sequences. Science 196:1313–1319
62. Unger ER, Budgeon LR, Myerson D, Brigati DJ (1986) Viral diagnosis by in situ hybridization. Am J Surg Pathol 10:1–8
63. Van den Berg F, Schipper M, Jiwa M, Rook R, van de Rijke F, Tigges B (1989) Implausibility of an aetiological association between cytomegalovirus and Kaposi's sarcoma shown by four techniques. J Clin Pathol 42:128–131
64. Wahl GM, Stern M, Stark GR (1979) Efficient transfer of large DNA fragments from agarose gels to diazobenzyloxymethyl-paper and rapid hybridization by using dextran sulfate. Proc Natl Acad Sci USA 76:3683–3687
65. Wilson MB, Nakane PK (1978) Immunofluorescence and related staining technique. Elsevier/North-Holland, Amsterdam, p 215
66. Yoytas D (1987) Resolution and recovery of large DNA fragment: agarose gel electrophoresis. In: Ausubel FM, Brent R, Kingston RE et al. (eds) Current protocols in molecular biology. Wiley, New York, pp 2.5.1–2.5.9
67. Yuan CF, Kao SM, Wang DC, Ng HT, Pao CC (1990) Detection of human cytomegalovirus in cervicovaginal cells by culture, in situ DNA hybridization and DNA amplification methods. Mol Cell Probes 6:475–483

Chapter 14 The Control of Cytomegalovirus Infection: Chemotherapy

Jonathan S. Serody and Charles M. van der Horst

Abstract

The pharmacokinetic profile, efficacy and toxicity of the two principal chemotherapeutic agents, ganciclovir and foscarnet, utilized in the treatment of cytomegalovirus infection in the immunocompromised host are reviewed. In addition, the efficacy, cost and safety of the various prophylactic regimens for prevention of cytomegalovirus disease is examined. Recommendations for treatment and prophylaxis in HIV infected and transplant recipients are given.

Introduction

In the immunocompetent host, primary cytomegalovirus (CMV) infection rarely causes disease. In those patients who develop disease, this is a self-limited mononucleosis type syndrome. However, in the immunosuppressed host, especially patients infected with the HIV virus and transplant recipients, CMV infection may result in life-threatening disease. Most of these immunosuppressed patients have evidence of CMV *infection*, as demonstrated by shedding of virus in urine, saliva or stool or the presence of virus in the leukocyte buffy coat. Investigators have distinguished CMV infection from CMV *disease*, in which patients have, in addition to serologic or culture evidence of CMV, symptoms and signs such as fever, myalgias, lethargy, leukopenia and thrombocytopenia and the presence of organ damage from CMV such as retinitis, pneumonitis, hepatitis, pancreatitis, esophagitis and colitis.

Since such high morbidity and mortality is associated with CMV disease in patients with defects in cell-mediated immunity, many different chemotherapeutic regimens have been utilized in an attempt to treat it. Leukocyte interferon, vidarabine, iododeoxyuridine, fluorodeoxyuridine, cytosine arabinoside and adenine arabinoside have been used with little clinical benefit and or high toxicity [1, 20, 57, 90, 102]. Acyclovir has been utilized with very limited success in the treatment of CMV infections [4, 131]. The antiviral compounds

Division of Infectious Disease, University of North Carolina, Campus Box #7030, Chapel Hill, NC 27599-7030, USA ganciclovir and foscarnet have demonstrated the most activity against CMV both in vivo and in vitro. In this chapter, we describe the clinical and pharmacokinetic data of acyclovir, ganciclovir and foscarnet in the treatment of CMV disease. We discuss the literature on the treatment and prevention of the different manifestations of CMV disease in AIDS patients and transplant recipients and the role of CMV-hyperimmune globulin in the prevention of CMV infection and disease.

Acyclovir

Acyclovir (9-(2-hydroxyethoxymethyl)guanine) is a guanine nucleoside analog in which the sugar moiety side chain has been removed. A viral thymidine kinase acts to phosphorylate acyclovir to the monophosphate form [35]. Cellular enzymes then act to phosphorylate the monophosphate form to the active triphosphate moiety. In vitro the susceptibility of each herpesvirus to inhibition by acyclovir is related to the ability of the infected cell to anabolize acyclovir to the triphosphate [47]. CMV lacks a viral thymidine kinase and thus only low levels of acyclovir triphosphate are formed in CMV-infected cells. In human CMV-infected WI38 cells the level of acyclovir triphosphate is 0.3 pmol/10^6 cells [47]. This compares with acyclovir triphosphate levels of 22.1 to 90.4 pmol/10^6 cells for HSV-1 infected Vero cells. Acyclovir triphosphate lacks the 3′ hydroxyl group and thus blocks viral DNA replication by chain termination [87]. In addition, acyclovir appears to inhibit the viral DNA polymerase [48].

One other critical factor in the activity of a drug is the K_i of the triphosphate for the viral DNA polymerase. Despite little phosphorylation in some cells, a drug that is a more effective inhibitor (lower K_i) of a virus could possibly overcome the low intracellular levels obtained. Thus the kinetic values for competitive inhibition of the AD169 strain of human CMV for acyclovir triphosphate is 0.33 μM, or five times lower than that for ganciclovir triphosphate (1.4 μM) [10].

Acyclovir is very active in vitro against Epstein-Barr virus, herpes simplex viruses 1 and 2 and varicella-zoster virus. However, much higher serum levels are required to inhibit CMV. The mean inhibitory dose in one study for acyclovir was 63.1 μM/l or 14 mg/l [23].

Pharmacokinetics

Bioavailability of the oral form of acyclovir is poor and decreases as the dose escalates. Peak levels after an oral dose of 200 mg range from 0.3 to 0.9 mg/l approximately 1.5 h after the dose [29]. After the 800-mg dose, levels of 1.8 mg/l are achieved [88]. The 600-mg pediatric suspension dose achieves even lower levels than the capsule form [127]. Levels achieved after intravenous administration are much greater. Peak and trough levels of 9.8 mg/l and 0.7 mg/l respectively are achieved after 5 mg/kg given every 8 h. Administration of 10 mg/kg every 8 h results in peak and trough levels of 20.7 mg/l and 2.3 mg/l respectively [12]. The volume of distribution is dependent on total body water.

Renal Dosing

The half-life of acyclovir is approximately 3 h, and 60%–90% of the drug is excreted by glomerular filtration and tubular excretion [26, 129]. The intracellular half-life of acyclovir triphosphate is 1.8–2.4 h [47]. In anuric patients, the half-life of acyclovir increases to approximately 20 h [82]. Dose adjustments of oral acyclovir are necessary if the creatinine clearance is less than 25 ml/min/per 1.73 m^2. Thus, acyclovir 800 mg given every 4 h would be changed to every 8 h for a creatinine clearance from 10–25 ml/min/per 1.73 m^2 and to every 12 h for clearance below 10 ml/min per 1.73 m^2. For intravenous acyclovir the dosing interval is increased to 12 h for a creatinine clearance of 25–50 ml/min per 1.73 m^2 and to 24 h for 10–25 ml/min/per 1.73 m^2. In the case of anuria the dose itself is also reduced by 50%. Intravenous acyclovir is readily hemodialyzable [82], with approximately 60% of this being dialyzed in a routine dialysis. Thus an additional dose should be given after dialysis. No additional doses are needed however, after peritoneal dialysis.

Toxicity

Intravenous acyclovir is a well-tolerated drug, with renal toxicity being the most common adverse event. Crystalluria has been demonstrated in both children and adults [104, 113]. Pre-existing renal dysfunction, dehydration and bolus delivery appear to increase the likelihood of crystalluria and tubular obstruction. Approximately 5% of patients on acyclovir have reversible renal dysfunction at dosage of 5 mg/kg every 8 h [82]. Using the higher doses of intravenous acyclovir to treat herpes zoster, 500 mg/m^2, 6%–25% of patients developed worsening renal function as manifested by an increase in serum creatinine [5, 8]. This was also reversible. Acyclovir has also caused neurotoxicity in approximately 1% of patients receiving the intravenous form, most commonly in patients with impaired renal function. The concomitant use of probenecid increases the plasma levels of acyclovir.

Clinical Activity

In clinical trials, acyclovir has shown very limited efficacy in the treatment of active CMV infection. In a study by Balfour et al. there was no statistically significant difference in mortality between immunocompromised patients treated with acyclovir and those who received placebo [4]. Wade et al. found similar results in a study of bone morrow transplant recipients [131].

Ganciclovir

Ganciclovir, 9-(2-hydroxy-1-(hydroxymethyl)ethoxy)methyl)guanine, is a guanine nucleoside analog that is very similar to acyclovir. Structurally, ganciclovir differs from acyclovir by an additional hydroxymethyl group on the ribose ring. Ganciclovir is also triphosphorylated to its active form, ganciclovir triphosphate, but the intracellular levels achieved are 10 times higher than those of acyclovir triphosphate [10]. The initial step of this process does not appear to require the presence of a viral thymidine kinase [41]. Ganciclovir triphosphate acts to terminate DNA chain elongation and inhibit the viral DNA polymerase. The ID_{50} ranges from 0.5 to 3 μM/l (0.125–0.75 mg/l) [21].

Pharmacokinetics

Ganciclovir is poorly absorbed orally, with only approximately 3% of an oral dose being bioavailable [68]. Increases in the dose of ganciclovir result in a decrease in the bioavailability, suggesting a dose-dependent mode of absorption. In one study oral ganciclovir 10 or 20 mg/kg every 6 h in four patients resulted in maximum ganciclovir plasma concentrations of 0.5 and 0.74 mg/l, respectively, 30–60 min after administration [68]. Another study dosed patients with 1 g every 8 h by mouth for 28 days [44]. Peak levels were 1.2 mg/l with a trough of 0.67 mg/l. The drug was well tolerated. These levels were sufficient to suppress CMV excretion in four of six patients treated [36]. With intravenous doses of 5 mg/kg twice each day, peak and trough levels of 5.3 mg/l and 1.1 mg/l are achieved after 14 days [122].

There is penetration of ganciclovir into the cerebrospinal fluid (CSF), with a CSF : plasma ratio of 0.24–0.67 in four patients after an infusion of 2.5 mg/kg [43].

Since ganciclovir has been used in the treatment of CMV retinitis, there have been several studies investigating intraocular levels of ganciclovir. In one patient with AIDS, subretinal and aqueous humor levels of 0.9 and 0.6 mg/l of ganciclovir were measured 2.5 h after a 1-h infusion of 6 mg/kg. The corresponding plasma level was 1.5 mg/l [67]. In the same patient, the vitreous humor concentration of ganciclovir 21 h after the same infusion, when ganciclovir could no longer be detected in plasma – was 0.8 μmol/l [67].

Ganciclovir has also achieved high intraocular concentrations when administered directly into the vitreous humor, and was successful in the treatment of a patient with CMV retinitis when used in this manner [56].

Renal Dosing

Ganciclovir has an elimination half-life of approximately 2.5 h with an intracellular half-life of 12 h [10]. Ganciclovir is cleared by glomerular filtration and tubular secretion, with approximately 90% of the native drug being excreted in the urine in 24 h [83]. No metabolites of ganciclovir have been isolated. Because of its renal excretion, most investigators have reduced the dose of ganciclovir by 50% if the creatinine clearance falls below 80 ml/min. For a creatinine clearance from 25–50 ml/min the interval is increased to 24 h. For a creatinine clearance less than 25 ml/min the dose is again reduced by 50%, to 25% of the standard dose given every 24 hours. Ganciclovir appears to be hemodialyzed, so a dose should be given after dialysis.

Toxicity

The safety of ganciclovir was initially examined in 5283 patients with sight- or life-threatening CMV disease and underlying immunodeficiency [65]. Of these patients 69% had AIDS. The most common adverse events were thrombocytopenia and granulocytopenia. A more detailed analysis of 1000 patients, of whom 50% had AIDS, was performed. As demonstrated in Table 1, absolute neutrophil counts less than 1000 cells/mm^3 occurred in 29% of the patients; 20% had platelet counts less than 50 000/mm^3. Since CMV itself can lead to

Table 1. (unpublished data April 14, 1992)

	Uncontrolled trials		Controlled trials – transplant recipients			
	Persons w. AIDS	Transplant recipients	Heart allograft *		Bone marrow allograft **	
	GCV ($n=532$)	GCV ($n=207$)	GCV ($n=76$)	Placebo ($n=73$)	GCV ($n=57$)	Control ($n=55$)
Granulocytopenia/neutropenia						
ANC <500/μl	18%	11%	4%	3%	12%	6%
ANC 500–1000 /μl	24%	10%	3%	8%	29%	17%
Total ANC ≤1000 μl	42%	21%	7%	11%	41%	23%
Thrombocytopenia						
Platelet counts <25 000/μl	4%	22%	3%	1%	32%	28%
Platelet counts 25 000–50 000/μl	9%	23%	5%	3%	25%	37%
Total platelets ≤50 000 μl	13%	45%	8%	4%	57%	65%

* Mean duration of treatment = 28 days
** Mean duration of treatment = 45 days

granulocytopenia we have noticed a rise in granulocyte count in some HIV patients and transplant recipients treated with ganciclovir.

Granulocytopenia was more common in AIDS patients than in patients with other immunosuppressive disorders. The frequency of severe granulocytopenia (< 500 cells/mm^3) was not different in the two groups. In the largest randomized treatment trial of CMV retinitis in AIDS patients, 32% (41 patients) developed a granulocyte count of less than 500 cells/mm^3 [126]. Thus ganciclovir is not recommended in patients with an absolute granulocyte count less than 500 cells/mm^3. Ganciclovir can not be given with azidothymidine since both drugs are bone-marrow toxic [58]. Other adverse events observed in patients who received ganciclovir included anemia, fever, rash and elevated liver enzymes (LFTs), found in approximately 2% of recipients. Less common adverse events included nausea, vomiting, diarrhea, abdominal pain, ataxia, dizziness, headache, nervousness, paresthesia, psychosis, somnolence, tremor, pruritis, urticaria, worsening renal function and phlebitis at the injection site. There have been case reports of pancreatitis associated with both oral and intravenous ganciclovir (Karen Helfert, personal communication, 1991).

Resistance

Approximately 8%–14% of AIDS patients with CMV retinitis who receive long-term maintenance therapy develop ganciclovir-resistant strains of CMV [37]. The ID_{50} of these resistant strains ranges from greater than 6 μM (1.5 mg/l) to greater than 12 μM, with an ID_{90} of over 30 μM. Resistant virus was associated with progression of retinitis. This resistance appears to be due to an inability of the ganciclovir-resistant strains to induce ganciclovir phosphorylation in virus-infected cells [124].

Foscarnet

Foscarnet, also identified as trisodium phosphonoformate, phosphonoformate, phosphonoformic acid, and foscarnet sodium, represents a new class of antiviral compounds. Unlike acyclovir and ganciclovir, foscarnet directly inhibits the DNA polymerase of members of the herpesvirus family, including CMV. Huang demonstrated in 1975 that an analog of foscarnet, phosphonoacetic acid, inhibited the viral DNA polymerase of CMV [63], with little effect on human fibroblast enzymes. Subsequently, in 1982, Eriksson demonstrated that foscarnet had the greatest inhibitory effect of 17 pyrophosphate analogs on the CMV DNA polymerase [40]. In addition, foscarnet appears to have an effect on HIV replication, possibly by inhibiting the viral reverse transcriptase.

In vitro data suggest that most strains of CMV are inhibited, with a mean ID_{50} of 720 μmol/l [105]. In addition HIV replication can be inhibited at 132 pM [112].

Pharmacokinetics

Foscarnet is poorly absorbed when given by mouth [117]. The pharmacokinetics of intravenous foscarnet were investigated in eight patients with AIDS being treated for CMV retinitis [2]. These patients received 60 mg/kg foscarnet in a 2-h infusion every 8 h for 14 days. Drug adjustments were made for patients with diminished creatinine clearance according to guidelines from the manufacturer. The mean peak concentration after 3 days of treatment was 509 ± 200 pM and 495 ± 149 pM on day 14. Patients with impaired renal function did not have an appreciable change due to dose reduction [2]. Plasma concentrations 23 h after the infusion were negligible. The mean half-life in plasma was 4.5 ± 1.2 h. There are no known metabolites.

Foscarnet appears to penetrate into the CNS in patients with impaired blood-brain barriers. In a study using continuous infusion of foscarnet, a mean foscarnet concentration of 68.5 μmol/l was detected in the CSF of six patients infected with HIV. This represented 43% of the plasma level of foscarnet [117]. In animal studies, foscarnet appears to be sequestered in bone and cartilage [54].

Renal Dosing

Approximately 80% of the drug is excreted unchanged by the kidney and therefore dose modification for patients with impaired renal function is necessary. Table 2 lists the renal dosing guidelines for foscarnet [100].

Table 2. Foscarnet dosing in patients with renal disease

CrCl (ml/min/kg) [a]	Induction dose (mg/kg every 8 h)	CrCl	Maintenance dose (mg/kg per day)
>1.6	60	>1.4	120
1.5	57	1.2–1.4	104
1.4	53	1.0–1.2	100
1.3	49	0.8–1.0	94
1.2	46	0.6–0.8	84
1.1	42	0.4–0.6	76
1.0	39		
0.9	35		
0.8	32		
0.7	28		
0.6	25		
0.5	21		
0.4	18		

[a] Creatinine clearance (CrCl) is calculated as follows: $\frac{140 - \text{age (years)}}{\text{serum Cr (mg/dl)} \times 72}$. For females multiply by 0.85

Toxicity

Side effects associated with the administration of foscarnet include worsening creatinine clearance, hematuria, proteinuria, changes in Ca^{2+} and PO_4^- metabolism, hypomagnesemia, hypokalemia, anemia, leukopenia, seizures, and nausea and vomiting. In 82 patients with AIDS treated for CMV retinitis or resistant HSV infection [33, 69, 71], 11 [13%] had a worsening of renal function (increase of 0.5–1.2 mg/dl creatinine) after taking foscarnet 60 mg/kg every 8 h or 120 mg/kg every 12 h. However, this deterioration was usually reversible and no patients had to stop therapy prematurely because of it. In a study in which foscarnet was infused continuously at 3.24–7.14 mg/kg/h six of 13 patients (46%) had a worsening of renal function and three (23%) had to have the drug discontinued for this reason [132]. Hydration with normal saline on the night prior to the administration of foscarnet throughout the period of administration of the drug appears to decrease the incidence of renal side effects [27, 28]. Eight percent of the foscarnet-treated patients (nine patients) in a recently completed trial had a rise in creatinine, and 20% (22 patients) had to switch to ganciclovir when they developed either nephrotoxicity or electrolyte disturbances [126]. In AIDS patients, coadministration of foscarnet with acyclovir, pentamidine or trimethoprim/sulfamethoxazole appears to increase the incidence of renal dysfunction [132].

Another important toxicity is transient hypocalcemia associated with the infusion. Jacobson et al., in a set of in vitro experiments, demonstrated that there is an inverse correlation between foscarnet levels and ionized calcium concentration [73]. The same results were found in patients treated with foscarnet. There was no difference in total serum calcium. Coadministration of intravenous pentamidine with foscarnet was been implicated in the severe hypocalcemia and paresthesias that developed in four patients [136]. Foscarnet has also been associated with penile ulcers [50, 128], congestive heart failure and gastrointestinal bleeding. One recent study of 40 patients treated with foscarnet at 100–120 mg/kg daily found that 15% had nausea, 8% hypophosphatemia, 5% paresthesia, 5% genital ulcers, 5% increased creatinine levels and 3% hypocalcemia [34].

Treatment: AIDS

Retinitis

Approximately 5% of patients infected with the HIV virus will have CMV retinitis as the initial opportunistic infection defining an AIDS diagnosis. The prevalence of CMV retinitis in HIV-infected patients is approximately 25% [95, 97]. Spontaneous remission in AIDS patients is unusual, and the majority of patients have progressive destruction of the retina and eventual blindness. Retinal detachment occurs in approximately 14%–29% of patients with CMV retinitis [18, 46, 49, 89]. As a result, the most extensive experience with the use of chemotherapeutic compounds for the treatment of CMV disease has been in the treatment of retinitis. Table 3 summarizes the induction and maintenance regimens for the treatment of CMV retinitis with ganciclovir that have been described in the literature. In these studies neutropenia, defined by an absolute neutrophil count less than 1000 cells/mm^3, developed in 24% of the patients. Some of the failures may have been related to low doses of ganciclovir.

Gross et al. evaluated 67 patients with AIDS and CMV retinitis who were treated with 5 mg/kg/12 h for two weeks followed by 5 mg/kg/5 days a week [51]. Fifty-four patients were available for follow-up for a mean of 15.6 weeks. Unilateral retinitis was observed at presentation in 39 patients, primary foveal retinitis was not observed. Serial visual acuity data was available for 77 eyes. In 56 eyes (73%), final visual acuity of 20/40 or better was obtained; 14 eyes (18%) had visual acuity worse than 20/200. Twenty-six percent of patients had a loss of visual acuity of two lines of vision or better, 68% remained the same and 6% improved. Progression of retinitis occurred in 21 (36%) of the 58 patients who received maintenance therapy, with a mean time to progression of 21 weeks. Breakthrough retinitis occurred in 14 patients, while smoldering retinitis was found in seven. By Kaplan-Meier analysis the mean survival after the diagnosis of CMV retinitis was 8 months. This survival was better than that of 6 weeks to 6 months reported in earlier studies [55, 59].

In a retrospective analysis of survival in AIDS patients with CMV retinitis, Holland et al. found a similar increase in patients receiving ganciclovir: mean survival after diagnosis was 2 months in untreated patients and 7 months in treated patients [61]. This held true when patients diagnosed in 1984–1985 were compared to patients diagnosed in 1986–1987, and was not confounded by the use of zidovudine.

Ganciclovir appears to have a virostatic effect in the treatment of CMV retinitis in AIDS patients, as demonstrated by the high rate of relapse after

Table 3. Induction regimens for ganciclovir therapy of CMV retinitis

No. of patients	Dose (mg/kg per day)	Duration (days)	Clinical response *n*	Clinical response %	Reference
18	10	14–21	14	78	66
2	15	19	2	100	42
6	3– 7.5	5–24	6	100	111
40	5–14	9–26	31	97	60
8	3–10	12–36	7	88	101
23	7.5	10–14	23	100	55
41	7.5	21	26	88	99
31	10	14–21	25	81	66
169	3–15	5–36	144	85	

therapy with ganciclovir. Jacobson et al. [70] evaluated 25 AIDS patients with CMV retinitis who were treated with a 10-day induction course and randomized to either immediate maintenance with 5 mg/kg on 5 days a week or deferment of further ganciclovir until progression of the disease. There was a marked difference in the time to progression of retinitis: 42 days in patients given immediate maintenance therapy compared with 16 days in those allocated to deferred treatment. Spector et al., in a similar study of 42 patients randomized to immediate induction therapy along with maintenance ganciclovir 5 mg/kg/day or delayed therapy, found that the mean time to progression was 69 days for the immediate therapy patients compared with 23 days for the delayed therapy patients ($p=0.01$) [123]. For this reason, most current studies utilize a maintenance regimen of 5 mg/kg on 7 days per week.

Because of the high incidence of neutropenia in these studies, most investigators suggest the discontinuation of zidovudine during the induction phase of therapy with ganciclovir. In patients with a neutrophil count greater than 750 cells/mm^3, azidothymidine may be reintroduced at 100 mg five times a day after completion of induction. Patients with neutrophil counts between 500 and 750 cells/mm^3 should start at 100 mg three times a day, with an increase to 100 mg five times a day if the neutrophil count remains stable [19]. Patients with an absolute neutrophil count consistently less than 500 cells/mm^3 should not be treated with the combination of azidothymidine and ganciclovir, and consideration ought to be given to initiating therapy with foscarnet. The use of colony-stimulating growth factors such as GM-CSF or G-CSF may allow a greater proportion of patients to be treated with a full course of ganciclovir. Hardy et al. treated patients given ganciclovir with GM-CSF 5 μg/kg daily subcutaneously [53, 135]. They found improved tolerance to ganciclovir, with 23 episodes of neutropenia in untreated patients against eight episodes of neutropenia in treated patients. The results of a blinded trial are still being analyzed. The cost of a year-long course of this dose of GM-CSF for a 70-kg person would be over $ 48 000 at our hospital. Most patients would not require daily dosing.

The experience with foscarnet in the treatment of CMV retinitis in AIDS patients is much less extensive. Jacobsen et al. described 10 patients with AIDS and CMV retinitis who were treated with foscarnet at 60 mg/kg every 8 h for 14 days [71]. Seven patients had stable retinitis while two patients improved with this regimen. One patient had progression. Patients who responded to foscarnet were given a maintenance regimen of 60 mg/kg/day on 5 days per week. Of the seven patients who received the maintenance regimen one progressed immediately and the mean time to progression in the other six patients was 24.5 days. Another group gave foscarnet induction at a dose of 100 mg/kg twice each day with a good response [49]. Dohin et al. randomized patients to receive foscarnet 100 mg/kg daily or 120 mg/kg daily as maintenance therapy [33, 34]. The higher dose postponed progression by a mean of 3 weeks. In two studies comparing three different daily doses of foscarnet (60, 90 or 120 mg/kg), the mean time to progression was 30–42 days longer when the highest dose was given. There was no difference in toxicity [72, 74].

A recent report suggests that foscarnet is equivalent to ganciclovir in efficacy but with higher median survival, 12.6 months vs 8.5 months. This is perhaps explained by foscarnet's antiretroviral effect or by the ability of the patients to take azidothymidine simultaneously with foscarnet [126]. The dose of foscarnet given in that trial was 60 mg/kg three times daily for 2 weeks followed by 90 mg/kg per day. The ganciclovir dose was the standard 5 mg/kg twice daily for 14 days followed by 5 mg/kg daily. Sixty-two percent of foscarnet patients vs 36% of the ganciclovir patients were able to take azidothymidine. As supporting evidence that foscarnet had a survival advantage, the CD4 lymphocyte count increased in foscarnet patients and decreased in ganciclovir patients ($p=0.013$). The mean time to disease progression was 56 days for ganciclovir recipients and 59 days for foscarnet recipients [126].

The cost of foscarnet at a maintenance dose of 90 mg/kg per day for a 60-kg person would be $ 24 000 per year vs $ 7600 for ganciclovir 5 mg/kg/per day [45]. We recommend an initial induction course of ganciclovir of 5 mg/kg twice a day for 14 days in patients with normal renal function. All patients who respond should then be treated with 5 mg/kg daily as a maintenance regimen. Some investigators have used a maintenance regimen of 6 mg/kg on 5 days per week. There are no studies indicating which dosing regimen is superior. Those patients that do not tolerate ganciclovir, particularly because of neutropenia, can be effectively treated with foscarnet. The dose we use is 60 mg/kg every 8 h for 2 weeks followed by maintenance therapy of 120 mg/kg per day given in a 2-h infusion with 1 l normal saline.

For patients who tolerate neither foscarnet nor intravenous ganciclovir, intravitreal ganciclovir should be used at a dose of 200 μg twice weekly for 3 weeks followed by 200 μg intravitreally once each week. Using this regimen Polsky et al. were successful in treating the retinitis. Several patients, however, developed extraocular CMV disease, which limits the usefulness of this method of administration [103].

Gastrointestinal Disease

Cytomegalovirus colitis is a frequent problem in AIDS patients, with estimates that 15%–25% of patients with AIDS have some manifestation of gastrointestinal disease due to CMV. After the treatment of retinitis, the treatment of colitis in AIDS patients has been most extensively studied. Dieterich et al. evaluated 66 homosexual men with biopsy-proven CMV colitis and AIDS [29, 31]. These patients were randomized to treatment with ganciclovir 5 mg/kg twice daily for 14 days or placebo. All patients discontinued zidovudine upon entrance into the trial. There was a significant decrease in CMV-positive cultures in the treated patients, significant increase in weight and an improved appearance on colonoscopy. Nelson et al., in a study of 22 patients, found that although 11 of 18 patients who completed therapy no longer had colitis as assessed by colonoscopy and biopsy, their diarrhea continued due to pathogens other than CMV [96]. Dieterich and Rahmin continued 32 patients with

CMV colitis on maintenance therapy and recorded no relapses over 6 months. Four of 7 patients who did not receive maintenance therapy had recurrence a mean of 4.2 months after stopping ganciclovir [29].

A clinical response to ganciclovir was also seen in a smaller group of AIDS patients treated with ganciclovir for CMV esophagitis [30]. Another study found that 18 episodes of esophagitis in 15 patients all responded within 2 weeks to ganciclovir [96]. Three patients relapsed 1–7 months after stopping therapy and responded to retreatment.

Foscarnet (60 mg/kg every 8 h for 14 days) was used to treat 14 patients with gastrointestinal disease who failed to respond to standard therapy with ganciclovir [32]. Seventy-nine percent had a clinical response and 79% had a biopsy response, with 10 days being the mean time to respond. Median survival was 10 weeks.

Sclerosing cholangitis in AIDS patients can present with right upper quadrant abdominal pain and abnormal serum alkaline phosphatase and is confirmed by endoscopic retrograde cholangiography. A study of 14 patients with cholangitis by Delaroque et al. found that five had CMV inclusions seen in a biopsy specimen from the biliary tree and another three had CMV viremia [25]. Survival in ganciclovir-treated patients was 6–12 months, whereas the one untreated patient died in 2 months.

Myelitis

Ganciclovir has not proven to be effective in the treatment of patients with advanced polyradiculomyelitis thought to be secondary to CMV, although one patient with a minor paresis showed improvement [24].

Pneumonia

There have been several studies assessing the importance of CMV when it is cultured from bronchoalveolar lavage (BAL) fluid in AIDS patients. Millar et al. [94] and Bower et al. [16] have reported on the significance of CMV in BAL specimens. In the study by Bower, the presence of CMV in BAL specimens of AIDS patients had no impact on the short-term or long-term mortality, and survival was similar in the group that did not receive therapy, which was usually foscarnet. However, patients with CMV in BAL specimens did have a higher incidence of extrapulmonary CMV infection. In the retrospective study by Millar, none of the 31 patients with CMV isolated by BAL were given treatment and the mortality of this group was only 6.0%. There are anecdotal reports that the presence of CMV in tissue at open-lung biopsy in AIDS patients does correlate with invasive CMV pneumonitis and does respond to ganciclovir [130]. Currently, we do not treat AIDS patients that demonstrate CMV on only BAL specimens. Patients with evidence of pneumonitis on chest radiography in which only CMV can be isolated from BAL specimens should be strongly considered for transbronchial or open-lung biopsy. If CMV inclusion bodies are found, treatment with ganciclovir can be initiated.

Treatment: Transplantation

Cytomegalovirus infection and disease is a major cause of morbidity and mortality in transplant recipients. In transplant recipients who are serologically CMV negative prior to the transplant, CMV infection occurs through a CMV-positive transplanted organ or from the transfusion of CMV-positive blood products. Patients who are CMV positive by serology prior to the transplant may be infected by either a new strain of CMV from the transplanted organ or they may reactivate the previous infecting CMV strain. Of renal transplant patients who are CMV positive prior to transplant, 80%–100% will excrete CMV in urine or saliva [9]. More than 50% of all bone marrow transplant (BMT) recipients excrete CMV within 8 weeks of the transplant [92]. In BMT recipients, CMV infection and disease is leading cause of death, with approximately 17% of patients developing CMV pneumonitis, a disease that has a mortality rate of 85% [92]. Because of the high morbidity and mortality of CMV disease in transplant recipients, several approaches to treatment and prophylaxis have been developed.

Bone Marrow Transplantation: Pneumonitis

Early studies attempted to decrease the mortality of CMV disease by the use of ganciclovir in the treatment of CMV pneumonitis, but the results were not encouraging. In a study by Shepp et al. [116] ganciclovir reduced viral excretion and lung titers of CMV in BMT recipients; however, 90% (9/10) of these patients died. In another trial in BMT recipients the combination of ganciclovir and steroids also was associated with a high mortality [106]. Similarly, there are conflicting reports concerning the efficacy of immunoglobulin when given alone in the treatment of CMV pneumonitis in BMT recipients. In one study, nine of 18 BMT recipients treated with CMV IgG for CMV pneumonitis survived [11]. However, the Seattle group did not find a similar response, as only three of 16 of their patients treated with CMV IgG survived [107].

In 1988 Reed et al. [108] at the Hutchinson Cancer Research Center and Emanuel et al. [39] at Memorial Sloan-Kettering Cancer Center reported on the mortality of BMT patients given ganciclovir combined with passive immunoglobulin in a nonrandomized, open-label fashion. In the study by Reed, a specially enriched immunoglobulin preparation was used with high immunoglobulin titres to CMV (Cutter Biological). The dose given was 400 mg/kg on days 1, 2 and 7 and 200 mg/kg on day 14. The antibody titer to CMV in this preparation, measured by indirect hemagglutination was 1:6400. The group at Sloan-Kettering used Gammagard (Travenol; standard IgG) 500 mg/kg qod for 10 doses and then 500 mg/kg two times a week for another eight doses. The titer is not comparable since the Sloan-Kettering group used an enzyme-linked immunosorbent assay to measure the antibody. Usually, there is an eight- to 10-fold difference in CMV titer between the regular intravenous immunoglobulin and CMV immunoglobulin when measured simultaneously. The dosage of ganciclovir was 2.5 mg/kg tid for 14 days in one study and 20 days in the other. A maintenance phase of 5 mg/kg of ganciclovir on 3–5 days each week for 20 doses was used in the study by Emanuel and colleagues. The initial survival of the two studies combined was 66% (23/35). Of the 23 survivors, four had a relapse of CMV pneumonitis and died and three other patients died with death unrelated to CMV disease. There was a substantially higher relapse rate in the study by Reed et al., in which no maintenance therapy was given. Two other groups have presented confirmatory data on the treatment of CMV pneumonitis with ganciclovir and immunoglobulin at meetings [17, 80].

Only one preparation of CMV hyperimmune globulin is currently available in the United States. It is sold by Connought Laboratories under the name CytoGam for use in prophylaxis of CMV disease in renal transplant recipients. There is no published data on the use of this particular product in the treatment of CMV pneumonia in BMT. The dose for the treatment of CMV pneumonia would presumably be higher than that for prophylaxis or similar to the dose used in the Reed study. That preparation was not the same product as the Connought product. The current retail cost of Gammagard for a 70-kg patient treated with the course described above [39] at our institution would be $ 17 200 for 630 g. If one used CytoGam at the same dose as the Reed study the cost would be $ 17 640 for 98 g.

It is clear that these patients need simultaneous administration of ganciclovir and some form of immunoglobulin as well as long-term maintenance therapy with ganciclovir.

Solid Organ Transplantation: Pneumonitis

There has been much less experience with the use of ganciclovir in the treatment of CMV pneumonitis in solid organ transplant recipients. However, the results have been more encouraging. Keay et al. [77] reported on 12 heart or heart-lung transplant recipients who were treated with ganciclovir for CMV limited to the lung. Ten of 12 patients survived the initial infection and one of the deaths was due to rejection, not CMV disease. Four of nine long-term survivors relapsed a mean of 23 days after stopping initial therapy. Dunn et al. [38] described the treatment of 93 solid organ transplant recipients of whom 48% were renal transplant recipients. All were treated for CMV disease with ganciclovir, although there was no breakdown of those with pneumonitis. Some of these patients received acylovir as prophylaxis. Ganciclovir was given in dosages of 5 mg/kg bid adjusted for renal function. Eighty-nine percent of those treated with ganciclovir survived for 30 days after the onset of CMV disease. Interestingly, in the 24-month follow-up period 11 of the patients with CMV died. Rondeau et al. [110] demonstrated an improvement rate of 80% (12/15) in renal transplant recipients who received ganciclovir for the treatment of CMV pneumonitis. Others have confirmed this success [98]. Ganciclovir was well tolerated in these studies. The need for and duration of maintenance therapy have yet to be determined, although the heart-lung data suggest that prolonged maintenance therapy is necessary.

Bone Marrow Transplantation: Gastrointestinal Disease

The group at Seattle [109] demonstrated no benefit in CMV ulcer healing in BMT patients treated with only 2 weeks of ganciclovir. The treatment course was probably too short for efficacy to be demonstrated, and like CMV pneumonia in BMT, recipients may require immunoglobulin.

Solid Organ Transplantation: Gastrointestinal Disease

Ganciclovir has proven effective in the treatment of esophageal, gastric and colonic ulcers in solid organ transplant recipients. Kaplan et al. [75] reported on the treatment of 10 heart or heart-lung transplant recipients who were treated with ganciclovir 5 mg/kg bid for CMV gastrointestinal disease (gastritis, gastric ulcerations, duodenitis, esophagitis and colitis). Nine of the ten patients had healing of their lesions as demonstrated endoscopically, with the longest treatment course being 8 weeks (six patients required at least 4 weeks of treatment) and the time for healing to occur being 4–12 weeks. The length of treatment was determined by biopsy results obtained during follow-up endoscopy. In one patient with nodular gastritis the lesions did not completely heal. Four of nine surviving patients relapsed 2–12 months after completing therapy and readily responded to retreatment. The University of Minnesota group [86] had a similar response rate (13/14 patients) in ganciclovir treatment of solid organ transplant recipients with CMV gastrointestinal disease. Four patients relapsed a mean of 28 days after stopping therapy. Recently, several centers have recognized the need to give prolonged therapy (8–12 weeks) to solid organ transplant recipients with CMV gastritis. In this group of patients, there may be a role for passive immunoglobulin (M.L. Smiley, personal communication, 1992).

CMV hepatitis is a commonly encountered disease in liver transplant recipients [84]. In this population CMV disease, especially hepatitis, is difficult to diagnose as it mimics allograft rejection in its clinical presentation. Liver transplant patients incur the same risks for CMV infection and disease as other transplant patients; the risk of disease is increased in seronegative patients who receive a seropositive graft. As in other transplant recipients, the transplanted organ is especially susceptible to CMV disease.

Barkholt et al. [7] described the clinical course of CMV infection and disease in 33 patients who received orthotopic liver transplants. Eighty-five percent (28/33) developed CMV infection, of whom six had a primary infection and 22 either a reactivated or second primary infection. CMV disease occurred in 11 patients, of whom eight had hepatitis. Of the six with primary infection, four developed CMV disease and three of these had hepatitis. Treatment was not standardized; five patients with CMV hepatitis received ganciclovir (in three combined with Gammagard), and two patients received foscarnet and hyperimmune CMV IgG. In six of these seven patients (85%) the treatment was effective; the one death occurred in a patient given ganciclovir and IgG. Two other patients died of rejection. A retrospective study compared the results of 50 liver transplant recipients from the ganciclovir era to the outcome in the pre-ganciclovir era [84]. There was no difference in time to defervescence, but there was decreased mortality and extrahepatic CMV disease in the ganciclovir-treated patients.

In a pediatric study of CMV infection in liver allograft recipients, 54% of the patients (14/26) developed CMV infection, of whom six had fulminant CMV disease leading to death [78]. Severe disease occurred exclusively in two groups: seropositive recipients who received a seropositive graft and seronegative recipients who received a seropositive graft. All patients in this study received either CMV hyperimmune globulin or conventional IgG as prophylaxis. All patients with disseminated CMV disease were treated with ganciclovir or foscarnet plus CMV hyperimmune globulin (200 mg/kg to 1 g/kg every 1–3 days). Treatment was uniformly unsuccessful, as all of the patients with disseminated disease died.

There is much less experience with foscarnet in the treatment of organ transplant patients with CMV infection or disease. Much of the experience comes from transplantation centers outside of the United States. A group in Sweden [79] described the treatment of six transplant recipients, three BMT and three renal allograft recipients, who developed CMV disease. The diagnosis of CMV disease was not always tissue based, and concurrent antibiotic therapy was given to these patients. Continuous-infusion foscarnet was given to each patient for treatment. Two of the six patients survived CMV infection/disease. As is described above, in very small trials foscarnet has shown efficacy similar to that of ganciclovir. Due to its renal toxicity foscarnet may not be ideal for the treatment of CMV disease in renal transplant recipients. Conversely, as it has little bone marrow toxicity, unlike ganciclovir, foscarnet may prove efficacious in the treatment of CMV disease in BMT recipients.

Bone Marrow Transplant: Other Syndromes

Foscarnet (60 mg/kg every 8 h) has been used to treat CMV-associated marrow suppression, defined as a reduction of more than 50% in neutrophil count after engraftment [15]. In eight of 12 courses in 10 patients the neutrophil count doubled within 15 days, with suppression of CMV cultures within 2 days. The neutropenia recurred in six cases.

In summary, CMV disease can be effectively treated in transplant recipients using ganciclovir. Foscarnet may be an alternative effective agent, although extensive clinical data is lacking. In BMT recipients, immunoglobulin must be added to ganciclovir for effective treatment. Unfortunately, there are no studies that evaluate the benefit of immunoglobulin in addition to ganciclovir in the treatment of CMV disease in solid organ transplant recipients. Many centers currently use immunoglobulin and ganciclovir to treat CMV disease in these patients. Given the severe morbidity and mortality of CMV in this population, and the limited side effects associated with immunoglobulin administration, one can understand the enthusiasm for this combination. However, until clinical data are presented that compare this combination with ganciclovir alone, it remains a very costly, unproven therapeutic modality.

Prophylaxis

As stated above, the use of ganciclovir with and without immunoglobulin has been shown to vastly reduce the morbidity and mortality associated with CMV disease. However, CMV infection and disease still cause significant morbidity and mortality in transplant recipients. This is especially true in seronegative recipients who receive a positive graft and in seropositive recipients regardless of graft status. Several different centers have attempted to use various antiviral compounds or immunoglobulin prophylactically in an attempt to decrease the incidence of CMV disease, especially in these groups.

Acyclovir

Acyclovir has proven effective in the prophylaxis of patients receiving both renal transplants and allogeneic BMT. Balfour et al., in a double-blind, placebo-controlled study treated 104 patients receiving a cadaveric renal transplant with placebo or acyclovir 800 mg p.o. 6 h prior to surgery and 24 h after surgery and then 800 mg four times a day dose-adjusted for renal function for a total of 12 weeks [6]. Patients receiving acyclovir had a lower incidence of CMV infection than those receiving placebo: 36% vs 61% ($p=0.011$). More importantly, CMV disease occurred in 29% of placebo patients compared with 7.5% of those on acyclovir ($p=0.0002$). There was no significant difference in graft or patient survival between patients receiving acyclovir and those receiving placebo [6]. The cost of this course of prophylaxis at our hospital would be $ 937.

Meyers et al., in an open-label, nonrandomized study, treated 156 patients who were seropositive for both HSV and CMV with acyclovir 500 mg/m^2 i.v. every 8 h from day 5 before allogeneic BMT to day 30 after transplant. Patients who were only CMV seropositive served as controls [93]. Fifty-nine percent of the patients who received acyclovir developed CMV infection in the first 100 days, against 75% of the control patients ($p=0.0001$). CMV pneumonia developed in 19% of patients on acyclovir compared with 31% of controls within 100 days of transplant ($p=0.04$). Patients who received acyclovir had significantly better survival due to the decreased mortality from CMV disease ($p=0.0002$). The cost for this course of prophylaxis would be $ 7382 at our hospital.

As yet, there have been no large studies evaluating the efficacy of acyclovir prophylaxis alone for CMV in other solid organ transplants. These studies appear to confirm the in vitro suggestion that although acyclovir itself is not effective against CMV, the low levels of triphosphate formed are sufficient to at least suppress reactivation of CMV [10].

Ganciclovir

Because of its good activity against CMV compared with acyclovir, ganciclovir is an attractive candidate as a prophylactic agent for transplant recipients. Ganciclovir does, however, have some limitations. There currently is no effective oral form of the drug. Ganciclovir is a bone marrow toxin, which limits its widespread use in BMT recipients. However, recently Schmidt et al. [115] evaluated the use of ganciclovir in seropositive BMT recipients and seronegative recipients of a seropositive graft. One hundred four CMV seropositive patients who received an allogeneic BMT and had no evidence of active pulmonary disease were entered into the study. These patients underwent bronchoscopy at day 35. Forty patients had evidence of CMV infection by positive shell-vial culture or the presence of CMV inclusion bodies in BAL fluid and were randomized to receive either ganciclovir or placebo. Patients who received ganciclovir were treated with 5 mg/kg twice each day for 2 weeks and then 5 mg/kg per day for 5 days each week. Patients were treated for 120 days with ganciclovir. Only four of 18 evaluable patients (22%) treated with ganciclovir were found to have CMV pneumonitis, compared with 10 of 15 (67%) in the untreated group ($p=0.015$). When all 40 randomized patients were compared the incidence was similar; five of 20 (25%) in the treated group vs 14 of 20 (70%) in the untreated group ($p=0.010$).

In this study, none of the patients with negative bronchoscopy (no CMV inclusion bodies in BAL fluid) at both 35 and 49 days developed CMV pneumonitis. Risk factors associated with the occurrence of CMV pneumonitis included a positive shell-vial culture on day 35, positive bronchoscopy and a positive buffy coat. These data would suggest that BMT recipients who are asymptomatic yet CMV positive or receive a CMV positive marrow should undergo bronchoscopy at day 35 and again at day 49. Patients with CMV demonstrated by shell-vial culture or cytologic examination should be treated with ganciclovir. Furthermore, consideration ought to be given to administration of ganciclovir to all BMT patients who exhibit CMV-positive buffy coat.

Other studies have examined ganciclovir as a prophylactic agent. Seven lung transplant recipients were given prophylactic ganciclovir 5 mg/kg twice each day, along with immunoglobulin, for the first 14 days after transplantation [3]. There was no benefit. In another study 16 heart transplant recipients were treated with either hyperimmune globulin (six doses over 1 month) or ganciclovir 7.5 mg/kg for 14 days [81]. One of the ganciclovir-treated patients and five of the immunoglobulin-treated patients developed invasive CMV disease. Obviously the small number of patients and the short duration of prophylaxis render any conclusions suspect.

Immunoglobulin

Administration of immunoglobulin for prophylaxis and treatment has attracted intense interest in the last decade. The mode of action of immunoglobulin in the prevention and treatment of CMV infection/disease is not completely understood. Nor is it known whether the specific titer of immunoglobulin for CMV determines the efficacy of this product. It is known that the half-life of immunoglobulin in transplant recipients is much shorter than that in agammaglobulinemic hosts [52]. The half-life of intravenous immunoglobulin in BMT recipients is approximately 3 days, and in renal transplant recipients the immediate post-transplant half-life is 6–9 days, increasing to 15–22 days 60 days after the transplant [118]. The half-life of intravenous immunoglobulin in the agammaglobulinemic host is approximately 21 days.

Renal Transplant Recipients

Snydman et al. [119] described the clinical course of 59 CMV-seronegative patients who received seropositive renal allografts. These patients were randomized to treatment with CMV hyperimmune globulin (Cytogram) or no treatment. The doses given were 150 mg/kg at entry, 100 mg/kg 2 and 4 weeks after transplantation and 50 mg/kg 6, 8, 12 and 16 weeks after transplantation. There was a reduction in CMV-associated syndromes in the treated patients from 60% to 21% ($p<0.01$). CMV pneumonitis was reduced from 17% to 4% (not significant). There was also a reduction in fungal infections and infections due to *Pneumocystis carinii*. Rates of virus isolation and seroconversion did not differ in the two groups. The cost of this course of CMV IgG would be approximately $ 6930 at our hospital. An open-label study [20] confirmed the results of the previous trial. A smaller study using standard immunoglobulin showed no benefit [76].

Bone Marrow Transplant Recipients

Many groups [13, 91, 133, 134] have demonstrated that both hyperimmune plasma and conventional immunoglobulin can decrease the risk of CMV infection in BMT recipients. In addition, immunoglobulin decreases the incidence of graft-vs-host (GVH) disease. However, evidence of reduction of the occurrence of CMV disease has been elusive. An early paper on BMT recipients described a four-arm randomized study of seronegative blood products and CMV immunoglobulin (Cytogam) at a dose of 100–150 mg/kg for seven doses [13]. The numbers of subjects were not large enough to confirm a benefit of CMV-immunoglobulin in preventing CMV disease. More recently, a different formulation of CMV-immunoglobulin manufactured by Cutter but not yet approved by the FDA was used in a randomized trial at a dose of 200 mg/kg for 10 doses in BMT recipients. Although there was significantly less CMV excretion and viremia in the treated group there was no difference in incidence of CMV disease, survival or number of hospital days [14].

Heart/Lung/Liver Transplant Recipients

In a noncontrolled retrospective evaluation [114], immunoglobulin was found to have decreased the incidence of severe CMV disease in heart transplant recipients who were seronegative and received a seropositive graft.

Cofer et al. studied 50 liver transplant recipients who were randomized to receive nine doses of standard immunoglobulin 500 mg/kg (Sandoglobulin, Sandoz) or placebo over the first 84 days after transplantation [22]. There was no benefit. Another study which suggested a benefit used historical controls and was not randomized [125]. Finally, Snydman et al. used CMV immunoglobulin in a randomized blinded study to treat 146 liver recipients. Seven doses of 100–150 mg/kg were given. The rate of CMV disease was reduced from 30% to 18% ($p=0.06$). The rate of fungemia was also reduced [121].

The toxicity of the CMV immunoglobulin currently approved in the United States is minimal and is usually related to the amount of fluid given with the product. Of 205 infusions in one study [119], only 12 infusions in seven patients were associated with possible side effects. These included flushing (three episodes), anxiety, nausea, a metallic taste in the mouth, headache, shortness of breath (two episodes each), palpitations, backache and muscle cramps (one episode each). There was no evidence of HIV, hepatitis B or C seroconversion or development of abnormal liver enzymes suggestive of non-A, non-B hepatitis.

These studies suggest that immunoglobulin has a role in the prevention of CMV disease in renal transplant recipients but probably not in BMT recipients. Uncontrolled studies suggest that immunoglobulin is effective in the prevention of CMV disease in other solid-organ transplant recipients; however, a prospective randomized trial is needed for proof. Whether acyclovir, ganciclovir or immunoglobulin is the best and most cost-effective agent for the prevention of CMV disease in transplant recipients awaits further study.

Conclusion

Clinical trials are continuing to explore new combinations and new therapies for the treatment and prophylaxis of CMV disease. With evidence of in vitro synergy, a trial of foscarnet and ganciclovir given on alternate days or on the same day for maintenance therapy of CMV retinitis in AIDS patients is ongoing [85]. Phase II studies of the oral pyrimidine nucleoside analogs FIAU and FIAC have been completed and have shown that they are too toxic for HIV-infected patients [62]. Phase I studies of etoposide begin in spring 1992 at our hospital [64]. Oral ganciclovir enters phase II trials at the same time. The possibility of using oral agents for treatment, maintenance therapy and prophylaxis lends hope to the thousands of patients with CMV disease.

References

1. Alfred CA (1984) Chronic intrauterine and perinatal infections. In: Galasso GJ, Merigan TC, Buchanan RA (eds) Antiviral agents and viral diseases of man, 2nd edn. Raven, New York, pp 433–486
2. Aweeka F, Gambertoglio JG, Mills J, Jacobson MA (1989) Pharmacokinetics of intermittently administered intravenous foscarnet in the treatment of acquired immunodeficiency syndrome patients with serious cytomegalovirus retinitis. Antimicrob Agents Chemother 33:742–745
3. Bailey T, Ettinger N, Storch G, Cooper J et al. (1991) Failure of prophylactic ganciclovir to prevent cytomegalovirus pneumonitis in lung transplant recipients. Abstract 778 of the 1991 Interscience Conference on Antimicrobial Agents and Chemotherapy, Chicago
4. Balfour HH Jr, Bean B, Edelman CK et al. (1982) Acyclovir in immunocompromised patients with cytomegalovirus disease: a controlled trial at one institution. Am J Med 73:241–248
5. Balfour HH Jr, Bean B, Laskin OL (1983) Acyclovir halts progression of herpes zoster in immunocompromised patients. N Engl J Med 308:1448–1453
6. Balfour HH Jr, Chace BA, Stapleton JT et al. (1989) A randomized placebo-controlled trial of oral acyclovir for the prevention of cytomegalovirus disease in recipients of renal allografts. N Engl J Med 320:1381–1387
7. Barkholt LM, Ericzon BG, Ehrnst A et al. (1990) Cytomegalovirus infections in liver transplant patients: incidence and outcome. Transplant Proc 22:235–237
8. Bean B, Braun C, Balfour HH Jr (1982) Acyclovir therapy for acute herpes zoster. Lancet 2:118–121
9. Betts RF (1984) The relationship of epidemiology and treatment factors to infection and allograft survival in renal transplantation. In: Plotkin SA, Michelson S, Patano J, et al. (eds) CMV: pathogenesis and prevention of human infection, birth defects: original article series, vol 20. Liss, New York, pp 87–99
10. Biron KK, Stanat SC, Sorrell JB et al. (1985) Metabolic activation of the nucleoside analog 9-((2-hydroxy-1-(hydroxmethyl)ethoxy)methyl)guanine in human diploid fibroblasts infected with human CMV. Proc Natl Acad Sci USA 82:2473–2477
11. Blacklock HA, Griffiths P, Stirk P et al. (1985) Specific hyperimmune globulin for cytomegalovirus pneumonitis. Lancet 2:152–153
12. Blum RM, Liao SHT, de Miranda P (1982) Overview of acyclovir pharmacokinetic disposition in adults and children. Am J Med 73 (supp):186–192

13. Bowden RA, Sayers M, Flournoy N, Newton B et al. (1986) Cytomegalovirus immune globulin and seronegative blood products to prevent primary cytomegalovirus infection after marrow transplantation. N Engl J Med 314:1006–1010
14. Bowden RA, Fisher LD, Rogers K, Cays M, Meyers JD (1991) Cytomegalovirus-specific intravenous immunoglobulin for prevention of primary CMV infection and disease after marrow transplant. J Infect Dis 164:483–487
15. Bowden RA, Reusser P, Cays M, Meyers JD (1991) The use of foscarnet for treatment of cytomegalovirus-associated marrow suppression after marrow transplant. Abstract 777 of the 1991 Interscience Conference on Antimicrobial Agents and Chemotherapy, Chicago
16. Bower M, Barton SE, Nelson MR et al. (1990) The significance of the detection of cytomegalovirus in the bronchoalveolar lavage fluid in AIDS patients with pneumonia. AIDS 4:317–320
17. Bratanow NC, Ash RC, Casper J et al. (1987) Successful treatment of serious cytomegalovirus (CMV) disease with 9,(1,3-dihydroxy-2-propoxymethyl) guanine (ganciclovir, DHPG) and intravenous immunoglobulin (IVIG) in bone marrow transplant (BMT) patients (abstract 254). Exp Hematol 15:541
18. Broughton WL, Cupples HP, Parver LM (1978) Bilateral retinal detachment following cytomegalovirus retinitis. Arch Ophthalmol 96:618–619
19. Causey D (1991) Concomitant ganciclovir and zidovudine treatment for cytomegalovirus retinitis in patients with HIV infection: an approach to treatment. J Acquir Immun Defic Syndr 4 [Suppl 1]:S16–S21
20. Chou S, Dylewski JS, Gaynon MW, Egbert PR, Merigan TC (1984) Alpha-interferon administration in cytomegalovirus retinitis. Antimicrob Agents Chemother 25:25–28
21. Chrisp P, Clissold SP (1991) Foscarnet: a review of its antiviral activity, pharmacokinetic properties and therapeutic use in immunocompromised patients with cytomegalovirus retinitis. Drugs 41:104–129
22. Cofer JB, Morris CA, Sutker WL, Husberg BS et al. (1991) A randomized double-blind study of the effect of prophylactic immune globulin on the incidence and severity of CMV infection in the liver transplant recipient. Transplant Proc 23:1525–1527
23. Cole NL, Balfour HH Jr (1987) In vitro susceptibility of cytomegalovirus isolates from immunocompromised patients to acyclovir and ganciclovir. Diagn Microbiol Infect Dis 6:255–261
24. De Gans J, Portegies P, Tiessens G et al. (1990) Therapy for cytomegalovirus polyradiculomyelitis in patients with AIDS: treatment with ganciclovir. AIDS 4:421–425
25. Delaroque E, Masio C, Salmon-Ceron D, Girard PM et al. (1991) Sclerosing cholangitis in 14 AIDS patients: diagnosis and outcome. Abstract M.B. 2287, VII International Conference on AIDS, Florence
26. De Miranda P, Good SS, Laskin OL et al. (1981) Disposition of intravenous radioactive acyclovir. Clin Pharmacol Ther 30:662
27. Deray G, Katlama C, Dohin E (1990) Prevention of foscarnet nephrotoxicity (letter). Ann Intern Med 113:332
28. Deray G, Martinez F, Beufils H et al. (1990) Foscarnet nephrotoxicity, mechanism, incidence and prevention. Am J Nephrol 9:316–321
29. Dieterich DT, Rahmin M (1991) Cytomegalovirus colitis in AIDS: presentation in 44 patients and a review of the literature. J Acquir Immun Defic Syndr 4 [Suppl 1]:S29–S34
30. Dieterich DT, Chachoua A, Lafleur F et al. (1988) Ganciclovir treatment of gastrointestinal infections caused by cytomegalovirus in patients with AIDS. Rev Inf Dis 10 [Suppl 3]:S532–S537
31. Dieterich D, Kotler D, Busch D, Crumpacker C et al. (1990) Randomized, placebo-controlled study of ganciclovir treatment of cytomegalovirus colitis in AIDS patients. Abstract F.B.94, VI International Conference on AIDS, San Francisco, June 20–24
32. Dieterich D, Dicker M, Tepper R (1991) Foscarnet treatment of cytomegalovirus gastrointestinal infections in AIDS patients who have failed ganciclovir. Abstract W.B.2293, VII International Conference on AIDS, Florence

33. Dohin E, Katlama C, Hoang P et al. (1990) Intermittent and ambulatory treatment of CMV retinitis with foscarnet in AIDS. Abstract Th.B.434, VI International Conference on AIDS, San Francisco, June 20–24
34. Dohin E, Katlama C, Brancon C, Caumes E et al. (1991) Foscarnet in maintenance therapy of cytomegalovirus retinitis in AIDS. Abstract W.B.2285, VII International Conference on AIDS, Florence
35. Dorsky DI, Crumpacker CS (1987) Drugs five years later: acyclovir. Ann Intern Med 107:859–874
36. Drew WL, Lalezari J, Busch D, Follansbee S et al. (1991) *In vivo* antiviral efficacy of oral ganciclovir. Abstract W.B.2309, VII International Conference on AIDS, Florence
37. Drew WL, Miner R, Busch D, Follansbee S et al. (1991) Prevalence of resistance in patients receiving ganciclovir for serious CMV infection. J Infect Dis 716–719
38. Dunn DL, Mayoral JL, Gillingham KJ et al. (1991) Treatment of invasive cytomegalovirus disease in solid organ transplant patients with ganciclovir. Transplantation 51:98–106
39. Emanuel D, Cunningham I, Jules-Elysee K et al. (1988) Cytomegalovirus pneumonia after bone marrow transplantation successfully treated with the combination of ganciclovir and high-dose intravenous immune globulin. Ann Intern Med 109:777–782
40. Eriksson B, Oberg B, Wahren B (1982) Pyrophosphate analogues as inhibitors of DNA polymerases of cytomegalovirus, herpes simplex virus and cellular origin. Biochim Biophys Acta 696:115–123
41. Estes JE, Huang ES (1977) Stimulation of cellular thymidine kinases by human cytomegalovirus. J Virol 24:13–21
42. Felsenstein D, D'Amico DJ, Hirsch MS et al. (1985) Treatment of cytomegalovirus retinitis with 9(2-hydroxy-1-(hydroxymethyl)ethoxymethyl)guanine. Ann Intern Med 103:377–380
43. Fletcher C, Sawchuk R, Balfour HH Jr et al. (1986) Human pharmacokinetics of the antiviral drug DHPG. Clin Pharmacol Ther 40:281–286
44. Follansbee S, Busch D, Connor J, Jung D et al. (1990) Phase I study of the safety and pharmacokinetics of oral ganciclovir. Abstract F.B.91, VI International Conference on AIDS, San Francisco, June 20–24
45. Foscarnet (1992) Med Lett Drugs Ther 34 (861):3–4
46. Freeman WR, Henderly DE, Wan WL et al. (1987) Prevalence, pathophysiology, and treatment of rhegmatogenous retinal detachment in treated cytomegalovirus retinitis. Am J Ophthalmol 103:527–536
47. Furman PA, de Miranda P, St. Clair MH et al. (1981) Metabolism of acyclovir in virus-infected and uninfected cells. Antimicrob Agents Chemother 20:518–524
48. Furman PA, St. Clair MH, Spector T (1984) Acyclovir triphosphate is a suicidal inactivator of the herpes simplex virus DNA polymerase. J Biol Chem 259:9575–9579
49. Gentilini M, Dohin E, Cochereau I, Brancon C et al. (1991) Foscarnet in acute therapy of CMV retinitis: experience with a twice daily intermittent regimen. Abstract W.B.2257, VII International Conference on AIDS, Florence
50. Gilquin J, Weiss L, Kazatchkine MD (1990) Genital and oral erosions induced by foscarnet. Lancet 335:287
51. Gross JG, Bozzette SA, Matthews WC et al. (1990) Longitudinal study of cytomegalovirus retinitis in acquired immune deficiency syndrome. Ophthalmology 97:681–686
52. Hagenbeck A, Brummelhuis HGJ, Lowenberg B et al. (1987) Rapid clearance of cytomegalovirus-specific IgG after repeated intravenous infusions of human immunoglobulin into allogeneic bone marrow transplant recipients. J Infect Dis 155:897–902
53. Hardy D, Spector S, Polsky B, Heath-Chiozzi M et al. (1990) Safety and efficacy of combined ganciclovir and granulocyte-macrophage stimulating factor vs ganciclovir alone for cytomegalovirus retinitis in AIDS (ACTG 073): a preliminary report. Abstract F.B.92, VI International Conference on AIDS, San Francisco, June 20–24

54. Helgstrand E, Flodh H, Oberg B et al. (1980) Trisodium phosphonoformate: antiviral activities, safety evaluation and preliminary clinical results. Ber Dtsch Chem Ges 78:1023–1038
55. Henderly DE, Freeman WR, Causey DM, Rao NA (1987) Cytomegalovirus retinitis and response to therapy with ganciclovir. Ophthalmology 94:425–434
56. Henry K, Cantrill H, Fletcher C et al. (1987) Use of intravitreal ganciclovir (dihydroxy propoxymethyl guanine) for cytomegalovirus retinitis in a patient with AIDS. Am J Ophthalmol 103:17–23
57. Ho M (1982) Treatment and prevention of CMV infection. In: Greenough WB III, Merigan TC (eds) Cytomegalovirus, biology and infection: current topics in infectious disease. Plenum, New York, pp 205–213
58. Hochster H, Dieterich D, Bozzette S, Reichman RC, et al. (1990) Toxicity of combined ganciclovir and zidovudine for cytomegalovirus disease associated with AIDS. Ann Intern Med 113:111–117
59. Holland GN, Pepose JS, Pettit TH et al. (1983) Acquired immune deficiency syndrome: ocular manifestations. Ophthalmology 90:859–873
60. Holland GN, Sidikaro Y, Kreiger AE et al. (1987) Treatment of cytomegalovirus retinopathy with ganciclovir. Ophthalmology 94:815–823
61. Holland GN, Sison RF, Jatulis DE et al. (1990) Survival of patients with the acquired immune deficiency syndrome after development of cytomegalovirus retinopathy. Ophthalmology 97:204–211
62. Hooton TM, Dejarnette L, Tartaglione T, Paar D, et al. (1991) Serial phase II dose-escalation studies of the oral pyrimidine nucleoside analog FIAC and its metabolite FIAU in HIV-infected patients (ACTG 122). Abstract 1218. Program and Abstracts, 31st Interscience Conference on Antimicrobial Agents and Chemotherapy
63. Huang ES (1975) Human cytomegalovirus: specific inhibition of virus-induced DNA polymerase activity and viral DNA replication by phosphonoacetic acid. J Virol 16:1560–1565
64. Huang ES, Benson JD, Huong SM, Wilson B et al. (1992) Irreversible inhibition of human cytomegalovirus replication by topoisomerase II inhibitor, etoposide: a new strategy for the treatment of human cytomegalovirus infection. Antiviral Res 17:17–32
65. Investigational brochure, intravenous ganciclovir, 9th edn (1991) Syntex Research, Palo Alto, California
66. Jabs DA, Enger C, Bartlett JG (1989) Cytomegalovirus retinitis and acquired immunodeficiency syndrome. Arch Ophthalmol 107:75–80
67. Jabs DA, Newman C, De Bustros S, Polk BF et al. (1987) Treatment of cytomegalovirus retinitis with ganciclovir. Ophthalmology 94:824–830
68. Jacobson MA, De Miranda P, Cederberg DM et al. (1987) Human pharmacokinetics and tolerance of oral ganciclovir. Antimicrob Agents Chemother 31:1251–1254
69. Jacobson MA, Crowe S, Levy J et al. (1988) Effect of foscarnet therapy on infection with human immunodeficiency virus in patients with AIDS. J Infect Dis 158:862–865
70. Jacobson MA, O'Donnell JJ, Brodie HR (1988) Randomized prospective trial of ganciclovir maintenance therapy for cytomegalovirus retinitis. J Med Virol 25:339–349
71. Jacobson MA, O'Donnell JJ, Mills J (1989) Foscarnet treatment of cytomegalovirus retinitis in patients with the acquired immunodeficiency syndrome. Antimicrob Agents Chemother 33:736–741
72. Jacobson MA, Causey D, Polsky B, Hardy D et al. (1990) Dose-ranging study of daily intravenous maintenance foscarnet therapy for cytomegalovirus retinitis in AIDS patients (ACTG 015/915). Abstract F.B.96, VI International Conference on AIDS, San Francisco, June 20–24
73. Jacobson MA, Gambertoglio JG, Aweeka FT et al. (1991) Foscarnet-induced hypocalcemia and effects of foscarnet on calcium metabolism. J Clin Endocrinol Metab 72:1130–1135
74. Jacobson MA, Wulfsohn M, Feinberg J, Davis R et al. (1991) Phase 2 dose-ranging study of foscarnet salvage therapy for CMV retinitis in patients intolerant of or resis-

tant to ganciclovir therapy (ACTG 093). Abstract 296, 1991 Interscience Conference on Antimicrobial Agents and Chemotherapy, Chicago

75. Kaplan CS, Petersen EA, Icenogle TB et al. (1989) Gastrointestinal cytomegalovirus infection in heart and heart-lung transplant recipients. Arch Intern Med 149:2095–2100
76. Kasiske BL, Heim-Duthoy KL, Tortorice KL, Ney AL et al. (1989) Polyvalent immune globulin and cytomegalovirus infection after renal transplantation. Arch Intern Med 149:2733
77. Keay S, Petersen E, Icenogle TB et al. (1988) Ganciclovir treatment of serious cytomegalovirus infection in heart and heart-lung transplant recipients. Rev Inf Dis 10 [Suppl 3]: S563–S572
78. King SM, Petric M, Superina R et al. (1990) Cytomegalovirus infections in pediatric liver transplantation. Am J Dis Child 144:1307–1310
79. Klintmalm G, Lonnqvist B, Oberg B et al. (1985) Intravenous foscarnet for the treatment of severe cytomegalovirus infection in allograft recipients. Scand J Infect Dis 17:157–163
80. Kovacs A, Schmidt GM, Zaia JA et al. (1988) Ganciclovir (GCV) plus intravenous immunoglobulin (IVIG) treatment of human cytomegalovirus interstitial pneumonia (HCMV-IP) in recipients of allogeneic bone marrow transplantation (BMT). Abstract 738, Program and Abstracts, 28th Interscience Conference on Antimicrobial Agents and Chemotherapy, Washington, DC
81. Laske A, Gallino A, Mohacsi P, Bauer EP et al. (1991) Prophylactic treatment with ganciclovir for cytomegalovirus infection in heart transplantation. Transplant Proc 23:1170–1173
82. Laskin OL, Longstreth C, Whelton A et al. (1982) Effect of renal failure on the pharmacokinetics of acyclovir. Am J Med 73 [Suppl]: 197–201
83. Laskin OL, Cederberg DM, Mills J et al. (1987) Ganciclovir for the treatment and suppression of serious infections caused by cytomegalovirus. Am J Med 83:201–207
84. Linden P, Dummer S, Kusne S, Ho M et al. (1991) Cytomegalovirus hepatitis following orthotopic liver transplantation: effect of 9-(1,3 dihydroxy-2-propoxymethyl) guanine on CMV-related morbidity. Abstract 1241, 1991 Interscience Conference on Antimicrobial Agents and Chemotherapy, Chicago
85. Manischewitz JF, Quinnan GV, Lane HC, Wittek AE (1990) Synergistic effect of ganciclovir and foscarnet on cytomegalovirus replication in vitro. Antimicrob Agents Chemother 34:373–375
86. Mayoral JL, Loeffer CM, Fasola CG et al. (1991) Diagnosis and treatment of cytomegalovirus disease in transplant patients based on gastrointestinal tract manifestations. Arch Surg 126:202–206
87. McGuirt PV, Furman PA (1982) Acyclovir inhibition of viral DNA chain elongation in herpes simplex virus-infected cells. Am J Med 73 [Suppl]: 67–71
88. McKindrick MW, McGill JI, White JE et al. (1986) Oral acyclovir in acute herpes zoster. Br Med J 293:1529–1532
89. Meredith TA, Aaberg TM, Reeser FH (1979) Rhegmatogenous retinal detachment complicating cytomegalovirus retinitis. Am J Ophthalmol 87:793–796
90. Meyers JD, McGuffin RW, Neiman PE, Singer JW et al. (1980) Toxicity and efficacy of human leukocyte interferon for treatment of cytomegalovirus pneumonia after marrow transplantation. J Infect Dis 141:555–562
91. Meyers JD, Lescczynski J, Thomas ED et al. (1983) Prevention of cytomegalovirus infection by cytomegalovirus immune globulin after marrow transplantation. Ann Intern Med 98:442–446
92. Meyers JD, Flournoy N, Thomas ED (1986) Risk factors for cytomegalovirus infection after bone marrow transplantation. J Infect Dis 153:478–488
93. Meyers JD, Reed EC, Shepp DH et al. (1988) Acyclovir for prevention of cytomegalovirus infection and disease after allogeneic marrow transplantation. N Engl J Med 318:70–75
94. Millar AB, Patou G, Semple SJ et al. (1990) Cytomegalovirus in the lungs of patients with AIDS. Am Rev Respir Dis 141:1474–1477

95. Mintz L, Drew WL, Miner L et al. (1983) Cytomegalovirus infections in homosexual men: an epidemiological study. Ann Intern Med 99:326–329
96. Nelson M, Connolly G, Hawkins D, Gazzard B (1991) Foscarnet in the treatment of cytomegalovirus infection of the oesophagus and colon. Abstract W.B.2262, VII International Conference on AIDS, Florence
97. Nerurkar LS, Biggar RJ, Goedert JJ et al. (1987) Antiviral antibodies in the sera of homosexual men: correlation with their lifestyle and drug usage. J Med Virol 21:123–135
98. Nicholson ML, Veitch PS, Donnelly PK, Flower AJE, Bell PRF (1990) Treatment of renal transplant-associated cytomegalovirus infection with ganciclovir. Transplant Proc 22:1811–1812
99. Orellana J, Teich SA, Friedman AH, Lerebours F et al. (1987) Combined short- and long-term therapy for the treatment of cytomegalovirus retinitis using ganciclovir (BW B759U). Ophthalmology 94:831–838
100. Package insert for Foscarnet, Astra Pharmaceutical Products, Inc, Westborough, Mass.
101. Palestine AG, Stevens G, Lane HC et al. (1986) Treatment of cytomegalovirus retinitis with dihydroxy propoxymethylguanine. Am J Ophthalmol 101:95–101
102. Plotkin SA, Friedman HM, Fleisher GR et al. (1981) Prevention and treatment of cytomegalovirus infection. In: Nahmias A, Dowdle W, Schinazi R (eds) The human herpesviruses: an interdisciplinary perspective. Elsevier, New York, pp 403–413
103. Polsky B, Wolitz R, Chuang EL, Cantrill H et al. (1991) Intravitreal ganciclovir salvage therapy for CMV retinitis (ACTG 085): a preliminary report. Abstract 295, 31st Interscience Conference on Antimicrobial Agents and Chemotherapy, Chicago
104. Potter JL, Krill CE (1986) Acyclovir crystalluria. Pediatr Infect Dis 5:710–712
105. Prostegard C, Sjovall J, Arvidsson A et al. (1991) Pharmacokinetics of foscarnet – a review. Abstract W.B.2288, VII International Conference on AIDS, Florence
106. Reed EC, Dandliker PS, Meyers JD (1986) Treatment of cytomegalovirus pneumonia with 9-(2-hydroxy-1-(hydroxymethyl)-ethoxymethyl)guanine and high-dose corticosteroids. Ann Intern Med 105:214–215
107. Reed EC, Bowden RA, Dandliker PS et al. (1987) Efficacy of cytomegalovirus immunoglobulin in marrow transplant recipients with cytomegalovirus pneumonia. J Infect Dis 156:641–645
108. Reed EC, Bowden RA, Dandliker PS et al. (1988) Treatment of cytomegalovirus pneumonia with ganciclovir and intravenous cytomegalovirus immunoglobulin in patients with bone marrow transplants. Ann Intern Med 109:783–788
109. Reed EC, Wolford JL, Kopecky KJ et al. (1990) Ganciclovir for the treatment of cytomegalovirus gastroenteritis in bone marrow transplant patients. Ann Intern Med 112:505–510
110. Rondeau E, Farquet C, Ruedin P et al. (1990) Efficacy of early treatment of cytomegalovirus infection by ganciclovir in renal transplant recipients. Transplant Proc 22:1813–1814
111. Rosecan LR, Stahl-Bayliss CM, Kalman CM et al. (1986) Antiviral therapy for cytomegalovirus retinitis in AIDS with dihydroxy propoxymethylguanine. Am J Opthalmol 101:405–418
112. Sandstrom EG, Byington RE, Hirsch MS et al. (1985) Inhibition of human T cell lymphotropic virus type III in vitro by phosphonoformate. Lancet 2:1480–1482
113. Sawyer MH, Webb DE, Balow JE et al. (1988) Acyclovir-induced renal failure: clinical course and histology. Am J Med 84:1067–1071
114. Schafers HJ, Wahlers T, Haverich A et al. (1988) Hyperimmuneglobulin for cytomegalovirus prophylaxis following heart transplantation. J Hosp Infect 2 [Suppl D]:61–65
115. Schmidt GM, Horak DA, Niland JC (1991) A randomized controlled trial of prophylactic ganciclovir for cytomegalovirus pulmonary infection in recipients of allogeneic bone marrow transplants. N Engl J Med 324:1005–1011
116. Shepp DH, Dandliker PS, de Miranda P et al. (1985) Activity of 9-(2-hydroxy-1-(hydroxymethyl)ethoxymethyl)guanine in the treatment of cytomegalovirus pneumonia. Ann Intern Med 103:368–373

117. Sjovall J, Karlsson A, Ogenstad S et al. (1988) Pharmacokinetics and absorption of foscarnet after intravenous and oral administration to patients with human immunodeficiency virus. Clin Pharmacol Ther 44:65–73
118. Snydman DR, McIver J, Grady GF et al. (1984) A pilot trial of a novel cytomegalovirus immune globulin in renal transplant recipients. Transplantation 38:553–557
119. Snydman DR, Werner BG, Heinze-Lacey B et al. (1987) Use of cytomegalovirus immune globulin to prevent cytomegalovirus disease in renal-transplant recipients. N Engl J Med 317:1049–1054
120. Syndman DR, Werner BG, Heinze-Lacey B et al. (1988) A further analysis of primary cytomegalovirus disease prevention in renal transplant recipients with a cytomegalovirus immune globulin: interim comparison of a randomized and an open-label trial. Transplant Proc 20 [Suppl 8]:24–30
121. Snydman DR, Werner BG, Rubin RH (1991) The use of cytomegalovirus immune globulin for prevention of CMV disease in patients undergoing liver transplantation. Abstract 1242, 1991 Interscience Conference on Antimicrobial Agents and Chemotherapy, Chicago
122. Sommadossi JP, Bevan R, Ling T et al. (1988) Clinical pharmacokinetics of ganciclovir in patients with normal and impaired renal function. Rev Infect Dis 10 (Suppl 3):S507–S514
123. Spector SA, Barker C, Buhles W, Feinberg J et al. (1991) A randomized, controlled study of immediate vs deferred ganciclovir therapy in AIDS patients with cytomegalovirus peripheral retinitis. Abstract M.B.86, VII International Conference on AIDS, Florence
124. Stanat SC, Reardon JE, Erice A, Jordan MC et al. (1991) Ganciclovir-resistant cytomegalovirus clinical isolates: mode of resistance to ganciclovir. Antimicrob Agents Chemother 35:2191–2197
125. Stratta RJ, Shaefer MS, Cushing KA, Markin RS et al. (1991) Successful prophylaxis of cytomegalovirus disease after primary CMV exposure in liver transplant recipients. Transplantation 51:90–97
126. Studies of Ocular Complications of AIDS Research Group et al. (1992) Mortality in patients with the acquired immunodeficiency syndrome treated with either foscarnet or ganciclovir for cytomegalovirus retinitis. New Engl J Med 326:213–220
127. Sullender WM, Arvin AM, Diaz PS et al. (1987) Pharmacokinetics of acyclovir suspension in infants and children. Antimicrob Agents Chemother 31:1722–1726
128. Van Der Pijl JW, Frissen PHJ, Reiss P et al. (1990) Foscarnet and penile ulceration. Lancet 335:286
129. Van Dyke RB, Connor JD, Wyborny C et al. (1982) Pharmacokinetics of orally administered acyclovir in patients with herpes progenitalis. Am J Med 73 [Suppl]:172–175
130. Vasudevan VP, Mascarenhas DAN, Lomvaridias S et al. (1990) Cytomegalovirus necrotizing bronchiolitis with HIV infection. Chest 97:483–484
131. Wade JC, Hintz M, McGuffin RW et al. (1982) Treatment of cytomegalovirus pneumonia with high-dose acyclovir. Am J Med 73 [Suppl 1a]:249–256
132. Walmsley SL, Chew E, Reed SE et al. (1988) Treatment of cytomegalovirus retinitis with trisodium phosphonoformate hexahydrate (foscarnet). J Infect Dis 157:569–572
133. Winston DJ, Pollard RB, Ho WG et al. (1982) Cytomegalovirus immune plasma in bone marrow transplant recipients. Ann Intern Med 97:11–18
134. Winston DJ, Ho WG, Lin C-H, Bartoni K et al. (1987) Intravenous immune globulin for prevention of cytomegalovirus infection and interstitial pneumonia after bone marrow transplantation. Ann Intern Med 106:12–18
135. Wool M, Hardy D, Holland G, Chafey S et al. (1991) Phase III recombinant GM-CSF and ganciclovir in neutropenic AIDS patients with CMV retinitis. Abstract W.B.2273, VII International Conference on AIDS, Florence
136. Youle MS, Clarbour J, Gazzard B et al. (1988) Severe hypocalcaemia in AIDS patients treated with foscarnet and pentamidine (letter). Lancet 2:1455–1456

Chapter 15 Vaccine Strategies for the Prevention of Cytomegalovirus Disease

Gary S. Marshall[1] and Stanley A. Plotkin[2]

Summary

The theorectical basis for vaccine immunoprophylaxis against cytomegalovirus rests on observations that naturally immune hosts are protected from disease, even though they may not be protected from infection per se. Indirect support for the vaccine paradigm derives from experimental models in the mouse and guinea pig, although these models are imperfect since they necessarily involve infection with species-specific cytomegaloviruses. Direct evidence is now available with the completion of a randomized, double-blind, placebo-controlled trial of Towne strain live attenuated vaccine in renal transplant patients. In seronegative patients who received kidneys from seropositive donors, the vaccine was able to prevent severe disease, albeit not infection; this is analogous to the protection afforded by natural immunity. Because theoretical safety concerns about a live herpesvirus vaccine exist, there is interest in developing noninfectious subunits that would mimic or exceed the immunogenicity of live whole virus. The abundant envelope glycoprotein gB is currently the most promising candidate, but other subunits, including immediate early proteins and other surface glycoproteins, are being investigated. Future work will concentrate on further study of the protective immune response to natural infection, testing live vaccines in other susceptible populations, and developing optimal vectors for the delivery of immunogenic subunits.

Introduction

Cytomegalovirus (CMV), which is a relatively benign agent in the immunocompetent host, has its greatest impact in two segments of the population: congenitally infected infants and immunosuppressed individuals. It has been estimated that in the last 2 decades in the United States alone, 30 000–40 000 children have died or suffered significant neurodevelopmental consequences

---

[1] Department of Pediatrics, University of Louisville School of Medicine, Louisville, Kentucky, KY 40292, USA

[2] Pasteur-Merieux Serums et Vaccins, Marnes-la-Coquette, France; and Connaught Laboratories, Swiftwater, PA, USA and Willowdale, Ontario, Canada

from congenital CMV infection, and an additional 45 000–60 000 have incurred less severe sequelae [1]. This disease burden is comparable to that resulting from invasive *Haemophilus influenzae* infection and establishes CMV as the most significant microbial cause of birth handicap in this country and probably other developed nations. CMV is also the most common opportunistic viral cause of death in patients with the acquired immunodeficiency syndrome and a common cause of morbidity and mortality in allograft recipients as well [2–4]. Since established CMV infections in immunocompromised hosts are only suppressed by antiviral chemotherapy, and treatment of infected newborns is unlikely to reverse the damage incurred during embryogenesis, the need for preventive strategies to minimize the public health impact of CMV infection is clear.

In CMV-naive allograft recipients, infection can be prevented by avoiding parenteral exposures to the virus in the form of organs or blood products from seropositive donors [5]. However, this approach is not always practical given the limited availability of donor organs and the high prevalence of latent CMV infection in some populations. In these patients, vaccine-induced immunity might be beneficial. Likewise, symptomatic congenital infection would be drastically reduced if primary CMV infection during pregnancy could be prevented (see below). Unfortunately, the sociobehavioral measures that would be necessary to avoid exposures to this ubiquitous agent during pregnancy would be prohibitive, and since maternal infection is usually asymptomatic, primary infections would not be readily identified [6]. Even if a fetus were known to be infected, one cannot reliably discriminate between those infants destined to be clinically affected and those who will escape severe disease. Thus, a vaccine that could protect women from infection, or at least mitigate the effects of infection on the fetus, would be highly desirable.

Most congenital CMV infections (0.2 > 3.0% of all live births [7]) are due to reactivated maternal infections during pregnancy. Fortunately, infants infected in this setting only rarely exhibit symptoms of cytomegalic inclusion disease [8, 9]. The protectice effect that maternal immunity has on the fetus has been clearly delineated. In one study, 5 of 33 infants born to seronegative mothers experiencing primary infection were symptomatic at birth, compared with 0 of 27 born to mothers who were previously immune [10]. In a subsequent study of primary infection in 96 women, 3 of 37 congenitally infected infants were symptomatic at birth and had mild to severe handicaps after a mean follow-up of 3.1 years [11]. Disturbingly, five infants who were initially normal developed clinically significant sequelae later on, including mental retardation, cerebral palsy, and hearing loss. From this information, it might be inferred that many "silently" infected newborns who develop late sequelae are also the products of pregnancies in which primary infection took place. Thus, whereas prior maternal immunity does not protect the fetus from CMV infection per se, it does appear to prevent the more serious consequences of intrauterine infection.

These observations constitute a fundamental rationale for the vaccine approach to prevention of congenital CMV disease. Vaccine-induced immunity among previously CMV-seronegative women would be expected to reduce the fetal morbidity resulting from exogeneous maternal infection during pregnancy, even if infection of the mother were not altogether prevented. If, however, maternal infection and/or transmission to the fetus were prevented as well, the number of asymptomatically infected children would be reduced; this is the reservoir of infectious virus that is potentially harmful to the fetuses of other (seronegative) mothers [12]. Further, a vaccine that was incapable of inducing latency could not give rise to congenital infection by reactivation. The importance of targeting young seronegative women for vaccination is underscored by recent data which suggest increasing susceptibility to primary CMV infection in this age group [13].

In many ways, the rubella vaccination program, which has dramatically reduced the incidence of congenital rubella syndrome in the United States [14], serves as the model for a CMV vaccine initiative. Both rubella and CMV, while relatively benign in the normal host, have devastating consequences for the susceptible fetus. However, biological differences between these two viruses render the analogy incomplete and serve to underscore the problems inherent in developing a CMV vaccine (Table 1). Whereas rubella virus is antigenically homogeneous and epidemic in occurrence, CMV strains are heterogeneous and endemic to populations. Natural and vaccine-induced immunity to rubella are lifelong and protect against reinfection; in contrast, reinfection with CMV commonly occurs in the context of natural immunity [15–20]. Rubella rarely persists after postnatal infection, whereas latent infection with CMV and the lifelong potential for reactivation are the rule. "Herd immunity" to rubella minimizes the exposure risk to susceptible individuals by decreasing the circulation of wild strains, but this concept may not be applicable to CMV.

Both cellular and humoral immune responses are important in preventing and eliminating CMV infection. During acute infection, CMV suppresses the cellular arm of the immune system, but after recovery the persistence of specific cellular responses constitute a major form of lasting immunity [21, 22]. CMV-seropositive adults have readily detectable lymphocyte transformation responses to CMV, and these responses may be cross-strain specific [23]. Cytotoxic T lymphocytes (CTLs) and other cellular effectors such as natural killer cells clearly have a role in the defense against CMV infection [24, 25].

Although humoral immunity was once considered "nearly irrelevant" to the outcome of CMV infection [26], this concept is changing. Neutralizing

Table 1. Rubella vaccination as a model for cytomegalovirus vaccination to prevent congenital disease

Rubella	Cytomegalovirus
Single strain necessary	Antigenically heterogeneous
Epidemic in occurrence	Endemic
Long-lasting natural immunity	Natural immunity incomplete
Does not persist	Persistence is universal
"Herd immunity" is important	"Herd immunity" not relevant

antibody is induced during acute infection and complement-requiring cytolytic antibodies against infected-cell antigens have been detected [27]. Adoptive humoral immunity favorably modifies the course of acute murine CMV (MCMV) infection [28], and studies of passive immunization in renal transplant patients show clear benefit [29]. Similarly, premature neonates with transplacentally-derived antibody who are postnatally infected through blood products less frequently develop CMV disease than those who are born to CMV-seronegative women [30], suggesting that antibody alone is sufficient for protection.

Even after primary maternal infection the rate of maternal-fetal transmission is only 20%–40% [11, 31, 32]. At the present time, the factors which prevent transmission in some cases are not known. Paradoxically, it has been shown that infected women who transmit CMV to their offspring have higher levels of virus-specific antibody than do infected women who do not transmit [33]. In addition, higher levels of virus-binding antibodies are found in mothers delivered of infants with clinically apparent disease [34]. The reasons for these observations are not clear, but may relate to the timing of infection during pregnancy. There are data to suggest that cellular responses are important in preventing transmission. In a study of 14 primary infections during pregnancy, congenital infection did not occur in 8 cases where maternal lymphoproliferative responses to CMV were demonstrable, but occurred in 4 of 6 cases where cellular responses to CMV were absent [35]. Interestingly, none of these babies exhibited symptoms at birth.

In recent years it has become increasingly apparent that natural immune mechanisms only partially protect the host during subsequent CMV experiences. Some healthy individuals shed more than one strain of virus, indicating that reinfection with exogenous strains can occur despite a normal immunity [16, 19]. Similarly, normal organ donors can be latently infected with more than one CMV strain [36], and in challenge experiments natural immunity can be overcome with a sufficiently high inoculum [20]. In one study, reinfection was seen much more frequently than reactivation in seropositive renal allograft patients receiving organs from seropositive donors [18]. However, from this study and others [37], it is clear that primary infections in transplant recipients are associated with more severe disease than secondary infections (including reinfections and reactivations). Thus, natural immunity does appear to protect individuals during subsequent CMV exposures.

Animal Models

Since human CMV is severely restricted in its host range, much experimental vaccine data derives from small animal infection with species-specific CMVs. The MCMV and guinea pig CMV (GPCMV) are the best studied and most illuminating models in this regard. While MCMV differs from human CMV in certain physical characteristics and in vitro growth properties, infectious syndromes caused by MCMV are similar to human infections [38]. The virus is probably transmitted by close contact (although in most laboratories parenteral routes of inoculation are used), has a propensity to infect many different tissues, produces similar histopathologic lesions, and can establish chronic productive and latent infections. However, although MCMV infection of susceptible pregnant females can cause intrauterine fetal demise, it does not result in live-born infected progeny [39]. Extrapolation from this model to the problem of congenital human disease is therefore limited.

Immunization with live attenuated MCMV strains can protect mice from lethal challenge with wild-type virus [40–42]. However, attenuation of MCMV by passage in tissue culture occurs by unclear mechanisms at low passage levels, and reversion to virulence can be demonstrated after single back-passage in mice [40]. While this is a worrisome observation, it must be pointed out that attenuation of MCMV in tissue culture may be due to nonheritable changes in the virion rather than genetic mutation [43, 44]. Of additional concern, infant female mice inoculated with tissue-culture-passaged MCMV may exhibit wasting, presumably resulting from latent infection [45], and reversion to virulence may occur with immunosuppression [46]. Given the biological peculiarities of MCMV, extrapolation of these findings to vaccination against human CMV infection may not be justified.

Closer parallels have been drawn between human CMV and GPCMV, based principally on the fact that transplacental transmission resulting in generalized fetal infection does occur [47]. As with human CMV, fetal GPCMV *infection* in the face of preexisting maternal immunity can occur, but this immunity appears to be protective against *disease* [48]. Further, early gestational exposure to the virus results in the most severe outcomes in these animals [49], as is suspected for human disease [11].

Prior infection with tissue-culture-passaged GPCMV protects pregnant females from viremia and death upon challenge with virulent virus and virtually eliminates fetal infection [50]. Highly passaged (more attenuated) GPCMV strains do not reactivate during subsequent pregnancies [51], and therefore are analogous to the human vaccines discussed below.

Towne Live Attenuated Vaccine

The first human inoculations with a live CMV vaccine, derived from laboratory strain AD169, were reported in 1974 [52]. These preliminary experiments, as well as subsequent studies [53, 54], demonstrated safety and immunogenicity. Issues of efficacy were not addressed, and since then more substantial experience has been generated with the Towne virus. This strain was originally isolated from a congenitally infected infant (named Towne) in 1970 and passaged 125 times in WI-38 human diploid fibroblasts, including 3 clonings [55]. Standard tests for safety and oncogenicity failed to raise concern. The virus exhibits in vitro characteristics different from the wild-type, including greater release of extracellular virions, thermostability, and trypsin resistance (characteristics of high-passage viruses). In addition, it is antigenically related to other human CMV strains.

The first published report of Towne vaccination in adult volunteers appeared in 1975 [56]. Five subjects with preexisting CMV antibody who were inoculated intramuscularly showed no reactions to the vaccine and had no change in antibody titer. Of ten CMV-seronegative volunteers who were vaccinated, seven developed minor localized reactions and all developed measurable antibodies. Seven of nine developed specific IgM, whereas only four of nine developed neutralizing antibodies. None of the vaccinees excreted CMV in the urine. Although local viral replication has been demonstrated at the injection site, the lack of "take" after mucosal inoculation and the absence of virus excretion have been taken as markers of attenuation. By comparison, wild-type virus administered subcutaneously to previously immune individuals caused systemic illness with positive cultures [57]. In 1976, a paper describing an earlier investigation confirmed these findings [58].

It was subsequently demonstrated that CMV-specific lymphocyte responses were induced in seronegative vaccinees [59]. The response was biphasic in some subjects, with decreased responses between 2 and 6 months despite the fact that cell-mediated immunity was not generally depressed. Complement-fixing antibody titers were seen to decrease over a year, whereas immunofluorescent antibodies were persistent. In contrast, data from renal transplant candidates indicate a decline in immunofluorescent antibodies by 1 year [60]. In another study, lymphocyte responsiveness was persistent at 36 and 40 weeks and was comparable to that seen in healthy young adults with prior natural CMV infection [61]. CMV-seronegative renal transplant candidates had positive but generally delayed or impaired cellular and humoral responses to the vaccine, and the induced lymphocyte response was cross-reactive with other CMV strains. Persistence of neutralizing antibody for at least 1 year and consistent but variable cellular responses were also seen in ten vaccinated pediatric nurses [62]. Towne virus is unlikely to be immunosuppressive, since CD4 to CD8 lymphocyte subset ratios do not change after vaccination as they do during natural CMV infection [63]. Towne strain induces a CMV-specific CTL response but does not cause increased circulating interferon, as does wild-type virus administered to seropositive volunteers [57].

A recent study addressed the issue of efficacy by challenging vaccinees with wild-type virus [20]. Whereas wild-type virus induced infection and disease in CMV-seronegative volunteers at a dose of 10 plaque-forming units or less, Towne vaccinees and naturally seropositive individuals resisted such low dose challenges. Interestingly, larger challenges resulted in disease in some individuals with either natural infection or vaccination, illustrating that natural immunity itself is incomplete.

The first trials to prevent CMV disease in a specific target population have been carried out in renal transplant candidates. Early open trials demonstrated that Towne virus was immunogenic in these patients, did not produce significant morbidity, and failed to reactive with subsequent peritransplant immunosuppression [64]. A controlled trial involving 400 renal transplant candidates was subsequently reported from Minneapolis in 1985 [65]. The major findings involved 35 CMV-seronegative subjects who received seropositive kidneys and were followed for at least 6 months. The incidence of infection (76%–86%) and clinically defined CMV disease (38%–43%) was the same for vaccine- and placebo-treated subjects. However, severe or lethal disease occurred in two of eight vaccinees as compared to five of six placebo recipients, and one of the vaccinees sustained severe disease only after a second solid organ transplant.

The question of efficacy has now been addressed in a 10-year-long, randomized, double-blind, placebo-controlled trial [66]. Renal transplant candidates in the Philadelphia area (473) were enrolled in the study. The final analysis involved 237 patients who had received vaccine or placebo and who had received a transplant from a donor of known serostatus. The vaccine appeared to be safe and well tolerated: 75% of CMV-seronegative vaccinees developed minor local reactions to the injection. Patients were stratified into four groups based on the serological status of the recipient and donor. Within each group, vaccinees and placebo-treated subjects had equally high rates of CMV infection. However, the severity of CMV disease, as measured by a clinical scoring system, was lower for vaccinees. Vaccine effect was most apparent in the group of seronegative recipients who received transplanted kidneys from seropositive donors, in whom efficacy in preventing disease of at least moderate severity was estimated to be 85% (Table 2). The vaccine was probably as efficacious as preexisting natural immunity, since the incidence of severe disease in this group of vaccinees (5.5%) was similar to that in the group of placebo recipients who were seropositive at entry into the study and who also received a kidney from a seropositive donor. In addition, cadaveric graft survival was prolonged in seronegative patients who received kidneys from seropositive donors. Neutralizing antibody responses to vaccination were common, and 73% of vaccinees who were not exposed to natural CMV were seropositive an average of 28 months later. Extensive restriction endonuclease analysis of isolates from culture-positive vaccine recipients provided definitive evidence against vaccine strain reactivation [67]. In summary, Towne virus did not protect against

Table 2. Distribution of CMV disease scores among seronegative recipients of kidneys from seropositive donors (from [66])

Disease severity score	Towne vaccine [a] (%)	Placebo [b] (%)
0 (no disease)	61	45
1– 3	8	3
4– 7	25	23
8–11	3	13
≥12 (serious disease)	3	16

[a] $n=36$
[b] $n=31$

Table 3. Towne strain live attenuated cytomegalovirus vaccine

Safety	Does not induce latency No major systemic side effects No immunosuppressive effects No evidence of oncogenicity
Immunogenicity	Elicits neutralizing antibody responses Induces lasting lymphoproliferative responses Induces cytotoxic T-lymphocyte responses
Efficacy	Protects seronegative renal allograft recipients from disease Mimics natural immunity in challenge experiments

infection, but it did prevent severe disease, in analogy to prior natural infection.

Studies are currently underway to determine if Towne vaccine can protect women who are at high risk of infection due to day care center exposure. Of interest, a recent analysis concluded that routine immunization of healthy women aged 15–25 years would be cost-beneficial and effective even if the majority of such women were already immune to CMV [68]. The cumulative experience with Towne vaccine is summarized in Table 3.

Subunit Vaccines

Live viral vaccines provide an amplifying source of antigen and can thereby stimulate strong, lasting immunity. In addition, CTL responses are more likely to be generated when viral antigens are produced within infected cells, rather than exogeneously supplied [69]. Despite this potential for success, the human CMV vaccine studies discussed above have generated considerable controversy based on theoretical concerns regarding the potentials for oncogenicity, induction of latency or chronic disease, and immunosuppression. Therefore, despite the record of success outlined above, current efforts have centered on the development of a noninfectious subunit vaccine that would be immunogenic and protective but carry certain assurance against the above liabilities.

Envelope Glycoproteins

Glycoproteins of the CMV virion envelope are thought to be of prime immunological importance. By analogy with other viral systems, it is probable that these proteins are involved in the initiation of infection. Convalescent human sera readily recognize these glycoproteins, and since they carry epitopes recognized by neutralizing antibodies, they might serve to elicit protective immune responses. Further, the immunogenicity of CMV envelope glycoproteins in experimental animals was directly demonstrated several years ago [70]. Extrapolation from work done with herpes simplex virus (HSV) seems to hold promise for this approach. In this system, passive immunization of animals with antibodies directed against HSV envelope glycoproteins is protective [71], as is active immunization with purified glycoproteins [72]. Estimates of the number of CMV virion glycoproteins and their antigenic relatedness have varied widely. In the last few years, with the application of molecular techniques, CMV glycoproteins have been better characterized. At least three distinct families of envelope glycoproteins have been identified in CMV envelopes [73]; each of these exists as disulfide-linked complexes and each carries neutralizing epitopes as detected by monoclonal antibodies. Two of these glycoproteins, glycoprotein B (gB) and glycoprotein H (gH), exhibit amino acid homology with envelope glycoproteins of other herpesviruses, implying the existence of conserved functional epitopes. Both of these glycoproteins are immunogenic when administered as vaccines. A third glycoprotein, glycoprotein complex II (gcII) [74, 75], bears no homology to other herpesvirus proteins and has not been well studied as an immunogen.

gH was originally immunoprecipitated from CMV-infected cells using the neutralizing monoclonal antibody 1G6 [76]. This protein of molecular mass 86 kDa was subsequently purified by immunoaffinity column chromatography and administered to guinea pigs, where it was found to induce complement-independent neutralizing antibodies [77]. The gene for this glycoprotein was subsequently mapped and cloned into vaccinia virus [78]. Amino acid homology was detected between this glycoprotein and gH of HSV, varicella-zoster virus gpIII, and the Epstein-Barr virus (EBV) BXLF2 gene product, hence its designation as a gH homologue (although some investigators refer to it as glycoprotein complex III (gcIII) [73]). The gH sequence for Towne and AD169 are very similar [79], suggesting that divergence in wild strains may be minimal. gH has recently been found to play a role in the fusion of viral and cellular membranes [80].

Currently, the most promising candidate for inclusion in a subunit vaccine is an abundant disulfide-linked envelope glycoprotein complex which has major components in the range of 130–55 kDa. This complex, first characterized in the early 1980s using monoclonal antibodies, was originally referred to as "gA" [81]. Since then alternative designations, such as "gcI", have been proposed [73]. However, the cloning and sequencing of the gene for this glycoprotein provided a rational basis for its designation as "gB" since it bears homology to gB of HSV [82].

Monoclonal antibodies which recognize gB neutralize laboratory CMV strains as well as clinical isolates [83, 84]. When this protein was immunoaffinity-purified and administered to experimental animals as a vaccine, it induced neutralizing antibody and cellular responses [77, 85]. The predominant neutralizing response was complement-dependent and directed against the mature, fully glycosylated gB protein. However, low levels of complement-independent neutralizing antibodies were also produced, and these antibodies predominate when nonglycosylated, prokaryote-derived gB is used as the immunogen [86]. This suggests that conformational or discontinuous epitopes on gB (which are present when the protein is made in mammalian cells) require antibody and complement to neutralize virus infectivity. Two different recombinant viral vectors expressing gB, vaccinia [82, 86] and adenovirus [87], have been used in animal immunization experiments with the successful generation of neutralizing activity. Of particular note, adenovirus vectors have potential for use in humans given the demonstrated safety and efficacy of live, enterically administered adenovirus vaccines used in the United States military [88, 89]. In addition, this vector has the potential to generate mucosal immune responses which may be important in protection.

gB first appears in infected cells in fully glycosylated forms of 170–130 kDa from which the carboxy terminus of 58–52 kDa is cleaved [90–93]. This fragment, generally referred to as "gp55", is the immunodominant portion of the mature protein; most gB monoclonal antibodies that have been generated bind to gp55 and neutralizing epitopes have been mapped there [90, 94–96]. The amino-terminal cleavage product, referred to as "gp93" by some authors [90] and "gp116" by others [92], remains in association with gp55 in the form of multimeric disulfide-linked complexes [83, 84, 91, 93, 97–99]. gp93/116 is less abundant in virions but it is known to be immunogenic and carries a neutralizing epitope [100].

Using gB partially purified by anion-exchange high-pressure liquid chromatography as the antigen in immunological assays, consistent humoral responses were demonstrated in a small group of CMV-immune individuals [101]. More recently, recombinant-derived antigen has been used to study gB antibody in human sera. Using vaccinia virus recombinant-infected cells as a specific absorbent, 26%–100% of neutralizing activity was removed from specimens from 12 convalescents [102]. Using gB partially purified from cells infected with an adenovirus-gB recombinant, each of 48 serum samples from convalescents were seen to contain specific IgG antibody to gB [103]. Furthermore, quantitative radioimmunoprecipitation showed a strong correlation between gB antibody and neutralizing activity (Fig. 1). When gB antibody was specifically absorbed from 20 serum specimens, neutralizing antibody titer was reduced by a median of 48%. These data suggest that antibodies to gB are a large component of the neutralizing antibody response to CMV after natural infection. It should be mentioned, however, that cellular responses to envelope glycoproteins may be variable and may not correlate with specific antibody levels [101].

The first human inoculations with gB have now been reported [104]. Two naturally CMV-seropositive and three seronegative volunteers were immunized intramuscularly with immunoaffinity purified protein. The immune individuals developed booster responses in neutralizing antibody and lymphocyte proliferation to CMV antigens, and the seronegative volunteers developed neutralizing antibodies and cellular responses as well, although several injections were necessary. Taken together, the above data provide strong support for the potential of gB as a component of a subunit vaccine.

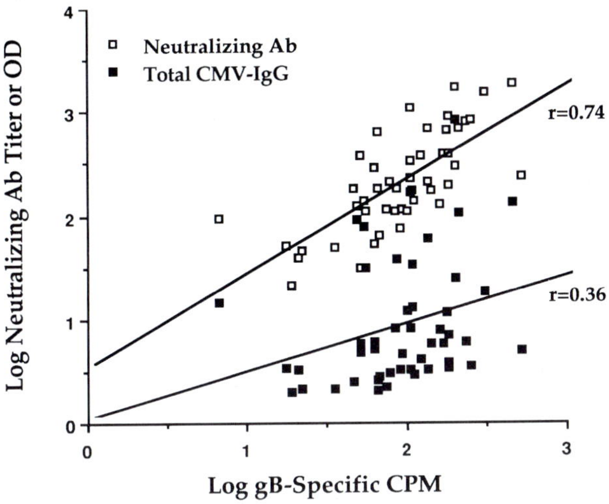

Fig. 1. Correlation between gB antibody (as counts per minute [CPM] in a radioimmunoprecipitation assay) and neutralizing antibody (Ab, as reciprocal titer) or total CMV-specific IgG (as optical density [OD] in an ELISA) in 48 naturally seropositive individuals. The correlation between gB antibody and neutralizing antibody exceeded that between gB antibody and total CMV-specific antibody, indicating that gB antibody was a relatively specific marker for neutralization (from reference 103 with permission [University of Chicago Press]). r = Spearman rank correlation coefficient

Other Structural Proteins

Two structural CMV proteins are highly immunogenic but at the present time their role in protection is not clear. High titer antibodies to a 66-kDa polypeptide, the lower matrix protein, appear very early during primary infection [105]. Since neutralizing antibodies are not apparent until much later [106], it is unlikely that the humoral response to this protein is protective. However, peripheral blood mononuclear cells from immune donors proliferate in response to this antigen as well as they do to whole virus; IL-2 production, IL-2 receptor expression, and interferon production are observed [107]. The in vivo significance of these responses remains to be determined.

Similarly, whereas a phosphorylated protein of 155–150 kDa is one of the most immunogenic polypeptides recognized by human sera [108], few data exist on its role in protection.

Immediate Early Proteins

The MCMV model has provided great insight into the role played by nonstructural proteins in the generation of cell-mediated immunity. Initial reports defined populations of CTLs that specifically recognize MCMV proteins expressed at immediate early (IE) times postinfection [109]; these proteins are regulatory in nature and are expressed prior to DNA replication. It was shown that a high proportion of CTL precursors generated in vivo recognize IE antigens [110]. Subsequent studies have shown that cloned CTLs recognize the 89-kDa IE-1 gene product expressed in cells after gene transfer [111] and that vaccination with a recombinant vaccinia virus expressing this IE protein protects against lethal MCMV challenge [112]. This protection is mediated by T lymphocytes of the CD8-positive, CD4-negative phenotype, although a role for CD4-positive cells has recently been defined [113, 114]. Infection per se is not prevented by IE-specific CTLs, since IE expression cannot take place until infection has already occurred. In addition, protection is incomplete inasmuch as morbidity is seen with high-challenge doses, reminiscent of the incomplete immunity seen in humans after natural infection and vaccination. There appears to be a single epitope on IE-1, amounting to nine amino acids encoded by the fourth exon of the gene, that is sufficient to induce protective immunity [115, 116].

IE gene products may be important in the generation of cellular immunity to human CMV as well. CMV-specific CTLs kill infected cells before viral DNA replication, indicating that they might be able to recognize regulatory viral proteins [117, 118]. In fact, limiting dilution analysis shows a high frequency of CTLs specific for the 72-kDa IE protein in CMV-seropositive individuals [119]. Although CTL responses to IE proteins appear to predominate, other proteins including gB can target infected cells for CTL lysis [119, 120]. In addition, there is recent evidence that IE-1 induces CD4-positive T cell responses in addition to classic CD8-positive CTLs [121]. CTLs from latently infected individuals can also lyse infected cells in the absence of viral gene expression, implicating as targets structural virion proteins that are introduced into cells after penetration [122].

In summary, both live attenuated whole virus and inert viral subunits are being considered in the development of a CMV vaccine. The rationale for vaccine immunoprophylaxis against CMV disease, largely theoretical until recently, has been greatly advanced by the demonstration of clinical efficacy using the Towne strain in one group of susceptible individuals. However, some safety issues still need to be addressed, and other populations at risk for CMV infection need to be examined. Subunit vaccines are probably safe, but there is uncertainty regarding efficacy. Optimal vectors for delivering these subunits will also need to be developed. Ultimately, vaccines may need to be more immunogenic than natural infection in order to be fully protective.

References

1. Yow MD (1989) Congenital cytomegalovirus disease: a NOW problem. J Infect Dis 159:163–167
2. Jacobson MA, Mills J (1988) Serious cytomegalovirus disease in the acquired immunodeficiency syndrome (AIDS): clinical findings, diagnosis and treatment. Ann Intern Med 180:585–594

3. Glenn J (1981) Cytomegalovirus infections following renal transplantation. Rev Infect Dis 3:1154–1178
4. Meyers JD (1984) Cytomegalovirus infection following marrow transplantation: risk, treatment, and prevention. Birth Defects 20:101–117
5. Davis CL (1990) The prevention of cytomegalovirus disease in renal transplantation. Am J Kidney Dis 16:175–188
6. Editorial (1989) Screening for congenital CMV. Lancet 2:599–600
7. Alford CA, Stagno S, Pass RF, Britt WJ (1990) Congenital and perinatal cytomegalovirus infections. Rev Infect Dis 12:S745–S753
8. Ahlfors K, Harris S, Ivarsson S, Svanberg L (1981) Secondary maternal cytomegalovirus infection causing symtomatic congenital infection. N Engl J Med 305:284
9. Rutter D, Griffiths P, Trompeter RS (1985) Cytomegalic inclusion disease after recurrent maternal infection. Lancet 2:1182
10. Stagno S, Pass RF, Dworsky ME et al. (1982) Congenital cytomegalovirus infection: the relative importance of primary and recurrent maternal infection. N Engl J Med 306:945–949
11. Stagno S, Pass RF, Cloud G et al. (1986) Primary cytomegalovirus infection in pregnancy: incidence, transmission to fetus, and clinical outcome. JAMA 256:1904–1908
12. Pass RF, Little EA, Stagno S et al. (1987) Young children as a probable source of maternal and congenital infection. N Engl J Med 316:1366–1370
13. White NH, Yow MD, Demmler GJ et al. (1989) Prevalence of cytomegalovirus antibody in subjects between the ages of 6 and 22 years. J Infect Dis 159:1013–1017
14. Bart KJ, Orenstein WA, Preblud SR, Hinman AR (1985) Universal immunization to interrupt rubella. Rev Infect Dis 7:S177–S184
15. Chou S (1986) Acquisition of donor strains of cytomegalovirus by renal-transplant recipients. N Engl J Med 314:1418–1423
16. Chandler SH, Handsfield HH, McDougall JK (1987) Isolation of multiple strains of cytomegalovirus from women attending a clinic for sexually transmitted diseases. J Infect Dis 155:655–660
17. Chou S (1987) Cytomegalovirus infection and reinfection transmitted by heart transplantation. J Infect Dis 155:1054–1056
18. Grundy JE, Lui SF, Super M et al. (1988) Symptomatic cytomegalovirus infection in seropositive kidney recipients: reinfection with donor virus rather than reactivation of recipient virus. Lancet 2:132–135
19. Collier AC, Chandler SH, Handsfield HH et al. (1989) Identification of multiple strains of cytomegalovirus in homosexual men. J Infect Dis 159:123–126
20. Plotkin SA, Starr SE, Friedman HM et al. (1989) Protective effects of Towne cytomegalovirus vaccine against low-passage cytomegalovirus administered as a challenge. J Infect Dis 159:860–865
21. Ho M (1984) Immunology of cytomegalovirus. Immunosuppressive effects during infections. Birth Defects 20:131–147
22. Rook AH (1988) Interactions of cytomegalovirus with the human immune system. Rev Infect Dis 10:S460–S467
23. Starr SE, Dalton B, Garrabrant T et al. (1980) Lymphocyte blastogenesis and interferon production in adult human leukocyte cultures stimulated with cytomegalovirus antigens. Infect Immun 30:17–22
24. Quinnan GV, Burns WH, Kirmani N et al. (1984) HLA-restricted cytotoxic T lymphocytes are an early immune response and important defense mechanism in cytomegalovirus infections. Rev Infect Dis 6:156–163
25. Rinaldo CR Jr, Ho M, Hamoudi WH et al. (1983) Lymphocyte subsets and natural killer cell responses during cytomegalovirus mononucleosis. Infect Immun 40:472–477
26. Osborn JE (1981) Cytomegalovirus: pathogenicity, immunology, and vaccine initiatives. J Infect Dis 143:618–630
27. Middledorp JM, Jongsma J, The TH (1986) Killing of human cytomegalovirus-infected fibroblasts by antiviral antibody and complement. J Infect Dis 153:48–55
28. Shanley JD, Jordan MC, Stevens JG (1981) Modification by adoptive humoral immunity of murine cytomegalovirus infection. J Infect Dis 143:231–237

29. Snydman DR, Werner BG, Heinze-Lacey B et al. (1987) Use of cytomegalovirus immune globulin to prevent cytomegalovirus disease in renal-transplant recipients. N Engl J Med 317:1049–1054
30. Yeager AS, Grumet FC, Hafleigh EG et al. (1981) Prevention of transfusion-acquired cytomegalovirus infections in newborn infants. J Pediatr 98:281–287
31. Griffiths PD, Baboonian C (1984) A prospective study of primary cytomegalovirus infection during pregnancy: final report. Br J Obstet Gynaecol 91:307–315
32. Yow MD, Williamson DW, Leeds LJ et al. (1988) Epidemiologic characteristics of cytomegalovirus infection in mothers and their infants. Am J Obstet Gynecol 158:1189–1195
33. Alford CA, Hayes K, Britt W (1988) Primary cytomegalovirus infection in pregnancy: comparison of antibody responses to virus-encoded proteins between women with and without intrauterine infection. J Infect Dis 158:917–924
34. Britt WJ, Vugler LG (1990) Antiviral antibody responses in mothers and their newborn infants with clinical and subclinical congenital cytomegalovirus infections. J Infect Dis 161:214–219
35. Stern H, Hannington G, Booth J, Moncrieff D (1986) An early marker of fetal infection after primary cytomegalovirus infection in pregnancy. Br Med J 292:718–720
36. Chou S (1989) Reactivation and recombination of multiple cytomegalovirus strains from individual organ donors. J Infect Dis 160:11–15
37. Smiley ML, Wlodaver CG, Grossman RA et al. (1985) The role of pretransplant immunity in protection from cytomegalovirus disease following renal transplantation. Transplantation 40:157–161
38. Hudson JB (1979) The murine cytomegalovirus as a model for the study of viral pathogenesis and persistent infections: brief review. Arch Virol 62:1–29
39. Johnson KP (1969) Mouse cytomegalovirus: placental infection. J Infect Dis 120:445–450
40. Osborn JE, Walker DL (1970) Virulence and attenuation of murine cytomegalovirus. Infect Immun 3:228–236
41. Minamishima Y, Eizuru Y, Yoshida A, Fukunishi R (1978) Murine model for immunoprophylaxis of cytomegalovirus infection. I. Efficacy of immunization. Microbiol Immunol 22:693–700
42. Howard RJ, Balfour HH Jr (1977) Prevention of morbidity and mortality of wild murine cytomegalovirus by vaccination with attenuated cytomegalovirus. Proc Soc Exp Biol Med 156:365–368
43. Chong KT, Mims CA (1981) Murine cytomegalovirus particle types in relation to sources of virus and pathogenicity. J Gen Virol 57:415–419
44. Ravindranath RMH, Graves MC (1990) Attenuated murine cytomegalovirus binds to N-acetylglucosamine, and shift to virulence may involve recognition of sialic acids. J Virol 64:5430–5440
45. Chantler JK, Misra V, Hudson JB (1979) Vertical transmission of murine cytomegalovirus. J Gen Virol 42:621–625
46. Jordan MC (1980) Adverse effects of cytomegalovirus vaccination in mice. J Clin Invest 65:798–803
47. Bia FJ, Griffith BP, Fong CKY, Hsiung GD (1983) Cytomegalovirus infections in the guinea pig. Experimental models for human disease. Rev Infect Dis 5:177–195
48. Kumar ML, Nankervis GA (1978) Experimental congenital infection with cytomegalovirus. A guinea pig model. J Infect Dis 138:650–654
49. Harrison CJ, Meyers MG (1990) Relation of maternal CMV viremia and antibody response to the rate of congenital infection and intrauterine growth retardation. J Med Virol 31:222–228
50. Bia FJ, Griffith BP, Tarsio M, Hsiung GD (1980) Vaccination for the prevention of maternal and fetal infection with guinea pig cytomegalovirus. J Infect Dis 142:732–738
51. Bia FJ, Miller SA, Lucia HL et al. (1984) Vaccination against transplacental cytomegalovirus transmission: vaccine reactivation and efficacy in guinea pigs. J Infect Dis 149:355–362

52. Elek SD, Stern H (1974) Development of a vaccine against mental retardation caused by cytomegalovirus infection in utero. Lancet 1:1–4
53. Neff BJ, Weibel RE, Buynak EB et al. (1979) Clinical and laboratory studies of live cytomegalovirus vaccine AD-169. Proc Soc Exp Biol Med 160:32–37
54. Stern H (1984) Live cytomegalovirus vaccination of healthy volunteers: eight-year followup studies. Birth Defects 20:263–269
55. Plotkin SA, Furukawa T, Zygraich N, Huygelen C (1975) Candidate cytomegalovirus strain for human vaccination. Infect Immun 12:521–527
56. Just M, Buergin-Wolff A, Emoedi G, Hernandez R (1975) Immunization trials with live attenuated cytomegalovirus Towne-125. Infection 3:111–114
57. Quinnan GV, Delery M, Rook AH et al. (1984) Comparative virulence and immunogenicity of the Towne strain and a nonattenuated strain of cytomegalovirus. Ann Intern Med 101:478–483
58. Plotkin SA, Farquhar J, Hornberger E (1976) Clinical trials of immunization with the Towne 125 strain of human cytomegalovirus. J Infect Dis 134:470–475
59. Gehrz RC, Christianson WR, Linner KM et al. (1980) Cytomegalovirus vaccine: specific humoral and cellular immune responses in human volunteers. Arch Intern Med 140:936–939
60. Sachs GW, Simmons RL, Balfour HH (1984) Cytomegalovirus vaccine: persistence of humoral immunity following immunization of renal transplant candidates. Vaccine 2:215–218
61. Starr SE, Glazer JP, Friedman HM et al. (1981) Specific cellular and humoral immunity after immunization with live Towne strain cytomegalovirus vaccine. J Infect Dis 143:585–589
62. Fleisher GR, Starr SE, Friedman HM, Plotkin SA (1982) Vaccination of pediatric nurses with live attenuated cytomegalovirus. Am J Dis Child 136:294–296
63. Carney WP, Hirsch MS, Iacoviello VR et al. (1983) T-lymphocyte subsets and proliferative responses following immunization with cytomegalovirus vaccine. J Infect Dis 147:958
64. Glazer JP, Friedman HM, Grossman RA et al. (1979) Live cytomegalovirus vaccination of renal transplant candidates. A preliminary trial. Ann Intern Med 91:676–683
65. Balfour HH Jr, Welo PK, Sachs GW (1985) Cytomegalovirus vaccine trial in 400 renal transplant candidates. Transplant Proc 17:81–83
66. Plotkin SA, Starr SE, Friedman HM et al. (1991) Effect of Towne live virus vaccine on cytomegalovirus disease after renal transplant. A controlled trial. Ann Intern Med 114:525–531
67. Plotkin SA, Huang E-S (1985) Cytomegalovirus vaccine virus (Towne strain) does not induce latency. J Infect Dis 152:395–397
68. Porath A, McNutt RA, Smiley LM, Weigle KA (1990) Effectiveness and cost benefit of a proposed live cytomegalovirus vaccine in the prevention of congenital disease. Rev Infect Dis 12:31–40
69. Ada GL (1990) The immunological principles of vaccination. Lancet 1:523–526
70. Furukawa T, Gonczol E, Starr S et al. (1984) HCMV envelope antigens induce both humoral and cellular immunity in guinea pigs. Proc Soc Exp Biol Med 175:243–250
71. Balachandran N, Bacchetti S, Rawls WE (1982) Protection against lethal challenge of BALB/c mice by passive transfer of monoclonal antibodies to five glycoproteins of herpes simplex virus type 2. Infect Immun 37:1132–1137
72. Berman PW, Gregory T, Crase D, Lasky LA (1985) Protection from genital herpes simplex virus type 2 infection by vaccination with cloned type 1 glycoprotein D. Science 227:1490–1492
73. Gretch DR, Kari B, Rasmussen L et al. (1988) Identification and characterization of three distinct families of glycoprotein complexes in the envelopes of human cytomegalovirus. J Virol 62:875–881
74. Kari B, Lussenhop N, Goertz R et al. (1986) Characterization of monoclonal antibodies reactive to several biochemically distinct human cytomegalovirus glycoprotein complexes. J Virol 60:345–352

75. Gretch DR, Kari B, Grehrz RC, Stinski MF (1988) A multigene family encodes the human cytomegalovirus glycoprotein complex gcII (gp 47–52 complex). J Virol 62:1956–1962
76. Rasmussen LE, Nelson RM, Kelsall DC, Merigan TC (1984) Murine monoclonal antibody to a single protein neutralizes the infectivity of human cytomegalovirus. Proc Natl Acad Sci USA 81:876–880
77. Rasmussen L, Mullenax J, Nelson M, Merigan TC (1985) Human cytomegalovirus polypeptides stimulate neutralizing antibody in vivo. Virology 145:186–190
78. Cranage MP, Smith GL, Bell SE et al. (1988) Identification and expression of a human cytomegalovirus glycoprotein with homology to the Epstein-Barr virus BXLF2 product, varicella-zoster virus gpIII, and herpes simplex virus type 1 glycoprotein H. J Virol 62:1416–1422
79. Pachl C, Probert WS, Hermsen KM et al. (1989) The human cytomegalovirus strain Towne glycoprotein H gene encodes glycoprotein p86. Virology 169:418–426
80. Keay S, Baldwin B (1991) Anti-idiotype antibodies that mimic gp86 of human cytomegalovirus inhibit viral fusion but not attachment. J Virol 65:5124–5128
81. Pereira L, Hoffman M, Tatsuno M, Dondero D (1984) Polymorphism of human cytomegalovirus glycoproteins characterized by monoclonal antibodies. Virology 139:73–86
82. Cranage MP, Kouzarides T, Bankier AT et al. (1986) Identification of the human cytomegalovirus glycoprotein B gene and induction of neutralizing antibodies via its expression in recombinant vaccinia virus. EMBO J 5:3057–3063
83. Britt WJ (1984) Neutralizing antibodies detect a disulfide-linked glycoprotein complex within the envelope of human cytomegalovirus. Virology 135:369–378
84. Rasmussen L, Mullenax J, Nelson R, Merigan TC (1985) Viral polypeptides detected by a complement-dependent neutralizing murine antibody to human cytomegalovirus. J Virol 55:274–280
85. Gonczol E, Hudecz F, Ianocone J et al. (1986) Immune responses to isolated human cytomegalovirus envelope proteins. J Virol 58:661–664
86. Britt WJ, Vugler L, Stephens EB (1988) Induction of complement-dependent and -independent neutralizing antibodies by recombinant-derived human cytomegalovirus gp55-116 (gB). J Virol 62:3309–3318
87. Marshall GS, Ricciardi RP, Rando RF et al. (1990) An adenovirus recombinant that expresses the human cytomegalovirus major envelope glycoprotein and induces neutralizing antibodies. J Infect Dis 162:1177–1181
88. Top FH Jr, Grossman RA, Bartelloni PJ et al. (1971) Immunization with live types 7 and 4 adenovirus vaccines. I. Safety, infectivity, and potency of adenovirus type 7 vaccine in humans. J Infect Dis 124:148–154
89. Top FH Jr, Buescher EL, Bancroft WH, Russell PK (1971) Immunization with live types 7 and 4 adenovirus vaccines. II. Antibody response and protective effect against acute respiratory disease due to adenovirus type 7. J Infect Dis 124:155–160
90. Spaete RR, Thayer RM, Probert WS et al. (1988) Human cytomegalovirus strain Towne glycoprotein B is processed by proteolytic cleavage. Virology 167:207–225
91. Britt WJ, Auger D (1986) Synthesis and processing of the envelope gp55-116 complex of human cytomegalovirus. J Virol 58:185–191
92. Britt WJ, Vugler LG (1989) Processing of the gp55-116 envelope glycoprotein complex of human cytomegalovirus. J Virol 63:403–410
93. Spaete RR, Saxena A, Scott PI et al. (1990) Sequence requirements for proteolytic processing of glycoprotein B of human cytomegalovirus strain Towne. J Virol 64:2922–2931
94. Lussenhop NO, Goertz R, Wabuke-Bunoti M et al. (1988) Epitope analysis of human cytomegalovirus glycoprotein complexes using murine monoclonal antibodies. Virology 164:362–372
95. Utz U, Britt W, Vugler L, Mach M (1989) Identification of a neutralizing epitope on glycoprotein gp58 of human cytomegalovirus. J Virol 63:1995–2001

96. Kneiss N, Mach M, Fay J, Britt WJ (1991) Distribution of linear antigenic sites on glycoprotein gp55 of human cytomegalovirus. J Virol 65:138–146
97. Law KM, Wilton-Smith P, Farrar GH (1985) A murine monoclonal antibody recognizing a single glycoprotein within a human cytomegalovirus virion envelope glycoprotein complex. J Med Virol 17:255–266
98. Farrar GH, Greenaway PJ (1986) Characterization of glycoprotein complexes present in human cytomegalovirus envelopes. J Gen Virol 67:1469–1473
99. Gretch DR, Gehrz RC, Stinski MF (1988) Characterization of a human cytomegalovirus glycoprotein complex (gcI). J Gen Virol 69:1205–1215
100. Meyer H, Masuho Y, Mach M (1990) The gp116 of the gp58/116 complex of human cytomegalovirus represents the amino-terminal part of the precursor molecule and contains a neutralizing epitope. J Gen Virol 71:2443–2450
101. Liu Y-N, Kari B, Gehrz RC (1988) Human immune responses to major human cytomegalovirus glycoprotein complexes. J Virol 62:1066–1070
102. Britt WJ, Vugler L, Butfiloski EJ, Stephens EB (1990) Cell surface expression of human cytomegalovirus (HCMV) gp55-116 (gB): use of HCMV-recombinant vaccinia virus-infected cells in analysis of the human neutralizing antibody response. J Virol 64:1079–1085
103. Marshall GS, Rabalais GP, Stout GG, Waldeyer SL (1992) Antibodies to recombinant-derived glycoprotein B after natural human cytomegalovirus infection correlate with neutralizing activity. J Infect Dis 165:381–384
104. Gonczol E, Ianacone J, Ho W et al. (1990) Isolated gA/gB glycoprotein complex of human cytomegalovirus envelope induces humoral and cellular immune-response in human volunteers. Vaccine 8:130–136
105. Landini MP, Rossier E, Schmitz H (1988) Antibodies to human cytomegalovirus structural polypeptides during primary infection. J Virol Methods 22:309–317
106. Spencer ES, Andersen HK (1972) The development of immunofluorescent antibodies as compared with complement-fixing and virus neutralizing antibodies in human cytomegalovirus infection. Scand J Infect Dis 4:109–112
107. Forman SJ, Zaia JA, Clark BR et al. (1985) A 64000 dalton matrix protein of human cytomegalovirus induces in vitro immune responses similar to those of whole viral antigen. J Immunol 134:3391–3395
108. Landini MP, Michelson S (1988) Human cytomegalovirus proteins. Prog Med Virol 35:152–185
109. Reddehase MJ, Keil GM, Koszinowski UH (1984) The cytolytic T lymphocyte response to the murine cytomegalovirus. II. Detection of virus replication stage-specific antigens by separate populations of in-vivo active cytolytic T lymphocyte precursors. Eur J Immunol 14:56–61
110. Reddehase MJ, Koszinowski UH (1984) Significance of herpes-virus immediate early gene expression in cellular immunity to cytomegalovirus infection. Nature 312:369–371
111. Koszinowski UH, Reddehase MJ, Keil GM, Schickedanz J (1987) Host immune response to cytomegalovirus. Products of transfected viral immediate-early genes are recognized by cloned cytolytic T lymphocytes. J Virol 61:2054–2058
112. Jonjic S, del Val M, Keil GM et al. (1988) A nonstructural viral protein expressed by a recombinant vaccina virus protects against lethal cytomegalovirus infection. J Virol 62:1653–1658
113. Reddehase MJ, Mutter W, Munch K et al. (1987) CD8-positive T lymphocytes specific for murine cytomegalovirus immediate-early antigens mediate protective immunity. J Virol 61:3102–3108
114. Jonjic S, Pavic I, Lucin P et al. (1990) Efficacious control of cytomegalovirus infection after long-term depletion of CD8+ T lymphocytes. J Virol 64:5457–5464
115. Del Val M, Volkmer H, Rothbard JB et al. (1988) Molecular basis for cytolytic T-lymphocyte recognition of the murine cytomegalovirus immediate-early protein pp89. J Virol 62:3965–3972

116. Del Val M, Schlicht H-J, Volkmer H et al. (1991) Protection against lethal cytomegalovirus infection by a recombinant vaccine containing a single nonameric T-cell epitope. J Virol 65:3641–3646
117. Borysiewicz LK, Morris S, Page JD, Sissons JGP (1983) Human cytomegalovirus specific cytotoxic T cells. Requirements for in vitro generation and specificity. Eur J Immunol 13:804–809
118. Borysiewicz LK, Graham S, Hickling JK, Sissons JGP (1988) Precursor frequency and stage specificity of human cytomegalovirus specific cytotoxic T cells. Eur J Immunol 18:269–275
119. Borysiewicz LK, Hickling JK, Graham S et al. (1988) Human cytomegalovirus-specific cytotoxic T cells. Relative frequency of stage-specific CTL recognizing the 72kd immediate early protein and glycoprotein B expressed by recombinant vaccinia viruses. J Exp Med 168:919–931
120. Liu Y-NC, Klaus A, Kari B et al. (1991) The N-terminal 513 amino acids of the envelope glycoprotein gB of human cytomegalovirus stimulates both B- and T-cell immune responses in humans. J Virol 65:1644–1648
121. Alp NJ, Allport TD, van Zanten J et al. (1991) Fine specificity of cellular immune responses in humans to human cytomegalovirus immediate-early 1 protein. J Virol 65:4812–4820
122. Riddell SR, Rabin M, Geballe AP et al. (1991) Class I MHC-restricted cytotoxic T lymphocyte recognition of cells infected with human cytomegalovirus does not require endogenous viral gene expression. J Immunol 146:2795–2804

Section IV Molecular Aspects of Human Cytomegalovirus

Chapter 16 Molecular Biology of Human Cytomegalovirus

Wade Gibson

Summary

This article presents a brief review of the molecular biology of human cytomegalovirus, with emphasis on the structure of the virion and events associated with its assembly.

Introduction

It has been over 35 years since the first reports appeared describing the isolation and characterization of cytomegalovirus (CMV, human herpes virus 5) [109, 117, 136]. During this period it has become apparent that there are many similarities at the molecular level between CMV and herpes simplex virus (HSV), the herpes group prototype (for review see [108]), but also many differences. Because these molecular differences are likely to underlie the different biological manifestations of these viruses, they are of particular interest and relevance as knowledge at the molecular level becomes applied at the clinical level.

Several comprehensive reviews of CMV molecular biology [51, 118, 129], transcription [88, 89, 123, 125], and protein coding [22, 78] have been published recently, and the reader is referred to them for a more thorough treatment of specific topics than will be presented here. The objective of this chapter is to consider aspects of CMV molecular biology that have not been as thoroughly described elsewhere, in particular, molecular events associated with virus assembly.

The Virion: General Considerations

The virion of CMV (Fig. 1) is similar in structure and composition to that of HSV. A major difference between the two is that the DNA genome of CMV

Virology Laboratories, Johns Hopkins School of Medicine, 725 North Wolfe Street, Baltimore, MD 21205, USA

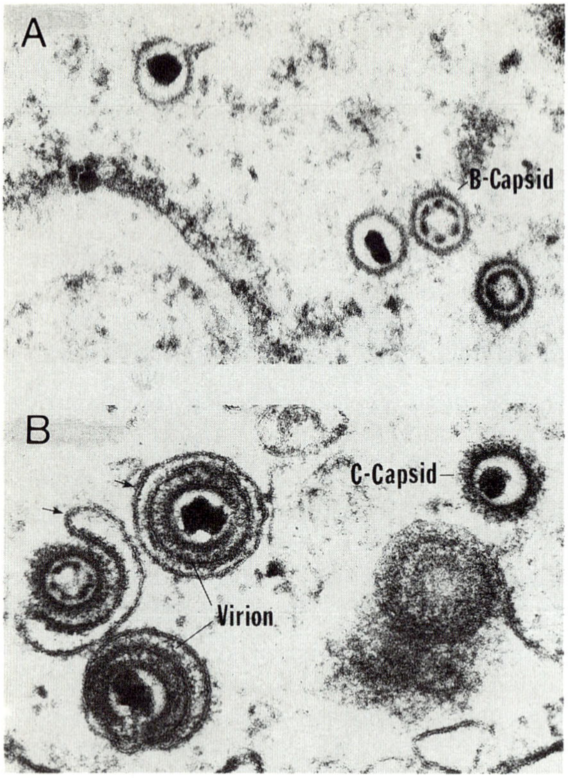

Fig. 1 A, B. Intracellular cytomegalovirus particles. **A** Nucleus contains capsids approximately 100 nm in diameter, some with heavily stained centers and others with a beaded-looking interior (*B-capsid*; also see Fig. 6 A, B). **B** Cytoplasm contains four types of particles: (1) nonenveloped capsids with heavily stained centers and a thick fibrillar exterior coating (*C-capsid*), frequently appearing to become enveloped at vesicle or tubule membranes (*arrows*), e.g., *far-left particle*, (2) virions contained within tubules or vesicles and therefore appearing to have a double membrane; (3) noninfectious enveloped particles with the general appearance of virions, but lacking DNA and having an interior more like that of B-capsids (e.g. *far-left particle*); and (4) dense bodies having the appearance of enveloped solid spheres approximately 200–400 nm in diameter (not shown)

is nearly 50% larger than that of HSV [30, 34, 36, 47, 69, 75, 77, 130]. Nevertheless, it is accommodated within a typical herpesvirus 100-nm icosahedral capsid (Fig. 1 A; B-capsid) composed of 162 capsomers [64, 116]. The CMV capsid appears to be lacking a counterpart for VP19 [38], one of the abundant HSV capsid proteins [43, 122], although the genome contains a positionally similar, smaller open reading frame (ORF, CMV UL46) [22]. The evolutionary or maturational loss of this protein may reflect the need for added space or flexibility in the capsid to contain the larger DNA molecule. It may also account for the reduced stability of the CMV nucleocapsid, as compared with that of HSV [38]. The capsid, which is surrounded by a tegument layer that can be visualized as a fibrillar coating on cytoplasmic nucleocapsids (e.g., C-capsids, Fig. 1 B) [38], contains only three abundant protein constituents [40, 61]. The mature particle is enveloped by a trilaminate membrane which contains most, if not all, of the virion glycoproteins [42, 70, 111, 128]. The high degree of size and charge heterogeneity that typifies many of the human CMV (HCMV) glycoproteins [9, 40] is not characteristic of HSV envelope glycoproteins. In addition to these DNA and protein constituents, purified extracellular virions of CMV contain: the polyamines spermine and spermidine [45]; the phospholipids phosphatidylcholine, phosphatidylethanolamine, phosphatidylserine, and phosphatidylinositol [106]; and several enzymatic activities, including protein kinase [83, 106, 119], deoxyribonuclease (DNase) [104], DNA polymerase [83], and topoisomerase II [13]. The location and requirement for these molecules in the virion is unknown.

DNA Structure and Replication

The virion DNA is a $\approx 150 \times 10^6$ M_r, linear, double-stranded molecule [30, 34, 36, 47, 69, 75, 77, 130]. It is composed of a long (L) and short (S) segment each bounded by terminal repeat elements [34, 77] that permit L and S to invert during replication and form four sequence isomers [107]. The complete nucleotide sequence of strain AD169 has been determined by Chee et al. [22], and the reader is referred to their recent review for a comprehensive description of sequence analyses. The nucleotide sequence of strain AD169 showed a G+C content of 57.2%, a length of 229 354 bp, and approximately 200 ORFs [22].

An interesting feature of the HCMV genome is that it contains a comparatively large number of related genes, or gene families, which tend to be clustered as homologous blocks of ORFs [22]. Nine such families have been identified, and most of them encode known (e.g., RL11 and US6 families) [21, 49] or predicted (e.g. US2 and GCR families) [23, 137] glycoproteins. Together these gene families (59 728 bp) represent about 26% of the AD169 nucleotide sequence and may in part account for the comparatively large size of the CMV genome. It is also interesting that the HCMV genome contains homologues of at least three cellular genes: class I major histocompatibility (MHC) antigens (CMV UL18), T-cell receptor gamma chains (TCRγ; CMV UL20), and G-protein-coupled receptors (GCR; CMV UL33 and US27) [28]. The fact that all of these are cell surface receptors raises interesting questions about the mechanism and chronology of their "hijacking" from the cell, and their function, if any, in the virus's life cycle. Though the protein products of the three HCMV GCR homologue genes have not yet been identified, it has been demonstrated that all are transcribed [133]. The US27 and UL33 genes are represented only as bigenic messenger RNAs (mRNAs) as a consequence of transcriptional readout of the US28 and UL34 genes, respectively, to the first downstream polyadenylation signals (Fig. 2) [22, 133]. The US28 and UL34 genes are also transcribed as monogenic mRNAs, presumably to enable their translation from otherwise international ATG start sites [73, 133].

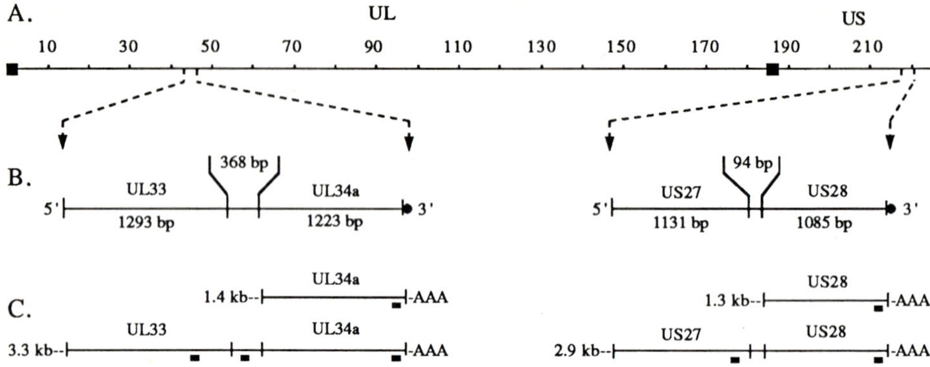

Fig. 2A–C. Human cytomegalovirus G-protein-coupled receptor (HCMV GCR) gene transcription. The genomic location (**A**) and genetic organization (**B**) of the three HCMV GCR genes (US27 and 28; UL33) is shown. Polyadenylation signals are indicated by *filled circles*. Transcripts from these genes (**C**) were identified by Northern blot assays by using ^{32}P-labeled antisense oligodeoxyribonucleotide probes. (From [133])

Synthesis of HCMV DNA initiates from a single origin during lytic replication (*ori*-Lyt), and this has been localized to a 3- to 4-kb region near the center of the unique L segment (i.e., AD169, *Eco*RI-V; Towne *Hin*dIII-A) by characterizing origin-proximal fragments made in the presence of ganciclovir (9-[1,3-Dihydroxy-2-propoxy)methyl]guanine) (DHPG) [55], an inhibitor of viral DNA synthesis, and by DNA transfection [5]. DNA synthesis appears to proceed bidirectionally from *ori*-Lyt and the nucleotide sequence of this region [22] has several interesting features (Fig. 3) [55]. First, *ori*-Lyt lies immediately upstream of the promoter for the early, single-strand DNA-binding protein, DB140 (CMV UL57). And second, there is a 2.5-kb region upstream which bears no homology to other described viral DNA replication origins. It contains duplications, inversions, consensus binding sequences for the cyclic AMP (cAMP) response element and other transcription factors, and a set of 23 copies of a consensus element AAAACACCGT that is conversed at the equivalent locus in simian CMV (SCMV) [5, 55]. Although the sequence of HCMV *ori*-Lyt differs from other described viral origins, its location adjacent to the 5′ end of the gene encoding the early single-strand DNA-binding protein is like that of *ori*-L, one of three duplicated origin sequences present in the HSV genome [108].

Cell Recognition and Early Events

Three virion proteins have been implicated in mediating virus attachment to host cells. The first of these is β_2-microglobulin, a host protein that is bound to the tegument [79] or to the surface of virions, and could promote interaction of the virus with cell surface MHC proteins [53, 54, 86]. A second protein that

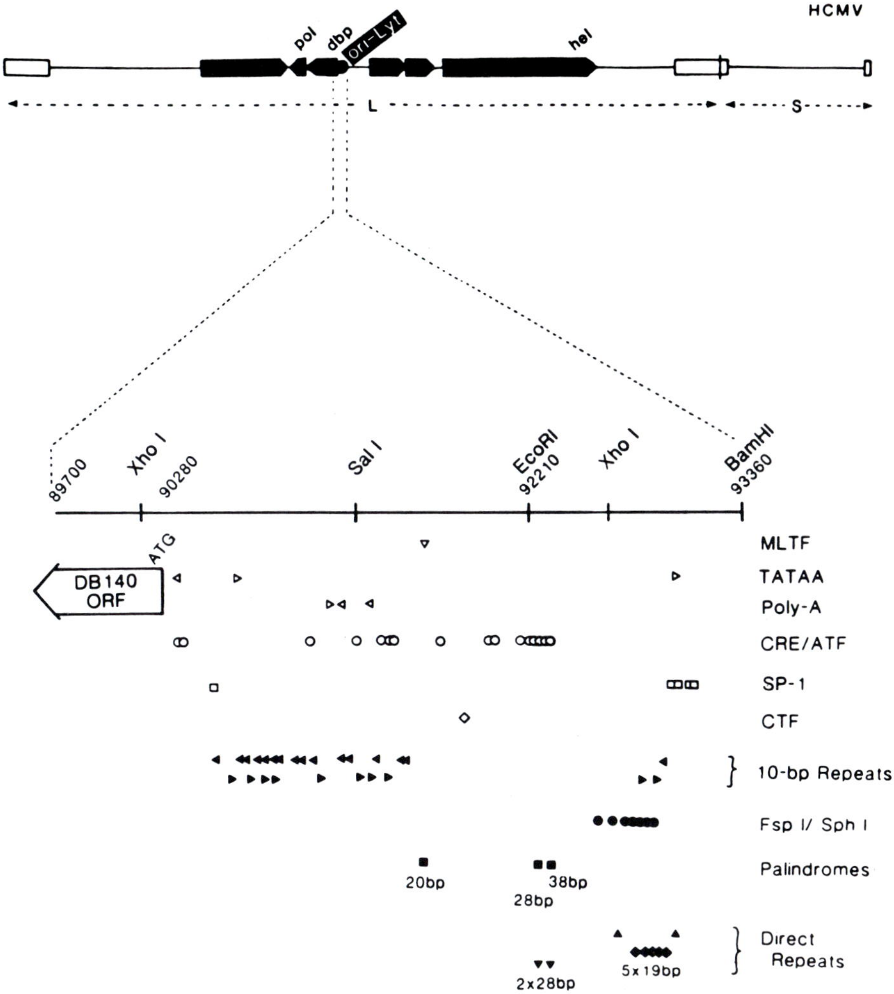

Fig. 3. Organization of human cytomegalovirus (HCMV) *ori*-Lyt. *Top* shows location of the origin of DNA synthesis during lytic replication of HCMV. Nearby genes include the DNA-binding protein (*dbp*) DB140, DNA polymerase (*pol*), and helicase (*hel*). Structural features of the 3660-bp region are indicated at bottom. *CRE/ATF,* cAMP response element binding site; *CTF,* CAAT transcription factor binding site; *MLTF,* adenovirus major late transcription factor binding site; *ORF,* open reading frame; *SP-I,* consensus SP-I factor binding site. (From [55])

may take part in virus entry is glycoprotein H (gH; CMV UL75). Anti-idiotype antibodies to CMV gH interfere with virus binding and react with a 90-kDa cellular protein, suggesting an involvement of both in the binding process [67, 102]. Glycoprotein B (gB; CMV UL55) also appears to participate in the virus–cell interaction, since purified gB binds to a 30-kDa host cell protein [102] corresponding in size to a previously identified CMV receptor [2, 132].

The specific involvement of each of these proteins in CMV binding and entry, and whether different host cells present different receptors, remains to be established.

Once inside the cell the viral DNA becomes transcriptionally active and a temporal pattern of gene expression ensues [129], which is generally similar to that of HSV [108]. An initial class of RNAs is synthesized from the input DNA. These are referred to as immediate-early (IE) or α transcripts and are operationally defined as being made in the absence of viral protein synthesis [58, 59]. The most abundant IE transcripts arise from a region between 0.732 and 0.751 map units, which contains ORF UL22 and exons UL123EX2-4 [22, 129]. These transcripts are related to each other by alternate splicing patterns, and encode IE1 and multiple forms of IE2 [88, 123, 125, 129]. The comparative strength of the CMV promoter/regulatory region is presumed to be due to its high content of consensus binding sequences for host cell transcription factors such as nuclear factor 1, CAAT binding protein, and SP1, and the large number of repeat sequences which contain cyclic-AMP response elements and which may interact with additional DNA binding proteins [88, 123, 125, 129]. The second class of transcripts, referred to as early or β, require preceding expression of the IE genes, but do not require viral DNA synthesis [58, 59]. Late or γ transcripts require preceding early gene expression and have been subgrouped in HSV according to whether their products are made in reduced amounts (γ_1) or not at all (γ_2) when viral DNA synthesis is inhibited [58, 59, 108]. At least one CMV protein, DB52 (CMV UL44), appears to be a "delayed-early" or γ_1 by this operational definition [40, 41, 44].

There is no evidence for generalized early shutoff of cell protein synthesis, as occurs in cells infected with HSV-1 [108]. There are, however, very early changes in the metabolism of CMV-infected cells. There is stimulated transcription of the genes for heat shock protein 70, ornithine decarboxylase, thymidine kinase, and creatine kinase [25, 110]; decreased transcription of the fibronectin gene [93]; and changes similar to those induced by the G protein signaling pathway, such as decreased intracellular Ca^{++} stores and increased levels of intracellular cAMP [1, 3, 16]. This last set of observations is of particular interest in connection with the three HCMV GCR genes [22]. The finding that all three of these viral genes are transcribed (Fig. 2) [133], and presumably translated, raises the possibility that one or more of them is involved in these early metabolic changes.

CMV Proteins: General Considerations

Only a small portion of the more than 200 proteins potentially encoded by HCMV [22] have been identified. Among these, however, are members of the IE, early, and late temporal classes, and both nonvirion and virion proteins. As a generalization, the number of abundant CMV-infected cell-specific proteins so far described is lower and their sizes are smaller than their HSV counterparts [39, 40]. Because the sizes of counterpart proteins can vary between human and simian isolates of CMV, as well as between different isolates from the same species, it has been simpler when possible to refer to counterparts by a common name rather than by their differing M_rs [40].

Nonvirion Proteins

Most of the nonvirion proteins so far identified have nuclear localizations and are synthesized at early times after infection. The first of these is the predominant IE protein IE1, an anomalously slow migrating 68- to 80-kDa (depending on conditions of sodium dodecyl sulfate polyacrylamide gel electrophoresis SDS-PAGE) phosphoprotein [15, 20, 39, 131, 138] that together with IE2 gene products [129] has the capacity to transactivate CMV early (β) promoter/regulators [31, 126]. Its association with chromosomes in selectively transformed cells [76] and detection in lymphocytes [113] has been suggested to have significance to latency [76]. A second IE gene, IE2, encodes a family of proteins ranging in size from 23- to 86-kDa, which are generated by alternate RNA splicing patterns and different translational start sites [57, 127]. IE2 proteins are able to repress the IE promoter [97] through a sequence located near the cap site, between nucleotides -12 and $+9$ [96], and act as nonspecific transactivators in vitro [57, 97]. Three additional IE proteins, coded for by UL36, UL37, and UL37 exon 1, have regulatory roles and can act synergistically with HCMV IE1 and the US3 protein to enhance transcription [26].

The early nonvirion proteins include the 140-kDa viral DNA polymerase (CMV UL54) [56, 60, 72], a nuclear DNA-binding protein referred to as DB140 or CMV ICP8 [4, 68], and a set of related nuclear phosphoproteins [123, 139]. DB140 (CMV UL57) is the counterpart of ICP8 [4, 68], one of seven HSV-1 proteins essential for viral DNA synthesis [85]. Like HSV ICP8, the DB140 gene is located adjacent to *ori*-Lyt (Fig. 3) [55]. The relatively increased levels of this protein and its SCMV counterpart DB129 in infected cells partially inhibited for viral DNA synthesis [4, 44] may be explained by an increased gene dosage effect resulting from the accumulation of origin-proximal fragments under such conditions [4, 55]. HCMV DB140 and SCMV DB129 localize to discrete foci within the nucleus, as does HSV ICP8, and accumulate in the cytoplasm when viral DNA synthesis is inhibited [6]. The set of four early, nuclear, DNA-binding phosphoproteins, of 84, 50, 43, and 34 kDa, was detected by using an antipeptide serum [123, 139]. These proteins share a common amino terminus and, like the IE2 products [129], appear to be generated by alternate RNA splicing patterns [123]. Their expression is under both transcriptional and posttranscriptional control [123], and they are differentially phosphorylated [123, 139]. Although the function of these proteins is not known, they bear some resemblance to the Epstein-Barr virus nuclear antigen (EBNA-1), suggesting a possible role in DNA replication or gene regulation [139].

Another nuclear DNA-binding phosphoprotein, referred to as DB52 or ICP36 [40, 41, 68], and DB51 in SCMV [40], is the product of CMV UL44 [87]. On the basis of its reduced but not eliminated synthesis under conditions of inhibited viral DNA replication, DB52 resembles a delayed early or γ_1 protein [44]. Its gene is transcribed at both early and late times, but under different promoter/regulatory control, and there is evidence that translation of early mRNA from this gene is also posttranscriptionally regulated [35, 80]. DB52 binds to DNA during affinity chromatography on single- or double-stranded DNA [44, 68] and when electrotransferred to nitrocellulose and probed with DNA [37]. It also binds DNA in vivo as evidenced by its copartitioning with chromatin [41] and its selective release along with DB140 from infected cell nuclei following their treatment with DNase [4]. The highly basic net charge of this molecule suggests that its interaction with DNA is electrostatic rather than sequence specific; however, the high content of glycine at its carboxyl end is a feature shared with EBNA-1, which does have sequence specificity and interacts with DNA through that glycine-rich domain [103]. The high abundance of DB52 in the infected cell nucleus is more consistent with a role in organizing DNA than enzymatically processing it. These properties point to an ancillary role in DNA replication or a histone-like function for DB52 [41]; however, direct support for these possibilities (e.g., demonstrating the presence of DB52 in a "replisome" or nucleosome-like association with viral or cellular DNA) has not been obtained.

Virion Proteins and the Assembly Pathway

Six virus particles have been recovered from CMV-infected cells and characterized with respect to their protein composition, DNA content, structure, and infectivity. Two of these are recovered from the nuclear fraction of infected cells and are referred to as A- and B-capsids (Fig. 1) [38, 39, 62]. A third is recovered from the NP-40 supernatant fraction of infected cells and is referred to as C-capsid (Fig. 1) [38]. The other three – virions, noninfectious enveloped particles (NIEPs) and dense bodies – are recovered from the extracellular growth medium [42, 61]. Figure 4 shows the virion protein composition of five strains of HCMV and the probable location of each protein within the particle.

A working model of the CMV assembly pathway is presented in Fig. 5 and summarizes the hypothetical interrelationship of these particles. The B-capsid is the earliest virus particle so far isolated and characterized; however, there is evidence [98] that it may have an immature form, indicated in the figure as "preB-capsid" and discussed below. CMV B-capsids are composed of: four abundant protein species, referred to as the major capsid protein (MCP, 153 kDa; CMV UL86), the assembly protein (AP, 36 kDa; CMV UL80), the minor capsid protein (mCP, 34 kDa), and smallest capsid protein (SCP, 10–12 kDa); and several less abundant proteins, including the assembly-protein-related 37-kDa protein and the 28-kDa protein [38, 40, 62]. When viral DNA synthesis is inhibited with hydroxyurea or phosphonoformate, only

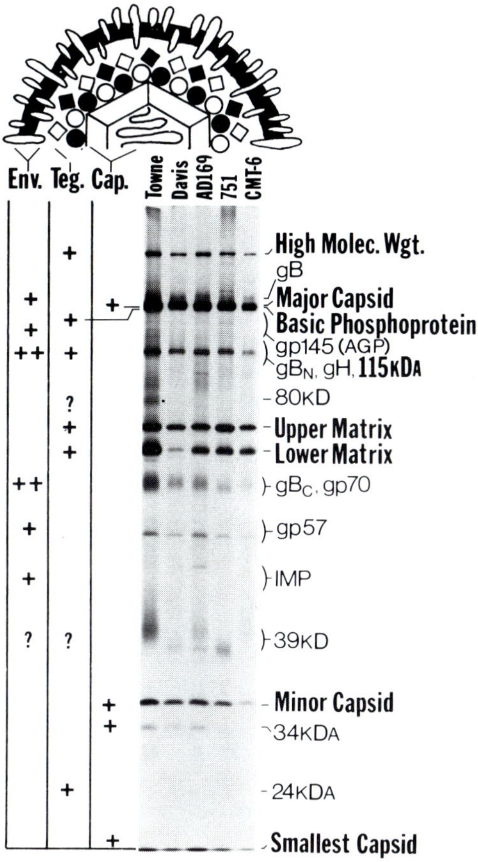

Fig. 4. Virion protein of human cytomegalovirus (HCMV). ^{14}C-amino-acid-labeled virions of five strains of HCMV were isolated [61] and subjected to sodium dodecyl sulfate polyacrylamide gel electrophoresis. This fluorogram of the resulting gel shows protein designations in the *right margin*. M_rs of the principal bands (*bold letters*) are: high molecular weight protein (212 kDa), major capsid protein (153 kDa), basic phosphoprotein (149 kDa), 115 kDa, upper matrix protein (74 kDa), lower matrix protein (69 kDa), minor capsid protein (34 kDa), smallest capsid protein (10–12 kDa). Several glycoproteins (*gp*) and other species are designated by M_r only; integral membrane protein, *IMP* (45 kDa); *AGP*, acidic glycoprotein. Assignment of proteins to the capsid (*Cap.*), tegument (*Teg.*), or envelope (*Env.*) is indicated at the *left* and is based on data from [38, 40, 42, 61] published results from other labs, and unpublished data from surface-labeling experiments with B- and C-capsids and virions. (Updated from [44])

B-capsids are seen (Fig. 6) and recovered [81] from the infected cells, suggesting that they are the immediate precursors of DNA-containing particles and the functional equivalent of the bacteriophage prohead [81]. By extension, the assembly protein would be the herpesvirus equivalent of the bacteriophage scaffolding protein – an abundant constituent of the empty prohead not found in the mature phage [14, 71].

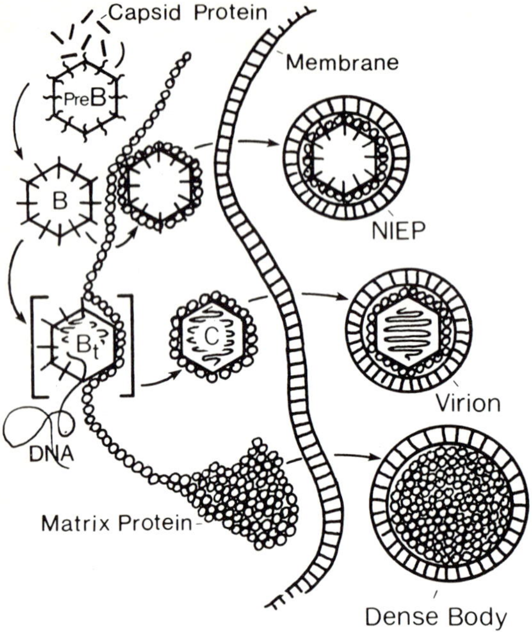

Fig. 5. Hypothetical assembly pathway for human cytomegalovirus. Putative B-capsid precursor (*PreB*) undergoes processing to become stable B-capsid (*B*) which can be enveloped to produce noninfectious enveloped particles (*NIEP*) or be filled with DNA and subsequently enveloped to become virions. A transition B-capsid (B_t) is suggested to be an intermediate in DNA packaging and entegumentation. C-capsids (*C*) are DNA-containing, tegument-coated nucleocapsids that are seen (Fig. 1) and recovered from the cytoplasmic fraction of infected cells [38]. Dense bodies are enveloped aggregates of lower matrix protein [42, 61]

Unlike the other capsid proteins, the assembly protein is derived from a precursor by proteolytic cleavage, is phosphorylated, and is not present in mature virions [38, 46, 62, 81, 105]. Recent studies have demonstrated that the gene encoding the assembly protein [105] is located at the 3′ end of a nested set of in-frame, 3′-coterminal genes [134]. The general organization of this region is the same in SCMV (Colburn strain) and HCMV (AD169) and gives rise to four mRNAs and four apparently corresponding proteins (Fig. 7). All four transcripts are late (i.e., not detected in phosphonoformate-treated infected cells) but their relative steady state amounts differ, possibly reflecting the different strengths of their respective TATA promoter/regulatory domains. The two most abundant transcripts are preceded by the sequences CGTGCGA*TATTAAA*G and ATCTG*TAATATTA*GATGATTGGC, respectively, in both HCMV and SCMV. These presumptive regulatory sequences are not similar to consensus binding domains for known host transcription factors, as might be expected for late genes. Neither are they conserved upstream of the assembly protein gene homologues of the other sequenced herpesviruses (i.e., HSV, varicella zoster virus, VZV; Epstein-Barr virus, EBV; and infectious

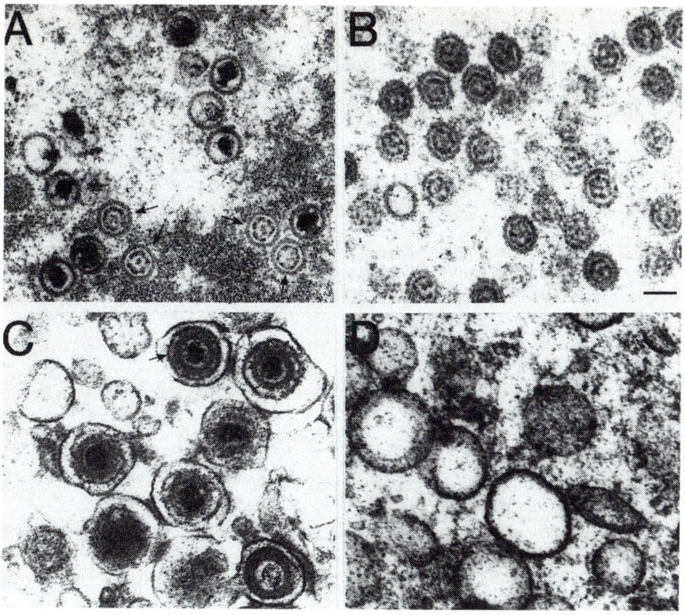

Fig. 6 A–D. Intracellular particles in hydroxyurea- (HU)-treated (**B, D**) and nontreated (**A, C**) cytomegalovirus infected cells. Cells treated with 5 m*M* HU or nontreated were processed 3 days after infection and examined by electron microscopy. Particles in the nucleus of HU-treated cells were uniform in appearance and had a beaded interior (**B**). Similar-looking particles (*arrows*) were present in the nucleus of nontreated cells (**A**). No cytoplasmic particles were present in HU-treated cells (**D**); nontreated cells (**C**) contained numerous cytoplasmic virions (*arrow*). (From [81])

laryngotracheitis virus, ILTV), suggesting that they are responsive to evolutionarily diverged viral regulatory factors. The phosphorylation and cleavage events that distinguish the assembly protein from the other abundant capsid proteins are likely to reflect its active role in the assembly process. Although the timing and consequences of these modifications have not been established, both occur by the time the assembly protein has become a B-capsid component [38, 81]. The report of an HSV temperature-sensitive mutant that fails to process its assembly protein (p40) precursor at the restrictive temperature, but nevertheless gives rise to empty capsids [98], suggests that B-capsids may have an immature form (preB-capsid [115], Fig. 5) which is similar in appearance but contains noncleaved assembly protein precursor.

Cleavage occurs at the carboxyl end of the SCMV and HCMV assembly protein precursors [46, 105, 112, 134, 135], and the cleavage site itself is conserved among all herpes group viruses examined (i.e., HCMV; SCMV; HSV-1; VZV; EBV; human herpes virus, HHV-6; ILTV) [135]. Interestingly, the proteinase responsible for this cleavage is coded for by the 5′ half of the same ORF that codes for the assembly protein precursor in it's 3′ half [135]. Figure

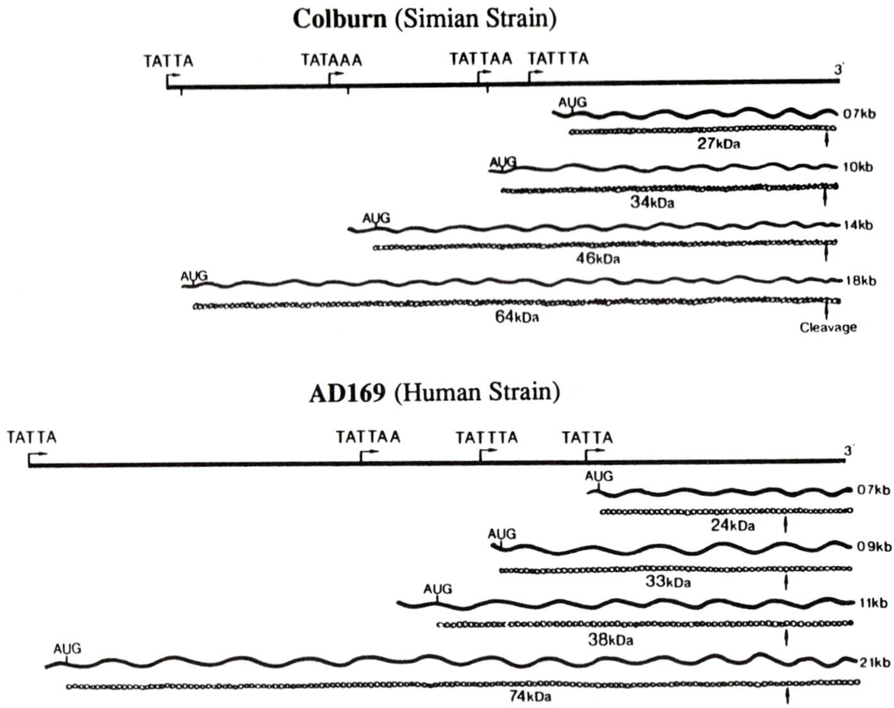

Fig. 7. Assembly protein nested genes, transcripts, and proteins of simian cytomegalovirus (SCMV, Colburn) and human CMV (AD169). The nucleotide sequence of the genomic region of strain Colburn encoding the assembly protein revealed a set of four, 3′-coterminal, in-frame open reading frames, each preceded by an upstream TATA element. Northern assays using specific antisense oligodeoxyribonucleotide probes detected all four predicted mRNAs (indicated by *wavy lines*); western assays using an antipeptide serum (Anti-C1) specific for the carboxy terminus of the assembly protein precursor detected four apparently corresponding proteins (indicated by *beaded lines*). Nuclease protection assays were used to determine the messenger RNA (nRNA) start sites (indicated as *tick marks under the line* representing gene at *top*). The organization of the AD169 assembly protein coding region [22] was similar, and parallel experiments identified the four predicted mRNAs and proteins. RNA sizes are indicated at *right*; protein sizes are indicated *below beaded lines*. The putative precursor cleavage sites (see text and [46, 105]) are indicated by *arrows*. (From [134])

8 presents a hypothetical model showing the synthesis and activities of this maturational proteinase, referred to as *assemblin*. The unusual nested organization of the assembly protein with the maturational proteinase responsible for its cleavage, and the posttranslational modifications that distinguish it from the other capsid proteins, suggest a central and potentially complex involvement in nucleocapsid formation and maturation.

Once formed, B-capsids are hypothesized to package viral DNA and mature into virions. Although this has been difficult to prove, evidence fully consistent with the model has been obtained from pulse-chase experiments using equine herpes virus [91], pseudorabies virus [74], and HSV [98]. HCMV

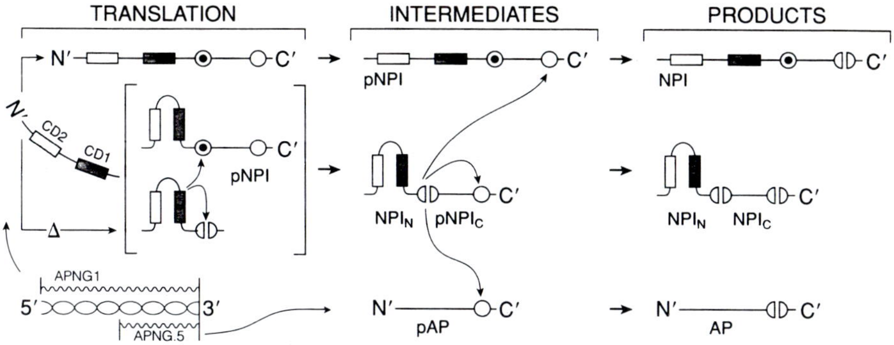

Fig. 8. Hypothetical model of the synthesis and function of the cytomegalovirus proteinase, *assemblin*: (1) The APNG1 transcript (*sawtooth line above double-stranded gene*) encodes the proteinase at its 5′ end and can be translated completely to yield pNP1 (85 kDa); (2) An undefined event (Δ) modifies the protein such that the proteinase is activated (indicated by *changed shape* in CD1/CD2 region); (3) Cotranslationally activated proteinase could free itself by cleaving in *cis* at a specific "release" site (*circle with dot*), and full length pNP1 would not be made. Alternatively, cleavage at this site could be made in *trans*. Both possibilities are indicated (see *brackets*); (4) Free proteinase ($NP1_N$) cleaves three substrates, all having the same sequence (*empty circle*) at their carboxyl ends – pNP1, $pNP1_C$ and pAP. Cleavage of these substrates eliminates an identical 33-amino acid fragment (*C′*). This model is based on the results of transfection assays; additional factors may modulate activity of the proteinase in the context of an infected cell. (From [135])

B-capsids devoid of DNA, unlike those of SCMV and HSV-1, can acquire a tegument and envelope and be shed from the cell as NIEPs (Fig. 5) [61]. NIEPs are similar to virions in composition and structure, but differ in two ways: (1) they do not contain DNA, and (2) they do contain assembly protein [61]. These particles demonstrate that removal or modification of the assembly protein is not required for – nor does it necessarily follow – acquisition of the tegument and envelope layers. They also show that the presence of viral DNA in the capsid is not a requirement for envelopment.

DNA packaging into preformed capsids, by analogy with bacteriophage, is expected to involve a cleavage/packaging enzyme to release unit length DNA from its concatameric replicating form [33]. In bacteriophage λ the enzyme that does this is called terminase and is a multimer, composed of small (Nu1) and large (A) subunits, whose genes are adjacent and in the order 5′-Nu1-A-3′ [7]. A likely candidate for this function has been identified in HSV-infected cells [24]. HSV ICP1 (HSV UL36) and a smaller protein possibly corresponding to ICP7 (HSV UL37) are part of a complex that recognizes the DR1-U_c sequence required for cleavage/packaging of viral DNA from concatamers [24, 29]. The CMV homologues of these genes are UL47 and UL48, respectively, which are predicted to encode proteins of $M_r \approx 110\,000$ and $\approx 253\,000$ [22]. The 212-kDa, high molecular weight protein (HMWP) is the largest CMV protein identified and has been shown to be the product of the largest CMV ORF, UL48 [17] (Bradshaw, Harmon, Gibson, unpublished results), and the counterpart of HSV ICP1. Interestingly, the CMV HMWP is present in virions as a multimer with the 115-kDa protein (Fig. 4; Roby and Gibson, unpublished data), consistent with the notion that these two proteins are part of a complex that represents the CMV counterpart of the HSV V4 complex [24] thought to be involved in DNA cleavage/packaging. Both of these CMV proteins are deduced to be in the virion tegument (Fig. 4) [42] and together constitute approximately 10% of the virion protein mass.

In this scheme, A-capsids, which lack the assembly protein but otherwise have the same protein composition as B-capsids [38], are formed after B-capsids. They may represent an obligate intermediate in the DNA-packaging pathway, possibly analogous to the DNA-packaging-competent, expanded prohead of bacteriophage. Alternatively, they may be byproducts of abortive DNA-packaging events or simply artifacts of the capsid isolation procedure [81, 91, 115].

Tegument Acquisition

It is unclear whether loss of the assembly protein, DNA packaging, and tegument acquisition occur sequentially or concomitantly. This transition phase is represented in Fig. 5 by a hypothetical "transition B-capsid," shown in brackets, that has a composition intermediate to those of empty B-capsids and fully entegumented nucleocapsids (e.g., C-capsids). Particles having such a composition have been recovered from the NP-40 supernatant of infected cells (Marcy and Gibson, unpublished data). They sediment close to the position of "empty" B-capsids but have a comparatively reduced amount of assembly protein. In addition, these particles contain viral DNA and tegument proteins, but in reduced amounts as compared with virions and C-capsids. DNA packaging in the nucleus and acquisition of tegument proteins at the nuclear membrane are assumed to occur as in HSV-infected cells [108], but this has not been demonstrated.

The virion of CMV has three predominant tegument proteins, the basic phosphoprotein (BPP, 149 kDa; pp 150; CMV UL32) and the upper (72 kDa; pp71; CMV UL82) and lower (69 kDa; pp 65 CMV UL83) matrix proteins (UM and LM, respectively) [38, 42, 61, 90]. Together they account for approximately 40% of the virion protein mass [61]. Of the three, the basic phosphoprotein is the most tightly associated with the nucleocapsid, as evidenced by its presence in the capsid pellet fraction following treatments that strip away the two matrix proteins (Roby and Gibson, unpublished data). Although there is no direct evidence for the relative locations of the upper and lower matrix proteins, the lower matrix protein is likely to be exposed at the periphery of the tegument because of its higher molar abundance [61]. The finding that dense bodies are essentially enveloped spheres of lower matrix protein (Fig. 6) [61], indicates that this protein possesses some, if not all, of the requisite amino acid sequence(s) to promode its own envelopment. Its presence at the surface of tegument-bearing capsids may similarly promote their envelopment.

All three of these tegument proteins are phosphorylated in vivo [83, 106], and peptide analyses have shown that each has multiple phosphorylation sites [106]. They are also the principal substrates in vitro for phosphorylation by a virion-associated protein kinase [83, 106], and two reports conclude that the lower matrix protein itself has protein kinase activity [19, 119]. The basic phosphoprotein additionally contains a single or tight cluster of O-linked *N*-acetylglucosamine residues [10, 12], but no other N- or O-linked carbohydrates are consistently detected on the three major tegument proteins [10, 12, 92]. At least two additional phosphoproteins are present in virions. One of these, 80 kDa, is also found in dense bodies [106]. The other, 24 kDa (pp28; CMV UL99), like the basic phosphoprotein is absent from dense bodies [106], suggesting a closer association with the nucleocapsid, or perhaps a different intracellular compartmentalization [79].

Envelopment

Envelopment of the nucleocapsid results in the addition of at least eight different glycoprotein species [9, 32, 50, 66, 82, 94, 95, 101, 128], which can be resolved by two-dimensional (charge/size) polyacrylamide gel electrophoresis (PAGE; Fig. 9) [40]. Three are homologue forms of HSV gB (e.g., gB, gB_N, gB_C) [9, 11, 18] and another is the homologue of HSV gH (e.g., gp86) [28, 101]. Like the HSV envelope glycoproteins, those of CMV are modified by both N- and O-glycosylation [9, 11, 65, 95]. CMV glycoproteins, however, exhibit a much greater degree of molecular heterogeneity in both size and charge [9, 40]. Because of their relative abundance and ability to elicit good infectivity-neutralizing antibodies [99, 100], gB and gH have been studied in the greatest detail. More recently these two glycoproteins have also been found to interact with putative cellular receptors for CMV [2, 67, 102, 132], underscoring their biological relevance.

As summarized in Fig. 10, gB is synthesized as a 130- to 160-kDa cotranslationally N-glycosylated precursor that undergoes at least four posttranslational modifications: First, its 17–19 predicted N-linked oligosaccharides [27] are converted from nontrimmed to trimmed high-mannose forms and then a portion are further modified to complex structures [9, 48, 95]; second, O-linked carbohydrates are added [11, Kari, cited in 48]; third, the carboxyl end of the molecule is phosphorylated [11]; and fourth, the protein is cleaved between Arg-460 and Ser-461 to yield a disulfide-linked heterodimer [18, 120, 121] composed of a highly glycosylated 115- to 130-kDa amino-terminal fragment (gB_N) [9, 11, 18, 121] and a less extensively modified 52- to 62-kDa carboxy-terminal fragment (gB_C) [9, 11, 121] (i.e., Complex A, Fig. 11). Upon exposure to oxidizing extracellular conditions, the intramolecularly disulfide cross-linked gB heterodimer (i.e., $gB_N{-}gB_C$) forms intermolecular disulfide cross-links, yielding a complex with the structure $(gB_N{-}gB_C)_2$ (Complex B, Fig. 11) [11]. The sole cysteine residue on the cytoplasmic side of the putative gB transmembrane domain [27, 120] appears to be responsible for the intermolecular disul-

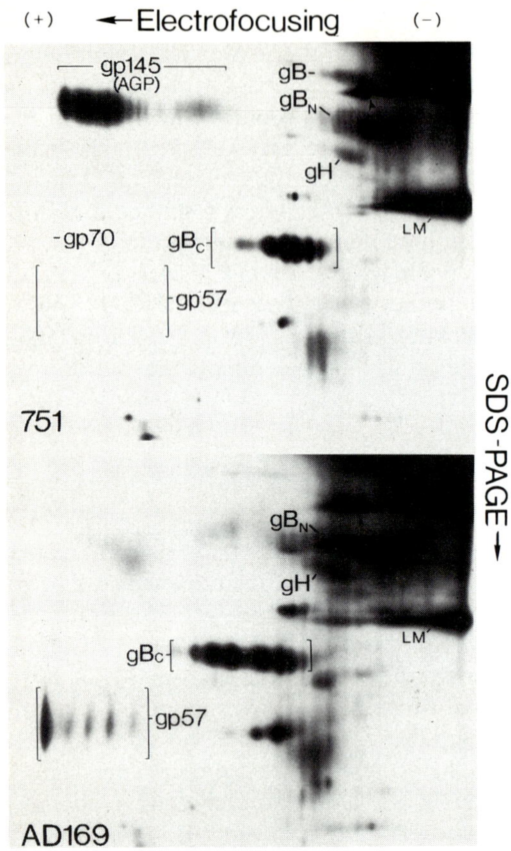

Fig. 9. Virion glycoproteins of HCMV strains 751 and AD169. Purified virions of HCMV strains 751 (*top*) and Ad169 (*bottom*) were labeled with ^{125}I and subjected to two-dimensional (charge/size) sodium dodecyl sulfate polyacrylamide gel electrophoresis (*SDS-PAGE*) [40]. Shown here are autoradiograms of the resulting gels. Seven of at least eight envelope glycoproteins can be seen: intact fully glycosylated *gB* (≈163 kDa), the amino portion of cleaved gB (*gB$_N$*, ≈130 kDa), the carboxyl portion of gB (*gB$_C$*, ≈62 kDa); *gH* (≈86 kDa); *gcII*, 52 kDa (gp57); gp70; and the nondisulfide cross-linked (i.e., Fig. 12) acidic glycoprotein (*AGP*) [40] gp145. Four proteins showed strain variability in amount: gB, gp145, gp70, and gp57. *gB$_C$* showed strain variability in size (AD169 homologue larger) and charge (AD169 homologue more heterogeneous). (From [11])

Fig. 11 A, B. Two-dimensional sodium dodecyl sulfate polyacrylamide gel electrophoresis ▶ separation of recombinant glycoprotein B (gB) expressed by CHO cell line 67.77. Immunoprecipitated [^{35}S]methionine-labeled gB was combined with unlabeled molecular mass markers and separated under nonreducing conditions followed by reducing conditions (**A**) or under reducing conditions in both dimensions (**B**). The second-dimension gel was stained with Coomassie brilliant blue, to visualize the marker proteins, and processed for fluorography. Shown here is a fluorogram of the resulting gel. *gB*, *gB$_N$*, and *gB$_C$* denote the noncleaved, N-terminal, and C-terminal gB cleavage products, respectively. The relative mobilities (M_r [10^{-3}]) of the marker proteins used to determine the *diagonal line* are shown on the *axis* for both dimensions. The doublet appearance of gB_N in **B** is due to its comigration with the unlabeled marker, phosphorylase b. Details of the experiment are in [121]

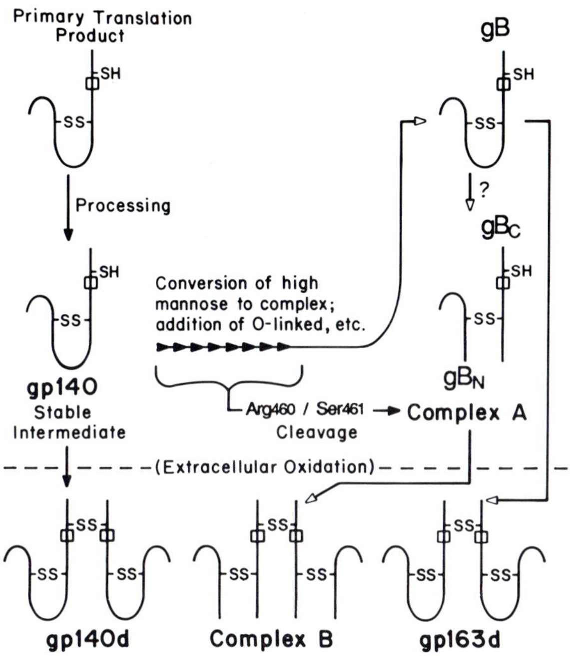

Fig. 10. Maturation pathway of human cytomegalovirus glycoprotein B (HCMV gB). A summary of modifications described for HCMV gB, as outlined in the text. Fully glycosylated, noncleaved gB (≈163 kDa) and its amino (gB_N, ≈130 kDa) and carboxyl (gB_C, ≈62 kDa) portions are indicated at *top right*. Oxidized forms, absent when N-ethylmaleimide is used to block oxidative disulfide formation [11], are shown at *bottom*. *Open box* at carboxyl end of gB_C indicates predicted transmembrane domain; *−SH* above it indicates position of cysteine residue on cytoplasmic side of membrane suspected to be responsible for intermolecular disulfide (*−SS−*) formation that cross-links Complex A dimers into Complex B tetramers. (Data from [11])

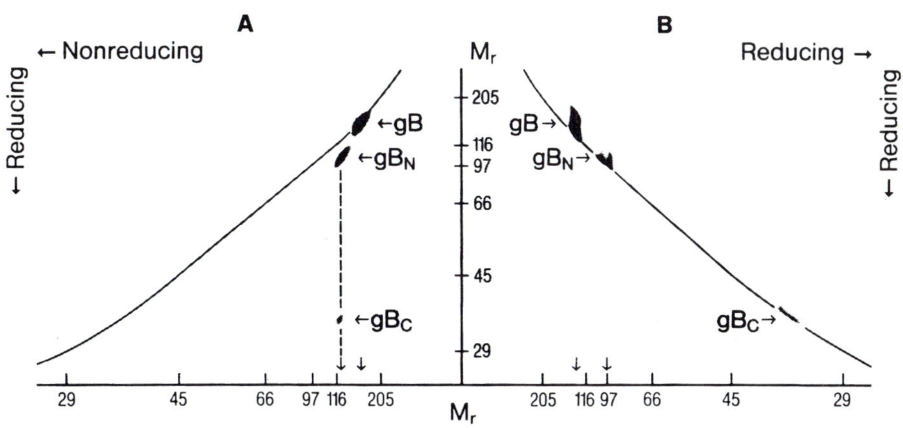

fide bonding, since a carboxyl truncation of gB which removed that cysteine eliminated formation of complex B, i.e., $(gB_N-gB_C)_2$ (Fig. 12).

Glycoprotein H is an N-glycosylated 86-kDa protein that is the CMV homologue of HSV-1 gH [28]. CMV gH induces complement-independent virus neutralizing antibodies [42], and may be involved in either intracellular spread or initiation of virus infection since monoclonal antibodies to gH can decrease CMV plaque size [102]. The finding that anti-idiotype antibodies bearing the internal image of a neutralizing epitope on gH inhibit the spread of CMV throughout the culture [67] is evidence that gH may be interacting with cellular receptors.

Two other envelope proteins of CMV and two disulfide-linked glycoprotein complexes have also been described. Glycoprotein complex II (gcII) has components of 93 kDa and 450 kDa in its nonreduced state [49]. After reduction the major species have M_rs of 50–52 kDa and more than 200 kDa. These proteins have similar peptide maps, indicating that they are closely related, and the 52-kDa component is comparatively highly O-glycosylated and sialylated [9, 11, 40, 65]; it corresponds to gp57 in Fig. 9. Glycoprotein complex III (gcIII) has an estimated size of 240 kDa under nonreducing conditions and, following reduction of disulfide bonds, was found to be composed of two glycoproteins, 145- and 86-kDa [50]. An additional highly sialylated, O-glycosylated virion glycoprotein, gp145 (Figs. 9, 12) [9, 11], originally referred to as the acidic glycoprotein (AGP) [40], differs from the 145-kDa gcIII protein in that it is not disulfide-linked (Fig. 12) [11]. The relative amounts of this protein and gp57 are more strain dependent than those of gB and gH: gp145 is more abundant in strain 751 and gp57 is more abundant in strain AD169 (Figs. 9, 12) [9, 11]. Another envelope protein, having an M_r, of approximately 45 kDa, has been detected and determined to have five potential N-glycosylation sites and eight possible membrane spanning domains [82]. It is referred to as the integral membrane protein (IMP) and has homologues in HSV-1 (UL10), VZV (ORF50), and EBV (BBRF3) [82].

The site of CMV envelopment has been assumed to be the inner nuclear membrane, as generally accepted for HSV [8, 108]. However, the apparent cytoplasmic envelopment commonly observed in CMV-infected cells (e.g., Fig. 1) may indicate that a different or additional envelopment mechanism is operative. It has been suggested that an envelopment/de-envelopment mechanism [124] may be used to cross the double nuclear membrane, and that final envelopment of HCMV nucleocapsids occurs at cytoplasmic membranes [114]. Experiments done using the ionophore monensin to inhibit carbohydrate processing in CMV-infected cells gave results compatible with such a pathway. Instead of producing an accumulation of enveloped particles in the Golgi region of the infected cell, as observed in a similar experiment with HSV-1 [63], large numbers of DNA-containing (i.e., darkly stained centers), tegument-bearing (i.e., thickened surface coating), nonenveloped particles accumulated in the cytoplasm (Fig. 13) [11]. These particles did not simply leak out of the nucleus through swollen membranes, because their appearance was completely different from that of nuclear capsids (e.g., larger diameter, more heavily

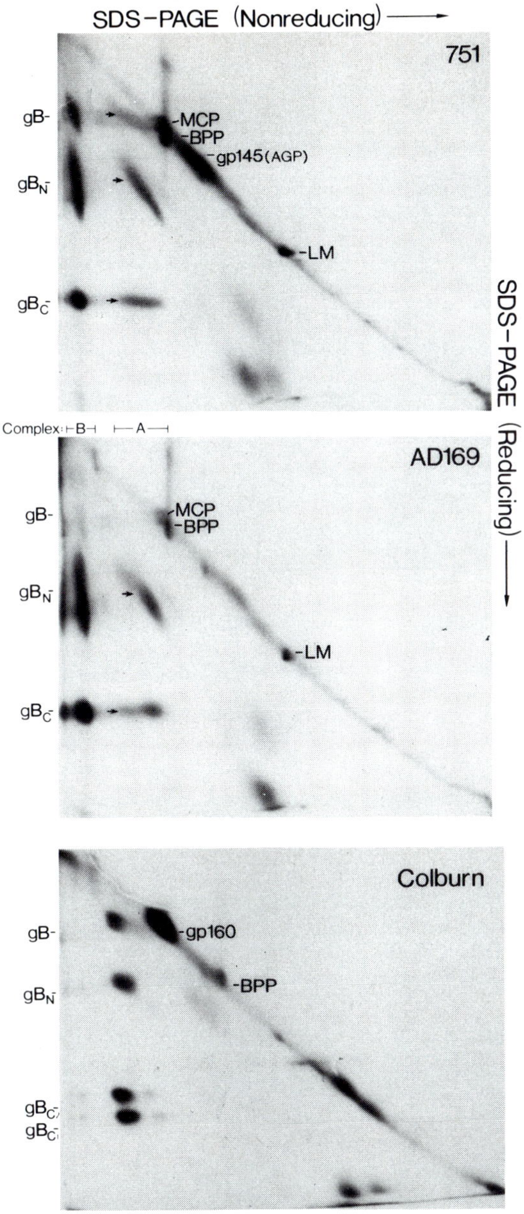

Fig. 12. Disulfide-linked virion proteins of strains 751 and AD169. Purified virions of strains 751 and AD169 were ^{125}I-labeled and subjected to two-dimensional (nonreducing/reducing) sodium dodecyl sulfate polyacrylamide gel electrophoresis (*SDS-PAGE*). Two gB disulfide-linked complexes were identified: Complex A, M_r 160–200 kDa, was a heterodimer of gB_N and gB_C; Complex B, M_r >280 kDa, was a dimer of Complex A, i.e., $(gB_NgB_C)_2$. Like the basic phosphoprotein (*BPP*) and major capsid protein (*MCP*), gp145 was not present in a disulfide cross-linked complex. It can be seen here that strain AD169 had less noncleaved gB and less gp145 than strain 751. *AGP*, acidic glycoprotein; *LM*, lower matrix protein; *arrows* indicate positions of corresponding glycoproteins. (From [11])

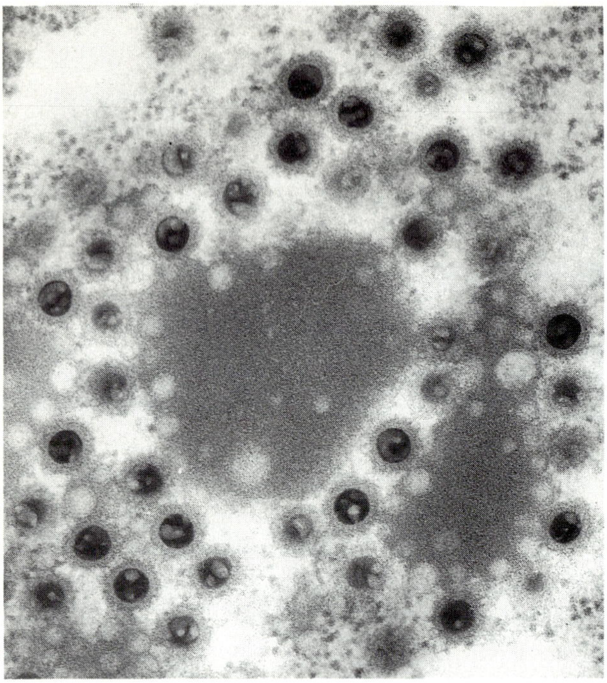

Fig. 13. Micrograph of virus particles in cytoplasm of monensin-treated human cytomegalovirus-(HCMV)-infected cells. Human foreskin fibroblasts were infected with HCMV strain 751 and incubated in 400 n*M* monensin, beginning 36 h after infection. Three days later the cells were processed for electron microscopy [81]. Nuclear capsids (not shown) were normal in number and appearance. Cytoplasmic capsids looked like C-capsids seen during the course of a normal infection (e.g., Fig. 1). They had densely stained centers and a thick fibrillar coating which distinguished them from the nuclear capsids (see Fig. 1). These cytoplasmic capsids were generally clustered around areas that had a homogeneous granular appearance similar to that of the tegument layer, and may represent large accumulations of some (e.g., abundant 69-kDa lower matrix protein) or all of those proteins (Fig. 4)

stained center, and fibrillar coating). A similar observation was reported for monensin-treated, VZV-infected cells [52], indicating that the phenomenon is not limited to CMV-infected cells.

Concluding Comment

This chapter was intended to update and supplement several excellent reviews that have been written recently on CMV molecular biology. Enormous progress has been made over the last decade in identifying the molecules elaborated by the virus during infection, and in determining their physical and chemical properties, but the challenge of unraveling their biological interactions at the molecular level has just begun.

References

1. AbuBaker S, Boldogh I, Albrecht T (1990) Human cytomegalovirus stimulates arachidonic acid metabolism through pathways that are affected by inhibitors of phospholipase A2 and protein kinase C. Biochem Biophys Res Commun 166:953–959
2. Adlish JD, Lahijani RS, St Jeor SC (1990) Identification of a putative cell receptor for human cytomegalovirus. Virology 176:337–345
3. Albrecht T, Boldogh I, Fons M, Lee CH, AbuBakar S, Russell JM, Au WW (1989) Cell-activation responses to cytomegalovirus infection relationship to the phasing of CMV replication and to the induction of cellular damage. Subcell Biochem 15:157–207
4. Anders DG, Gibson W (1988) Location, transcript analysis, and partial nucleotide sequence of the cytomegalovirus gene encoding an early DNA-binding protein with similarities to ICP8 of herpes simplex virus type 1. J Virol 62:1364–1372
5. Anders DG, Punturieri SM (1991) Multicomponent origin of cytomegalovirus lytic-phase DNA replication. J Virol 65:931–937
6. Anders DG, Kidd JR, Gibson W (1987) Immunological characterization of an early cytomegalovirus single-strand DNA-binding protein with similarities to the HSV major DNA-binding protein. Virology 161:579–588
7. Becker A, Murialdo H, Lucko H, Morell J (1988) Bacteriophage lambda DNA packaging. The product of the *FI* gene promotes the incorporation of the prohead to the DNA-terminase complex. J Mol Biol 199:597–607
8. Becker P, Melnick JL, Mayer HD (1965) A morphologic comparison between the developmental stages of herpes zoster and human cytomegalovirus. Exp Mol Pathol 4:11–23
9. Benko DM, Gibson W (1986) Primate cytomegalovirus glycoproteins: lectin-binding properties and sensitivities to glycosidases. J Virol 59:703–713
10. Benko DM, Gibson W (1988) A major tegument phosphoprotein of human cytomegalovirus contains O-linked GlcNAc. In: Compans R, Helenius A, Oldstone M (eds) Cell biology of virus entry, replication, and pathogenesis. Liss, New York, pp 57–66
11. Benko DM, Gibson W, Manuscript in preparation
12. Benko DM, Haltiwanger RS, Hart GW, Gibson W (1988) Virion basic phosphoprotein of human cytomegalovirus contains O-linked N-acetylglucosamine. Proc Natl Acad Sci USA 85:2573–2577
13. Benson JD, Huang E-S (1990) Human cytomegalovirus induces expression of cellular topoisomerase II. J Virol 64:9–15
14. Black LW, Showe MK (1984) Morphogenesis of the T4 head. In: Mathews CK, Kutter EM, Mosig G, Berget PB (eds) Bacteriophage T4. ASM, Washington, pp 219–245
15. Blanton RA, Tevethia M (1981) Immunoprecipitation of virus-specific immediate-early and early polypeptides from cells lytically infected with human cytomegalovirus strain AD169. J Virol 112:262–273
16. Boldogh I, AbuBakar S, Albrecht T (1990) Activation of protooncogenes: an immediate early event in human cytomegalovirus infection. Science 247:561–564
17. Bradshaw PA, Duran MR, Foung SKH (1991) Anti-CMV human monoclonal antibodies: epitope identification and immune response analysis. In: Landini MP (ed) Progress in cytomegalovirus research. Excerpta Medica, Amsterdam, pp 157–160
18. Britt WJ, Auger D (1986) Synthesis and processing of the envelope gp55-116 complex of human cytomegalovirus. J Virol 58:185–191
19. Britt WJ, Auger D (1986) Human cytomegalovirus virion-associated protein with kinase activity. J Virol 59:185–188
20. Cameron JM, Preston CM (1981) Comparison of the immediate early polypeptides of human cytomegalovirus isolates. J Gen Virol 54:421–424
21. Chang C-P, Vesole DH, Nelson J, Oldstone MBA, Stinski MF (1989) Identification and expression of a human cytomegalovirus early glycoprotein. J Virol 63:3330–3337
22. Chee MS, Bankier AT, Beck S, Bohni R, Brown CM, Cerny R, Horsnell T, Hutchison A, Kouzarider T, Martignetti JA, Preddie E, Satchwell SC, Tomlinson P, Weston KM,

Barrell BG (1990) Analysis of the protein-coding content of the sequence of human cytomegalovirus strain AD169. Curr Top Microbiol Immunol 154:125–169
23. Chee MS, Satchwell SC, Preddie E, Weston KM, Barrell BG (1990) Human cytomegalovirus encodes three G protein-coupled receptor homologues. Nature 344:774–777
24. Chou J, Roizman B (1989) Characterization of DNA sequence-common and sequence-specific proteins binding to *cis*-acting sites for cleavage of the terminal α sequence of the herpes simplex virus 1 genome. J Virol 63:1059–1068
25. Colberg-Poley AM, Santomenna LD (1988) Selective induction of chromosomal gene expression by human cytomegalovirus. Virology 166:217–228
26. Colberg-Poley AM, Santomenna LD, Hossle JP, Benfield P, Rüger R, Tenney DJ (1991) Interactions between human cytomegalovirus immediate early genes in *trans*-activation of cellular and viral promoters. In: Landini MP (ed) Progress in cytomegalovirus research. Excerpta Medica, Amsterdam, pp 259–262
27. Cranage MP, Kouzarides T, Bankier AT, Satchwell S, Weston K, Tomlinson P, Barrell B, Hart H, Bell SE, Minson AC, Smith GL (1986) Identification of the human cytomegalovirus glycoprotein B gene and induction of neutralizing, antibodies via its expression in recombinant vaccinia virus. EMBO J5:3057–3063
28. Cranage MP, Smith GL, Bell SE, Hart H, Brown C, Bankier AT, Tomlinson P, Barrell BG, Minson TJ (1988) Identification and expression of a human cytomegalovirus glycoprotein with homology to the Epstein-Barr virus BXLF2 product, varicella-zoster virus gpIII, and herpes simplex virus type 1 glycoprotein H. J Virol 62:1416–1422
29. Deiss LP, Chou J, Frenkel N (1986) Functional domains within the α sequence involved in the cleavage-packaging of herpes simplex virus DNA. J Virol 59:605–618
30. DeMarchi JM, Blankenship ML, Brown GD, Kaplan AS (1978) Size and complexity of human cytomegalovirus DNA. Virology 89:643–646
31. Depto AS, Stenberg RM (1989) Regulated expression of the human cytomegalovirus pp65 gene: octomer sequence in the promoter is required for activation by viral gene products. J Virol 63:1232–1238
32. Farrar GH, Oram JD (1984) Characterization of human cytomegalovirus envelope glycoproteins. J Gen Virol 65:1991–2001
33. Feiss M (1986) Terminase and the recognition, cutting and packaging of γ chromosomes. Trends Genet 2:100–104
34. Fleckenstein B, Muller I, Collins J (1982) Cloning of the complete human cytomegalovirus genome in cosmids. Gene 18:39–46
35. Geballe AP, Leach FS, Mocarski EM (1986) Regulation of cytomegalovirus late gene expression: γ genes are controlled by posttranslational events. J Virol 57:864–874
36. Geelen JLM, Walig C, Wertheim P, van der Noordaa J (1978) Human cytomegalovirus DNA. I. Molecular weight and infectivity. J Virol 26:813–816
37. Gergely L, Czegledy J, Vaczi L (1985) Detection of human cytomegalovirus-induced DNA-binding proteins on western blots. J Virol Methods 12:263–270
38. Gibson W (1981) Structural and nonstructural proteins of strain Colburn cytomegalovirus. Virology 111:516–537
39. Gibson W (1981) Immediate-early proteins of human cytomegalovirus strains AD169, Davis and Towne differ in electrophoretic mobility. Virology 112:350–354
40. Gibson W (1983) Protein counterparts of human and simian cytomegaloviruses. Virology 128:391–406
41. Gibson W (1985) Synthesis, structure and function of cytomegalovirus major nonvirion nuclear protein. In: Rapp F (ed) UCLA symposia on molecular and cellular biology, Vol 21. Liss, New York, pp 423–440
42. Gibson W, Irmiere A (1984) Selection of particles and proteins for use as human cytomegalovirus subunit vaccines. In: Plotkin SA, Michelson S, Pagano JS, Rapp F (eds) Birth defects. Liss, New York, pp 305–324
43. Gibson W, Roizman B (1972) Proteins specified by herpes simplex virus. VIII. Characterization and composition of multiple capsid forms of subtypes 1 and 2. J Virol 10:1044–1052

44. Gibson W, Murphy TL, Roby C (1981) Cytomegalovirus-infected cells contain a DNA-binding protein. Virology 111:251–262
45. Gibson W, van Breeman R, Fields A, LaFemina R, Irmiere AJ (1984) D,L-α-difluoromethylornithine inhibits human cytomegalovirus replication. Virology 50:145–154
46. Gibson W, Marcy AI, Comolli JC, Lee J (1990) Identification of precursor to cytomegalovirus capsid assembly protein and evidence that processing results in loss of its carboxy-terminal end. J Virol 64:1241–1249
47. Greenaway PJ, Oram JD, Downing RG, Patel K (1982) Human cytomegalovirus DNA: *Bam*HI, *Eco*RI and *Pst*I restriction endonuclease cleavage maps. Gene 18:355–360
48. Gretch DR, Gehrz RC, Stinski MF (1988) Characterization of a human cytomegalovirus glycoprotein complex (gcI). J Gen Virol 69:1205–1215
49. Gretch DR, Kari B, Gehrz RC, Stinski MF (1988) A multigene family encodes the human cytomegalovirus glycoprotein complex gcII (gp47-52 complex). J Virol 62:1956–1962
50. Gretch DR, Kari B, Rasmussen L, Gehrz RC, Stinski MF (1988) Identification and characterization of three distinct families of glcoprotein complexes in the envelopes of human cytomegalovirus. J Virol 62:875–881
51. Griffiths PD, Grundy JE (1987) Molecular biology and immunology of cytomegalovirus. Biochemistry 241:313–324
52. Gross C, Edwards DP, Weigle KA, Friedrichs WE, McGuire WL (1984) Varicella-zoster virus-specific gp140: a highly immunogenic and disulfide-linked structural glycoprotein. Virology 132:138–146
53. Grundy JE, McKeating JA, Griffiths PD (1987) Cytomegalovirus strain AD169 binds β_2 microglobulin in vitro after release from cells. J Gen Virol 68:777–784
54. Grundy JE, McKeating JA, Ward PJ, Sanderson AR, Griffiths PD (1987) β_2 microglobulin enhances the infectivity of cytomegalovirus and when bound to the virus enables class I HLA molecules to be used as a virus receptor. J Gen Virol 68:793–803
55. Hamzeh FM, Lietman PS, Gibson W, Hayward GS (1990) Identification of the lytic origin of DNA replication in human cytomegalovirus by a novel approach utilizing ganciclovir-induced chain termination. J Virol 64:6184–6195
56. Heilbronn R, Jahn G, Burkle A, Freese U-K, Fleckenstein B, zur Hausen H (1987) Genomic localization, sequence analysis, and transcription of the putative human cytomegalovirus DNA polymerase gene. J Virol 61:119–124
57. Hermiston TW, Malone CL, Witte PR, Stinski MF (1987) Identification and characterization of the human cytomegalovirus immediate-early region 2 gene that stimulates gene expression from an inducible promoter. J Virol 61:3214–3221
58. Honess RW, Roizman B (1974) Regulation of herpesvirus macromolecular synthesis. I. Cascade regulation of the synthesis of three groups of viral proteins. J Virol 14:8–19
59. Honess RW, Roizman B (1975) Regulation of herpesvirus macromolecular synthesis: sequential transition of polypeptide synthesis requires functional viral polypeptides. Proc Natl Acad Sci USA 72:1276–1280
60. Huang E-S (1975) Human cytomegalovirus III. Virus-induced DNA polymerase. J Virol 16:298–310
61. Irmiere A, Gibson W (1983) Isolation and characterization of a virion-like particle from cells infected with human strains of cytomegalovirus. Virology 130:118–133
62. Irmiere A, Gibson W (1985) Isolation of human cytomegalovirus intranuclear capsids, characterization of their protein consituents, and demonstration that the B-capsid assembly protein is also abundant in noninfectious enveloped particles. J Virol 56:277–283
63. Johnson DC, Spear PG (1983) O-linked oligosaccharides are acquired by herpes simplex virus glycoproteins in the golgi apparatus. Cell 32:987–997
64. Kanich RE, Craighead JE (1972) Human cytomegalovirus infection of cultured fibroblasts. II. Viral replicative sequence of a wild and an adapted strain. Lab Invest 27:273–282
65. Kari B, Gehrz R (1988) Isolation and characterization of a human cytomegalovirus glycoprotein containing a high content of O-linked oligosaccharides. Arch Virol 98:171–188

66. Kari B, Lussenhop N, Goertz R, Wakuke-Bunoti M, Radeke R, Gehrz R (1986) Characterization of monoclonal antibodies reactive to several biochemically distinct human cytomegalovirus glycoprotein complexes. J Virol 60:345–352
67. Keay S, Rasmussen L, Merigan T (1988) Syngeneic monoclonal anti-idiotype antibodies that bear the internal image of a human cytomegalovirus neutralization epitope. J Immunol 140:944–948
68. Kemble GW, McCormick AL, Pereira L, Mocarski ES (1987) A cytomegalovirus protein with properties of herpes simplex virus ICP8: partial purification of the polypeptide and map position of the gene. J Virol 61:3143–3151
69. Kilpatrick BA, Huang E-S (1977) Human cytomegalovirus genome: partial denaturation map and organization of genome sequences. J Virol 24:261–276
70. Kim KS, Sapienza VJ, Carp RI, Moon HM (1976) Analysis of structural polypeptides of purified human cytomegalovirus. J Virol 20:604–611
71. King J, Casjens S (1974) Catalytic head assembling protein in virus morphogenesis. Nature 251:112–119
72. Kouzarides T, Bankier AT, Satchwell SC, Weston K, Tomlinson P, Barrell BG (1987) Sequence and transcription analysis of the human cytomegalovirus DNA polymerase gene. J Virol 61:125–133
73. Kozak M (1981) An analysis of 5′-noncoding sequences from 699 vertebrate messenger RNAs. Nucleic Acids Res 15:8125–8148
74. Ladin BF, Ihara S, Hampl H, Ben-Porat T (1982) Pathway of assembly of herpesvirus capsies: an analysis using DNA^{+} temperature-sensitive mutants of pseudorabies virus. Virology 116:544–561
75. LaFemina RL, Hayward GS (1980) Structural organization of the DNA molecules from human cytomegalovirus. ICN UCLA Symp Mol Cell Biol 18:39–55
76. LaFemina RL, Pizzorno MC, Mosca JD, Hayward GS (1989) Expression of the acidic nuclear immediate-early protein (IE1) of human cytomegalovirus in stable cell lines and its preferential association with metaphase chromosomes. Virology 172:584–600
77. Lakeman AD, Osborn JE (1979) Size of infectious DNA from human and murine cytomegaloviruses. J Virol 30:414–416
78. Landini MP, Michelson S (1988) Human cytomegalovirus proteins. Prog Med Virol 35:152–185
79. Landini MP, Severi B, Furlini G, DeGiorgi LB (1987) Human cytomegalovirus structural components: intracellular and intraviral localization of p28 and p65-69 by immunoelectron microscopy. Virus Res 8:15–23
80. Leach FS, Mocarski ES (1989) Regulation of cytomegalovirus late-gene expression: differential use of three start sites in the transcriptional activation of ICP36 gene expression. J Virol 63:1783–1791
81. Lee JY, Irmiere A, Gibson W (1988) Primate cytomegalovirus assembly: evidence that DNA packaging occurs subsequent to B-capsid assembly. Virology 167:87–96
82. Lehner R, Meyer H, Mach M (1989) Identification and characterization of a human cytomegalovirus gene coding for a membrane protein that is conserved among human herpesviruses. J Virol 63:3792–3800
83. Mar E-S, Patel PC, Huang E-S (1981) Human cytomegalovirus-associated DNA polymerase and protein kinase activities. J Gen Virol 57:149–156
84. McGavran MH, Smith MG (1965) Ultrastructural, cytochemical, and microchemical observations on cytomegalovirus (salivary gland virus) infection of human cells in tissue culture. Exp Mol Pathol 4:1–10
85. McGeoch DJ, Dalrymple MA, Dolan A, McNab D, Perry L, Taylor P, Challberg MD (1988) Structures of herpes simplex virus type 1 genes required for replication of virus DNA. J Virol 62:444–453
86. McKeating JA, Griffiths PD, Grundy JE (1987) Cytomegalovirus in urine specimens has host β_2 microglobulin bound to the viral envelope: a mechanism of evading the host immune response? J Gen Virol 68:785–792
87. Mocarski ES, Pereira L, Michael N (1985) Precise localization of genes on large animal virus genomes: use of λgt11 and monoclonal antibodies to map the gene for a cytomegalovirus protein family. Proc Natl Acad Sci USA 82:1266–1270

88. Mocarski ES, Abenes GB, Manning WC, Sambudetti LC, Cherrington JM (1990) Molecular genetic analysis of cytomegalovirus gene regulation in growth, persistence and latency. Curr Top Microbiol Immunol 154:47–74
89. Nelson JA, Ganann JW, Ghazal P (1990) Regulation and tissue-specific expression of human cytomegalovirus. Curr Top Microbiol Immunol 154:75–100
90. Nowak B, Sullivan C, Sarnow P, Thomas R, Bricout F, Nicolas JC, Fleckenstein B, Levine AJ (1984) Characterization of monoclonal antibodies and polyclonal immune sera directed against human cytomegalovirus virion proteins. Virology 132:325–338
91. O'Callaghan DJ, Randall CC (1976) Molecular anatomy of herpesviruses: recent studies. Prog Med Virol 22:152–210
92. Pande H, Lee TD, Churchill MA, Zaia JA (1990) Structural analysis of a 64-kDa major structural protein of human cytomegalovirus (Towne): identification of a phosphorylation site and comparison to pp65 of HCMV (AD169). Virology 178:6–14
93. Pande H, Terramani T, Tressel T, Churchill MA, Hawkins GG, Zaia JA (1990) Altered expression of fibronectin gene in cells infected with human cytomegalovirus. J Virol 64:1366–1369
94. Pereira L (1985) Glycoproteins specified by human cytomegalovirus. In: Roizman B (ed) The herpesviruses, vol 3. Plenum, New York, pp 383–404
95. Pereira L, Hoffman M, Tatsuno M, Dondero D (1984) Polymorphism of human cytomegalovirus glycoproteins characterized by monoclonal antibodies. Virology 139:73–86
96. Pizzorno MC, Hayward GS (1990) The IE2 gene products of human cytomegalovirus specifically down-regulate expression from the major immediate-early promoter through a target sequence located near the cap site. J Virol 64:6154–6165
97. Pizzorno MC, O'Hare P, Sha L, LaFemina RL, Hayward GS (1988) Trans-activation and autoregulation of gene expression by the immediate-early region 2 gene products of human cytomegalovirus. J Virol 62:1167–1179
98. Preston VG, Coates JAV, Rixon FJ (1983) Identification and charaterization of a herpes simplex virus gene product required for encapsidation of virus DNA. J Virol 456:1056–1064
99. Rasmussen L (1990) Immune response to human cytomegalovirus infection. Curr Top Microbiol Immunol 154:221–254
100. Rasmussen L, Mullenax J, Nelson M, Merigan T (1985) Human cytomegalovirus polypeptides stimulate neutralizing antibody in vivo. Virology 145:186–190
101. Rasmussen L, Nelson M, Neff M, Merigan TC (1988) Characterization of two different human cytomegalovirus glyocproteins which are targets for virus neutralizing antibody. Virology 163:308–311
102. Rasmussen L, Resta S, Merigan T (1991) Human cytomegalovirus glycoprotein–receptor interactions. In: Zaia J, Hooper J (eds) Pathogenesis of human cytomegalovirus-associated diseases. Transplant Proc 23:60–63
103. Rawlins DR, Milman G, Hayward SD, Hayward GS (1985) Sequence-specific DNA binding of the Epstein-Barr virus nuclear antigen (EBNA-1) to clustered sites in the plasmid maintenance region. Cell 42:859–868
104. Ripalti A, Landini MP, LaPlace M (1988) A 46 kD polypeptide, present in purified human cytomegalovirus, is provided with DNase activity and is antigenically related to a higher molecular weight, enzymatically inactive, cellular protein. Microbiologica 11:69–76
105. Robson L, Gibson W (1988) Primate cytomegalovirus assembly protein: Genome location and nucleotide sequence. J Virol 63:669–676
106. Roby C, Gibson W (1986) Characterization of phosphoproteins and protein kinase activity of virions, noninfectious enveloped particles, and dense bodies of human cytomegalovirus. J Virol 59:714–727
107. Roizman B (1979) The structure and isomerization of herpes simplex virus genomes. Cell 16:481–494
108. Roizman B, Sears AE (1990) Herpes simplex viruses and their replication. In: Fields BN, Knipe DM, Chanock RM, Hirsch MS, Melnick JL, Monath TP, Roizman B (eds) Fields virology. Raven, New York, pp 1795–1841

109. Rowe WP, Hartley JW, Waterman S, Turner HC, Huebner RJ (1956) Cytopathogenic agent resembling human salivary gland virus recovered from tissue cultures of human adenoids. Proc Soc Exp Biol 92:418–424
110. Santomenna LD, Colberg-Polly AM (1990) Induction of cellular *hsp*70 expression by human cytomegalovirus. J Virol 64:2033–2040
111. Sarov I, Abady I (1975) The morphogenesis of human cytomegalovirus. Virology 66:464–473
112. Schenk P, Woods AS, Gibson W (1991) The 45-kDa protein of cytomegalovirus (Colburn) B-capsids is an amino terminal extension form of the assembly protein. J Virol 65:1525–1529
113. Schrier RD, Nelson JA, Oldstone MBA (1985) Detection of human cytomegalovirus in peripheral blood lymphocytes in a natural infection. Science 230:1048–1051
114. Severi B, Landini MP, Govoni E (1988) Human cytomegalovirus morphogenesis: An ultrastructural study of late cytoplasmic phases. Arch Virol 98:51–64
115. Sherman G, Bachenheimer SL (1988) Characterization of intranuclear capsids made by ts morphogenic mutants of HSV-1. Virology 163:471–480
116. Smith JD, DeHarven E (1974) Herpes simplex virus and human cytomegalovirus replication in WI-38 cells. II. An ultrastructural study of viral penetration. J Virol 14:945–956
117. Smith MG (1956) Propagation in tissue cultures of a cytopathogenic virus from human salivary gland virus (SGV) disease. Proc Soc Exp Biol 92:424–430
118. Somogyi T, Colimon R, Michelson S (1986) An illustrated guide to the structure of the human cytomegalovirus genome and a review of transcription data. Prog Med Virol 33:99–133
119. Somogyi T, Michelson S, Masse M-JO (1990) Genomic location of a human cytomegalovirus protein with protein kinase activity (PK68) Virology 174:276–285
120. Spaete RR, Thayer RM, Probert WS, Masiarz FR, Chamberlain SH, Rasmussen L, Merigan TC, Pachl C (1988) Human cytomegalovirus strain Towne glycoprotein B is processed by proteolytic cleavage. Virology 167:207–225
121. Spaete RR, Saxena A, Scott PI, Song GJ, Probert WS, Britt WJ, Gibson W, Rasmussen L, Pachl C (1990) Sequence requirements for proteolytic processing of glycoprotein B of human cytomegalovirus strain Towne. J Virol 64:2922–2931
122. Spear PG, Roizman B (1972) Proteins specified by herpes simplex virus V. Purification and structural proteins of the herpesvirion. J Virol 9:143–159
123. Spector DH, Klucher KM, Rabert DK, Wright DA (1990) Human cytomegalovirus early gene expression. In: McDougall JK (ed) Cytomegaloviruses. Springer, Berlin Heidelberg New York, pp 21–45 (Current topics in microbiology and immunology, vol 154)
124. Stackpole CW (1969) Herpes-type virus of the frog renal adenocarcinoma. I. Virus development in tumor transplants maintained at low temperature. J Virol 4:75–93
125. Stamminger T, Fleckenstein B (1990) Immediate-early transcription regulation of human cytomegalovirus. In: McDougall JK (ed) Cytomegaloviruses. Springer, Berlin Heidelberg New York, 3–19 (Current topics in microbiology and immunology, vol 154)
126. Staprans SI, Spector DH (1986) 2.2-kilobase class of early transcripts encoded by cell-related sequences in human cytomegalovirus strain AD169. J Virol 57:591–602
127. Stenberg RM, Witte PR, Stinski MF (1985) Multiple spliced and unspliced transcripts from human cytomegalovirus immediate-early region 2 and evidence for a common initiation site within immediate-early region 1. J Virol 56:665–675
128. Stinski MF (1976) Human cytomegalovirus: glycoproteins associated with virions and dense bodies. J Virol 19:594–609
129. Stinski MF (1990) Cytomegalovirus and its replication. In: Fields BN, Knipe DM, Chanock RM, Hirsch MS, Melnick JL, Monath TP, Roizman B (eds) Fields virology. Raven, New York, pp 1959–1980
130. Stinski MF, Mocarski ES, Thomsen DR (1979) DNA of human cytomegalovirus: size heterogeneity and defectiveness resulting from serial undiluted passage. J Virol 31:231–239

131. Stinski MF, Thomsen DR, Stenberg RM, Goldstein LC (1983) Organization and expression of the immediate early genes of human cytomegalovirus. J Virol 46:1–14
132. Taylor HP, Cooper NR (1990) The human cytomegalovirus receptor on fibroblasts is a 30-kilodalton membrane protein. J Virol 64:2484–2490
133. Welch AR, McGregor LM, Gibson W (1991) Cytomegalovirus G protein receptor homologue genes transcribed late. J Virol 65:3915–3918
134. Welch AR, McNally LK, Gibson W (1991) Cytomegalovirus assembly protein nested gene family: four 3′ coterminal transcripts encode four in-frame, overlapping proteins. J Virol 65:4091–4100
135. Welch AR, Woods AS, McNally LM, Cotter RJ, Gibson W (1991) A herpesvirus maturational proteinase, *assemblin*: identification of its gene, putative active site domain, and cleavage site. Proc Natl Acad Sci 88:10792–10796
136. Weller TH, Macaculey JE, Craig JM, Wirth P (1957) Isolation of intranuclear inclusion producing agents from infants illnesses resembling cytomegalic inclusion disease. Proc Soc Exp Biol 94:4–12
137. Weston K (1988) An enhancer element in the short unique region of human cytomegalovirus regulates the production of a group of abundant immediate early transcripts. Virology 162:406–416
138. Wilkinson GWG, Akrigg A, Greenaway PJ (1984) Transcription of the immediate early genes of human cytomegalovirus strain AD169. Virus Res 1:101–111
139. Wright DA, Staprans SI, Spector DH (1988) Four phosphoproteins with common amino termini are encoded by human cytomegalovirus AD169. J Virol 62:331–340

Chapter 17 Immediate-Early Genes of Human Cytomegalovirus: Organization and Function *

Richard M. Stenberg

Summary

Immediate-early (IE) genes of human cytomegalovirus are the first genes expressed after the virus infects the cell. The most extensively characterized of the IE genes is the major IE gene region. Originating from this gene is a series of overlapping mRNAs which encode proteins that have common and unique domains. Functionally, at least three IE proteins, IE 72, IE 55, and IE 86, are responsible for regulation of viral promoters. These proteins interact to enhance and repress expression of the major IE promoter resulting in a coordinate regulation that affects the balance of IE gene expression. In addition, IE proteins interact with cell factors during regulation of viral gene expression to activate early promoters. Therefore, the coordinate regulation of IE genes and their corresponding proteins, by cellular proteins in the infected cell, is likely to be the single most important determinant influencing the outcome of human cytomegalovirus infection.

Introduction

During the past decade, a great deal of new information has been generated concerning the organization, structure, and function of the immediate-early (IE) genes of human cytomegalovirus (HCMV). By definition, expression of IE genes requires no prior protein synthesis since these genes are transcribed in the presence of protein synthesis inhibitors such as cycloheximide. Consequently, IE genes are the first genes expressed after the virus infects the host cell and are thought to regulate subsequent viral and cellular gene expression. These genes are transcribed from a limited region of the HCMV genome and are comprised of at least four transcription units. The most widely studied IE gene is transcribed from the most abundantly expressed or major IE promoter (MIEP) and consists of IE coding regions one (IE 1) and two (IE 2). This

---

Department of Microbiology and Immunology, Eastern Virginia Medical School, 700 West Olney Road, Norfolk, VA 23501-1980, USA

* This work was supported by Public Health Service Grant AI-23313 from the National Institutes of Health

chapter presents information currently available concerning the genomic location of the IE genes, the structure of the IE proteins, and the potential role(s) of IE proteins in regulating gene expression in the infected cell.

Immediate-Early Protein Synthesis

Early studies of CMV gene expression, using cycloheximide to inhibit protein synthesis, demonstrated that a restricted class of proteins was synthesized immediately after removal of the drug [3, 26, 73]. The most abundant protein migrates as a heterogeneous band of approximately 72 kDa on sodium dodecyl sulfate-polyacrylamide gels. Two other proteins are also evident at approximately 55 and 38 kDa. Because the kinetics of appearance of these proteins differed from that of other infected cell proteins produced later in infection, they were proposed to be a separate class of proteins and were referred to as immediate-early [73].

Further kinetic analysis of IE protein synthesis, using human convalescent sera to immune precipitate viral proteins, demonstrated that complicated levels of regulation exist during synthesis of IE proteins [3]. The first proteins synthesized are the 72-kDa (77 kDa-) and the 55-kDa (52-kDa) proteins (Fig. 1). These proteins appear within 1 h after virus adsorption and clearly precede the appearance of other IE proteins. By 2.5 h, the 38-kDa (41-kDa) protein appears as well as two other proteins of 86 (87 kDa) and 97 kDa. As infection proceeds, the mobility of the 72-kDa protein changes to a faster moving form (68 kDa), indicating that posttranslational modification may occur after the onset of IE protein synthesis. This shift in mobility may be due to changes in phosphorylation since the 72-kDa protein is modified by phosphate [26]. However, Tsutsui and coworkers [80, 81] presented evidence that the 68-kDa protein was primarily associated with the cytoplasm and suggested that this protein is not a modification of the 72-kDa protein. Clearly, there is variation in the appearance of IE proteins or forms of IE proteins during the initial phase of infection. These data indicate that an additional level of regulation may exist within the IE phase of replication, or that several of these proteins, by definition, are not IE.

Immediate-Early Gene Expression

Historical studies on IE transcription demonstrated that a limited region of the viral genome is expressed [17, 47, 82, 83] (Fig. 2). The most abundantly expressed region is located in the long unique component of the viral genome within the *Xba*I E fragment (map units, mu, 0.68–0.77). Another region that is transcribed at high levels exists in the adjacent *Xba*I N fragment (mu 0.66–0.68). At least two other regions of the genome are transcribed at IE times, one

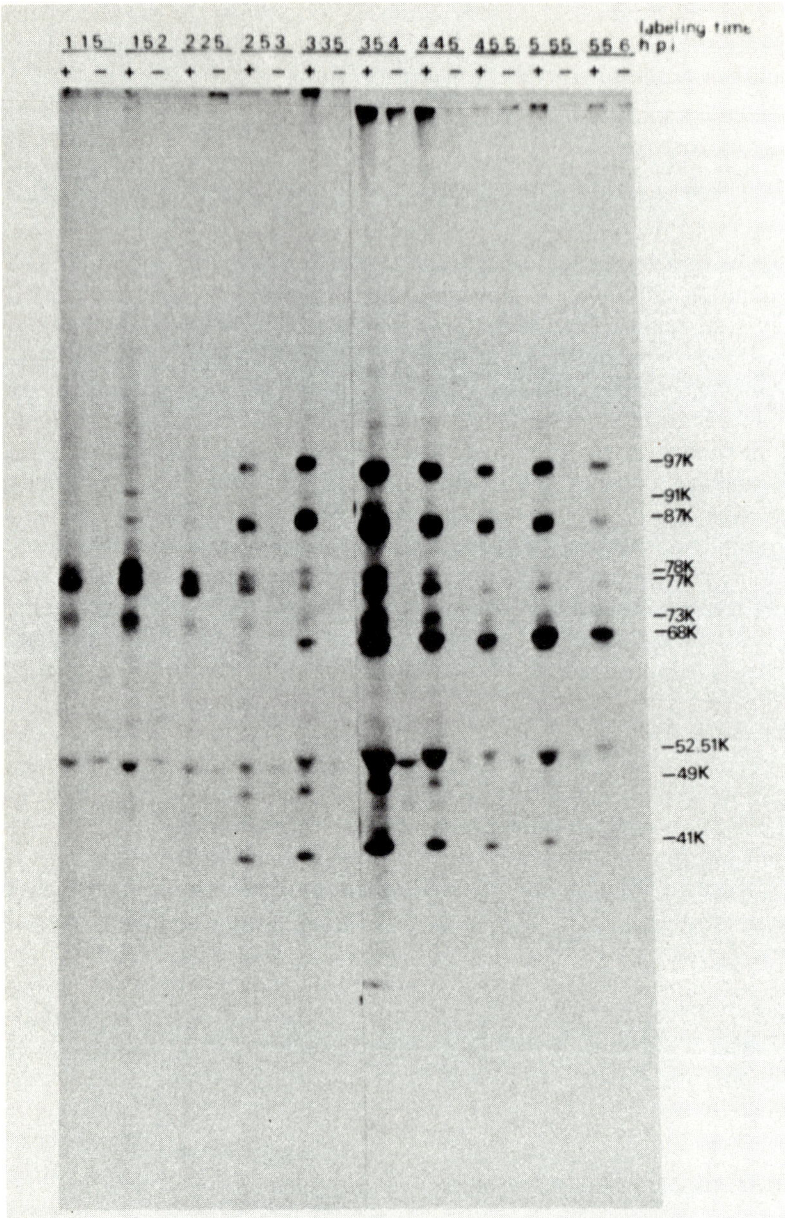

Fig. 1. Time course of appearance of immunoprecipitable ICSPs. Infected cells were pulse-labeled for ten sequential 30-min intervals beginning 1 h after virus adsorption. Cell extracts were made following each labeling period, and cleared extracts were analyzed by immunoprecipitation with 10 µl CMV positive (+) or CMV negative (–) serum. Immunoprecipitates were electrophoresed on 5%–12% gradient SDS-PAGE. ICSPs are labeled as to their apparent molecular weight. (Reprinted with permission from [3])

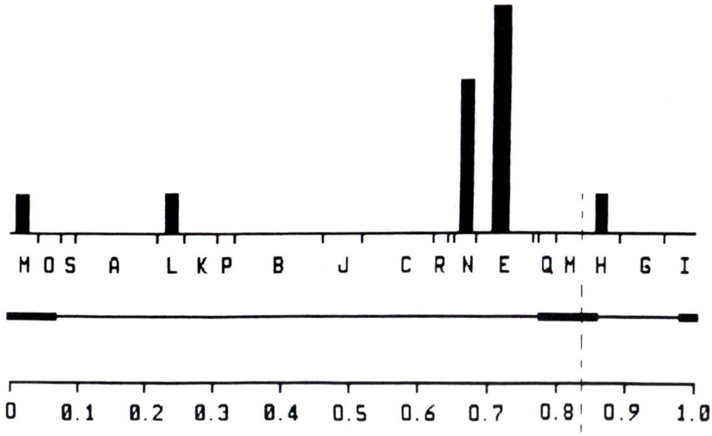

Fig. 2. Relative level of gene expression from the HCMV genome under IE conditions. *Solid bars*, relative level of gene expression. *Below*, the *Xba*I restriction endonuclease map and the map coordinates (Adapted from [82])

in the short unique (*Xba*I H) and the other in the long unique (*Xba*I L, mu 0.22–0.26). After IE protein synthesis, the pattern of CMV gene expression switches from limited to extensive transcription with RNAs originating from virtually every region of the viral genome [17, 47, 82, 83]. This was the first evidence that IE proteins were important regulatory molecules for the expression of HCMV genes.

Organization and Expression of Immediate-Early Genes

Analysis of mRNA produced under IE conditions demonstrated that two size classes are predominantly associated with polysomes, one of 4.8–5.2 kb (mu 0.66–0.68) and another of 1.9–2.2 kb (mu 0.68–0.77) [17, 82, 83]. Also associated with polysomes under IE conditions are less abundant RNAs of 2.0 kb (mu 0.22–0.26) and 0.9 kb (short unique) [82, 83]. These transcription units are discussed individually below.

Major IE Gene Region

More detailed studies on IE transcription revealed that the region located between mu 0.68 and 0.77 actually consists of several subregions capable of encoding proteins [33, 75, 85] (Fig. 3). The most abundant RNA associated with the polysomes is a species of 1.9 kb that originates from mu 0.739–0.751. This is commonly referred to as immediate early region 1 (IE 1) or the major immediate early gene [75]. This is also referred to as UL 123 based on the new

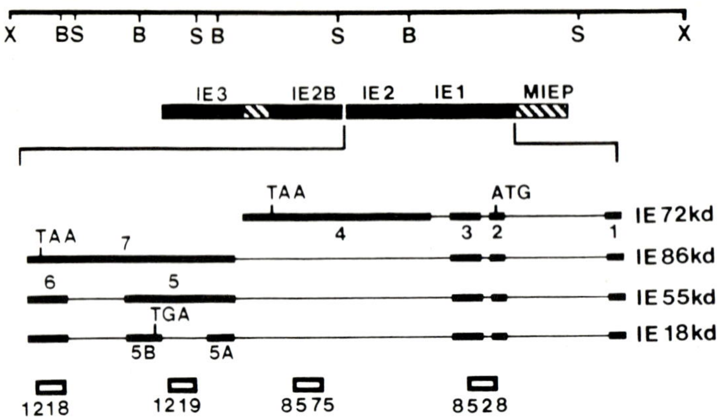

Fig. 3. Structure of the IE gene region. *Heavy black lines*, IE genes located within *Xba*I E, labeled accordingly; *hatched boxes*, promoters. *Below*, IE RNAs of known structure including the locations of introns (*light lines*) and exons (*bold lines*); exons are numbered as described elsewhere [70]; initiation (ATG) and termination (TAA) codons are indicated. *Above*, map of *Xba*I E and its corresponding *Xba*I (*X*), *Bam*HI (*B*) and *Sal*I (*S*) sites. Antibodies are indicated with respect to peptide location [70]

nomenclature employed since the HCMV genome was completely sequenced [8]. Translation of IE1 mRNA in cell-free systems demonstrated that this gene codes for the predominant IE protein of 72 kDa [33, 75, 85], also referred to as the major IE protein [75].

Adjacent and 3′ to IE1 is another coding region that expresses protein under IE conditions, and which is referred to as IE region 2 (IE2) [75] (Fig. 3). Analysis of polysome-associated RNA isolated from cells infected with HCMV Towne demonstrated that IE2 is capable of coding for several RNAs that range from 1.1 to 2.2 kb. These RNAs, when translated in cell-free systems, are capable of synthesizing several proteins which range from 16 to 56 kDa [75]. It is important to note that analysis of polysome-associated RNA revealed that IE1 is expressed in significantly greater quantities than IE2, and that IE2 mRNAs are present in approximately equal proportion [75] relative to each other.

Studies on RNA isolated from cells infected with HCMV strain AD169 demonstrated striking differences in IE2 RNA abundance [33, 85]. Examination of whole cell RNA originating from IE2 indicated that the predominant species is 2.2 kb, and that other previously described IE2 RNAs were undetectable [33]. In a second study, examination of cytoplasmic RNA demonstrated that the 2.2-kb and the 1.7-kb transcripts are present in relatively equal proportions [85]. However, in both of these studies, the smaller IE2 RNAs (1.4 and 1.1 kb) were not evident. It has been proposed that these differences might be due to variation between strains Towne and AD169. However, recent studies suggest that the observed differences are due to the types of RNA isolated (polysomal versus cytoplasmic versus whole cell) and are likely a consequence of compartmentalization of selected IE mRNAs. Subsequent examination of cytoplasmic RNA from cells infected with the Towne strain revealed equal levels of the 1.7- and 2.2-kb species, and these species were abundant relative to the IE1 1.9-kb mRNA [70]. These data are consistent with the data obtained with AD169 and imply that the 2.2-kb mRNA is preferentially excluded from polysomes at IE times. Consistent with this, Tenney and Colberg-Poley [77] recently compared polysome associated and cytoplasmic RNA from IE1 and 2 at 4 h after infection. They demonstrated that while the 1.9-kb mRNA was abundantly expressed on polysomes, the 2.2-kb mRNA was virtually undetectable on polysomes. Analysis of cytoplasmic RNA demonstrated that both species were readily detectable, and that the 2.2-kb mRNA was actually present in higher relative quantities. Taken together, these studies confirm and extend our studies and demonstrate that posttranscriptional regulation occurs during the IE phase, and that certain species of RNA are selectively associated with polysomes under IE conditions. This is not surprising since posttranscriptional regulation has been proposed as a means to regulate HCMV gene expression [21, 22, 27, 70]. The expression of the major IE gene region at early and late times is discussed in more detail below.

Translation of AD169 IE2 mRNAs in cell-free systems revealed similar patterns of protein synthesis as Towne mRNAs [85]. However, it is interesting to note that the 2.2-kb mRNA, which encodes the 86-kDa protein (see below), is not translated in any of the in vitro studies reported [5, 75, 85]. Also, this protein appears after the other IE proteins during pulse labeling experiments [2] (Fig. 1). Together, these data suggest that IE protein synthesis is necessary prior to translation of the 86-kDa protein.

Studies on the structure of the major IE gene region by Stinski et al. [75] demonstrated that the major IE mRNA, although only 1.9 kb in length, is capable of hybridizing across a 2.7-kb region of the CMV genome. This indicated the presence of intervening sequences within IE1. Studies on the structure of polysome-associated RNA demonstrated that IE1 mRNA is composed of four exons totaling 1741 nucleotides [68] (Fig. 3). DNA sequence analysis demonstrates that the major IE protein (72 kDa, IE72) contains 491 amino acids and has a theoretical molecular weight of 55 kDa.

Structural analysis of IE region 2 demonstrates that IE2 mRNAs share sequences with IE1 mRNAs [69]. The 5′ end of the IE region 2 coding domain is located 35 n 3′ of IE1 and consists of spliced and unspliced exons. The predominant IE2 related mRNAs are spliced onto the first three exons of IE1 and consequently are transcribed from the same promoter, initiate translation at the same AUG methionine residue, and share amino terminal sequences through the first 85 amino acids. The 1.7- and 2.2-kb mRNAs differ due to a splice in the 3′ region of the gene which effectively removes a protein domain from IE55, thereby distinguishing it from IE86 [69, 70]. The structures of the IE RNAs have been recently confirmed by cDNA analysis and are depicted in Fig. 3.

Analysis of IE proteins using specific peptide antibodies demonstrated that (a) IE2 related proteins IE86 and IE55 originate from the 2.2- and 1.7 kb mRNAs, respectively, (c) IE1 codes for 38- and 31 kDa proteins which arise from minor spliced RNAs, and (c) two additional IE proteins originate from IE2 (27 and 23 kDa) [70] (Fig. 4). These latter IE2 proteins may originate from the 1.4- and 1.1-kb IE2 mRNAs [69, 70, 75].

More recently, a fourth RNA from the major IE gene region has been characterized (Stenberg et al., unpublished data). Nuclease analysis of

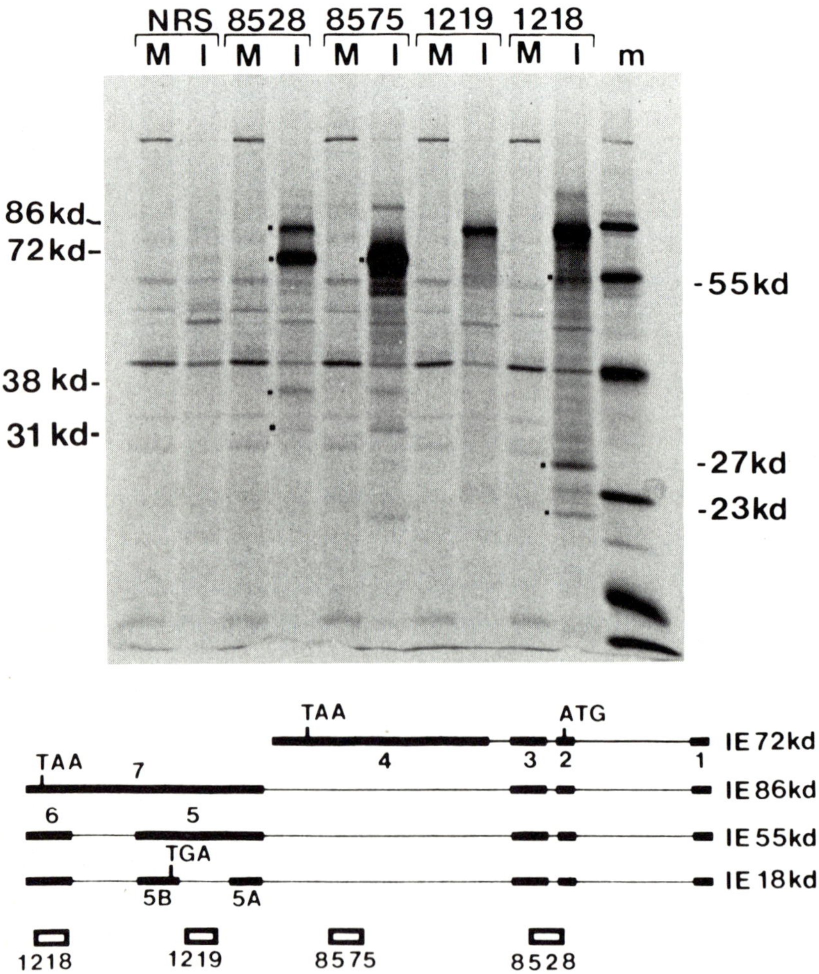

Fig. 4. Peptide mapping of IE proteins. Infected (*I*) and mock-infected (*M*) cells were treated with cycloheximide, reversed, and labeled with [^{35}S]-methionine for 2 h. Extracts were prepared and reacted with anti-peptide antibodies or normal rabbit serum (*NRS*). Precipitated products were subjected to SDS-PAGE [70]. The peptide antibodies and the locations of the corresponding peptides are indicated. IE proteins are indicated in kilodaltons (*kd*). *Below*, map of the major IE gene region (described in the legend to Fig. 3). (Adapted from [70])

polysome-associated RNA as well as cDNA analysis has demonstrated a previously uncharacterized splice within exon 5. The results in a premature termination of the reading frame and a truncated version of IE 55 and IE 86. The structure of this mRNA is shown in Fig. 3.

An additional IE gene region exists 3′ to IE 2 and has been referred to as IE region 2 B [31] (Fig. 3). Evidence suggests that IE RNAs from region 2 B are spliced onto region 2 specific sequences [69]. However, this gene is expressed at low levels under IE conditions, and to date it has not been conclusively shown that this region codes for any viral proteins during the IE phase of HCMV infection.

UL 119-115

This transcription unit was formerly referred to as IE region 3 (see Fig. 3) but has recently been more extensively characterized and is now referred to as UL 119-115 [41, 75]. This region contains multiple promoters that function at IE and late times after infection and codes for a series of complex spliced mRNAs [41]. As is the case for the major IE gene region, this IE region contains internal nested promoters that function at late times allowing for amplified expression of downstream reading frames. The reasons that HCMV employs these types of mechanisms remains unclear. The protein products encoded by this region and their potential functions are unknown at this time.

UL 36-38

Wathen and Stinski [82] originally described a 1.9- to 2.0-kb polysomal mRNA that originates from the *Xba*I L fragment between mu 0.22 and 0.26. Wilkinson et al. [85] also demonstrated IE RNA originating from this region although their examination of cytoplasmic RNA revealed two species of 1.7 and 3.8 kb. These mRNAs appear to code for translation products of approximately 40 and 50 kDa, respectively. More recent studies have demonstrated several mRNAs which are expressed throughout the HCMV replicative cycle [39, 76, 77]. The mRNAs from this region are generated by alternative splicing and consist of two mRNAs in the 1.8- to 1.9-kb size range, a 1.3-kb mRNA, and a minor RNA of 3.4 kb which is poorly expressed on polysomes. These mRNAs are temporally regulated throughout the HCMV replicative cycle and also contain internal nested promoters that function at different times [77].

Recently, products of this region have been shown to work with IE 1 or IE 2 gene products to activate homologous or heterologous promoters in permissive human fibroblasts [11]. However, individually these proteins work poorly implying that they may act as cofactors for transcription activation during HCMV infection. More detailed studies on the role of individual proteins are necessary prior to drawing conclusions as to their functional role.

US3

Wathen and Stinski [82] described a low-abundance, polysome-associated RNA of 0.9 kb originating from the *Xba*I D region of the viral genome. More recently, Weston [84] demonstrated that several IE RNAs are transcribed from the short unique component of the viral genome, and that expression occurs throughout infection. Weston [84] also demonstrated that this region is transcribed from a promoter that has homology with the MIEP enhancer sequence [4, 79], thereby suggesting a common mechanism for transcription of IE genes. RNAs are expressed from this region during the IE and early phase but are apparently repressed later in infection [77].

As in the case of UL36-38, vectors capable of expressing US 3 gene products have been shown to activate a HCMV early promoter in permissive cells, but only in the presence of IE 2 constructs [11]. This implies that these proteins may exist as components of larger transcription complexes capable of regulating HCMV gene expression.

Map Units 0.66–0.68

A region of abundant IE transcription resides adjacent to IE 1 and 2 between mu 0.66 and 0.68. This region codes for two RNAs of 4.8 and 5.0 kb that are abundantly expressed at both IE and late times after infection [82, 83]. However, this gene does not have a significant open reading frame, and by all criteria these RNAs do not appear to encode proteins [57]. RNA from this region is present in both the nucleus and cytoplasm as well as the poly A+ and poly A– fractions [57]. In addition, this region has been shown to transform cells in vitro [52]. To date, it is not clear what role this gene plays during HCMV infection.

Expression of RNA and Protein from the Immediate-Early Gene Region at Early and Late Times After Infection

As stated above, early studies by Blanton and Tevethia (1981) demonstrated that IE proteins vary in their time of appearance after infection (Fig. 1). The first proteins detected in the infected cell are IE 72 and IE 55, which are evident within 1 h after virus adsorption. However, appearance of IE 86 is delayed relative to other IE proteins and does not appear until 2.5 h after infection. This is consistent with the finding that the majority of the 2.2-kb mRNA, which codes for IE 86, is absent from polysomes under IE conditions [70, 77]. These data indicate that gene expression from the IE gene region is regulated post-IE.

Synthesis of IE 72 reaches a maximum within a few hours after infection and subsequently declines [3] (Fig. 1). However, steady-state levels continue to

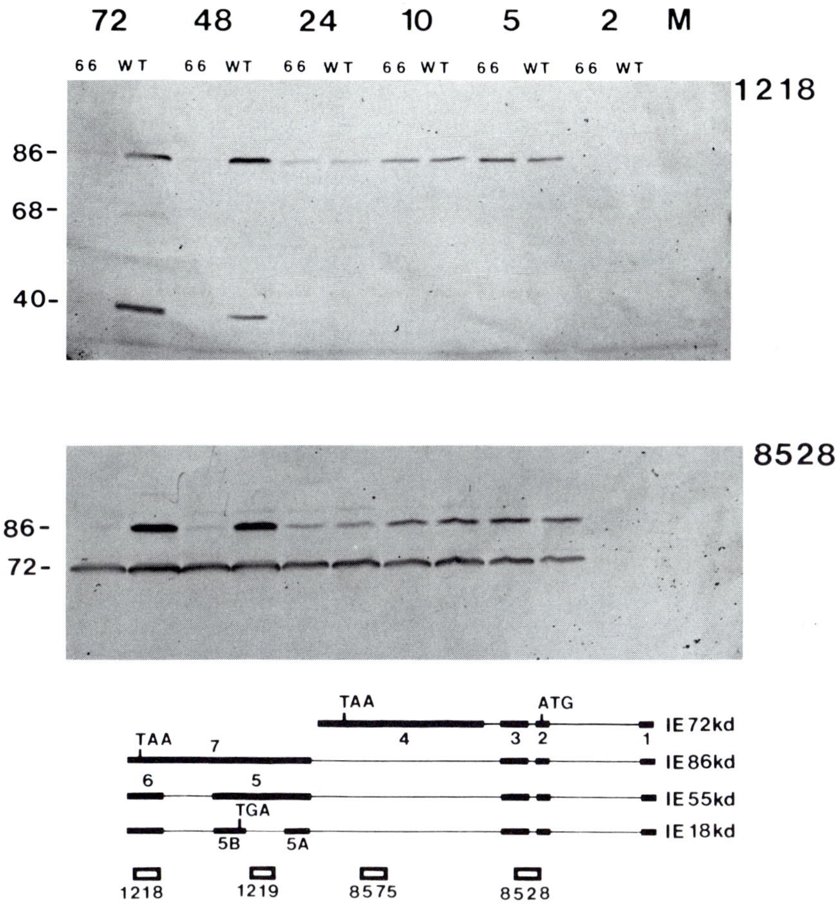

Fig. 5. Steate-state levels of region 1 and 2 proteins. Human fibroblast cells were infected with wild type (*WT*) HCMV or ts66 (*66*) at 39.5 °C and harvested at the indicated times. Samples were subjected to SDS-PAGE and western blot analysis using anti-peptide antibodies 1218 or 8528 (see Fig. 3). *Below,* map of the major IE gene region (described in the legend to Fig. 3). (Adapted from [70])

increase slowly throughout infection, suggesting that IE 72 is quite stable [70] (Fig. 5). Synthesis of IE 86 reaches a maximum by 4 h after infection [3], but the steady state levels decrease until the onset of DNA replication, after which IE 86 expression increases dramatically [70] (Fig. 5).

An investigation of RNA originating from IE 1 and 2 during the course of infection demonstrates that (a) the level of RNA present at late times is significantly higher than that at IE times [70], (b) IE 1 RNA is repressed post-IE although detectable levels exist throughout infection [67] (Fig. 6), (c) IE 2 RNAs increase throughout the course of infection [69, 70] (Fig. 6), (d) RNA which codes for IE 86 (2.2 kb) is down-regulated through 24 h and reexpressed

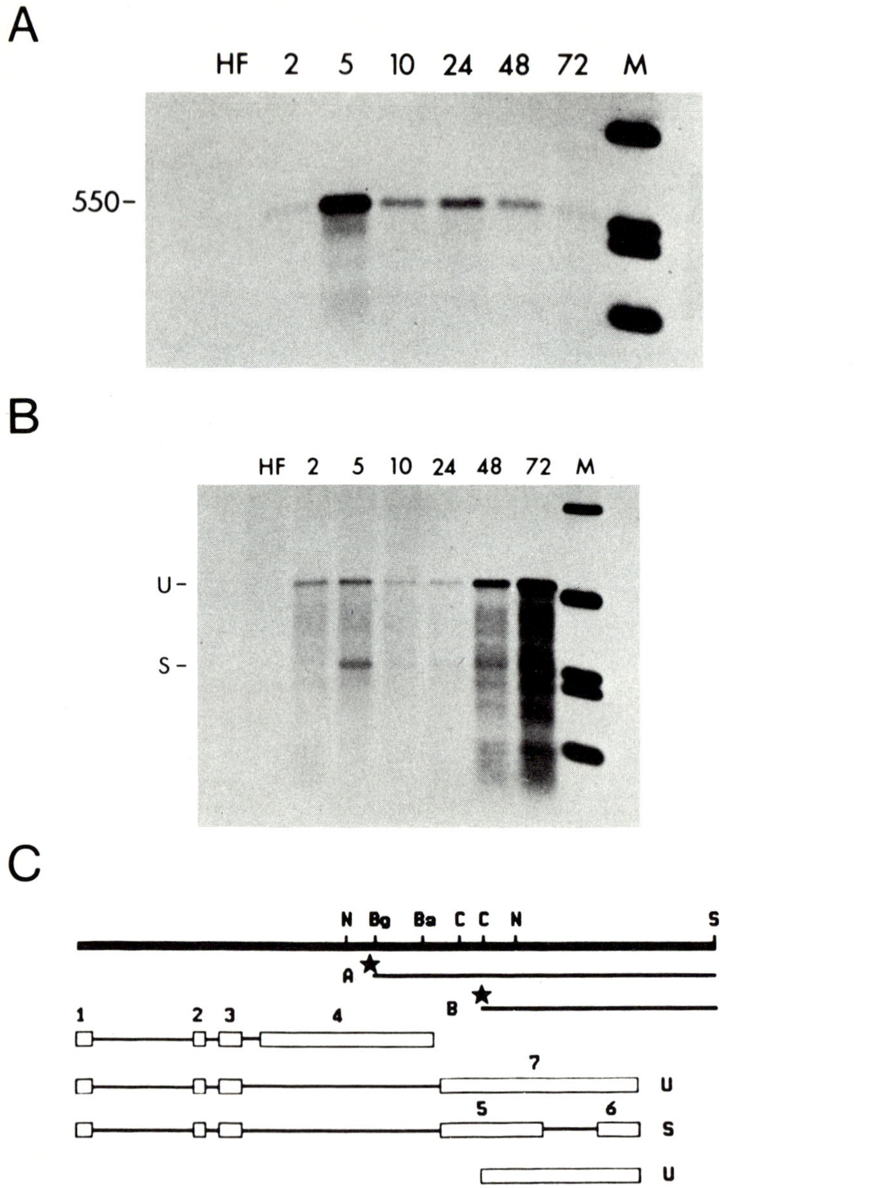

Fig. 6. Steady-state levels of region 1 and 2 RNAs. Whole-cell RNA was isolated from CMV-infected cells at the indicated times and subjected to mung bean nuclease analysis. IE 1 (*A*) and IE 2 (*B*) specific RNA was analyzed using the probes indicated in *panel C*. IE 1 RNA is indicated by the 550-nucleotide band in *panel A* and IE 2 RNAs are represented by the spliced (*S*) and unspliced (*U*) exons. *Panel C*, IE gene region and the corresponding RNAs [70]. *HF*, Uninfected human fibroblast RNA; *M*, molecular weight markers; *N*, *Nco*I; *Bg*, *Bgl*II; *Ba*, *BAM*HI; *C*, *Cla*I; *N*, *Nco*I; *S*, *Sal*I; *asterisks*, 3′ end-label. (Adapted from [67, 69])

late in infection but only after DNA replication [70], and (e) an unspliced RNA from region 2 is expressed late in infection, only after DNA replication, and encodes a 40-kDa late protein [70].

As discussed above, posttranscriptional regulation appears to play a major role during HCMV infection, especially with respect to regulation of IE genes. This is supported by the fact that all the IE RNAs from IE1 and 2 are transcribed from the MIEP [69, 70]. Because of this, the eventual translation of individual IE mRNAs on polysomes depends on posttranscriptional regulatory events such as (a) 3′ end addition, (b) splicing of a primary transcript into one of the many IE RNAs, (c) nuclear transport, or (d) selective association or exclusion of certain RNA species with the polysomes. While it is possible and even likely that regulation of IE RNA could occur at each level, to date there is little information on this subject. In addition, because the MIEP functions throughout infection, and because the relative level of individual IE RNAs changes over time, these posttranscriptional regulatory events must continue through early and late times to affect the level of RNA originating from this region [70].

Regulation of the MIEP by IE Gene Products

Early studies on IE protein function demonstrated that IE72 is capable of regulating IE1 mRNA levels in non-permissive cells [69]. Other studies using nonpermissive cells demonstrated that IE2 proteins can repress MIEP function [56]. The MIEP contains a number of repeated elements as well as discrete sequences that are involved in regulating IE transcription [4, 23, 30, 53, 57, 64, 74, 79]. To date it is not clear how IE proteins function to affect MIEP activity, but the cell probably plays a major role in determining the outcome. Interaction of the MIEP with virus- and cell-specific regulatory proteins likely dictates the level of IE gene expression and consequently could determine the outcome of infection. Clearly, studies by Nelson et al. [53] demonstrate that MIEP function differs under permissive and nonpermissive conditions, and that the difference is independent of viral proteins. This area is covered in greater depth in the chapter by Ghazal and Nelson (this volume).

Studies in permissive human fibroblast cells demonstrate that IE proteins greatly affect MIEP function in a coordinated and balanced manner. IE72 causes an increase in MIEP function [9, 71], as does IE55 [2]. In contrast, IE86 represses MIEP function [71]. This is consistent with previous studies which demonstrated that IE2 genomic clones were capable of repressing MIEP function in nonpermissive cells [55]. The *cis* repression signal (CRS) of the MIEP has been mapped and shown by three separate groups to span the CAP site although interaction of IE proteins with this element has not been demonstrated [10, 44, 55]. Mutations in IE2, which fail to repress the MIEP, result in increased levels of all the IE proteins [71] (Fig. 7). Together, IE72 and IE86 interact to regulate the MIEP to obtain an intermediate level of promoter

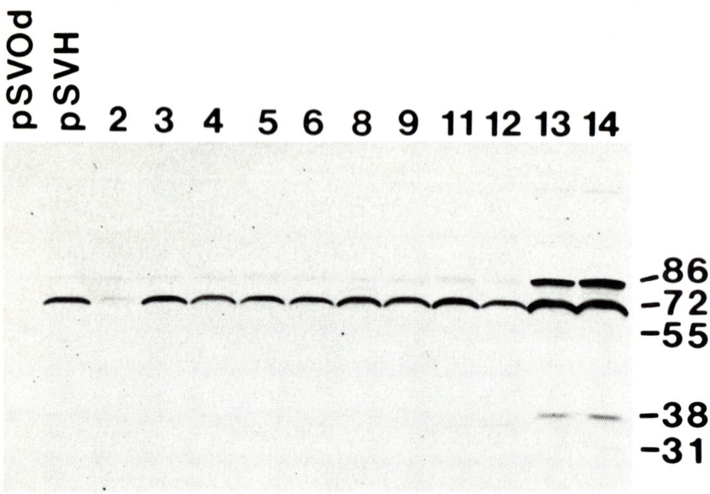

Fig. 7. Proteins expressed by IE insertion mutants. Human fibroblast cells were transfected with 10 μg of the indicated mutant and cells harvested after 48 h. Samples were subjected to western blot analysis using anti-peptide antibody 8528 (see Fig. 3). Protein molecular weights are expressed in kilodaltons. (Reprinted from [71] with permission)

activity [71]. Consequently, any perturbation of IE protein function may cause an imbalance of IE proteins which could result in an abortive infection.

Regulation of HCMV Early Gene Expression

For many years it has been assumed that IE proteins function to regulate gene expression in HCMV-infected cells. Initial studies on IE protein function demonstrated that IE1 and 2 can (a) activate heterologous viral and cellular promoters [15, 19, 20, 31, 56, 78], (b) complement adenovirus E1A deletion mutants and allow for the growth of defective virus [78], and (c) repress expression of IE gene products in nonpermissive cells [56, 69]. Spaete and Mocarski [62], using the promoter for the major early gene coupled to a reporter gene, demonstrated that an early promoter can be activated by superinfecting virus. Although viral protein synthesis was necessary for this effect, the role of IE proteins in early gene activation was not addressed.

To completely understand how IE proteins function to regulate HCMV early gene expression, one must consider the definition of an early gene. Historically, HCMV early genes are transcribed in the absence of viral DNA replication. However, this is probably an oversimplification of a complex class of genes that are regulated both transcriptionally and posttranscriptionally. Recently, a number of early genes have been mapped, allowing for specific analysis of individual genes [12–14, 28, 29, 32, 34, 37, 45, 48, 60, 65]. Also, the use of a temperature-sensitive, DNA negative mutant of HCMV demonstrates that various HCMV early RNAs are regulated differently after the onset of viral DNA replication. Figure 8 represents a comparison of the relative level of viral gene expression at early (ts 66) and late (WT) times after infection. This study demonstrates that early genes can be grouped into three classes. The first class is transcribed early and repressed late (E 1), the second class is transcribed at similar levels at early and late times (E 2), and the third class is transcribed at low levels early and at significantly higher levels late (E 3). Examples of these classes of early genes, as well as potential mechanisms involved in their regulation, are discussed below.

Activation of CMV Early Promoters by IE Gene Products

Recent studies have demonstrated that IE proteins are capable of activating HCMV early promoters [6, 18, 46, 66, 71], and that both IE 1 and 2 are required for maximal activity [6, 18, 46, 71]. A comparison of the relative expression of two early genes is shown in Fig. 9. The gene for HCMV DNA polymerase (pol) is expressed soon after infection, and the level of expression remains relatively constant throughout the course of infection [72]. In contrast, the gene for the major virion component (pp 65) is expressed at low levels at early times (5–24 h), but expression increases significantly later in infection [18].

Analysis of the pol and pp 65 promoters coupled to the CAT reporter gene demonstrates that both are activated by superinfecting virus, and that both IE 1 and 2 are required for maximal expression [18, 71]. IE 1 and 2, when separated and cotransfected, reconstruct the activation effect [18, 71], and mutations in IE 1 or 2 disrupt early gene activation [71]. Mutations in the common amino terminal region (exons 2 and 3), within exon 4 of IE 1, and within the carboxy terminus of IE 2 result in a decreased ability to activate HCMV early promoters (Fig. 10).

Analysis of individual IE gene products demonstrated that within IE 2, IE 86 is responsible for activation of early genes [71]. Use of cDNA expression vectors capable of expressing IE 86 (pIE 86) or IE 55 (pIE 55) demonstrated that IE 55 has no effect on activation of the pol promoter whereas IE 86 fully reconstructs the IE 2 effect (Fig. 11). The synergistic interaction of IE 72 and IE 86 indicates that complex formation by these two proteins may enhance their activation potential relative to what occurs when they act independently and suggests that the balance of IE proteins may be important to the regulation of virus gene expression.

Because the IE proteins influence MIEP expression, they may ultimately control their own level in the infected cell. In fact, cDNA expression vectors capable of expressing the individual IE proteins under the control of the MIEP generate high levels of IE 72 and IE 55 and low levels of IE 86 [71]. This is consistent with their relative influences on MIEP function. The inability of

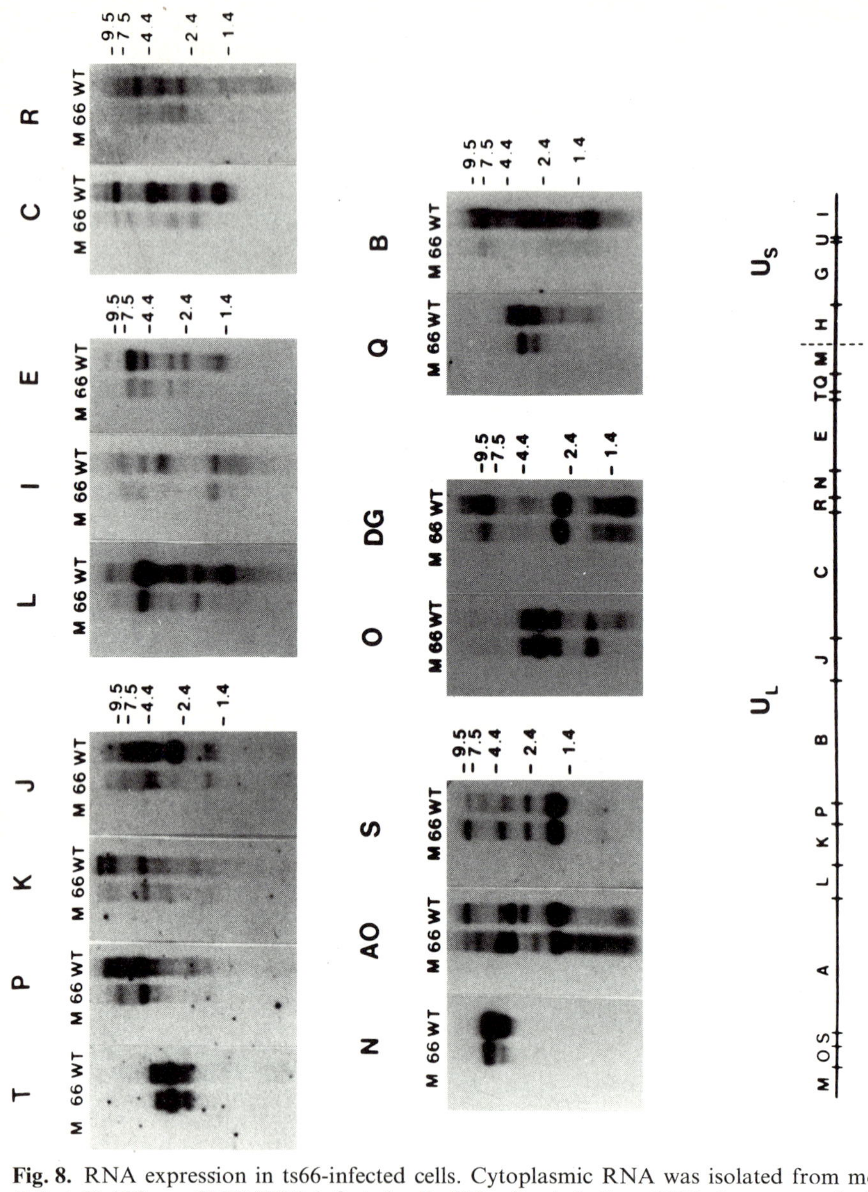

Fig. 8. RNA expression in ts66-infected cells. Cytoplasmic RNA was isolated from mock (*M*), ts66 (*66*), or CMV (*WT*) infected cells 72 h after infection. RNA from an equivalent number of infected cells was subjected to northern blot analysis and hybridized to the *Xba*I fragment indicated at the top of each blot. Molecular weights are indicated in kilobases. *Below*, *Xba*I restriction endonuclease map of the HCMV genome

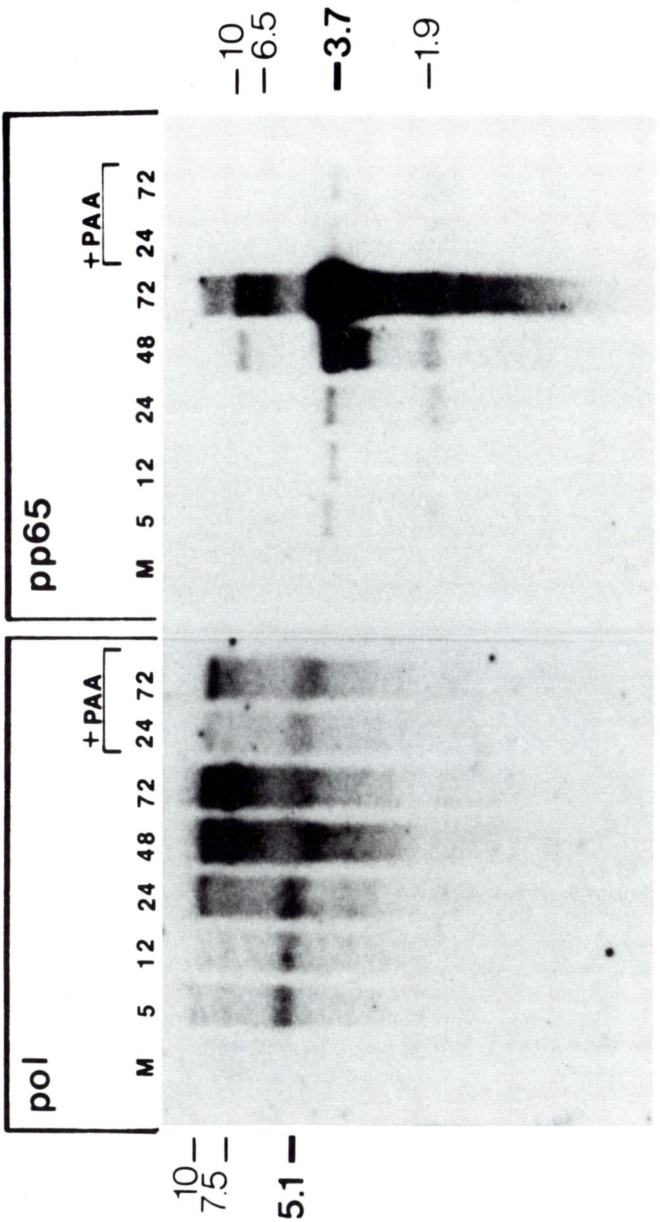

Fig. 9. Expression of DNA polymerase (*pol*) and pp65 genes. Whole-cell RNA was isolated at the indicated times (hours) from mock-infected cells (*M*) or cells infected in the presence or absence of phosphonoacetic acid (*PAA*) [40]. RNAs were subjected to northern blot analysis using single-strand RNA probes specific for pol or pp65. pol (*5.1*) and pp65 (*3.7*) RNAs are indicated

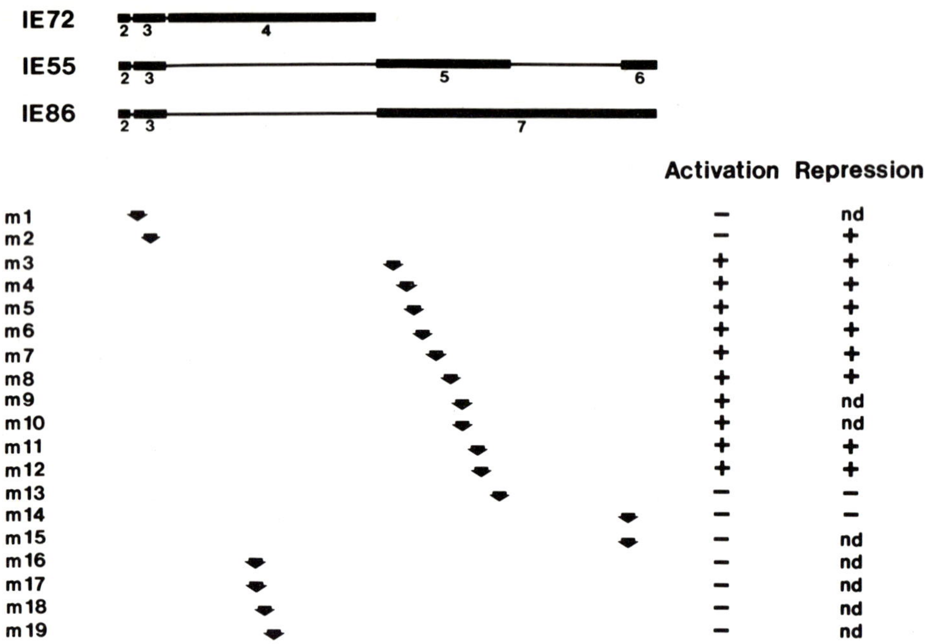

Fig. 10. Activation/repression by IE insertion mutants. The ability (+) or inability (–) of each mutant to activate the polymerase promoter or repress the MIEP is indicated. Activation and repression are based on CAT activity obtained as compared to the parental IE 1 and 2 plasmid pSVH. *Arrows*, locations of IE mutants. *nd*, Not determined (Reprinted from [71] with permission)

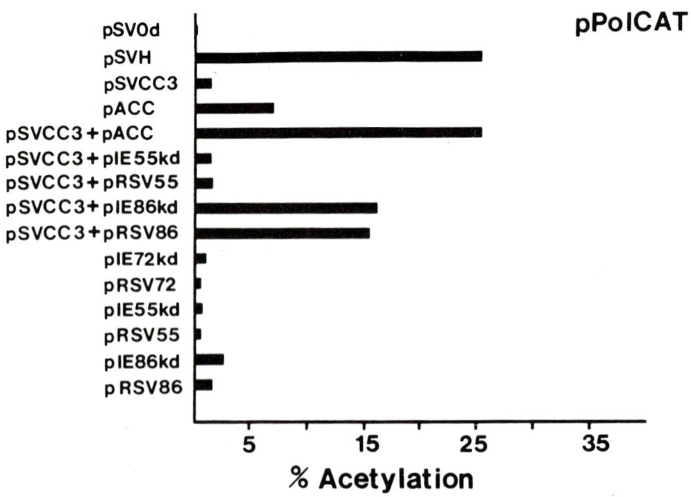

Fig. 11. IE cDNA activation of pPolCAT. Human fibroblast cells were transfected with pPolCAT (5 μg) and the indicated expression plasmids (5 μg) and subsequently assayed for CAT. Expression constructs are as described [25, 71]. CAT values are expressed as % acetylation

IE 86 to efficiently activate HCMV early promoters could be explained by insufficient levels of IE 86 protein. By expressing IE 86 independent of the MIEP and under the control of the Rous sarcoma virus (RSV) promoter this problem can be circumvented. Figure 11 demonstrates that pIE 86 and RSV 86 are identical in their actions on the DNA polymerase promoter, indicating that both IE 72 and IE 86 are necessary for synergistic activation of early promoters.

Functional Domains Within the IE Gene Region

The IE proteins of HCMV contain domains that are common or unique depending on the splicing of their corresponding RNAs. Consequently, these proteins contain potentially overlapping or unique functions depending on the presence or absence of a given functional domain. Early studies on IE protein function using nonpermissive cells demonstrated that IE 2 proteins are sufficient for activation of heterologous promoters [15, 20, 56] and repression of the MIEP [56]. However, other studies on IE protein function in non-permissive cells demonstrated a role for IE 72 in negative regulation of IE 1 [69]. The ambiguities of these studies probably reflect variation in cell type as well as differences in the assays employed. It should be noted however, that these studies are important since the ability or inability of HCMV to replicate in various cell types or tissues can ultimately determine whether the virus causes disease (see chapter by Ghazal and Nelson, this volume).

To date, only a limited number of studies have been performed to assess functional domains in permissive cells. Recent evidence demonstrates that within the IE gene region multiple functional regions are involved in activation of early promoters and/or repression of the MIEP [43, 46, 71]. Figure 10 shows the location of a series of linker insertion mutations within the IE gene region as well as the effect of those mutations on IE and early promoter function. The amino terminus of IE 1 and 2 is important for the activation of early promoters and possibly IE promoters. This region is characterized by two potential functional motifs, a proline-rich region between amino acids 11 and 25 and a leucine-rich stretch located in exon 3 (see Fig. 12). Studies on the transcription factor CTF/NF 1 have also implicated a proline-rich region as a transcriptional activator domain [49]. The significance of the leucine residues remains to be determined. Because exons 2 and 3 are common to many of the IE proteins, it is not surprising that this region should encode a potential activator domain. This is especially true since IE 72, IE 55, and IE 86 are capable of activating IE and/or early promoters [2, 71].

Exon 4 is also important for early promoter activation as mutations disrupt *trans*-activation potential. Within exon 4 exist two putative structures that resemble a zinc finger [50] and a leucine zipper [40] (Fig. 12). However, it should also be noted that IE 72 is hypersensitive to mutation, as all mutations tested to date abrogate function [71, 72]. The role of these domains in regulating HCMV gene expression remains to be tested.

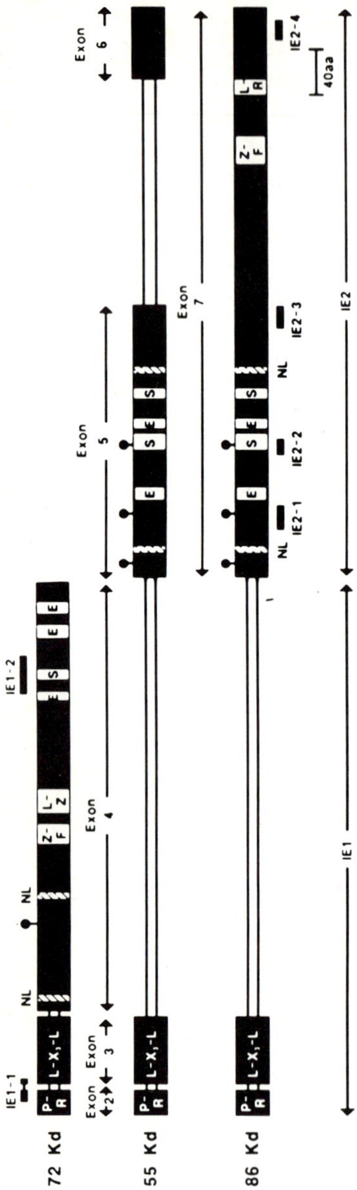

Fig. 12. Linear representations of the structures of IE 72, IE 55, and IE 86. *Large black boxes*, primary coding structures; *interconnecting bars*, intergenic regions (not to scale); *horizontal arrows*, exons of the IE 1 and IE 2 regions; *small black boxes*, location of peptides. The scale indicates amino acid number; structural features of interest are indicated within the coding region. *P-R*, Proline-rich region; *L-X3-L*, leucine repeat unit; *NL*, nuclear localization sequence; *Z-F*, putative zinc finger; *L-Z*, putative leucine zipper; *L-R*, leucine-rich region; *E*, polyglutamic acid region; *S*, polyserine region; *P*, potential glycosylation sites; *Kd*, kilodaltons

Finally, the carboxy terminus of IE 2 is involved in both activation of early promoters and repression of the MIEP in permissive cells [43, 46, 71]. Mutations in the carboxy terminus fail to repress the MIEP, cause an increase in promoter activity relative to basal levels, and result in increased production of IE proteins (Figs. 7, 10). This domain also contains a putative zinc finger structure as well as a leucine-rich stretch within the IE 2 intron. Consequently, these functional regions are unique to IE 86 and are consistent with its associated functions of early promoter activation and MIEP repression.

Sequence-Specific Activation of CMV Early Promoters

From recent studies, it is clear that IE proteins function to regulate early gene expression by activating early promoters. Analysis of sequences responsible for promoter-specific activation demonstrate the involvement of discrete sequences containing direct and inverted repeats [6, 18, 36, 46, 66, 71]. However, upon close inspection of these sequences, there appears to be little to no homology between HCMV promoters or their respective repeats. In addition, the number and types of repeats vary among the different promoters.

A comparative analysis of two early promoters, an E 2 promoter (pol) and an E 3 promoter (pp 65) demonstrates that sequences 5′ to the CAP site are responsible for the differential regulation of these genes. Deletion studies of the pol promoter indicate the presence of an attenuator sequence between –268 and –128 relative to the CAP site [72] (Fig. 13). Sequential removal of these

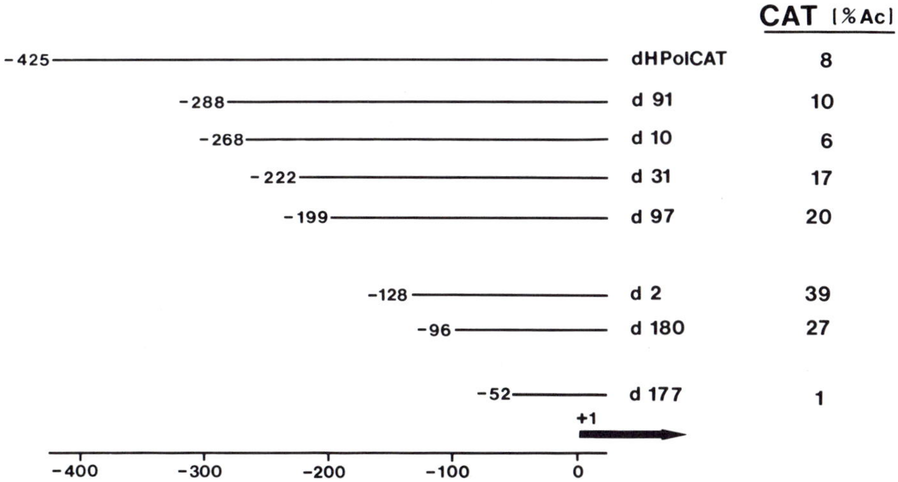

Fig. 13. Deletion analysis of the DNA polymerase promoter. Deletion mutants of pPolCAT were generated by partial restriction endonuclease digestion with *Hae*III or *Nla*IV. Mutants were transfected with pSVH (IE 1 and 2) as described [71] and CAT activity (*%Ac*) assessed after 48 h

sequences results in a gradual increase in promoter function that eventually reaches fivefold. However, deletion of sequences 3′ to this region (–128) results in abrogation of pol promoter function. Within this region exists a discrete sequence (DR 1/ATF) that contains a 12n direct repeat adjacent to an ATF consensus binding site (Fig. 14). This element can be transferred to a promoter that is poorly responsive to IE proteins and subsequently confer responsiveness, indicating that DR1/ATF can mediate synergistic activation by IE proteins (Fig. 15).

Similar studies on pp65 promoter function demonstrate that deletion of upstream sequences (–306 to –61) has no effect on promoter activity [18]. However, deletion to –52 results in dramatic reduction of promoter function and this response is identical for either superinfecting virus or cotransfected plasmids capable of expressing IE proteins [18]. Inspection of the sequence reveals the presence of an octamer repeat which appears responsible for activation.

These studies taken together indicate that some early genes may have attenuator sequences that repress or modulate expression late in infection. Chang et al. [6] suggested that an early gene located in the *Xba*I O fragment contains an inhibitory sequence since deletion within the promoter resulted in increased activity. By our definition, the gene in that study is an E 1 early gene as the expression of its RNA (1.5–1.7 kb) is repressed late in infection [6] (Fig. 7). In contrast, E 3 genes such as pp 65 do not appear to have sequences that attenuate expression. E 3 genes could then be expressed at higher levels at late times due to (a) increased available template, (b) additional proteins involved in late gene expression, or (c) a combination of the two effects. Further studies are necessary to resolve these possibilities.

```
-425 GAATTCAACT CGTACAAGCA GCGGGTAAAG TACGTGGAGG ACAAGGTAGT CGACCCGCTA
     EcoRI
-365 CCGCCCTACC TCAAGGGTCT GGACGACCTC ATGAGCGGCC TGGGCGCCGC GGGAAAGGCC
                       d91                        d10
-305 GTTGGCGTAG CCATTGGGGC CGTGGGTGGC GCGGTGGCCT CCGTGGTCGA AGGCGTTGCC
                           d31                         d97
-245 ACCTTCCTCA AAAACCCCTT CGGAGCCTTC ACCATCATCC TCGTGGCCAT AGCCGTAGTC
                            IR1                                    d2
-185 ATTATCACTT ATTTGATCTA TACTCGACAG CGGCGTCTGT GCACGCAGCC GCTGCAGAAC
                                 d180                         Pst I
-125 CTCTTTCCCT ATCTGGTGTC CGCCGACGGG ACCACCGTGA CGTCGGGCAG CACCAAAGAC
                d177                   DR1         Aat II        CAAT
 -65 ACGTCGTTAC AGGCTCCGCC TTCCTACGAG GAAAGTGTTT ATAATTCTGG TCGCAAAGGA
        +1→        IR1                            TATA
  -5 CCGGGACCAC CGTCGTCTGA TGCAT
        DR1               Nsi I
```

Fig. 14. Sequence of the pol promoter. Sequences from –425 to +20 are indicated. Direct (*DR*) and inverted (*IR*) repeats are indicated, as are the location of the deletion mutants. Sequences of interest are indicated. *+1*, CAP site

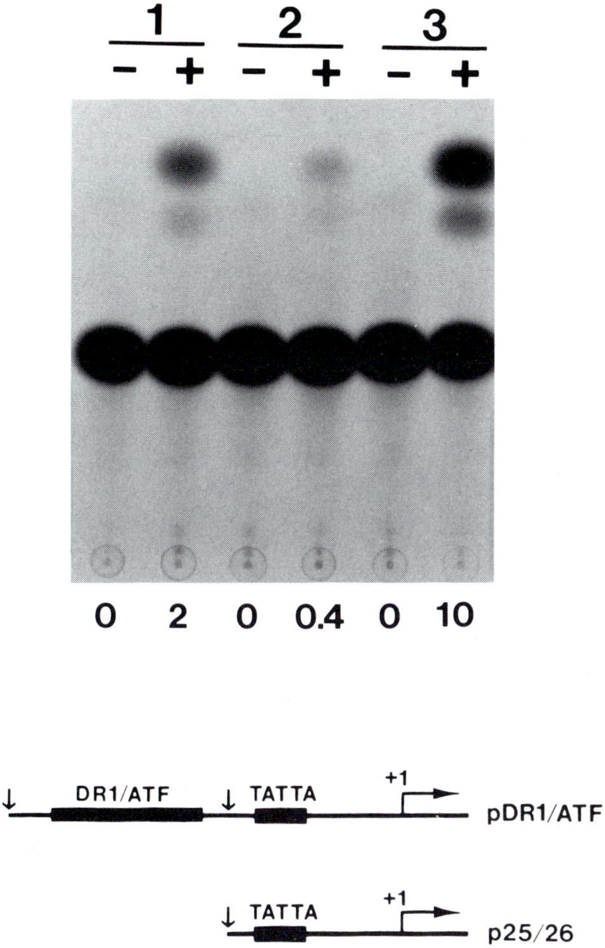

Fig. 15. Activation of pDR1/ATFCAT by IE proteins. Target promoter-CAT plasmids were cotransfected in the presence (+, pSVH) or absence (–, pSVOD) of IE proteins and assayed for CAT. *Lane 1*, pDR1/ATFCAT; *lane 2*, p25/26CAT; *lane 3*, pPolCAT. Values are expressed as % acetylation. pDR1/ATFCAT and p25/26CAT are shown at the bottom of the figure. *Vertical arrows, Hin*dIII sites and the Dr1/ATF site. TATA homology and CAP site (+*1*) are shown

Interaction of Proteins with CMV Early Promoters

It is now clear that HCMV IE proteins function to activate early promoters, and that IE 72 and IE 86 proteins function to activate these promoters through discrete sequences. These proteins could accomplish this effect by (a) direct binding to the sequences, (b) interaction with cellular proteins to stimulate promoter function, or (c) a combination of these two possibilities. Clearly,

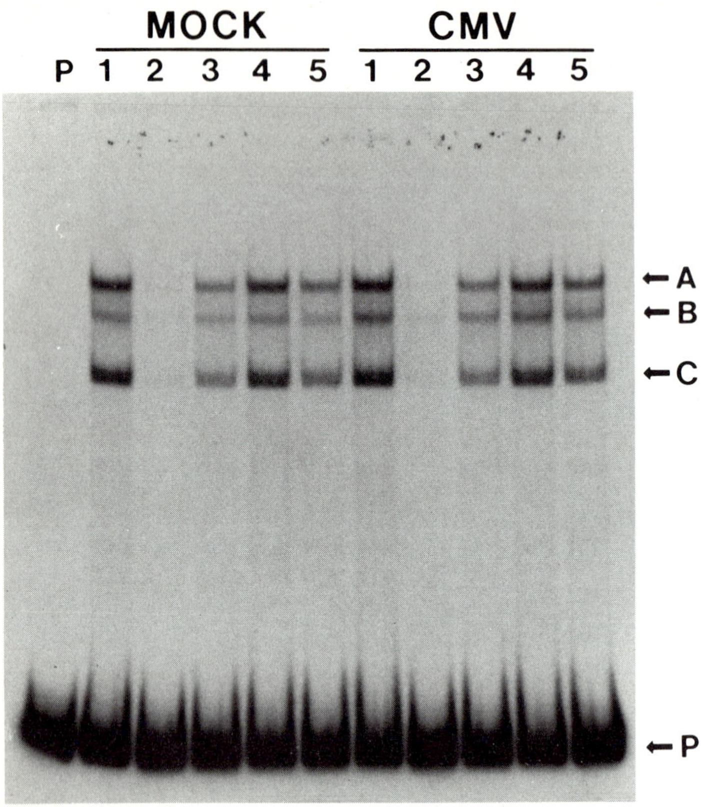

Fig. 16. Binding of IE-infected cell proteins to pol activator element. Radiolabeled pol activator element (–128 to +20) was incubated with infected (*CMV*) and mock-infected (*MOCK*) nuclear extracts isolated 4 h after infection. Protein from an equivalent number of infected cells or uninfected cells was used in each assay. Reactions were incubated in the presence or absence of competitor DNAs. *Lane 1*, No competitior; *lane 2*, 50-fold excess unlabeled pol activator element; *lane 3*, 50-fold excess unlabeled pol repressor element; *lane 4*, 50-fold excess of a 147-basepair nonspecific competitor fragment; *lane 5*, 50-fold excess of a 250-basepair nonspecific competitor fragment. Location of the bands (A, B, C) and probe (P) are indicated

because HCMV is host restricted and replicates efficiently only in a limited number of human cell types in vitro, the cell must play a major role in determining the outcome of infection. Also, because there is little to no homology between the regulatory motifs of the different early genes studied, it reduces the possibility of a common binding sequence for IE proteins.

Studies on proteins interacting with HCMV promoters demonstrated that cell proteins can specifically bind to regulatory elements within early promoters (Fig. 15) [36, 72]. Analysis of the pol activator domain reveals specific binding by proteins present in uninfected cells (Fig. 16). This binding could be successfully competed with excess specific competitor DNA but not with nonspecific DNA of equivalent size. This binding also occurred to an oligonucle-

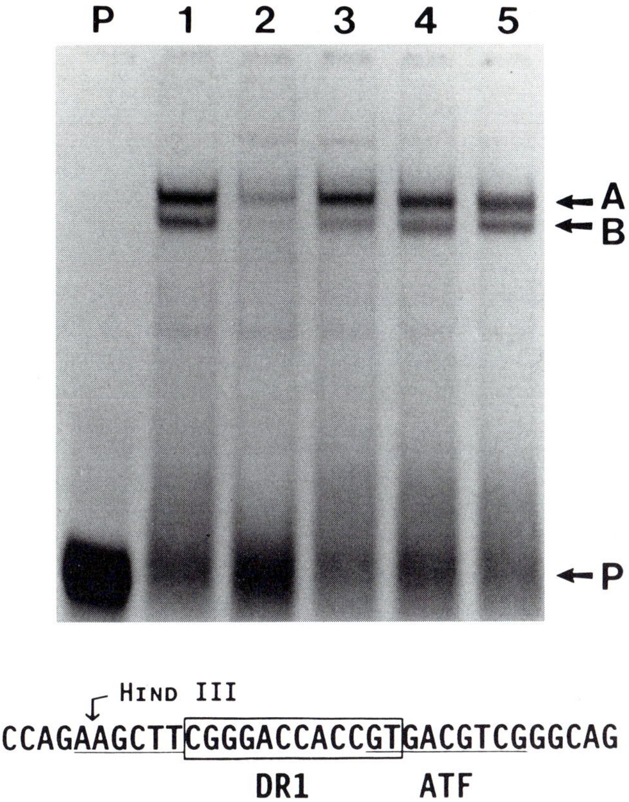

Fig. 17. Binding of infected cell proteins to DR1/ATF. Nuclear extracts from cells infected for 4 h were incubated with the DR1/ATF oligonucleotide shown at the bottom of the figure. Reactions were as described in the legend to Fig. 16. *Lane 1*, No competitor; *lane 2*, 100-fold excess unlabeled DR1/ATF; *lane 3*, 100-fold excess of an IR1-specific oligonucleotide; *lane 4*, same as *lane 1* but with 1 μl normal rabbit serum; *lane 5*, same as *lane 1* but with IE peptide antibody 8528. Location of the bands (A, B) and probe (P) are indicated

otide specific for DR 1/ATF but not unrelated oligonucleotides (Fig. 17). Because the DR 1/ATF element is involved in the synergistic activation of the early DNA polymerase promoter by IE 72 and IE 86, these data suggest that IE proteins interact with cell regulatory proteins in complex to drive early promoters.

Analysis of proteins that bind to the major early gene promoter also demonstrated a role for the cell transcription factor USF in early promoter function [35]. Also, Staprans and Spector [65] implied that the transcription factor E2F may play a role in activation of the UL 112–113 early promoter. As stated above, early promoters contain regulatory elements with little to no homology. Therefore, it is likely that they interact with various cell proteins, in complex with IE 72 and IE 86, to regulate CMV gene expression. This is consistent with our recent studies on the HIV LTR, which demonstrate that IE 72 and IE 86 can mediate synergistic activation through the USF site [25]. Taken together, these findings are interesting because each of these cell transcription factors is influenced by E1A protein [1, 7, 42, 43, 54, 59, 61]. This implies that IE 72 and IE 86 activate early promoters in an E1A-like manner. This is supported by the studies of Spector and Tevethia [63] who demonstrated that DNA capable of encoding IE 1 and 2 proteins can complement adenovirus early region 1 deletion mutants. However, fragments that could encode only IE 1 or 2 proteins were incapable of this complementation. Also, these authors subsequently demonstrated that IE 1 and 2 proteins could synergistically activate the adenovirus E2A promoter, which is consistent with the hypothesis that HCMV IE proteins and particularly IE 72 and IE 86 can work in an E1A-like manner.

It must be remembered that HCMV early promoters are not activated in uninfected cells or cells lacking IE proteins. This is consistent with the observation that early promoters are not expressed in the infected cell until after the IE phase of gene expression is underway. Clearly, cell transcription factors are insufficient for activation of HCMV early genes. This would indicate that (a) transcription factor complexes are modified in HCMV-infected cells thereby influencing the transcriptional machinery, (b) sequences that mediate repression are influenced in a dominant manner until IE proteins release the inhibitory effect, or (c) IE proteins act as coactivators that work through numerous cellular proteins in conjunction with TFIID and related TATA binding proteins. This latter mechanism would be most consistent with available data and could explain how HCMV IE proteins act through a diverse series of regulatory sequences to control HCMV gene expression.

Conclusions

Expression of IE genes throughout the course of HCMV infection occurs in a complicated, yet coordinated manner. While IE 1 and 2 are involved in regulation of subsequent virus gene expression, other IE genes of unknown function are also expressed. How these additional IE genes and gene products influence HCMV replication, both in vivo and in vitro, remains an important question. Clearly the host cell plays a major role in determining the outcome of HCMV infection, and cell transcription factors are important for interacting with IE proteins to regulate HCMV early gene expression.

Specifically, IE 72 and IE 86 interact to activate HCMV early promoters and to regulate the MIEP (Fig. 18). With respect to early promoter activation, IE proteins and cell proteins interact with specific promoter sequences in order to accomplish this effect. In addition, IE proteins directly influence their own levels in a coordinated manner. IE 72 plays a role in activation of both IE and early promoters. Also, IE 72 dominantly suppresses the repressive effect of

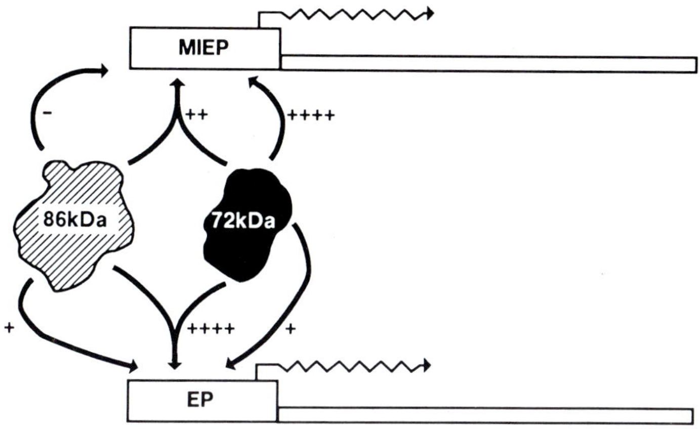

Fig. 18. Model of IE protein function. Influence of IE 72 (*72 kDa*) and IE 86 (*86 kDa*) on the MIEP and an early promoter is depicted. *Offset arrows*, direction of transcription from the promoters; *arrows from the proteins*, interaction of proteins and their subsequent influence on the promoters. The relative levels of activation (+) and repression (–) are indicated. (Reprinted with permission from [71])

IE 86 on IE expression. Clearly, the differential effect of IE proteins on IE and early gene expression in various cell types must influence the outcome of infection.

Acknowledgements. I would like to express my sincere thanks to Alison Depto, Jay Nelson, Peter Ghazal, Scott Barlow, James Fortney, Catherine Kohler, Brian Magrane, and Ann Campbell for their contributions to this work.

References

1. Bagchi S, Raychaudhuri P, Nevins JR (1989) Phosphorylation-dependent activation of the adenovirus inducible E2F transcription factor in a cell free system. Proc Natl Acad Sci USA 86:4352–4356
2. Baracchini E, Glezer E, Fish K, Stenberg RM, Nelson JA, Ghazal P (1992) Cytomegalovirus immediate-early (IE) IE 55 isoform of the IE 86 auto-repressor functions as a transcriptional activator and targets a unique response element. Virology 188:518–529
3. Blanton RA, Tevethia MJ (1981) Immunoprecipitation of virus-specific immediate-early and early polypeptides from cells lytically infected with human cytomegalovirus strain AD 169. Virology 112:262–273
4. Boshart M, Weber F, Jahn G, Dorsch-Hasler K, Fleckenstein B, Schaffner W (1985) A very strong enhancer is located upstream of an immediate early gene of human cytomegalovirus. Cell 41:521–530
5. Cameron JM, Preston CM (1981) Comparison of the immediate early polypeptides of human cytomegalovirus isolates. J Gen Virol 54:421–424
6. Chang CP, Malone CP, Stinski MF (1989) A human cytomegalovirus early gene has three inducible promoters that are regulated differentially at various times after infection. J Virol 63:281–290

7. Chang LS, Shi Y, Shenk T (1989) Adenovirus associated virus P5 promoter-containing an adenovirus E1A-inducible element and a binding site for the major late transcription factor. J Virol 63:3479–3488
8. Chee MS, Bankier AT, Beck S, Bohni R, Brown CM, Cerny R, Hornsnell T, Hutchinson CA III, Kouzarides T, Martignetti JA, Preddie E, Satchwell SC, Tomlinson P, Weston KM, Barrell BG (1990) Analysis of the protein-coding content of the sequence of human cytomegalovirus strain AD169 p125–170. In: McDougall JK (ed) Cytomegaloviruses. Springer, Berlin Heidelberg New York. Current topics in microbiology and immunology, vol 154
9. Cherrington JM, Mocarski ES (1989) Human cytomegalovirus ie1 transactivates the promoter-enhancer via an 18-base-pair repeat element. J Virol 63:1435–1440
10. Cherrington JM, Khoury EL, Mocarski ES (1991) Human cytomegalovirus ie2 negatively regulates alpha gene expression via a short target sequence near the transcription start site. J Virol 65:887–896
11. Coldberg-Poley AM, Santomenna LD, Harlow PP, Benfield PA, Tenney DJ (1992) Human cytomegalovirus US3 and UL36-38 immediate-early proteins regulate gene expression. J Virol 66:95–105
12. Cranage MP, Kouzarides T, Bankier AT, Satchwell S, Weston K, Tomlinson P, Barrell B, Hart H, Bell SE, Minson T (1986) Identification of the human cytomegalovirus glycoprotein B gene and induction of neutralizing antibodies via its expression in recombinant vaccinia virus. EMBO J 5:3057–3063
13. Cranage MP, Smith GL, Bell SE, Hart H, Brown C, Bankier AT, Tomlinson P, Barrell BG, Minson TC (1988) Identification and expression of a human cytomegalovirus glycoprotein with homology to the Epstein-Barr virus BXLF2 product, varicella-zoster virus gpIII, and herpes simplex virus type 1 glycoprotein H. J Virol 62:1416–1422
14. Davis MG, Huang ES (1985) Nucleotide sequence of a human cytomegalovirus DNA fragment encoding a 67-kilodalton phosphorylated viral protein. J Virol 56:7–11
15. Davis MG, Kenney SC, Kamine J, Pagano TS, Huang E-S (1987) Immediate-early gene region of human cytomegalovirus *trans*-activates the promoter of human immunodeficiency virus. Proc Natl Acad Sci USA 84:8642–8646
16. DeMarchi JM, Blankship ML, Brom GD, Kaplan AS (1978) Size and complexity of human cytomegalovirus DNA. Virology 89:653
17. DeMarchi JM, Schmidt GA, Kaplan AS (1980) Patterns of transcription of human cytomegalovirus in permissively infected cells. J Virol 35:227–286
18. Depto AS, Stenberg RM (1989) Regulated expression of the human cytomegalovirus pp65 gene: octamer sequence in the promoter is required for activation by viral gene products. J Virol 63:1232–1238
19. Depto AS, Stenberg RM (1992) Functional analysis of the true late human cytomegalovirus pp28 upstream promoter: *cis* acting elements and viral *trans* acting proteins necessary for promoter activation. J Virol 66:3241–3246
20. Everett RD (1984) *Trans*activation of transcription by herpes virus products: requirement for two HSV-1 immediate early polypeptides for maximum activity. EMBO J 3:3135–3141
21. Geballe AP, Mocarski ES (1988) Translational control of cytomegalovirus gene expression is mediated by upstream AUG codons. J Virol 62:3334–3340
22. Geballe AP, Spaete RR, Mocarski ES (1986) A *cis*-acting element within the 5′ leader of a cytomegalovirus β transcript determines kinetic class. Cell 46:865–872
23. Ghazal P, Lubon H, Reynolds-Kohler C, Henninghausen L, Nelson JA (1990) Interactions between cellular regulatory proteins and a unique sequence region in the human cytomegalovirus major immediate-early promoter. Virology 174:18–25
24. Ghazal P, Nelson JA (1991) Enhancement of RNA polymerase II initiation complexes by a novel DNA control domain downstream from the cap site of the cytomegalovirus major immediate early promoter. J Virol 65:2299–2307
25. Ghazal P, Young J, Giulietti E, DeMattei C, Garcia J, Gaynor R, Stenberg RM, Nelson JA (1991) A discrete *cis* element in the human immunodeficiency virus long terminal

repeat mediates synergistic *trans* activation by cytomegalovirus immediate-early proteins. J Virol 65:6735–6742
26. Gibson W (1981) Immediate early proteins of human cytomegalovirus strains AD169, Davis and Towne differ in electrophoretic mobility. Virology 112:350–354
27. Goins WF, Stinski MF (1986) Expression of a human cytomegalovirus late gene is posttranscriptionally regulated by a 3′ end processing event occurring exclusively late after infection. Mol Cell Biol 6:4202–4213
28. Greenaway PJ, Wilkinson WG (1987) Nucleotide sequence of the most abundantly transcribed early gene of human cytomegalovirus strain AD169. Virus Res 7:17–31
29. Heilbronn R, Jahn G, Burkle A, Freese U, Fleckenstein B, zur Hausen H (1987) Genomic location, sequence analysis, and transcription of the putative human cytomegalovirus DNA polymerase gene. J Virol 61:119–124
30. Henninghausen L, Fleckenstein B (1986) Nuclear factor 1 interacts with five DNA elements in the promoter region of the human cytomegalovirus major immediate early gene. EMBO J 5:1367–1371
31. Hermiston T, Malone C, Witte P, Stinski M (1987) Identification and characterization of the human cytomegalovirus immediate-early region 2 gene that stimulates gene expression from an inducible promoter. J Virol 61:3214–3221
32. Hutchinson NI, Sondermeyer RT, Tocci MJ (1986) Organization and expression of the major genes from the long inverted repeat of the human cytomegalovirus genome. Virology 155:160–171
33. Jahn G, Knust E, Schmolla H, Sarre T, Nelson JA, McDougall TK, Fleckenstein B (1984) Predominant immediate early transcripts of human cytomegalovirus AD169. J Virol 49:363–370
34. Kemble GW, McCormick L, Pereira L, Mocarski ES (1987) A cytomegalovirus protein with properties of herpes simplex virus ICP8: partial purification of the polypeptide and map position of the gene. J Virol 61:3143–3151
35. Klucher KM, Spector DH (1990) The human cytomegalovirus 2.7-kilobase RNA promoter contains a functional binding site for the adenovirus major late transcription factor. J Virol 64:4189–4198
36. Klucher KM, Rabert DK, Spector DH (1989) Sequences in the human cytomegalovirus 2.7-kilobase RNA promoter which mediate its regulation as an early gene. J Virol 63:5334–5343
37. Kouzarides T, Bankier AT, Satchwell SC, Weston K, Tomlinson P, Barrell BG (1987) Large scale rearrangement of homologous regions in the genomes of HCMV and EBV. Virology 157:397–413
38. Kouzarides T, Bankier AT, Satchwell SC, Weston K, Tomlinson P, Barrell BG (1987) Sequence and transcription analysis of the human cytomegalovirus DNA polymerase gene. J Virol 61:125–133
39. Kouzarides T, Bankier AT, Satchwell SC, Preddie E, Barrell BG (1988) An immediate early gene of human cytomegalovirus encodes a potential membrane glycoprotein. Virology 165:151–164
40. Landschults WH, Johnson PF, Mcknight SL (1988) The leucine zipper: a hypothetical structure common to a new class of DNA binding proteins. Science 240:1759–1764
41. Leatham MP, Witte PR, Stinski MF (1991) Alternate promoter selection within a human cytomegalovirus immediate early and early transcription unit (UL 119-115) defines true late transcripts containing open reading frames for putative viral glycoproteins. J Virol 65:6144–6153
42. Lin YS, Green MR (1988) Interaction of a common cellular transcription factor, ATF, with regulatory elements in both E1A- and cyclic AMP-inducible promoters. Proc Natl Acad Sci USA 85:3396–3400
43. Liu F, Green MR (1990) A specific member of the ATF transcription factor family can mediate transcription activation by the adenovirus E1A protein. Cell 61:1217–1224
44. Liu B, Hermiston TW, Stinski MF (1991) A *cis*-acting element in the major immediate-early (IE) promoter of human cytomegalovirus is required for negative regulation by IE 2. J Virol 65:897–903

45. Mach M, Utz U, Fleckenstein B (1986) Mapping of the major glycoprotein gene of human cytomegalovirus. J Gen Virol 67:1461–1467
46. Malone CL, Vesole DH, Stinski MF (1990) Transactivation of a human cytomegalovirus early promoter by gene products from the immediate-early gene IE 2 and augmentation by IE 1: mutational analysis of the viral proteins. J Virol 64:1498–1506
47. McDonough SH, Spector DH (1983) Transcription in human fibroblasts permissively infected by human cytomegalovirus strain AD 169. Virology 125:31–46
48. McDonough SH, Staprans DI, Spector DH (1985) Analysis of the major transcripts encoded by the long repeat of human cytomegalovirus strain AD 169. J Virol 53:711–718
49. Mermod N, O'Neill EA, Kelly TJ, Tjian R (1989) The proline-rich transcriptional activator CTF/NF1 is distinct from the replication and DNA binding domain. Cell 58:741–753
50. Miller J, McLachlan AD, Klug A (1985) Repetive zinc-binding domains in the protein transcription factor III A from *Xenopus* oocytes. EMBO J 4:1609–1614
51. Nelson JA, Groudine M (1986) Transcriptional regulation of the human cytomegalovirus major immediate early gene is associated with induction of DNaseI-hypersensitivity sites. Mol Cell Biol 6:452–461
52. Nelson JA, Fleckenstein B, Jahn G, Galloway DA, McDougall JK (1984) Structure of the transforming region of human cytomegalovirus AD 169. J Virol 49:109–115
53. Nelson JA, Reynolds-Kohler C, Smith BA (1987) Negative and positive regulation by a short segment in the 5′ flanking region of the human cytomegalovirus major immediate-early gene. Mol Cell Biol 7:4125–4129
54. Pei R, Berk AJ (1989) Multiple transcription factor binding sites mediate adenovirus E1A transactivation. J Virol 63:3499–3506
55. Pizzorno MC, Hayward GS (1990) The IE 2 gene products of human cytomegalovirus specifically down-regulate expression from the major immediate-early promoter through a target sequence located near the Cap site. J Virol 64:6154–6165
56. Pizzorno MC, O'Hare O, Sha L, LaFemina RL, Hayward GS (1988) *trans*-Activation and autoregulation of gene expression by the immediate-early region 2 gene products of human cytomegalovirus. J Virol 62:1167–1179
57. Plachter B, Traupe B, Albrecht J, Jahn G (1988) Abundant 5 kb RNA of human cytomegalovirus without a major translational reading frame. J Gen Virol 69:2251–2266
58. Rando RF, Srinivasan A, Feingold J, Gonczol E, Plotkin S, Characterization of multiple molecular interactions between human cytomegalovirus (HCMV) and human immunodeficiency virus type-1 (HIV-1). Virology 176:87–97
59. Raychaudhuri P, Rooney R, Nevins JR (1987) Identification of an E1A-inducible cellular factor that interacts with regulatory sequences within the adenovirus E4 promoter. EMBO J 6:4073–4081
60. Ruger B, Klages S, Walla B, Albrecht J, Fleckenstein B, Tomlinson P, Barrell B (1987) Primary structure and transcription of the genes coding for the two virion phosphoproteins pp 65 and pp 71 of human cytomegalovirus. J Virol 61:446–453
61. SivaRamon L, Thimmappaya B (1987) Two promoter specific host factors interact with adjacent sequences in an E1A-inducible adenovirus promoter. Proc Natl Acad Sci USA 84:6112–6116
62. Spaete RR, Mocarski ES (1985) Regulation of cytomegalovirus gene expression: α and β promoters are *trans* activated by viral functions in permissive human fibroblasts. J Virol 56:135–143
63. Spector DJ, Tevethia MJ (1986) Identification of a human cytomegalovirus DNA segment that complements an adenovirus 5 immediate early mutant. Virology 151:329–338
64. Stamminger T, Fickenscher H, Fleckenstein B (1990) Cell type-specific induction of the major immediate-early enhancer of human cytomegalovirus. J Gen Virol 71:105–113
65. Staprans SI, Spector DH (1986) 2.2-Kilobase class of early transcripts encoded by cell-related sequences in human cytomegalovirus strain AD 169. J Virol 57:591–602
66. Staprans SI, Rabert DK, Spector DH (1988) Identification of sequence requirements and *trans*-acting functions necessary for regulated expression of a human cytomegalovirus early gene. J Virol 62:3463–3473

67. Stenberg RM, Stinski MF (1985) Autoregulation of the human cytomegalovirus major immediate-early gene. J Virol 56:676–682
68. Stenberg RM, Thomsen DR, Stinski MF (1984) Structural analysis of the major immediate early gene of human cytomegalovirus. J Virol 49:190–199
69. Stenberg RM, Witte PR, Stinski MF (1985) Multiple spliced and unspliced transcripts from human cytomegalovirus immediate-early region 2 and evidence for a common initiation site within immediate-early region 1. J Virol 56:665–675
70. Stenberg RM, Depto AS, Fortney J, Nelson JA (1989) Regulated expression of early and late RNAs and proteins from the human cytomegalovirus immediate-early gene region. J Virol 63:2699–2708
71. Stenberg RM, Fortney J, Barlow SW, Magrane BP, Nelson JA, Ghazal P (1990) Promoter-specific *trans* activation and repression by human cytomegalovirus immediate-early proteins involves common and unique protein domains. J Virol 64:1556–1565
72. Stenberg RM, Depto AS, Kohler CP, Fortney J (1992) Activation of the human cytomegalovirus DNA polymerase promoter by immediate early proteins is mediated through a discrete sequence containing a direct repeat (DR1) and an ATF binding site. (submitted)
73. Stinski MF (1978) Sequence of protein synthesis in cells infected by human cytomegalovirus: early and late virus induced polypeptides. J Virol 26:686–701
74. Stinski MF, Roehr TJ (1985) Activation of the major immediate early gene of human cytomegalovirus by *cis*-acting elements in the promoter-regulatory sequence and by virus-specific *trans*-acting components. J Virol 55:431–441
75. Stinski MF, Thomsen DR, Stenberg RM, Goldstein LC (1983) Organization and expression of the immediate early genes of human cytomegalovirus. J Virol 46:1–14
76. Tenney DJ, Colberg-Poley AM (1991) Expression of the human cytomegalovirus UL36-38 immediate early region during permissive infection. Virology 182:199–210
77. Tenney DJ, Colberg-Poley AM (1991) Human cytomegalovirus UL36-38 and US3 immediate early genes: temporally regulated expression of nuclear, cytoplasmic, and polysome-associated transcripts during infection. J Virol 65:6724–6734
78. Tevethia MJ, Spector DJ, Leisure KM, Stinski MF (1987) Participation of two human cytomegalovirus immediate early gene regions in transcriptional activation of adenovirus promoters. Virology 161:276–285
79. Thomsen DR, Stenberg RM, Goins WF, Stinski MF (1984) Promoter regulatory region of the major immediate early gene of human cytomegalovirus. Proc Natl Acad Sci USA 81:659–663
80. Tsutsui Y, Nogami-Satake T (1990) Differential expression of the major immediate-early gene of human cytomegalovirus. J Gen Virol 71:115–124
81. Tsutsui Y, Yamazaki Y (1991) Subcellular distribution of the major immediate-early proteins of human cytomegalovirus changes during infection. J Gen Virol 72:1415–1419
82. Wathen MW, Stinski MF (1982) Temporal patterns of human cytomegalovirus transcription: mapping the viral RNAs synthesized at immediate early, early, and late times after infection. J Virol 41:462–477
83. Wathen MW, Thomsen DR, Stinski MF (1981) Temporal regulation of human cytomegalovirus transcription at immediate early and early times after infection. J Virol 38:446–459
84. Weston K (1988) An enhancer element in the short unique region of the production of a group of abundant immediate early transcripts. Virology 162:406–416
85. Wilkinson GWG, Akrigg A, Greenaway PJ (1984) Transcription of the immediate early genes of human cytomegalovirus strain AD169. Virus Res 1:101–116

Chapter 18 Transcription Factors and Viral Regulatory Proteins as Potential Mediators of Human Cytomegalovirus Pathogenesis

Peter Ghazal [1,2] and Jay A. Nelson [1]

Summary

The mechanism(s) of pathogenesis caused by persistent viruses such as the human cytomegalovirus (HCMV) are strongly associated with the control of transcription. In this chapter we explore in vitro systems which suggest the interplay of both viral and cellular regulatory factors as major determinants in controlling the expression state of HCMV. Importantly, we address the issue of both cellular transcription factors and viral regulatory proteins as possible mediators in the pathogenesis associated with HCMV infection.

Introduction

A primary infection by human cytomegalovirus (HCMV) results in a lifetime persistence of virus in the host [37]. Infected individuals who are immunocompetent remain asymptomatic with the viral genome demonstrating either an undetectable presence or restrictive expression in a limited number of cells. However, when an infected individual's immune system is compromised, extensive expression of the viral genome may occur leading to disseminated infection and death. Therefore, the key to understanding the pathogenesis caused by HCMV is the elucidation of factors involved in the activation of the viral genome from a restrictive state to one of extensive expression.

A pictorial representation of the HCMV life cycle is shown in Fig. 1. In this scheme virus is absorbed and uncoated, releasing a linear double-stranded genome which migrates to the nucleus. Upon entry into the nucleus, expression of the HCMV genome is sequentially regulated and is initially dependent on cellular factors for activation. The genes encoded by HCMV have been subdivided into three kinetic classes: immediate-early (IE), early (E), and late (L) genes [100]. The expression of the IE genes is dependent on host-cell factors while both early and late gene expression are interdependent on cellular and viral factors. The synthesis of IE proteins is required for the initiation of early

[1] Department of Immunology and [2] Department of Neuropharmacology, Division of Virology, The Scripps Research Institute, Clinic, La Jolla, CA 92037, USA

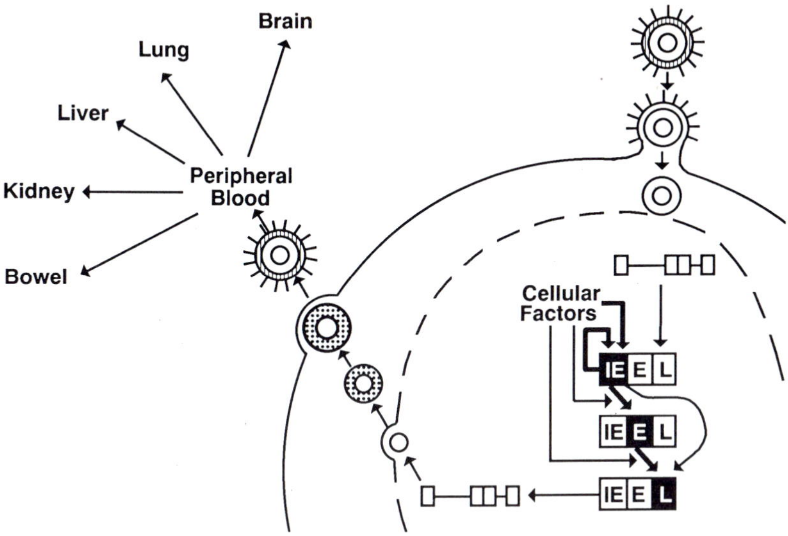

Fig. 1. Representation of the life cycle of human cytomegalovirus (see "Introduction" for details). *IE*, immediate-early genes; *E*, early genes; *L*, late genes

gene expression since infection in the presence of inhibitors of protein synthesis prevents subsequent viral gene expression [21, 64, 106, 107]. Studies to date have demonstrated that three distinct segments of the CMV genome are predominantly transcribed during IE expression [43, 50, 96–98, 108, 111]. Two regions of abundant IE gene expression designated IE region one (IE-1) [96, 102] and IE region two (IE-2) originate from one of these segments [97, 102]. Together IE-1 and IE-2 constitute the major IE gene that is under the control of a single promoter regulatory region located upstream of IE-1 [97], which has been referred to as the major IE promoter (MIEP) [12, 104]. The level of the major IE gene products synthesized in an infected cell are predicted to switch the viral genome from restrictive to extensive expression [74]. Therefore, the transcription control of the MIEP describes a primary target for determining the state of the virus within a cell. If the genome is extensively expressed then virions are assembled and exported out of that cell to repeat the cycle.

A variety of cell types are infected by HCMV in vivo. These include: epithelial cells [70] from lung and rectum; large artery and capillary endothelial cells [70, 110]; astrocytes [110], neurons, and oligodendrocytes [110]; and T-cells [88] and monocyte/-macrophage cells [42, 85]. As depicted in Fig. 1, the peripheral blood mononuclear cells (PBMNs) are important cellular vectors for the dissemination of the virus throughout the body [13, 46, 54, 78, 83, 85, 88]. We have previously reviewed the involvement of PBMNs in the biology of HCMV [74, 75] and therefore will not discuss this aspect further. However, it is important to note that HCMV expression and replication in PBMNs is restricted in immunocompetent individuals and that either mitogenic or antigenic stimulation of the cells increases viral expression. Therefore, we have proposed that the state of either activation or cellular differentiation may be a critical determinant of viral replication.

In this chapter, we will discuss model cell culture systems used to explore HCMV activation and transcription factor interactions in vitro which may identify HCMV–host-cell interactions that regulate expression of the virus. In addition, we will discuss the possible structure and function of the major IE proteins with HCMV promoters as well as with the cellular regulatory network.

Teratocarcinoma Cells as a Model for HCMV Activation

A major determinant controlling reactivation of HCMV is likely to involve changes in cellular transcription factors utilized by the virus. These changes may occur upon either activation or differentiation of an infected cell. Teratocarcinoma cell systems have provided a unique in vitro tool to dissect molecular events involved in the regulation of viral genes after cellular differentiation. These cells are derived from embryonal carcinomas which can be stimulated to differentiate into a wide variety of somatic cell types. HCMV has been shown to replicate in a differentiated human teratocarcinoma cell (Tera-2), but there was an unidentified block in viral replication in undifferentiated cells [33]. This cell line, therefore, provided a unique system to analyze the cellular events which occur when a cell is activated and allows HCMV replication.

To test directly the hypothesis that the expression level of the IE proteins is an important determinant of permissiveness of HCMV in a cell, we studied the regulation of expression of the IE genes in undifferentiated and differentiated Tera-2 cells. By comparison of steady-state RNA levels and in vitro run-on transcription of nuclei, we demonstrated that the major IE gene is inactive in undifferentiated but active in differentiated Tera-2 cells. Thus, the block in HCMV replication in these cells is at the transcriptional level of the MIEP [72].

Analysis of chromatin characteristics of active and inactive genes has identified hypersensitive sites to nuclease attack which correlate with important cis-acting regulatory elements. A comparison of the structural features of chromatin on the promoter regulatory region with the active and inactive major IE gene demonstrated the presence of constitutive and inducible deoxyribonuclease I (DNaseI) hypersensitive sites. The majority of the constitutive sites existed between –175 and –525 relative to the start of transcription (Fig. 2) [72]. This region was shown to have simian virus 40 (SV40) enhancer function [12]. In contrast, the inducible DNaseI hypersensitive sites were located outside this region between –650 and –975 as well as an area within the first exon [72] (Fig. 2). Since this is one of the primary viral genes to be turned on when the virus enters the cell, the increased nuclease hypersensitivity in the active gene may reflect an altered chromatin conformation which is favorable for the binding of transcription factors. Furthermore, altered DNA conformations may also be involved. Altered DNA structures were detected in se-

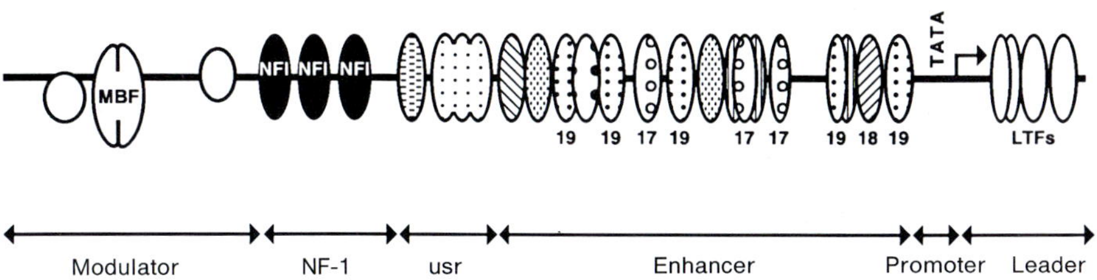

Fig. 2. Structure of the major immediate-early promoter regulatory region. The *line* represents the 5′-flanking sequences with the *ovals* marking regions of in vitro deoxyribonuclease I protection. The *differently coded ovals* positioned over these protected areas illustrate the distinctive nature and multiplicity of interacting nuclear proteins. The *numbers* refer to the repeat elements protected. *NF1*, nuclear factor 1 protein; *MBF*, modulator binding factor; *LTFs*, leader transcription factor; *usr*, unique sequence region

quences distal to the enhancer during the active transcription of these genes using a chemical carcinogen (chloracetaldehyde) as a probe [48].

To test the significance of the upstream inducible DNaseI hypersensitive sites, reporter constructs under the control of variously deleted portions of MIEP were assayed in transient transfection experiments using differentiated and undifferentiated Tera-2 cells. These experiments identified a novel regulatory region between –750 and –1145. Deletion of this region causes a tenfold increase in MIEP activity in undifferentiated Tera-2 cells [73]. However, in permissive differentiated Tera-2 cells, removal of this regulatory region results in a decrease in activity. Therefore, the MIEP is a complex element which contains a dual function cis-regulatory element between –750 and –1145 which negatively modulates expression in undifferentiated cells but positively influences expression in differentiated cells. On the basis of these observations we have designated this region as the "modulator".

Therefore, by utilizing this in vitro cell culture system we have shown that the state of the virus within the cell is dependent on the level of IE gene expression. In addition, the corresponding regulatory cis-acting sequences and their respective *trans*-acting factors are functionally dependent on the differentiation state of the cell. The importance of cellular transcription factor interactions with cis-acting regulatory elements of the MIEP will be discussed in the next section.

Cellular Transcription Factor Interactions with the MIEP

The regulatory sequences of MIEP offer a complex spectrum of distinct control domains encompassing: an RNA polymerase II promoter between +1 and –50; a downstream promoter proximal transcription control domain within exon 1 (between +1 and +112); a strong enhancer between –50 and –530; a unique sequence region (between –530 and –640) adjacent to a cluster of nuclear factor 1 protein (NF1)/CCAAT binding transcription factor (CTF) binding sites between –650 and –750; and the modulator sequence between –750 and –1145. Consideration of the cellular involvement with the complete MIEP regulatory region is important in understanding the mechanism(s) of virus-host-cell transcriptional regulation. It is our hope that specific cellular transcription factors will be linked to the pathogenesis of viral disease. Therefore, we will summarize our current understanding about the dependence of transcriptional control of the MIEP on host-cell transcription factors.

Promoter

The promoter of the major IE gene of HCMV utilizes the host's RNA polymerase II and associated general factors for transcription [28, 29]. A basic eukaryotic RNA polymerase II promoter consists of at least two kinds of cis-acting DNA sequences. These motifs are upstream elements positioned at around –100 and TATA elements. TATA elements consist of a ubiquitous sequence of 7 bp, TATAWAW, located between 19 and 34 bp upstream from the initiation site of transcription [14]. The sequence between –29 and –23 of MIEP is identical to the 7-bp consensus TATA box sequence. This *cis* element plays an important role in control of gene expression and interacts with a general transcription initiation factor, designated TFIID [63]. The binding of TFIID represents the first step in core-promoter activation [71] and promotes the stepwise interactions of RNA polymerase II and other general initiation factors [15, 38, 105].

Immediately upstream of the MIEP TATA box between nucleotides –72 and –53 is a sequence that is similar to the 19-bp palindromic elements located within the enhancer region (see below). This redundant form of the 19-bp palindromic element binds a sequence-specific transcription factor that resembles or is identical to the 19-bp enhancer binding factor(s) [29] (Fig. 3). The extent of this interaction is distinct from the interaction of the factors with the enhancer 19-bp elements, as shown by DNaseI protection analysis [29]. Nevertheless, the sequence is important for transcription from MIEP and appears to function equivalently in a wide variety of different cell types [29, 59].

Leader Transcription Control Domain

Recently a novel regulating domain associated with the MIEP downstream from the initiation site of transcription has been characterized [27]. This downstream regulatory region was first identified by analyzing a series of mutations in the 5′ untranslated leader exon. This regulatory domain was shown to enhance the number of functional initiation complexes without significantly altering the apparent elongation rate by RNA polymerase II. In addition, run-off in vitro transcription and DNA-binding experiments identified two distinct downstream elements that specify the interaction of cellular transcrip-

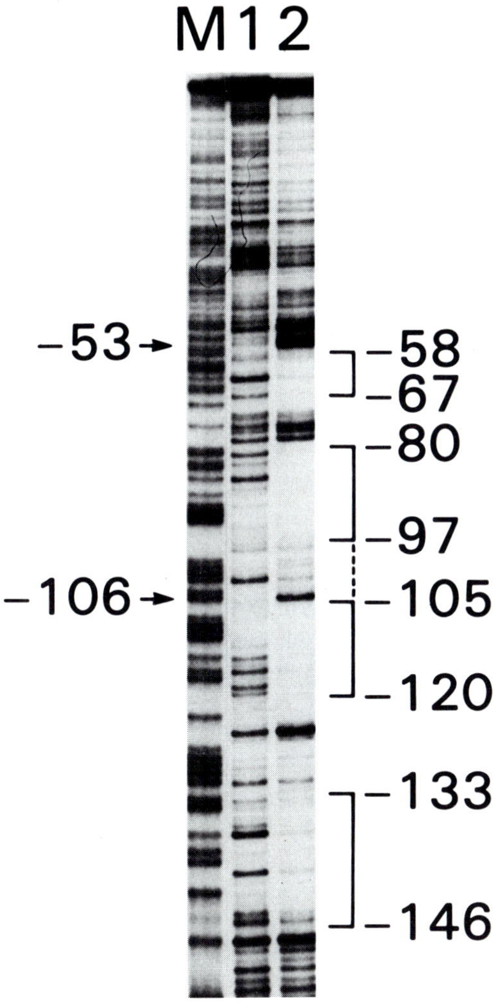

Fig. 3. Deoxyribonuclease I (DNase I) protection analysis of the sense strand of major immediate-early promoter region using HeLa cell nuclear proteins. *Lane M* represents A + G maxam and Gilbert sequence reaction of the fragment. *Lane 1*, partial DNase I digestion of the promoter fragment in the presence of bovine serum albumin. *Lane 2*, partial DNase I digestion of the promoter fragment in the presence of HeLa nuclear proteins eluted from a single-stranded DNA cellulose chromatography column with 0.6 *M* KCl step wash. The conditions used for footprinting were as described by Ghazal et al. [28]. *Numbers* represent the distance in base pairs located upstream of the transcription start site (+1). Sequences protected from DNase I cleavage are marked by the *brackets*. *Arrows* mark sites of enhanced DNase I cleavage

tion factors. One of these elements contains a reiterated sequence motif, present twice within the leader exon between nucleotides +53 and +92. The second element located between nucleotide position +33 and +52 represents sequences that are conserved between strains of CMV from different species. The binding of factors to the conserved box was shown to be important for mediating the level of transcription from the MIEP [27]. Two discrete cellular nuclear proteins, designated LTFA and B (for leader transcription factor A and B binding factors), were found to specifically recognize overlapping sequences in the conserved element. The leader transcription control domain of the MIEP describes the first example of a transcription control domain, outside overlapping transcription units, internal to a gene encoded by HCMV. We propose that this leader control domain may constitute a key target for regulating viral activation.

Enhancer

A remarkable array of short repetitive sequences ranging in size from 16 or 17 to 21 nucleotides occur between –510 and –50 [1, 12, 104]. This region is an important regulatory region [101] and possesses strong enhancer activity [12]. These repetitive sequence motifs are thought to represent potential regulatory elements. A similar highly repetitive arrangement of short sequences also exists in the 5′-flanking sequence of the major IE genes of murine and simian CMV (SCMV) [24, 44]. Some of the mouse and SCMV repetitive elements are identical to repetitive sequences of HCMV.

The activity of MIEP enhancer has been reproduced partially in vitro using nuclear extracts [28]. In vitro run-off transcription offers an experimentally amenable system to investigate the functional relevance of the relationship between MIEP regulatory elements and potential interacting cellular transcription factors. A competition assay was used to determine whether the stimulation of transcription by the enhancer sequences could be due to specific DNA-binding transcription factors. In vitro transcription of templates either with or without enhancer sequences in the presence of various fragments from the MIEP regulatory region has shown directly that enhancer activity is mediated by binding cellular transcription factors [28]. Using the technique of in vitro DNaseI footprinting with transcriptionally active nuclear proteins, we have demonstrated the existence of multiple distinct cellular proteins that bind sequence-specifically to the various repeat sequences as well as to the unique sequences [28, 29]. Complete protection of all 19- and 17-bp repeat elements was observed while only partial and/or weak interactions were observed for the 18- and 21-bp repeats (see Fig. 4). Recently, Fickenscher et al. [25] and Sambucetti et al. [86], using a mobility shift assay, have also detected binding to the 19-, 18-, and 17-bp repeat elements from the MIEP. In the case of the 21-bp repeats, protection extended from the 3′-end half of the repeat and sequences immediately adjacent. A comparison of these protected sequences revealed a common motif of $TGGCN_5GCCCA$ [28]. In addition, unique se-

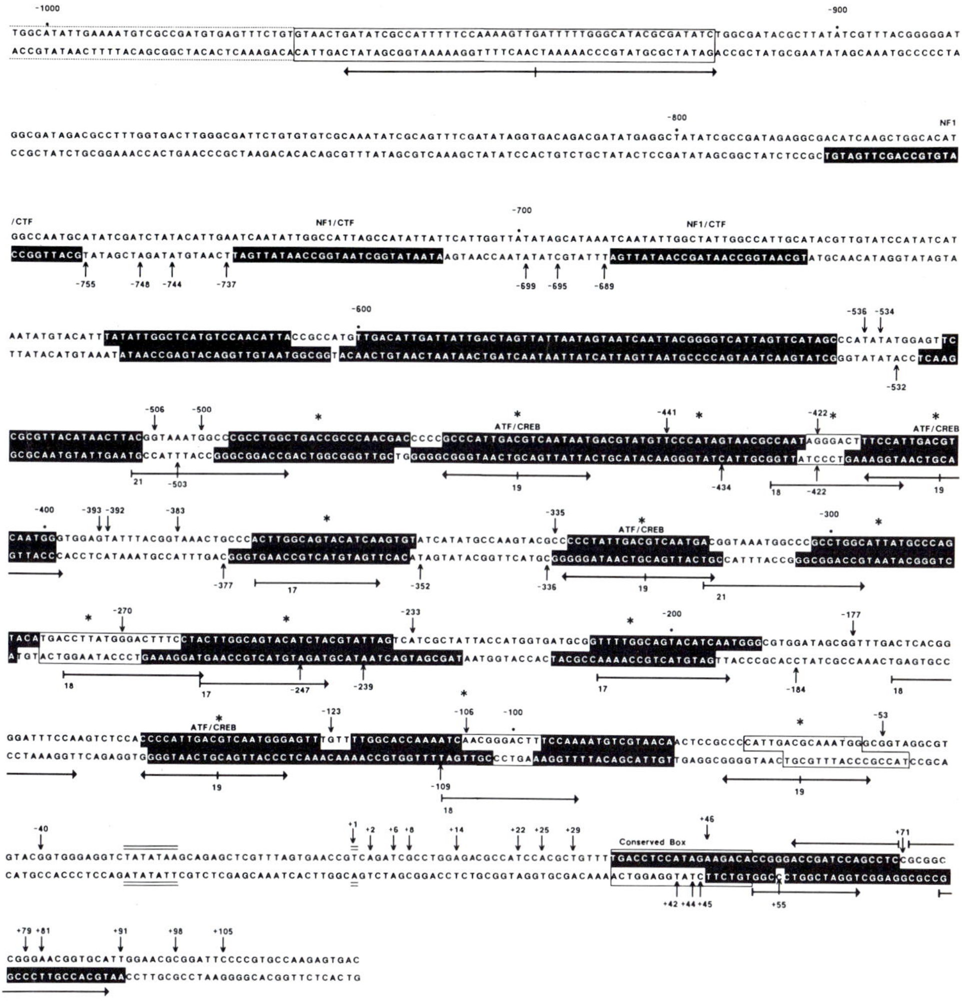

Fig. 4. Sites of protein-DNA interaction on the major immediate-early promoter (MIEP) regulatory region. *Numbers* represent the distance in base pairs located upstream of the transcription start site (+1). Sequences protected from deoxyribonuclease I (DNase I) cleavage are marked by *reverse printing* (strong protection) or a *box* (weak protection). *Vertical arrows* denote positions of enhanced protein-induced DNase I cleavage in vitro. Repeated sequence elements are designated by *horizontal arrows* with the respective repeat size indicated *below*. Those binding sites shown to be functional (see text) are marked with an *asterisk*

quences outside the repeat elements were also bound by nuclear proteins. A summary of the sequences contacted by sequence-specific nuclear proteins is depicted in Figs. 2 and 4.

The function of the repeat elements as well as the unique sequences bound by their sequence-specific DNA-binding proteins was shown by developing an in vitro transcription oligonucleotide-competition assay [30]. This technique involves the use of synthetic double-stranded oligonucleotides corresponding to the target sequences of the DNA-binding proteins in an in vitro transcription competition assay. These experiments clearly demonstrated the requirement for the 18-bp repeat, the 19-bp repeat, the unique sequence, and the 21-bp associated binding sites and their cognate sequence-specific transcription factors to provide enhancer function. The 17-bp repeat only marginally contributed to the action of the enhancer; however, it should be noted that the activities of different enhancer-binding proteins are unlikely to be equivalent under all circumstances. Importantly, this work suggests that the enhancer requires the coordinated action of several distinct elements, some of which are reiterated while others only occur once. Those binding sites shown to be functional so far are marked with an asterisk in Fig. 4. Intriguingly, the 5′-end halves of many of the binding sites thus far determined by MIEP have a common sequence motif, (T)TG(G/A)C. This homology may suggest a particular class of nuclear factor(s) associated with this sequence, while the 3′-end half of the binding site may associate with distinct factors [29]. Thus, nonsymmetrical sites may involve heterodimer binding sites with a common protomer (Fig. 5). Whether a common protomer exists with these binding sites is currently not known.

Many of the sequence-specific transcription factor binding sites are also represented within the simian and murine MIEP 5′-flanking sequences (Table 1), such as the 19-bp repeat and the 21-bp repeat associated binding site, TGGCN$_5$GCCCA. However, some sequence motifs appear to be absent, such as the 18-bp repeat (including the 10-bp core GGGACTTTCC) in the simian MIEP and the 17-bp repeat in the murine MIEP. Differences in the modular arrangement and combinations of sequence elements between species-specific strains of CMV may confer unique programs of cell-type or tissue-specific regulation. Indeed, the wide variety of control elements may enable the virus to adapt to a variety of cell types which are restricted in the expression of particular transcription factors.

A number of the transcription factor sites are also known to mediate induction responses to various signals. For example, a rapid increase in the RNA

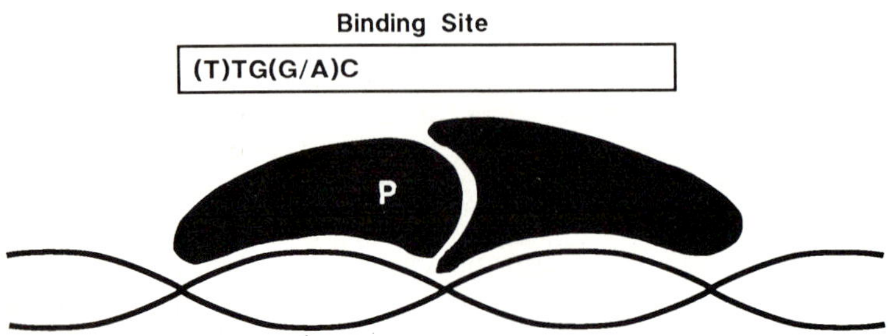

Fig. 5. Model for either a particular class or a protomer of nuclear factors associated with the common sequence motif (T)TG(G/A)C at the 5′ end of the binding site. Nonsymmetrical sites may involve heterodimer binding sites and symmetrical sites, homodimer binding sites, with a common protomer (*P*)

Table 1. Nuclear protein binding sites associated with repeat elements in the MIEP of HCMV and homologous sequences in the simian and murine CMV MIEP regions

Repeat	HCMV		SCMV		MCMV	
17/16	−373	ACTTGGCAGTACATCAA	−253	ACTTGGCAGTACATCAA		NDI
	−260	ACTTGGCAGTACATCTA	−220	ACTTGGCAAGTACATTAC		
	−209	TTTTGGCAGTACATCAA	−203	TATTGGCAAGTACGCCAA		
	−122	(TTTTGGCACCAAAATCAA)				
18	−428	CCAATAGGGACTTTCCAT		NDI	−767	TCAATAGGGACTTTCCAT
	−277	CCTTATGGGACTTTCCTA			−674	TCAATAGGGACTTTCCAT
	−109	ATCAACGGGACTTTCCAA			−581	TCAATAGGGACTTTCCAA
					−488	TCATTAGGGACTTTCCAA
					−396	TCAATAGGGACTTTCCAT
19	−469	GCCCATTGACGTCAATAAT	−488	CCCCATTGACGTCAATGGT	−236	CACCATTGACGTCAATGGG
	−416	TTCCATTGACGTCAATGGG	−453	TCCTATTGACGTCATATGG		
	−333	CCCTATTGACGTCAATGAC	−430	TCCTATTGACGTATATGGC		
	−147	CCCCATTGACGTCAATGGG	−406	CCCCATTGACGTCAATTAC		
	−73	CCCCATTGACGCAAATGGG	−303	GCCCATTGACGTCAATAGG		
			−338	CACCATTGACGTCAATGGG		
			−284	CCCTATTGACGTCAATGAC		
			−167	TCCCATTGACGTCAATGGC		
			−113	CCCCATTGACGTCAATGGG		
			−91	GGGCAATGACGCAAATGGG		
			−70	TTCCATTGACGTAAATGGC		
(21)	−495	GCCTGGCTGACCGCCCA	−417	ATATGGCGCCTCCCCCA	−515 (Rev)	CATTGGCTTACCACCCA
	−302	GCCTGGCATTATGCCCA	(21) −375	GCCTGGCTCAATGCCCA		
			−321	GGATGGCTCATTGCCCA		

(21), 21 – bp repeat element associated binding site consensus $TGGCN_5GCCCA$; (Rev), reverse sequence; NDI, no detectable identity; SCMV, simian CMV; MCMV, murine CMV levels of the proto-oncogenes c-*fos*, c-*jun*, and c-*myc* occurs after HCMV infection by the interaction of viral particles with the cell surface [10, 11]. The nuclear proteins *jun* and *fos* are components of the transcription factor, AP-1 [9]. The MIEP contains a number of putative AP-1 binding sites [28, 77] and may consequently be involved in the initiation and progression of HCMV replication. Infection with HCMV also increases a variety of secondary messengers including cyclic adenosine 3′,5′-monophosphate (cAMP) [2]. The 19-bp repeat is related to the AP-1 binding site but binds a distinct transcription factor(s) that is responsible in part for mediating the effects of cAMP [16, 40, 76, 93]. The core of the 19-bp palindromic sequence, TGACGTCA, occurs within cAMP-regulated genes [68]. A nuclear protein family, ATF/CREB (mol. wt. 43–47 kDa), binds to this sequence [34, 41, 67] and suggests the 19-bp repeat binding factor(s) is likely to be a member(s) of this family of proteins. Moreover, ATF/CREB has been implicated in mediating the trans-activation of the adenovirus early E2 promoter in combination with the E1A protein [57]. This observation may be of some significance since the HCMV IE genes can complement trans-activation functions of adenovirus E1A defective mutants [103].

Another example of an inducible sequence motif within the enhancer is the 10-bp core sequence of the 18-bp repeat (GGGACTTTCC). This core sequence binds a nuclear protein designated NF-$\varkappa$B and confers phorbol ester inducibility as well as B-cell preference for expression [56, 89, 90]. In most cells, with the exception of the mature B-cell, NF-$\varkappa$B forms a reversible heterodimer with I$\varkappa$B (60–70 kDa), an inhibitory molecule in the cytosol [4]. Phorbol esters that are mediated by protein kinase C are thought to activate a dissociation event leading to the nuclear translocation of the factor and activation of transcription. An important characteristic of NF-$\varkappa$B is its capacity to function as a pleiotropic mediator for many signals [55]. The activation of MIEP by IE-1 product(s) has been suggested to be predominantly mediated by inducing the binding of NF-$\varkappa$B to the 18-bp repeat [17, 86]. Furthermore, other ubiquitously available nuclear proteins also bind functionally to this sequence [5]. We have also detected the functional binding of HeLa cell nuclear proteins to the 18-bp repeat [28, 29]. These inducible sequence elements illustrate, in addition to the modulator, other regions of the MIEP that may subtly alter the levels of expression of the virus within the cell.

Unique Sequence Region

Immediately 5′ to the repetitive sequence structure of the enhancer exists a 100-bp stretch of unique sequence. Recently, the unique sequence region (usr) has been shown to contribute to the transcriptional activity from the MIEP in both permissive and nonpermissive cells [31]. Whether this region represents an extension of the enhancer domain or whether it constitutes an independent transcription control domain is not known. In addition, the usr may play a role in communicating neighboring effects between the enhancer and modulator domains. Nevertheless, in the context of the MIEP, usr provides a target region for a complex binding arrangement of sequence-specific nuclear proteins. A minimum of five sequence-specific DNA-binding interactions were detected between –632 and –602, –602 and –557, –602 and –590, –563 and –540, and –602 and –582 [31]. The simplest interpretation of these results is that each of the binding sites represents a distinct protein. Alternatively, the different binding sites may result from the binding of either a modified or a multisubunit(s) protein(s). One of these binding sites (between –632 and –602) corresponds to a previously characterized putative NF-1 binding site; however, this site does not bind NF-1 but instead strongly interacts with a distinct cellular factor. These observations add further complexity to the already highly complicated regulatory region of MIEP.

NF1/CTF Binding Domain

There exist within MIEP four consensus binding sequence motifs for the family of proteins involved in replication (NF-1) and transcription (CTF) [45]. Earlier studies suggested that all four consensus sequences were bound by NF1/CTF [35]; however, as discussed above, one of these sites lies within the usr between –632 and –602, and appears not to interact with NF1/CTF [31]. However, this NF1/CTF consensus binding sequence does interact strongly with a sequence-specific nuclear protein which is distinct from the NF1/CTF proteins [31].

SCMV, which constitutively expresses a homologous IE gene in undifferentiated Tera-2 cells [51], contains a region in the regulatory sequence 5′ to the enhancer that is composed of 23 NF-1 binding sites [44], compared with three in HCMV. The presence of 20 more NF-1 sites in SCMV relative to HCMV suggests that the protein may have a role in activation. Hayward et al. [44] have argued that the large cluster of NF-1 sites in SCMF may act by overcoming the effects of repressors. However, there are perhaps many more functionally relevant differences. For example, the HCMV MIEP 18-bp repeat or the unique sequence elements are absent in the SCMV regulatory region (above, and Table 1). In addition, the presence of the HCMV modulator sequence that is absent in SCMV may also contribute to the differences in viral expression in Tera-2 cells. The functional significance of the NF-1 binding sites is unknown. However, the occurrence of two inducible in vivo DNaseI hypersensitive sites near these sequences (Fig. 2) suggests the NF-1/CTF proteins may be involved in the regulation of MIEP.

Modulator

The modulator region as described above negatively affects MIEP function in undifferentiated nonpermissive Tera-2 cells while positively influencing transcription from MIEP in the differentiated cells. We have examined whether the modulator sequences confer cell specificity for expression in other types of cells [60]. CAT reporter constructs containing the MIEP with and without the modulator were assayed in several different cell types (epithelial, T-cells, and B-cells). The constructs were either transiently transfected and analyzed or transcriptionally active extracts prepared and assayed. The effect of the modulator sequence on CAT activity in the transient transfection experiments or levels of transcription from MIEP in the in vitro transcription assays differed depending on the cell type. A negative effect was observed in H-9 (T-cell), CEM (T-cell), and SW480 (epithelial) cells, but expression in Jurkat (T-cell), 293 (kidney), Raji (B-cell), Namalwa (B-cell), and U937 (monocyte/macrophage) cells were unaffected by the presence of the modulator sequence. These results indicate that the HCMV modulator sequence can influence MIEP activity in cell types other than teratocarcinoma cells. In particular, the modulator negatively affects expression in cell types, T-cells and epithelial cells, that are important during natural infection.

To determine whether protein–DNA complexes in the modulator region correlated with transcriptional activity, the nuclear extracts described above were utilized in mobility shift assays. Similar migrating nuclear protein–DNA complexes formed between the modulator region and the various nuclear extracts were detected. A simple correlation was not observed between modulator activity and a specific migrating nucleoprotein complex [60]. Nucleoproteins from these extracts were found to interact with distinct regions of the modulator. A major complex (Complex C in [60]) mapped to sequences containing a large "dyad symmetry" using the mobility shift assay with different and overlapping restriction fragments (Fig. 6).

Interestingly, Shelbourn et al. [91] have shown that undifferentiated Tera-2 cells contain a nuclear factor that binds the dyad symmetry. The differentiation of Tera-2 cells is associated with a decrease in this factor binding, and deletion of the dyad symmetry results in increased levels of expression in undifferentiated cells. Furthermore, this factor binds to the 21-bp repeat in the enhancer, which also negatively regulates the MIEP in undifferentiated Tera-2 cells [49]. This factor, termed modulator binding factor-1 (MBF-1), has been proposed to be a differentiation-specific negative regulator of the MIEP. Together these studies demonstrate that the modulator sequence exerts differential activities in a variety of cells. We suggest that the unequal pattern of activity of the modulator sequence may be an important determinant toward viral latency and reactivation.

Summing our current knowledge of the MIEP region, we conclude that the 5′-flanking sequence of the MIEP is highly complex and appears to be composed of several domains. These domains interface with a wide variety of cellular transcription factors. The known regulatory domains and protein–DNA interactions of the HCMV MIEP are summarized in Fig. 4. The elements appear to be acting coordinately to contribute to chromatin conformations important for accessibility to these transcription factors and subsequent gene expression. We think that the overall activity of the negative and positive domains of the HCMV MIEP within any given cell determines the final level

A

-962 GATATCGCCATTTTTCCAAAAGTTGATTTTTGGGCATACGCGATATC

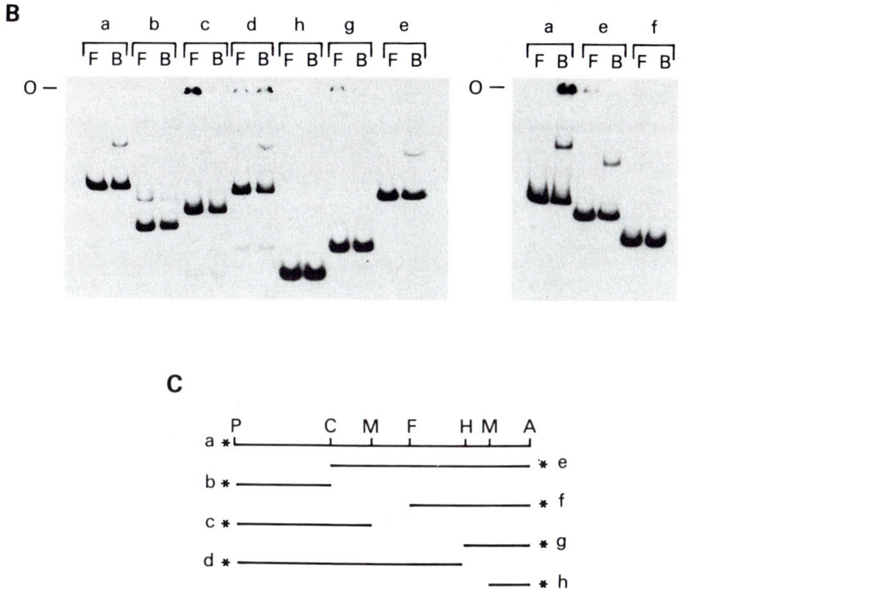

Fig. 6. **A** Primary sequence of the dyad symmetry within the modulator region. **B** Mobility shift assay using various DNA fragments from the modulator region (*a–h*). Conditions used in the mobility shift assay were as previously described [29]. *O* indicates the origin of the gel; *F*, free DNA fragment in the absence of nuclear protein; *B*, bound DNA fragment in the presence of crude HeLa nuclear proteins. **C** The labeled fragments *a–h* with the ^{32}P-labeled end indicated by *asteriks*. *Capital letters* mark the location of restriction endonuclease cleavage sites used to generate the fragments. *P*, PstI; *C*, ClaI; *M*, MaeIII; *F*, FokI; *H*, HaeIII; *A*, AluI. The cleavage sites are located at nucleotide positions –1145, –1022, –969, –875, –867, –820, –775, respectively. Only fragments a, d and e were observed to bind the major nuclear protein complex, thus mapping the binding site between –969 and –875. Sequences between –969 and –875 contain a large dyad symmetry (**A**)

of IE expression. The importance of the IE regulatory factors' interactions will be discussed in the next section.

Role of IE Regulatory Proteins in Pathogenesis

The MIEP regulates transcription of several different transcripts that have been divided into two regions, IE-1 and IE-2 (Fig. 7) [97]. These two regions encompass the major IE gene which codes for a family of mRNAs that differ due to differential splicing and polyadenylation and consequently code for a

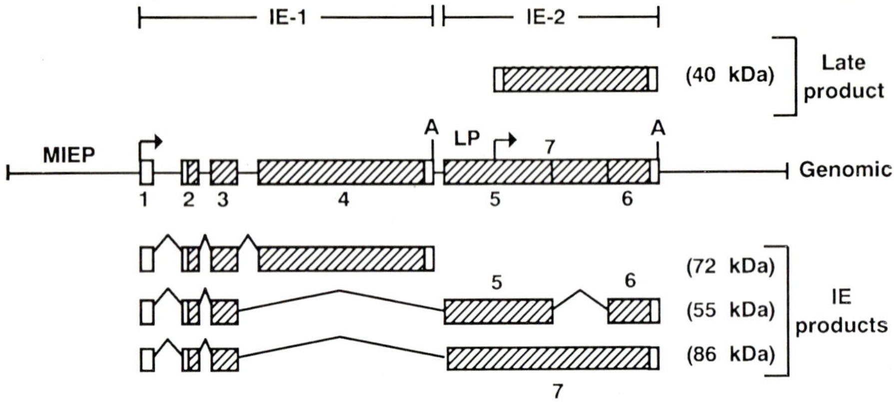

Fig. 7. Predominant proteins encoded by the HCMV major IE gene. A schematic representation of the genomic region and the splicing pattern resulting in the different IE gene products. *Arrows* indicate the transcriptional start site for major IE promoter (*MIEP*) and the late promoter (*LP*). The *clear and hatched boxes* represent the noncoding and coding exons, respectively. *Numbers above exons* represent the different exons. The three most predominant IE proteins wth molecular weights of 72, 55, and 86 kDa are shown. A 40-kDa protein which had been characterized as a late protein originates from a promoter located within exon 5.

series of unique and related proteins [97, 98]. The IE-1 codes for the major IE protein (72 kDa, IE 72) which originates from a 1950 nt mRNA [96]. The IE-2 codes for several proteins, some of which share sequences with IE-1 [97, 98]. The predominant IE proteins that contain the IE-2 polyadenlyation site are the 86-kDa (IE 86) and the 55-kDa (IE 55) proteins. At late times, a 40-kDa protein is expressed from region 2 [98]. Numerous studies [6, 7, 17, 18, 20, 22, 32, 36, 58, 61, 74, 80–82, 86, 92, 94, 95, 99, 103] have shown that viral protein products from these regions are capable of trans-activating heterologous promoters. The details of these studies in relation to the IE proteins are presented in the chapter by Dr. Richard Stenberg and will not be discussed in this chapter. However, it is important to note that these proteins are essential for subsequent viral gene expression and are therefore a key determinant in the pathogenesis of viral disease.

Examination of the primary sequence structure of the IE 72, IE 55, and IE 86 proteins reveals several interesting features characteristic of nuclear proteins and transcription factors (Fig. 8). All three proteins share a repeated motif of proline-*N*-proline at the N-terminus which is characteristic of other transcription factors including CTF/NF-1, C/EBP, AP-1, c-Fos, Fra1, AP-2, and tat [3, 9, 19, 52, 88]. In the case of CTF/NF-1 this proline-rich stretch maps to a domain in the protein which is important for transcriptional activation [65].

Exon 3 of the MIE gene codes for amino acid sequences that are also common to the IE 72, IE 55, and IE 86 proteins. These amino acid sequences are predicted by the Chou-Fasman algorithm to have the potential to form three amphipathic α-helices (Fig. 9). The linker sequence between helix II and helix III are also predicted to contain one putative β turn. Thus, hypothetically, exon 3 coding sequences would predict to topographically fold into helix I-loop-helix II-turn-helix III structure. This predictive form is a potentially common feature of numerous transcription control proteins [69].

Another amino acid sequence motif found in transcription factors is the "zinc finger" [66]. This motif, which recognizes specific DNA sequences, was first identified in the transcription factor TFIII-A from *Xenopus laevis* and later in a variety of factors that influence RNA polymerase II transcription [84]. The zinc is either coordinated by two Cys and two His ligands (TFIIIA-type) or by four Cys ligands (steroid receptor type [8]). In general, sequence-specific DNA-binding proteins with the TFIIIA-type motif have the zinc finger tandemly repeated a minimum of twice with a 7- to 8-amino-acid linker. The other classes of metal-binding proteins have a variable number of conserved Cys available for metal chelation. For example, the steroid receptors contain two unrelated fingers encoded by separate exons with four to five conserved Cys [39]. The HCMV IE72 and IE86 proteins each contain a distinct single putative zinc finger motif of the TFIIIA-type shown in Fig. 10. The significance of a single zinc finger motif in the separate IE proteins is unknown. However, these structures may facilitate interactions of the IE proteins with viral nucleic acids.

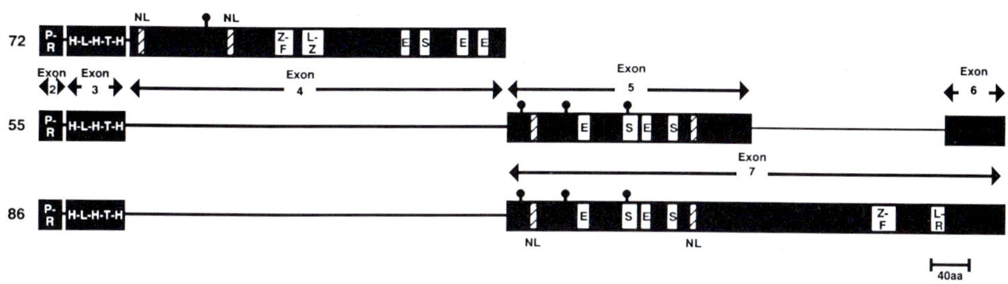

Fig. 8. A linear representation of the structure of the 72-, 55-, and 86-kDa IE proteins. Primary coding structure is represented by *large black boxes,* while intergenic regions (not to scale) are shown by *interconnecting bars. Horizontal arrows* delineate the exons of the IE-1 and -2 region. The location of the peptide antibodies IE1-1, 2 and IE2-1, 2, 3, 4 are shown by *small black boxes*. The *scale* indicates amino acid number. Structural features of interest are marked within the coding sequences. *P-R*, proline-rich region; *H-L-H-T-H*, helix-loop-helix-turn-helix; *NL*, nuclear localization sequence; *Z-F*, putative "zinc finger" modif; *L-Z*, putative leucine-zipper motif; *L-R*, leucine-rich region; *E*, polyglutamic acid segment; *S*, polyserine segment; ●, potential N-linked glycosylation sites

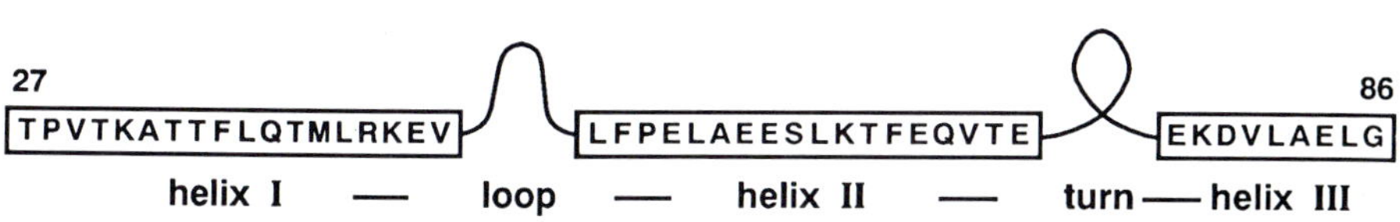

Fig. 9. Predicted α-helical protein domains encoded by exon 3. *Numbers* refer to the amino acid position for IE55, IE72, and IE86

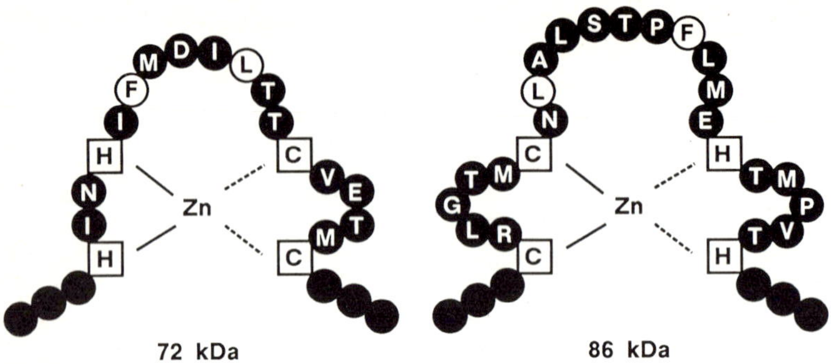

Fig. 10. Two-dimensional folding scheme for a linear arrangement of putative "zinc fingers" of IE72 asnd IE86 proteins. *White*-coded amino acids indicate conserved residues, including the Cys and His zinc ligands

Another sequence motif present in the IE 72 and IE 86 proteins of HCMV that is present in other gene regulatory proteins is a structure called the "leucine zipper" [53]. Landschulz et al. [52, 53] proposed that a heptad repeat of leucine side chains may interdigitate with those of another to hold two proteins together. This interaction would facilitate DNA-binding domains of two proteins to attach to DNA at specific sites. Our current understanding of the leucine zipper complex is that of a parallel, heterodimeric, coiled coil [79]. The interaction surface between helices in a coiled coil is formed from two interspersed heptad repeats of hydrophobic residues known as the 4-3 repeat. The IE 72 protein contains a 4-3 repeat of leucine residues (a putative leucine zipper) in the fourth exon adjacent to the zinc finger (Fig. 8). Interestingly, adjacent to the putative zinc finger of the 86-kDa protein exists a leucine-rich region that contains a single 4-3 repeat motif. On the basis of these observations we propose that the IE 72 and IE 86 proteins may interact with each other through their proposed leucine zippers, bringing their putative DNA-binding zinc fingers in close proximity, and thereby facilitate specific interaction at the DNA level. Alternatively and most likely, cellular elements may also mediate these interactions.

An additional similarity of the IE 72, IE 55, and IE 86 sequence motifs to other DNA-binding proteins and transcription factors is the presence of polyglutamic acid and polyserine stretches. These polyamino acid stretches may form potential "acidic activation domains." Similar stretches of these amino acids are found in the transcription factor ACE-1 [26], Sp1 [47], Ap-2 [112], and HSTF [109]. Also, both proteins contain at least two nuclear localization sequences that are characterized by the clustering of four to six basic residues [23, 82]. Finally, these proteins contain asparagine-X-threonine/serine motifs that are potential sites of N-linked glycosylation [62]. No other major amino acid sequence similarities of the IE proteins were detected in a comparative analysis with the Doolittle protein databank (Doolittle, personal communication).

These homologies may indicate that several distinct and shared modular units exist in these proteins that enable these factors to interact with cellular and viral components to modulate HCMV gene expression. However, comparative analysis of amino acid sequence similarities only infers potential functions of these IE proteins. Nevertheless, we predict that these IE proteins represent viral transcription factors which can modulate both viral and cellular gene expression and ultimately pathogenesis.

Conclusion

In this chapter we have described model tissue culture systems that were utilized to study how the differentiation state may regulate viral gene expression. These studies strongly indicate the importance of cellular factors influencing transcription of the IE gene and the subsequent viral state. The interactions of cellular transcription factors with the MIEP region, encompassing the promoter, the leader, the enhancer, the unique sequence region, the NF-1/CTF cluster, and the modulator sequences have been investigated using a functional in vitro biochemical approach. This work has revealed a highly complex arrangement of distinct sequence-specific transcription factor interactions with each region that appears to act in a coordinated manner to control the level of IE gene expression. The products of this major IE region regulate expression from heterologous cellular and viral promoters and constitute an early event directing the activation of the virus. We predict that it is the level and combinations of these cellular and viral proteins which dictate the fate of the virus within its host. Therefore, identification of the *cis* and *trans* regulatory elements controlling the expression of these IE genes is predicted to be the key for unlocking the mechanisms of latency and reactivation.

Acknowledgements. This is publication no. 6138-IMM from the Department of Immunology, The Scripps Research Institute, La Jolla, CA 92037.

This work was supported by United States Public Health Service grants from the National Institute of Allergy and Infectious Diseases, and a grant from the Universitywide Task Force on AIDS. J.A. Nelson is a recipient of a Faculty Award from the American Cancer Society. We thank Catherine Kohler, Emi Giulietti, Emilia Glezer, and Richard Landes for valuable technical assistance, and Drs. Henryk Lubon, Clayton Wiley, and Carlos Ibanez for valuable discussions. We thank Margaret Stone for the excellent preparation and typing of this chapter.

References

1. Akrigg A, Wilkinson GWG, Oram JD (1985) The structure of the major immediate-early gene of human cytomegalovirus strain AD169. Virus Res 2:107–121
2. Albrecht T, Boldogh I, Fons M, Lee CH, AbuBakar S, Russell JM, Au WW(1989) Cell-activation responses to cytomegalovirus infection: relationship to the phasing of CMV replication and to the induction of cellular damage. Subcell Biochem 15:157–202
3. Arya SK, Guo C, Joseph SF, Wong-Staal F (1985) Transactivator gene of human T lymphotropic virus type III (HTLV-III). Science 229:69–73
4. Baeuerle PA, Baltimore D (1988) IκB: a specific inhibitor of the NF-κB transcription factor. Science 242:540–546
5. Baldwin AS, Sharp PA (1987) Binding of a nuclear factor to a regulatory sequence in the promoter of the mouse H-2K^b class I major histocompatibility gene. Mol Cell Biol 7:305–313
6. Baracchini E, Glezer E, Fish K, Stenberg RM, Nelson JA, Ghazal P (1992) An isoform variant of the cytomegalovirus immediate-early auto-repressor functions as a transcriptional activator. Virol 138 (in press)
7. Barry PA, Pratt-Lowe E, Peterlin BM, Luciw PA (1990) Cytomegalovirus activates transcription directed by the long terminal repeat of human immunodeficiency virus type 1. J Virol 64:2932–2940
8. Berg J (1986) Potential metal-binding domains in nucleic acid binding proteins. Science 232:485–487
9. Bohmann DT, Bos TJ, Adman A, Nishimura T, Vogt PK, Tjian R (1987) Human proto-oncogene c-*jun* encodes a DNA binding protein with structural and functional properties of transcription factor AP1. Science 238:1386–1392
10. Boldogh I, AbuBakar S, Albrecht T (1990) Activation of proto-oncogenes: an immediate early event in human cytomegalovirus infection. Science 247:561–563
11. Boldogh I, AbuBakar S, Deng CZ, Albrecht T (1991) Transcriptional activation of cellular oncogenes *fos, jun,* and *myc* by human cytomegalovirus. J Virol 65:1568–1571
12. Boshart M, Weber F, Jahn G, Dorsch-Hassler K, Fleckenstein B, Schaffner W (1985) A very strong enhancer is located upstream of an immediate-early gene of human cytomegalovirus. Cell 41:521–530
13. Braun RW, Reiser HC (1986) Replication of human cytomegalovirus in human peripheral blood T cells. J Virol 60:29–36
14. Breathnach R, Chambon P (1981) Organization and expression of eukaryotic split genes coding for protein. Annu Rev Biochem 50:349–383
15. Buratowski S, Hahn S, Guarente L, Sharp PA (1989) Five intermediate complexes in transcription initiation by RNA polymerase II. Cell 56:549–561
16. Chang Y-N, Crawford S, Stall S, Rawlins DR, Jeang K-T, Hayward GS (1990) The palindromic series I repeats in the simian cytomegalovirus major immediate-early promoter behave as both strong basal enhancers and cyclic AMP response elements. J Virol 64:264–277
17. Cherrington JM, Mocarski ES (1989) Human cytomegalovirus ie1 transactivates the α promoter-enhancer via an 18-base-pair repeat element. J Virol 63:1435–1440
18. Cherrington JM, Khoury EL, Mocarski ES (1991) Human cytomegalovirus ie2 negatively regulates a gene expression via a short target sequence near the transcription start site. J Virol 65:887–896
19. Cohen DR, Curran T (1988) *Fra*1: a serum-inducible, cellular immediate-early gene that encodes a *Fos*-related antigen. Mol Cell Biol 8:2063–2069
20. Davis MG, Kenney SC, Kamine J, Pagano JS, Huang E-S (1987) Immediate-early gene region of human cytomegalovirus *trans*-activates the promoter of human immunodeficiency virus. Proc Natl Acad Sci USA 84:8642–8646
21. DeMarchi JM (1981) Human cytomegalovirus DNA: restriction enzyme cleavage maps and map locations for immediate-early, early, and late RNAs. Virology 114:23–28

22. Depto AS, Stenberg RM (1989) Regulated expression of the human cytomegalovirus pp65 gene: octamer sequence in the promoter is required for activation by viral gene products. J Virol 63:1232–1238
23. Dingwall C, Laskey RA (1986) Protein import into the cell nucleus. Annu Rev Cell Biol 2:367–390
24. Dorsch-Hasler K, Keil GM, Weber F, Jasin M, Schaffner W, Koszinwoski UH (1985) A long and complex enhancer activates transcription of the gene coding for the highly abundant immediate-early mRNA in murine cytomegalovirus. Proc Natl Acad Sci USA 82:8325–8329
25. Fickenscher H, Stamminger T, Ruger R, Fleckenstein B (1989) The role of a repetitive palindromic sequence element in the human cytomegalovirus major immediate early enhancer. J Gen Virol 70:107–123
26. Furst P, Hu S, Hackett R, Hamer D (1988) Copper activates metallothionein gene transcription by altering the conformation of a specific DNA binding protein. Cell 55:705–717
27. Ghazal P, Nelson JA (1991) Enhancement of RNA polymerase II initiation complexes by a novel DNA control domain downstream from the cap site of the cytomegalovirus major immediate-early promotor. J Virol 65:2299–2307
28. Ghazal P, Lubon H, Fleckenstein B, Hennighausen L (1987) Binding of transcription factors and creation of a large nucleoprotein complex on the human cytomegalovirus enhancer. Proc Natl Acad Sci USA 84:3658–3662
29. Ghazal P, Lubon H, Hennighausen L (1988) Specific interactions between transcription factors and the promoter-regulatory region of the human cytomegalovirus major immediate-early gene. J Virol 62:1076–1079
30. Ghazal P, Lubon H, Hennighausen L (1988) Multiple sequence-specific transcription factors modulate cytomegalovirus enhancer activity in vitro. Mol Cell Biol 8:1809–1811
31. Ghazal P, Lubon H, Reynolds-Kohler C, Hennighausen L, Nelson JA (1990) Interactions between cellular regulatory proteins and a unique sequence region in the human cytomegalovirus major immediate-early promoter. Virology 174:18–25
32. Ghazal P, Young Y, Giulietti E, DeMattei C, Garcia J, Gaynor R, Stenberg RM, Nelson JA (1991) A discrete *cis*-element in the HIV-LTR mediates synergistic *trans*-activation by cytomegalovirus immediate-early proteins. J Virol 65:6735–6742
33. Gonczol E, Andres PW, Plotkin SA (1984) Cytomegalovirus replicates in differentiated but not undifferentiated human embryonal carcinoma cells. Science 224:159–161
34. Hai T, Liu F, Allegretto EA, Karin M, Green MR (1988) A family of immunologically related transcription factors that includes multiple forms of ATF and AP-1. Genes Dev 1:1216–1226
35. Hennighausen L, Fleckenstein B (1986) Nuclear factor 1 interacts with five DNA elements in the promoter region of the human cytomegalovirus major immediate-early gene. EMBO J 5:1367–1371
36. Hermiston T, Malone C, Witte P, Stinski MJ (1987) Identification and characterization of the human cytomegalovirus immediate-early region 2 gene that stimulates gene expression from an inducible promoter. J Virol 61:3214–3221
37. Ho M (1982) Cytomegalovirus biology and infection. Plenum, New York, pp 119–129
38. Horikoshi M, Hai T, Lin YS, Green MR, Roeder RG (1988 b) Transcription factor ATF interacts with the TATA factor to facilitate establishment of a preinitiation complex. Cell 54:1033–1042
39. Huckaby CS, Connelly OM, Beattie WG, Dabron AW, Tsai MJ, O'Malley BW (1987) Structure of the chromosomal chicken progesterone receptor gene. Proc Natl Acad Sci USA 84:8380–8384
40. Hunninghake GW, Monick MM, Liu B, Stinski MF (1989) The promoter-regulatory region of the major immediate-early gene of human cytomegalovirus responds to T-lymphocyte stimulation and contains functional cyclic AMP-response elements. J Virol 63:3026–3033

41. Hurst HC, Jones N (1987) Identification of factors that interact with the E1a-inducible adenovirus E3 promoter. Genes Dev 1:1121–1146
42. Ibanez C, Schrier R, Ghazal P, Wiley CA, Nelson JA (1991) Human cytomegalovirus productively infects primary differentiated macrophages. J Virol 65:6581–6588
43. Jahn G, Knust E, Schmolla H, Sarre T, Nelson JA, McDougall JK, Fleckenstein B (1984) Predominant immediate-early transcripts of human cytomegalovirus AD169. J Virol 49:363–370
44. Jeang K, Rawlins DR, Rosenfeld PJ, Shero JH, Kelly TJ, Hayward GS (1987) Multiple tandemly repeated binding sites for cellular nuclear factor I that surround the major immediate-early promoters of simian and human cytomegalovirus. J Virol 61:1559–1570
45. Jones KA, Kadonaga JT, Rosenfeld PJ, Kelly T, Tjian R (1987) A cellular DNA binding protein that activates eukaryotic transcription and DNA replication. Cell 48:79–89
46. Jordan MC, Shanley JD, Stevens JG (1977) Immunosuppression reactivates and disseminates latent murine cytomegalovirus. J Gen Virol 37:419–423
47. Kadonaga JT, Cavner KR, Masiarz FR, Tjian R (1987) Isolation of cDNA encoding transcription factor Sp1 and functional analysis of the DNA binding domain. Cell 51:1079–1090
48. Kohwi-Shigematus T, Nelson JA (1988) The chemical carcinogen, chloracetaldehyde, modifies a specific site within the regulatory sequence of human cytomegalovirus major immediate gene in vivo. Mol Carcinog 1:20–25
49. Kothari S, Baillie J, Sissons JGP, Sinclair JH (1991) The 21bp repeat element of the human cytomegalovirus major immediate early enhancer is a negative regulator of gene expression in undifferentiated cells. Nucleic Acids Res 19:1767–1771
50. Kouzarides T, Bankier AT, Satchwell SC, Preddy E, Barrell BG (1988) An immediate-early gene of human cytomegalovirus encodes a potential membrane glycoprotein. Virology 165:151–164
51. LaFemina R, Hayward GS (1986) Constitutive and retinoic acid-inducible expression of cytomegalovirus immediate-early genes in human teratocarcinoma cells. J Virol 58:434–440
52. Landschulz WH, Johnson PF, Adashi EY, Graves BJ, McKnight SL (1988) Isolation of a recombinant copy of the gene encoding C/EMP. Genes Dev 2:786–800
53. Landschulz WH, Johnson PF, McKnight SL (1988) The leucine zipper: a hypothetical structure common to a new class of DNA binding proteins. Science 240:1759–1764
54. Lang DJ, Ebert PA, Rodgers BM, Boggess HP, Rixse RS (1977) Reduction of post perfusion CMV infections following the use of leukocyte depleted blood. Transplantation 17:391–395
55. Lenardo MJ, Baltimore A (1989) NF-κB: a pleiotropic mediator of inducible and tissue-specific gene control. Cell 58:227–229
56. Lenardo MJ, Kuang A, Gifford A, Baltimore D (1988) NF-κB protein purification from bovine spleen: nucleotide stimulation and binding site specificity. Proc Natl Acad Sci USA 85:8825–8829
57. Lin YS, Green MR (1988) Interaction of a common transcription factor, ATF, with regulatory elements in both E1a and cyclic AMP-inducible promoters. Proc Natl Acad Sci USA 85:3396–3400
58. Liu B, Hermiston TW, Stinski MF (1991) A *cis*-acting element in the major immediate-early (IE) promoter of human cytomegalovirus is required for negative regulation by IE2. J Virol 65:897–903
59. Lubon H, Ghazal P, Nelson JA, Hennighausen L (1988) Cell-specific activity of the human immunodeficiency virus enhancer repeat in vitro. AIDS Res Hum Retroviruses 4:381–391
60. Lubon H, Ghazal P, Hennighausen L, Reynolds-Kohler C, Lockshin C, Nelson JA (1989) Cell-specific activity of the modulator region in the human cytomegalovirus major immediate-early gene. Mol Cell Biol 9:1342–1345

61. Malone CL, Vesole DH, Stinski MF (1990) Transactivation of a human cytomegalovirus early promoter by gene products from the immediate-early gene IE 2 and augmentation by IE 1: mutational analysis of the viral proteins. J Virol 64:1498–1506
62. Marshall RD (1972) Glycoproteins. Annu Rev Biochem 41:673–701
63. Matsui T, Segall J, Weil PA, Roeder RG (1980) Multiple factors required for accurate iniation of transcription by purified RNA polymerase II. J Biol Chem 255:11992–11996
64. McDonough S, Spector D (1985) Transcription in human fibroblasts permissively infected by human cytomegalovirus strain AD 169. Virology 125:31–46
65. Mermod N, O'Neill EA, Kelly TJ, Tjian R (1989) The proline-rich transcriptional activator CTF/NF1 is distinct from the replication and DNA binding domain. Cell 58:741–753
66. Miller J, McLachlan AD, Klug A (1985) Repetitive zinc-binding domains in the protein transcription factor IIIa from *Xenopus* oocytes. EMBO J 4:1609–1614
67. Montminy MR, Bilezsikjian LM (1987) Binding of a nuclear protein to the cyclic AMP response element of the somatostatin gene. Nature 328:175–178
68. Montminy MR, Sevarino KA, Wagner JA, Mandel G, Goodman RH (1986) Identification of a cyclic-AMP-responsive element within the rat somatostatin gene. Proc Natl Acad Sci USA 83:6682–6686
69. Murre C, McCaw PS, Baltimore D (1989) A new DNA binding and imerization motif in immunoglobulin enhancer binding, *daughterless, MyoD,* and *myc* proteins. Cell 56:777–783
70. Myerson D, Hackman RC, Nelson JA, Ward DC, McDougall JK (1984) Widespread presence of histologically occult cytomegalovirus. Hum Pathol 15:430–439
71. Nakajima N, Horikoshi M, Roeder RG (1988) Factors involved in specific transcription by mammalian RNA polymerase II: purification, genetic specificity, and TATA box-promoter interactions of TFIID. Mol Cell Biol 8:4028–4040
72. Nelson JA, Groudine M (1986) Transcriptional regulation of the human cytomegalovirus major immediate-early gene is associated with induction of DNaseI hypersensitive sites. Mol Cell Biol 6:452–461
73. Nelson JA, Reynolds-Kohler C, Smith B (1987) Negative and positive regulation by a short segment in the 5′-flanking region of the human cytomegalovirus major immediate-early gene. Mol Cell Biol 7:4125–4129
74. Nelson JA, Gnann JW, Ghazal P (1990) Regulation and tissue specific expression of human cytomegalovirus. Curr Top Microbiol Immunol 154:77–103
75. Nelson JA, Ibanez C, Schrier R, Wiley C, Ghazal P (1991) Expression of cytomegalovirus in mononuclear cells. In: Fan HY et al. (eds) Viruses that affect the immune system. American Society for Microbiology, Washington, pp 231–246
76. Niller HH, Hennighausen L (1990) Phytohemagglutinin-induced activity of cyclic AMP (cAMP) response elements from cytomegalovirus is reduced by cyclosporine and synergistically enhanced by cAMP. J Virol 64:2388–2391
77. Niller HH, Hennighausen L (1991) Formation of several specific nucleoprotein complexes on the human cytomegalovirus immediate early enhancer. Nucleic Acids Res 19:3715–3721
78. Olding LB, Jensen FC, Oldstone MBA (1975) Pathogenesis of cytomegalovirus infection. I. Activation of virus from bone marrow-derived lymphocytes by in vitro allogenic reaction. J Exp Med 141:561–572
79. O'Shea EK, Rutkowski R, Stafford WF III, Kim PS (1989) Evidence that the leucine zipper is a coiled coil. Science 243:538–542
80. Pizzorno MC, Hayward GS (1990) The IE 2 gene products of human cytomegalovirus specifically down-regulate expression from the major immediate-early promoter through a target sequence located near the cap site. J Virol 64:6154–6165
81. Pizzorno MC, O'Hare P, Sha L, La Femina RL, Hayward GS (1988) Transactivation and autoregulation of gene expression by the immediate-early region 2 products of human cytomegalovirus. J Virol 62:1167–1179

82. Pizzorno MC, Mullen M-A, Chang Y-N, Hayward GS (1991) The functionally active IE2 immediate-early regulatory protein of HCMV is an 80-kD polypeptide that contains two distinct activator domains and a duplicated nuclear localization signal. J Virol 65:3839–3852
83. Prince AM, Szmuness W, Millian SJ, David DS (1971) A serologic study of cytomegalovirus infections associated with blood transfusions. N Engl J Med 284:1125–1131
84. Rhodes D, Klug A (1988) "Zinc fingers": a novel motif for nucleic acid binding. Nucleic Acids Mol Biol 2:149–166
85. Rice GPA, Schrier RD, Oldstone MBA (1984) Cytomegalovirus infects human lymphocytes and monocytes: virus expression is restricted to immediate-early gene products. Proc Natl Acad Sci USA 81:6134–6138
86. Sambucetti LC, Cherrington JM, Wilkinson GWG, Mocarski ES (1989) NF-kB activation of the cytomegalovirus enhancer is mediated by a viral transactivator and by T cell stimulation. EMBO J 8:4251–4258
87. Santoro CN, Mermod N, Andrews PC, Tjian R (1988) A family of human CCAAT box-binding proteins active in transcription and DNA replication: cloning and expression of multiple cDNAs. Nature 334:218–224
88. Schrier RD, Nelson JA, Oldstone MBA (1985) Detection of human cytomegalovirus in peripheral blood lymphocytes in a natural infection. Science 230:1048–1051
89. Sen R, Baltimore D (1986) Multiple nuclear factors interact with the immunoglobulin enhancer sequences. Cell 46:705–716
90. Sen R, Baltimore D (1987) Inducibility of k immunoglobulin enhancer-binding protein NK-$\varkappa$B by a post-translational mechanism. Cell 47:921–928
91. Shelbourn SL, Kothari SK, Sissons JGP, Sinclair JH (1989) Repression of human cytomegalovirus gene expression associated with a novel immediate-early regulatory region binding factor. Nucleic Acids Res 17:9165–9171
92. Spaete R, Mocarski E (1985) Regulation of cytomegalovirus gene expression: alpha and beta promoters are transactivated by viral functions in permissive human fibroblasts. J Virol 56:135–143
93. Stamminger T, Fickenscher H, Fleckenstein B (1990) Cell type-specific induction of the major immediate early enhancer of human cytomegalovirus by cyclic AMP. J Gen Virol 71:105–113
94. Staprans SI, Rabert DK, Spector DH (1988) Identification of sequence requirements and *trans*-acting functions necessary for regulated expression of a human cytomegalovirus early gene. J Virol 62:3463–3473
95. Stenberg RM, Stinski MF (1985) Autoregulation of the human cytomegalovirus major immediate-early gene. J Virol 56:676–682
96. Stenberg RM, Thomsen DR, Stinski MF (1984) Structural analysis of the major immediate-early gene of human cytomegalovirus. J Virol 49:190–199
97. Stenberg RM, Witte PR, Stinski MF (1985) Multiple spliced and unspliced transcripts from human cytomegalovirus immediate-early region two and evidence for a common initiation site within immediate-early region. J Virol 56:665–675
98. Stenberg RM, Depto AS, Fortney J, Nelson JA (1989) Regulated expression of early and late RNA and protein from the human cytomegalovirus immediate-early gene region. J Virol 63:2699–2708
99. Stenberg RM, Fortney J, Barlow SW, Magrane BP, Nelson JA, Ghazal P (1990) Promoter-specific *trans*activation and repression by human cytomegalovirus immediate-early proteins involves common and unique protein domains. J Virol 64:1556–1565
100. Stinski MF (1983) The molecular biology of cytomegaloviruses. In: Roizman B (ed) The herpes viruses, vol 2. Plenum, New York, pp 67–113
101. Stinski MF, Roehr TS (1985) Activation of the major immediate-early gene of human cytomegalovirus by cis-acting elements in the promoter-regulatory sequence and by virus-specific *trans*-acting components. J Virol 55:431–441

102. Stinski MF, Thomson DR, Stenberg RM, Goldstein LC (1983) Organization and expression of the immediate-early genes of human cytomegalovirus. J Virol 46:1–14
103. Tevethia MJ, Spector DJ, Leisure KM, Stinski MF (1987) Participation of two human cytomegalovirus immediate-early gene regions in transcriptional activation of adenovirus promoters. Virology 161:276–285
104. Thomson DR, Stenberg RM, Goins WF, Stinski MF (1984) Promoter-regulatory region of the major immediate-early gene of human cytomegalovirus. Proc Natl Acad Sci USA 81:659–663
105. Van Dyke MW, Roeder RG, Sawadogo M (1988) Physical analysis of transcription preinitiation complex assembly in a class I gene promoter. Science 241:1335–1338
106. Wathen MW, Stinski MF (1982) Temporal patterns of human cytomegalovirus transcription: mapping the viral RNAs synthesized at immediate-early, early, and late times after infection. J Virol 41:462–477
107. Wathen MW, Thomson DR, Stinski MF (1981) Temporal regulation of human cytomegalovirus transcription at immediate-early and early times after infection. J Virol 38:446–459
108. Weston K (1988) An enhancer element in the short unique region of human cytomegalovirus regulates the production of a group of abundant immediate-early transcripts. Virology 162:406–416
109. Wiederrecht G, Steo D, Parker CS (1988) Isolation of the gene encoding the *S. cerevisiae* heat shock transcription factor. Cell 54:841–853
110. Wiley CA, Schrier RD, Denaro FJ, Nelson JA, Lampert PW, Oldstone MBA (1986) Localization of cytomegalovirus proteins and genome during fulminant central nervous system infection in an AIDS patient. J Neuropathol Exp Neurol 45:127–139
111. Wilkinson GWG, Akrigg A, Greenaway PJ (1984) Transcription of the immediate-early genes of human cytomegalovirus strain AD169. Virus Res 1:101–116
112. Williams T, Admon A, Luscher B, Tjian R (1988) Cloning and expression of AP-2, a cell-type-specific transcription factor that activates inducible enhancer elements. Genes Dev 2:1557–1569

Chapter 19 Activation of Proto-oncogenes and Cell Activation Signals in the Initiation and Progression of Human Cytomegalovirus Infection

T. Albrecht[1], I. Boldogh[1,2], M.P. Fons[1], and T. Valyi-Nagy[1,3]

Summary

Human cytomegalovirus (HCMV) activates cells through a signal cascade that shares components with the activation mechanisms induced by serum or growth factors. Moreover, HCMV infection appears to perturb cellular control of the signal cascade protracting some cellular responses. These cellular responses may be divided into three phases. Immediate early (IE) cellular signals include increased metabolism of phosphoinositides and arachidonic acid and activation of cellular oncogenes *fos*, *jun*, and *myc*. These IE cellular responses appear to result from the interaction of the virus particle with the plasmalemma, since they do not appear to be related to virus infectivity, do not require cellular or viral protein synthesis, occur when virus particles are located at the plasma membrane, and appear to be related to the activity of membrane-associated enzymes. Our preliminary findings suggest that the IE cellular responses are related to initiation and regulation of HCMV IE gene expression. Early cellular responses include increases in the cellular levels of inositol 1,4,5-trisphosphate (IP_3), 1,2-diacylglycerol (DG), cyclic nucleotides, release of arachidonic acid (AA), a substantial and protracted increase in cytosolic $[Ca^{2+}]$, and a decrease in Na^+/K^+ adenosine triphosphatase (ATPase) activity that may be related to changes in intracellular pH. Early cellular responses appear to be related to virus infectivity, ongoing cellular RNA and protein synthesis, and to the development and progression of cytopathology. Ca^{2+} signals are protracted into the late phase, which is most notably characterized by a sustained increase in Na^+/K^+ ATPase activity that is presumably related to Na^+ entry. As interference with the cellular responses results in substantial reductions in infectious yields of HCMV, it is likely that these cellular changes are related to efficient HCMV replication. Furthermore, the cellular signals provoked by HCMV appear to be related to cell cycle perturbation and induction of chromosome damage.

---

[1] Department of Microbiology, University of Texas Medical Branch, Galveston, TX 77550, USA
[2] Department of Microbiology, Medical University of Debrecen, 4012 Debrecen, Hungary
[3] The Wistar Institute, 36th and Spruce Streets, Philadelphia, PA, USA

Introduction

Our understanding of the processes by which human cytomegalovirus (HCMV) alters cellular metabolism to support the pathogenic mechanisms associated with acute and persistent infections is improving. Viruses, including HCMV, have adapted to replicate in tissues that have ready access to one or more portals of entry and/or exit (e.g., the upper respiratory tract and the bowel) as well as in other tissues. A number of obstacles must be overcome for a virus to produce abundant progeny. One of the principal obstacles is that many of the cells that are located in these sites are differentiated and predisposed to the expression of a limited repertoire. If productive replication is to take place in these cells, then one of the molecular strategies that could prove advantageous for virus replication is activation of certain cell functions, so that the cells' metabolism is stimulated and the synthesis of macromolecules useful in virus replication is increased.

Although HCMV is widely recognized for its induction of a mitogenic signal and its stimulatory effects on cellular macromolecular synthesis, until recently our understanding of the role of these stimulatory effects in HCMV replication was confounded by the early observations that stimulation of cellular DNA synthesis was limited to abortively infected cells [31]. Thus, it was difficult to reconcile how the stimulatory effect of HCMV infection on the cell could be involved in virus replication. Recently, we suggested an explanation for the involvement of HCMV-induced activation of cells through mitogenic signaling and stimulatory effects on cellular metabolism in productive infection that accounts for the observed inhibition of cellular DNA synthesis in acutely infected cells. Our findings suggest that the HCMV particle activates cells through preexisting cellular pathways, resulting in broad stimulation of the cell [8–10]. The mechanisms utilized by HCMV to stimulate cells seem to be related to cellular pathways for activation of cells to work or to proliferate [29, 44, 47, 50, 61, 63, 69]. The process of cell activation promotes rapid metabolic changes that occur within minutes and that are potentially related to the initiation of HCMV replication. As HCMV replication progresses, control over the activation process is perturbed and some of the cellular activation signals are protracted. These protracted signals lead to further changes in the cell (associated with the development of cytomegaly) that promote efficient HCMV replication.

This perspective of the pathologic activation of cells by HCMV has several potentially important implications. First, if cell activation and perturbation of the activation process are related to the initiation and progression of HCMV replication, respectively, then they may be necessary steps in the production of high yields of HCMV that have been largely overlooked. Second, this view suggests that HCMV can profoundly modify and damage cells without necessarily synthesizing new virus and completing its replication cycle. Third, if cell activation, and particularly perturbation of activation signals, is necessary for high yields of infectious HCMV, then these pathologic activation signals are potential targets for novel antiviral therapeutic approaches that have yet to be exploited appropriately.

Activation of Cells to Work or to Proliferate by Serum, Growth Factors, or Tumor Promoters

A particular strength of the view that HCMV activates cells through preexisting signal transduction pathways is that the molecular and cellular events involved in the activation of cells to work or to proliferate are the subject of intensive investigation. Indeed, much progress has been made recently in understanding the cascade of events required for cell activation by serum, growth factors, and viruses [8–10, 12, 29, 47, 50, 61, 63, 67, 69]. Figure 1 presents a scheme illustrating some of the major events involved in this cascade. The activation process begins with a ligand binding to a membrane-bound receptor, which may lead to substantial modification of the cell through a rapid activation of membrane-bound enzymes (e.g., phospholipase C, PLC; phospholipase A_2, PLA_2; protein kinase C, PKC; and adenylate cyclase) which mediate increases in the cellular levels of a number of secondary messengers (e.g., inositol 1,4,5-triphosphate, IP_3; 1,2-diacylglycerol, DG; intracellular free Ca^{2+}, $[Ca^{2+}]_i$; arachidonic acid, AA; AA metabolites; cyclic AMP, cAMP; and cyclic guanosine monophosphate, cGMP). Some of these messengers, such as DG, remain in the plane of the membrane, while others (e.g., $[Ca^{2+}]_i$) function within the cytosol to activate specific protein kinases. The activated protein kinases phosphorylate specific proteins, some of which affect regulatory factors within the nucleus, leading to activation of cellular genes, including in some instances cell-cycle-associated genes (e.g., proto-oncogenes). The changes in the activity of specific cellular proteins and/or genes may lead to cellular work or DNA synthesis, depending on the specific stimulus, physiological state of the cell, and cell type [29, 47, 50, 61, 69, 73].

Activation of Cells by HCMV

We have previously reviewed in some detail the evidence that HCMV activates cells, inducing both cellular work, in the form of a contractile-like response, and a proliferative response [8]. Findings which suggest that HCMV is activating cells through a molecular pathway that is similar to that involved in signal transduction for activation of cells by serum, growth factors, tumor promoters, or hormones are summarized in Table 1. Even though some of the same signal components are involved in activation of cells by HCMV and soluble growth factors, it is noteworthy that in cells productively infected with HCMV the activation process is pathologically modified as illustrated by the time courses for some of these responses (Fig. 2). That is, in productive HCMV

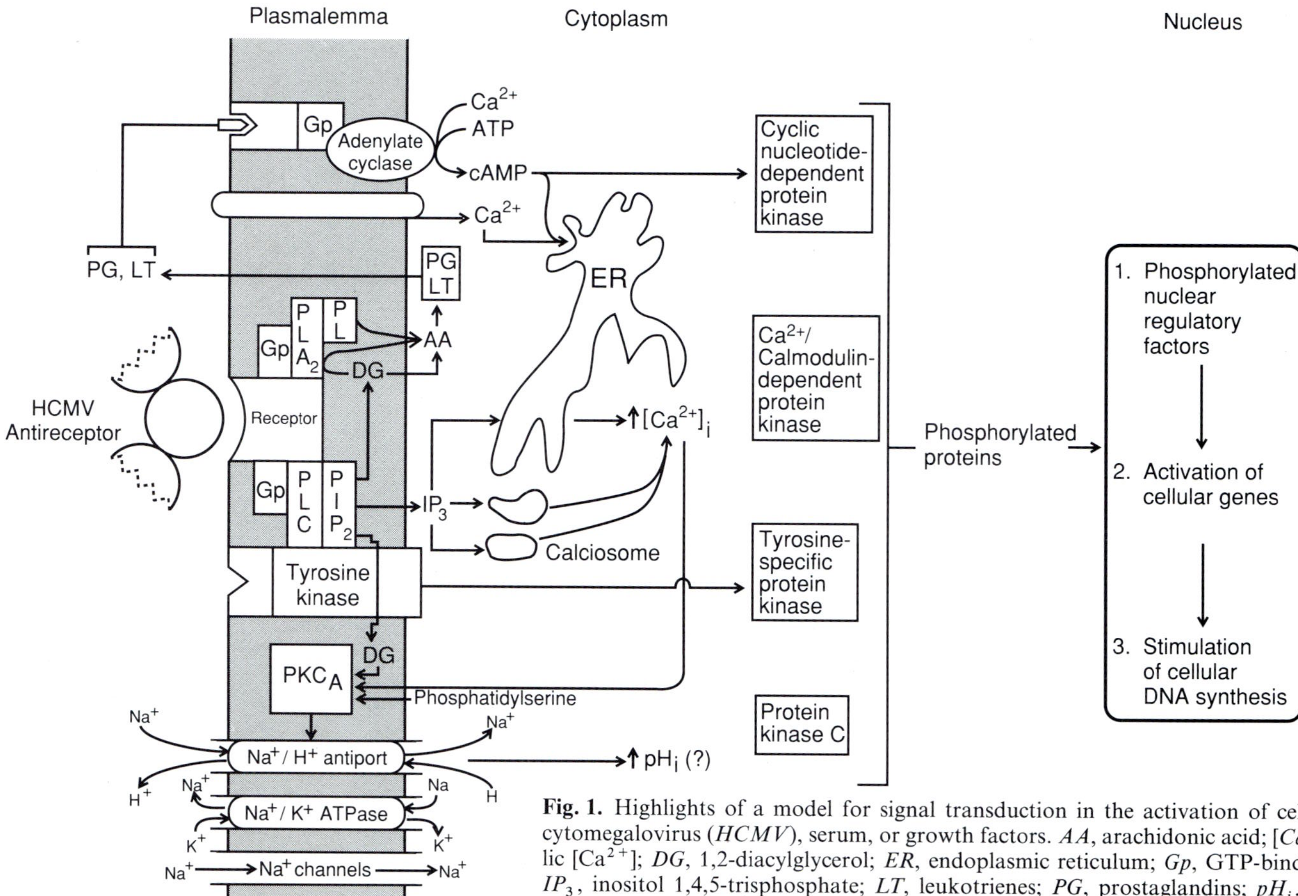

Fig. 1. Highlights of a model for signal transduction in the activation of cells by human cytomegalovirus (*HCMV*), serum, or growth factors. *AA*, arachidonic acid; $[Ca^{2+}]_i$, cytosolic $[Ca^{2+}]$; *DG*, 1,2-diacylglycerol; *ER*, endoplasmic reticulum; *Gp*, GTP-binding proteins; IP_3, inositol 1,4,5-trisphosphate; *LT*, leukotrienes; *PG*, prostaglandins; pH_i, intracellular pH; PIP_2, phosphatidylinositol 4,5-bisphosphate; *PKC*, protein kinase C; *PL*, phospholipids; PLA_2, phospholipase A_2; *PLC*, phospholipase C; *cAMP*, cyclic AMP

Table 1. Biochemical and physiologic cellular responses associated with HCMV infection

Response	Phase *	Time of response after infection: Initial	Time of response after infection: Maximum	Cellular location	Requirement for infectious virus
Increased IP_3	IE	10 min	20 min	Plasmalemma	No
Increased DG	IE	10 min	20 min	Plasmalemma	No
Increased AA	IE	10 min	20 min	Plasmalemma	No
Increased transcription of					
c-*fos*	IE	20 min	40 min	Nucleus	No
c-*jun*	IE	20 min	40 min	Nucleus	No
c-*myc*	IE	20 min	60 min	Nucleus	No
Increased Ca^{2+} influx	?	60 min	120 min	Plasmalemma	?
Increased IP_3	E	4 h	6 h	Plasmalemma	Yes
Increased DG	E	4 h	6 h	Plasmalemma	Yes
Increased AA	E	5 h	7 h	Plasmalemma	Yes
Increased total cellular Ca^{2+}	E	6 h	9 h	Cell	?
Increased $[Ca^{2+}]_i$	E	7 h	49?h	Cytosol	Yes
Decreased Na^+/K^+ ATPase	E	6 h	25 h	Plasmalemma	Yes
Increased cAMP	E	3 h	7 h	Cytosol	Yes
Increased cGMP	E	7 h	13 h	Cytosol	Yes
Increased $[Ca^{2+}]_i$	L	7 h	49?h	Cytosol	Yes
Increased total cellular Ca^{2+}	L	49 h	96?h	Cell	?
Increased cAMP	L	49 h	73 h	Cytosol	Yes
Increased Na^+/K^+ ATPase	L	37 h	97?h	Plasmalemma	Yes

* IE, immediate early; E, early; L, late; ATPase, adenosine triphosphatase; ?, unknown

infection, the cellular biochemical and physiologic responses are protracted and at least three phases are apparent (Table 1, Fig. 2).

HCMV-Induced Immediate Early Activation Signals

Biochemical and Physiologic Cellular Responses to HCMV Infection

Activation signals of the immediate early (IE) phase are associated with initiation of HCMV infection and replication. These biochemical and physiologic responses include increases in the cellular levels of IP_3, DG, AA, and its metabolites, and possibly Ca^{2+} influx (discussed in "early Ca^{2+} Responses to HCMV Infection"). Increases in these secondary messengers occur within 10 min of exposing cells to HCMV at 37 °C (PI[1]) and attain their maximum

[1] PI, the time after infection, is noted beginning with either the addition of virus to cells at 37 °C (0 h) or upon the rapid warming of cells to 37 °C after virus is adsorbed for 30 min at 4 °C. For data reported using the older convention with 0 h established following 1 h adsorption at 37 °C, 1 h has been added to each time.

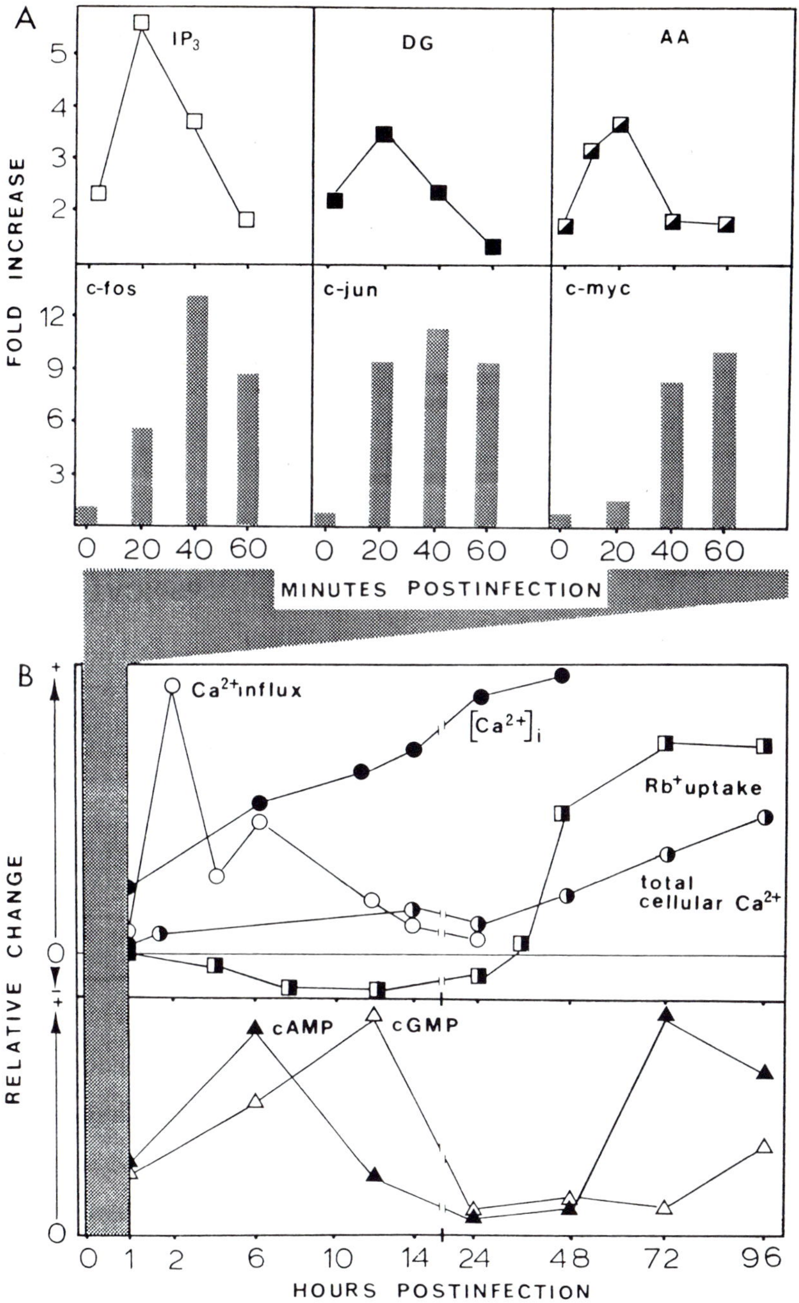

Fig. 2 A, B. Immediate early (**A**), and early and late (**B**) physiologic and biochemical cellular responses to HCMV infection in human fibroblasts (LU). **A** Increases in the cellular levels of inositol 1,4,5-trisphosphate (*IP*$_3$), 1,2-diacylglycerol (*DG*), and arachidonic acid (*AA*), and in RNA derived from the cellular (c-) oncogenes *fos*, *jun*, and *myc*. **B** Changes in Ca^{2+} metabolism including the intracellular free $[Ca^{2+}]$ ($[Ca^{2+}]_i$), ouabain-sensitive Rb^+ uptake (a measure of Na^+/K^+ adenosine triphosphatase activity), and cellular cyclic nucleotide levels (*cAMP*, *cGMP*)

levels by 20 min PI (Fig. 2). In addition to their similar time courses, a number of other features are shared by these cellular responses. Those identified thus far seem to be induced by the interaction of the HCMV particle with the cytoplasmic lamella and, accordingly, neither virus infectivity nor the synthesis of HCMV IE antigens appear to be necessary for induction of these IE cellular responses [2, 3]. Furthermore, neither transcription nor translation appears to be required for induction of these responses [2, 3].

Increases in these secondary messengers suggest that HCMV infection is broadly affecting membrane-associated enzymes whose activity is often related to cell activation [15, 61, 69]. In a recent study of the IE increase in AA metabolism AbuBakar et al. [3] investigated this possibility. They observed that interference with the activity of PLA_2, PKC, or diacylglycerol lipase inhibited the release of ^3H from [^3H]AA-prelabeled cells, suggesting that the activity of these enzymes was related to HCMV-induced increased AA metabolism. In addition, involvement of PLC in the IE responses is suggested by the inhibitory effect of diacylglycerol lipase on the release of ^3H from [^3H]AA-prelabeled cells, since the former enzyme effects the hydrolysis of phosphatidylinositol 4,5-bisphosphate (PIP_2) yielding IP_3 and DG, the substrate for diacyclglycerol lipase. It may be noteworthy that in this study inhibition of an individual arm of the pathways leading to release of AA was insuffient to completely block the HCMV-stimulated release of ^3H from [^3H]AA-prelabelled cells. Complete inhibition was achieved, however, when PKC was desensitized and PLA_2 activity was blocked with quinacrine. These findings are consistent with the view that the interaction of the HCMV particle with the cell membrane rapidly affects the activity of a number of enzymes associated with cell activation signaling induced by serum or growth factors [15, 47, 61, 63, 69].

Transcriptional Activation of Cellular Oncogenes *fos*, *jun*, and *myc*

As noted previously, cells activated by serum or growth factors often demonstrate rapid and transient increases in the transcription of proto-oncogenes [29, 37, 38, 50, 69]. Indeed, in HCMV-infected cells transcriptional activation of cellular oncogenes (c-oncogenes) *fos*, *jun*, and *myc* follows rapidly after increases in the cellular levels of secondary messengers (Table 1). Increases in the cellular levels of RNA [23] or rate of transcription [24] for these nuclear proto-oncogenes are first observed from 20 (c-*fos*, c-*jun*) to 40 min (c-*myc*) PI and reach their maximum levels from 40 (c-*fos*, c-*jun*) to 60 min (c-*myc*). The HCMV-induced increases in proto-oncogene RNAs are quantitatively similar to those induced in cells stimulated by fetal calf serum (FCS, 10%), but the increases in RNA levels occur somewhat more rapidly in the FCS-stimulated cells, reaching their maximum values by 20 (c-*fos*, c-*jun*) or 40 min (c-*myc*). The increases in proto-oncogene RNAs are transient in cells exposed to either HCMV or FCS. By 90 (c-*fos*, c-*jun*) or 150 min (c-*myc*), the RNA levels in HCMV-infected cells return to values similar to those for unstimulated or mock-infected cells.

The similar findings for serum and HCMV suggest that the increase in c-oncogene RNAs observed after HCMV infection might be a result of serum components present in the HCMV stocks. Induction of increased proto-oncogene RNAs by HCMV, however, does not appear to be a result of contamination of the HCMV stocks with serum components. Two observations support this view. First, serum induces increased rates of transcription and levels of RNA from the *β*-actin gene, while HCMV does not [24]. If the stimulation of proto-oncogene transcription observed in HCMV-infected cells resulted from serum contamination, then increases in transcription and RNA from the *β*-actin gene would be likely to be detected in the HCMV-infected cells. Second, purified serum-free stocks of HCMV stimulate increased transcription and RNA levels to about the same extent as unpurified serum-free stocks. If contaminating serum components were responsible for the changes in cellular oncogene expression observed after HCMV infection, then as the virus stocks were purified a decrease in their stimulatory effect would be expected. In fact, no decrease was observed in the studies by Boldogh et al. [23, 24]. Thus, the increases in transcription and RNAs from the c-oncogenes appear to be induced by HCMV. Furthermore, the absence of an effect on expression of the *β*-actin gene and the slower induction of expression for c-*fos*, c-*jun*, and c-*myc* by HCMV relative to serum suggest that some aspects of the activation of cells by HCMV are unique.

The increase in proto-oncogene RNAs could result from either stabilization of RNAs produced at a relatively constant low level or from transcriptional activation of the cellular genes. The increased levels of proto-oncogene RNAs in the HCMV-infected cells do not appear to result from stabilization of the RNA species, since half-lives (monitored by dactinomycin chase) for the RNAs were not changed significantly after HCMV infection. The half-life for c-*fos* or c-*jun* RNA was about 20 min and for c-*myc* about 40 min in the study by Boldogh et al. [24]. Results of transcriptional rate analysis indicate that the rapid increases in RNA levels for these oncogenes in HCMV-infected cells are controlled at the transcriptional level and are related to enhanced transcription (Fig. 3). Consistent with these findings, inclusion of either dactinomycin or *α*-amanitin essentially eliminated the HCMV-induced increases in either the transcriptional rate or cellular levels of RNA for c-*fos*, c-*jun*, or c-*myc*. Since these compounds are effective inhibitors of DNA-dependent RNA synthesis through inhibition of RNA elongation or of the activity of RNA polymerase II, respectively, it is likely that the HCMV-induced increases in proto-oncogene RNAs are the result of increased transcription by RNA polymerase II.

HCMV-Induced Increases in Nuclear Oncoproteins

Although transcriptional activation of c-*fos*, c-*jun*, and c-*myc* is consistent with the IE responses induced by other mitogenic stimuli [29, 50, 69], the findings of increased rates of transcription and increased levels of RNA do not necessarily indicate enhanced levels of oncoproteins. Transcriptional rate analysis using selected c-oncogene DNA fragments from the beginning and from the

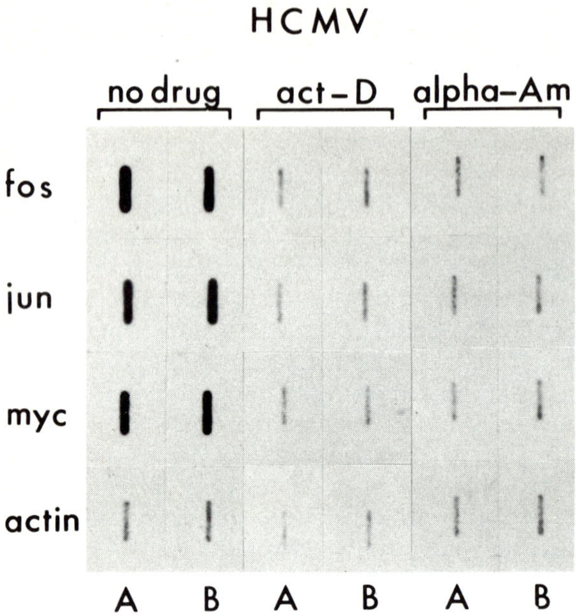

Fig. 3. Transcriptional rate analysis of cellular (c-) oncogenes (*fos*, *jun*, *myc*) after human cytomegalovirus (HCMV) infection of quiescent LU cells. The effect of actinomycin-D (*act-D*, dactinomycin) and alpha-amanitin (*alpha-Am*), inhibitors of RNA elongation or the activity of RNA polymerase II, respectively, is illustrated. *Panels A and B* represent hybridization of ^{32}P-labeled nuclear RNA obtained at 40 (*fos*, *jun*) or 60 min (*myc*) PI to the first and last exon of each of the c-oncogenes, respectively. Transcription from β-actin was monitored as an internal control

end of c-*fos*, c-*jun*, or c-*myc* gene reveals hybridization to both the first and last exons of the three proto-oncogenes. Furthermore, similar transcription rates were observed for both the first and last exons. Thus, the increases in proto-oncogene RNAs represent transcription from the entire gene and are consistent with a potential for increased expression of the corresponding oncoproteins. Indeed, oncoproteins derived from c-*fos*, c-*jun*, and c-*myc* genes are observed by immunofluorescence using appropriate antisera (e.g., Fig. 4).

Lack of Dependence of IE Cellular Responses on the Expression of HCMV-Specific IE Proteins

HCMV IE proteins can accumulate within an hour after infection [55, 80] and have been found to regulate transcription from the promoters of homologous and several heterologous genes, including, for example, the human immunodeficiency virus long terminal repeat (LTR) [14, 30]. Furthermore, it has been reported that the *ie1* gene product specifically binds to the promoters for

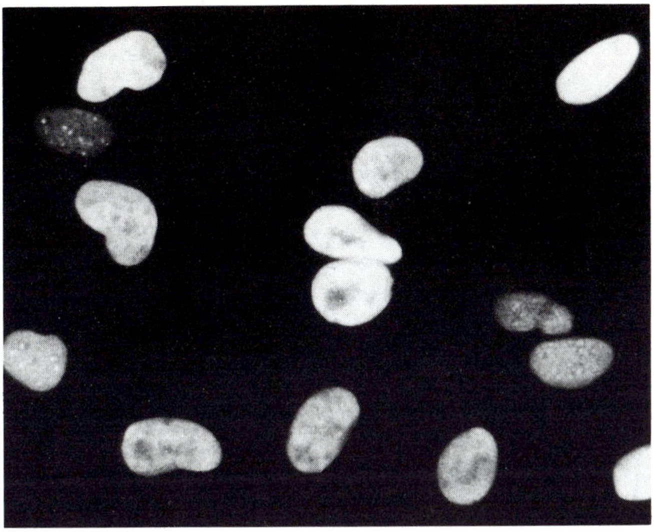

Fig. 4. Detection of oncoprotein in the nuclei of human cytomegalovirus-infected LU cells by immunofluorescence with affinity-purified hyperimmune rabbit serum to Jun/AP-1

c-oncogenes (c-*fos*, c-*myc*) [40] and to the gene encoding the heat shock protein (HSP) 70 [68]. Accordingly, it would not be particularly surprising if the rapid transcriptional activation of proto-oncogenes induced by HCMV resulted from the activity of the HCMV IE gene products.

Boldogh et al. [25] have recently evaluated this possibility. Careful examination of the relationship between HCMV IE gene expression and the induction of increased proto-oncogene RNAs by several approaches has suggested that the transcriptional activation of the c-oncogenes is not dependent on de novo synthesis of HCMV IE gene products. Even though there is a considerable temporal correlation between the detection of either HCMV IE transcripts or proteins and RNAs from c-*fos*, c-*jun*, and c-*myc*, this correlation is not complete. Substantial increases in the transcription rates and RNA levels for c-*fos* and c-*jun* and detectable increases in transcription and RNA for c-*myc* are observed by 20-min PI, indicating that transcriptional activation of these proto-oncogenes occurs prior to 20 min. At 20 min, however, substantial amounts of IE proteins are not detectable. Thus, there is not a convincing correlation between the detection of HCMV IE gene products and the IE transcriptional activation of proto-oncogenes.

More rigorous methods have been used to evaluate the possibility that small amounts of HCMV IE proteins that escaped detection are present in sufficient amounts at this very early time to activate transcription of the c-oncogenes. A considerable decrease in infectious yields is observed with serial passage of HCMV at high multiplicity of infection and is accompanied by an increase in defective HCMV particles [32]. These defective virus stocks demonstrate a significant reduction in the induction of early protein synthesis and, accordingly, have proven useful for examining the association of de novo HCMV IE protein synthesis with the transcriptional activation of c-oncogenes.

Infection with purified infectious (IVS) or defective (DVS) virus stocks at multiplicities from 10 to 0.1 PFU/cell and analysis of the increase in c-oncogene RNAs (Table 2) strongly suggests that the infectivity of the virus stock is not quantitatively related to the mangitude of the proto-oncogene induction. Additionally, a strong correlation is not evident between the expression of HCMV IE antigens and the induction of c-oncogenes. For example, RNA levels for c-oncogenes were as high for cells infected with DVS at a multiplicity of 1 or 5 plaque-forming units (PFU) per cell (with as few as 1.4% of the cells demonstrating straining for HCMV IE proteins) as for cells infected with IVS at a multiplicity of 10 PFU/cell (where 34% of cells appeared to contain IE proteins). Thus, there does not appear to be a good quantitative correlation between the increases in c-oncogene RNAs and the expression of HCMV IE antigens.

Table 2. The relationship of virus infectivity, multiplicity of infection, and IE viral protein synthesis to c-oncogene activation by HCMV

PFU/cell	UV[a] irradiation	Cells demonstrating fluorescence (%)[b]		Fold increase in RNA levels for[c]		
		40 min	60 min	c-*fos*[d]	c-*jun*[d]	c-*myc*[e]
Infectious virus stock						
10	–	34	90	12	10	7
	+	<0.01	<0.01	14	11	7
5	–	28	80	5	6	3
	+	<0.01	<0.01	6	5	4
1	–	18	26	1	1	1
	+	<0.01	<0.01	2	1	1
0.1	–	3	5	<1	<1	<1
	+	<0.01	<0.01	<1	<1	<1
Defective virus stock[f]						
5	–	5.4	17	12	12	9
	+	<0.01	<0.01	14	14	8
1	–	1.4	5	12	12	8
	+	<0.01	<0.01	14	14	8
0.1	–	0.01	0.3	3	3	1
	+	<0.01	<0.01	3	4	2

[a] At a dose of 19.2×10^4 ergs/mm^2
[b] The percentage of cells demonstrating fluorescence is the average of three parallel experiments
[c] Determined relative to mock-infected cells
[d] Determined at 40 min PI
[e] Determined at 60 min PI
[f] Propagated by serial undiluted passage at a high multiplicity of infection

Although the above-noted experiments provide data indicating the lack of a quantitative correlation between HCMV IE protein synthesis and the IE activation of c-oncogene expression, they provide only one datum point for conditions where HCMV IE protein synthesis is undetectable. Reduction of HCMV IE protein synthesis also can be achieved by ultraviolet (UV) light irradiation of HCMV stocks or by drugs such as cycloheximide or anisomycin. As summarized in Table 2, HCMV IE antigens were not detected by immunofluorescence ($<0.01\%$) in cells infected with either IVS (at multiplicities of 10–0.1 PFU/cell) or DVS (at multiplicities of 5–0.1 PFU/cell) after UV-irradiation at 19.2×10^4 ergs/mm^2. UV-irradiation, however, had no adverse effect on the HCMV-induced increase in c-oncogene RNAs. Furthermore, DVS stimulated increased levels of proto-oncogenes as well as, or better than, IVS. Consistent with these findings, the synthesis of HCMV IE antigens was undetectable in the presence of cycloheximide (100 µg/ml) or anisomycin (100 µg/ml), while the magnitude of the increase in proto-oncogene RNA levels exceeded those measured in parallel cultures in the absence of either protein synthesis inhibitor and resembled the superinduction reported for cells activated by serum [38]. Thus, neither HCMV infectivity nor the synthesis of HCMV IE antigens may be required for the rapid induction of increased c-oncogene expression.

Mechanism of Induction of IE Cellular Responses to HCMV Infection

Since HCMV IE proteins can be phosphorylated [36], demonstrate DNA binding activity [45], form homodimers through a "leucine zipper" [46, 57], and activate transcription of cellular genes, including proto-oncogenes (*fos*, *myc*) in chloramphenicol acetyltransferase (CAT) assays [40], it is reasonable to propose that HCMV IE proteins may also stimulate the transcriptional activation of proto-oncogenes *fos*, *jun*, and *myc* observed rapidly after HCMV infection [23–26]. As noted above, however, examination of the relationship between the expression of HCMV IE genes and transcriptional activation of IE c-oncogenes suggests that the very early induction of proto-oncogene transcription is not related to de novo synthesis of HCMV IE proteins [25].

Other explanations for the activation of c-oncogene transcription by HCMV are more consistent with our findings. It is possible that similar mechanisms involving the same cellular transcription factors could be involved in the activation of both c-oncogenes and HCMV IE genes, with the slight delay in the appearance of the HCMV IE transcripts resulting from the time required for HCMV DNA to enter the nucleus. It is also possible that some of the products of the proto-oncogenes activated by HCMV (e.g., Jun/AP-1) may contribute to the activation of HCMV IE gene transcription. The discrepancy in the coincidence of appearance of HCMV IE transcripts and those for the c-oncogenes suggests that transcriptional activation of HCMV IE genes could be related to the *trans*-acting effect of proto-oncogene products, since the promoter-regulatory region of the HCMV IE genes contains AP-1/CRE response elements (Fig. 5). These two possibilities are not mutually exclusive and both may contribute to the initial regulation of HCMV IE gene transcription.

Neither of these hypotheses explains how HCMV infection in general, and defective HCMV particles in particular, trigger an increase in the levels of cellular transcription factors. The results of studies of the IE increase in c-oncogene transcription [23–26] and of other IE cellular responses, including increased cellular levels of IP_3 and DG [80], and increased AA metabolism [2, 3], are consistent with the possibility that these IE phenomena are a result of the HCMV particle interacting with the cell and are not directly related to the infectivity of the virus stock.

This view is supported further by findings suggesting that the activities of a number of membrane-associated cellular enzymes are involved in the IE cellular responses to HCMV infection, including the transcriptional activation of proto-oncogenes. For example, as mentioned previously, the findings from a study of the mechanisms involved in the release of ^3H from [^3H]AA prela-

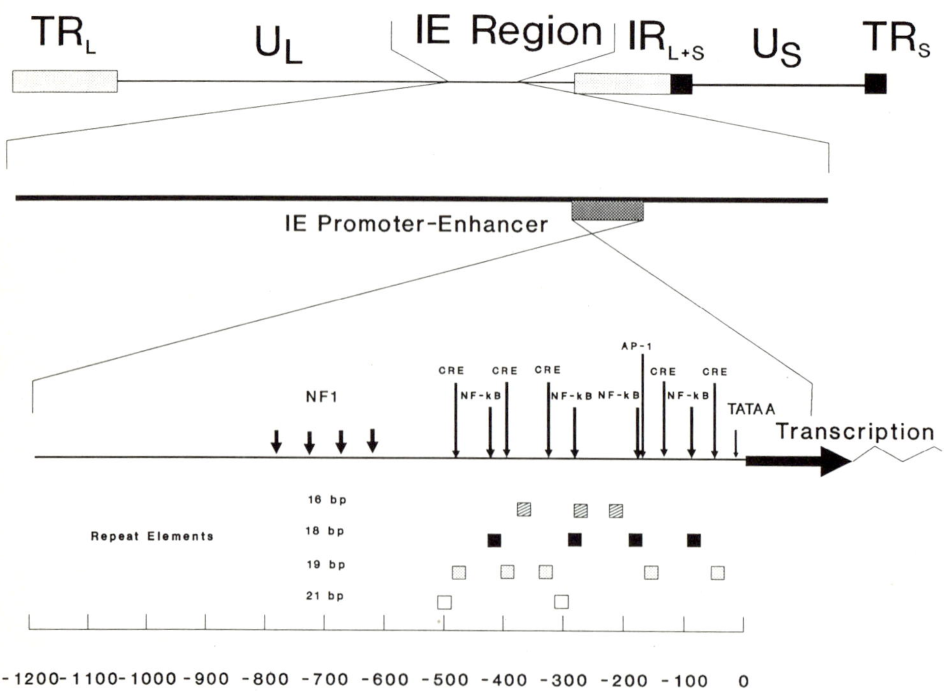

Fig. 5. Representation of the human cytomegalovirus (HCMV) immediate early (*IE*) promoter/enhancer region. The entire 235-bp genome is shown at the *top*, consisting of a unique long (U_L) and a unique short (U_S) region flanked by repeats at the termini of the long (TR_L) and short (TR_S) regions. The major IE promoter/enhancer region contains consensus sequences for nuclear factor 1 (NF1) binding and a series of 16-, 18-, 19-, and 21-bp repeat elements [56, 57, 75]. Within these repeat elements are consensus sequences for binding of nuclear factors including cyclic nucleotide response factors (*CREB*), nuclear factor-kappa B (*NF-κB*) and Jun/AP-1

beled cells suggest that the HCMV-induced IE stimulation of AA metabolism is mediated by pathways that are associated with activation of PLA_2 and PKC. A similar evaluation was undertaken for the induction c-oncogene transcription. Prolonged treatment of cells with 12-0-tetradecanoylphorbol 13-acetate (TPA) to desensitize PKC, prior to infection resulted in a significant reduction and delay in the appearance of c-oncogene transcripts and viral gene products. On the other hand, brief exposure of cells to TPA increased c-oncogene transcription.

The possibility that protein kinase activity was involved in activation of IE transcription was investigated further by blocking protein kinase activity with inhibitors (H-7 or H-8). In the presence of either drug, we noted a significant reduction in c-oncogene and viral IE RNA levels with Northern blot analysis and a delay in the appearance and reduction in the quantity of HCMV IE proteins measured by immunofluorescence and Western blot analysis, respectively (Boldogh et al., unpublished observations). In the presence of both drugs, the increase in IE cellular (*fos*, *jun*, *myc*) and viral gene products was not detectable through 180 min, while in nontreated cells IE gene products were present by 20 min PI. These and other data suggest strongly that protein kinases may be involved in the activation of transcription of c-oncogenes and HCMV IE genes. Furthermore, since the expression of cellular and viral genes appear to be equally sensitive to TPA or drug treatment (H-7, H-8) and their expression is temporally similar, it is possible that the same cellular factors are involved in the initiation of their transcription. c-oncogenes *fos*, *jun*, and *myc* [57, 60, 78], and the HCMV IE enhancer (Fig. 5) contain similar recognition sequences for DNA-binding proteins (AP-1, NF-$\varkappa$B, CREB). Accordingly, the drug treatments may have inhibited the activation of cellular transcription factors which are present in an inactive form in the cytoplasm of quiescent cells.

There are several other mechanisms that could explain how the interaction of HCMV particles with the cell is related to the induction of IE cellular responses, including c-oncogene transcription, independent of de novo HCMV IE gene expression or HCMV infectivity. The possibility has not been excluded that HCMV IE proteins as components of the virion could be involved in transcriptional activation of proto-oncogenes or other IE cellular responses. Although the presence of HCMV IE proteins in the virion has not been demonstrated and is currently under investigation, IE proteins of HSV-1 (ICP0 and 4) have been identified in virions [54, 83]. Also, increases in RNA levels for c-*fos*, c-*jun*, and c-*myc* and/or other IE cellular responses could be related to the activity of other structural components of the virion (e.g., those with protein kinase activity [52, 64]).

Possible Functions of IE Cellular Responses in the Pathogenesis of HCMV Infections

It appears that the HCMV particle in the absence of de novo protein synthesis can induce rapid (within minutes) cellular changes that are associated with cell activation. Precisely how these cellular changes are involved in the pathogenesis and replication of HCMV are presently the subjects of intensive investigation. Although the possibility that the IE activation of c-oncogene transcription may be related to the initiation and regulation of HCMV IE gene expression is attractive (e.g., Fig. 5), it is likely that the IE cellular responses are involved in additional ways in the pathogenesis of HCMV infections. The data available at this time suggest that regulation of the HCMV-induced cell activation signals is perturbed relative to activation responses induced by other mitogenic stimuli (e.g., serum) leading to protracted biochemical and physiologic activation responses. The protracted responses are associated with cellular changes that may permit efficient HCMV replication and may be involved in various disease processes even in the absence of HCMV replication as described below.

HCMV-Induced Early Physiologic and Biochemical Cellular Responses

The early HCMV-induced biochemical and physiologic cellular responses identified thus far are primarily the result of membrane-related events that produce changes in the levels and activities of constituents of the cytoplasm (Table 1). These responses include a decrease in the rate of Ca^{2+} uptake from the initial Ca^{2+} influx, presumably the release of Ca^{2+} from stores, a substantial and protracted increase in $[Ca^{2+}]_i$, increases in the cellular levels of cAMP and cGMP, and changes in Na^+ flux (Fig. 2). These responses occur later than IE cellular responses and are typically first seen after about 3 h PI with the maximum levels reached from about 7 to 13 h or later (Table 1).

Although these early responses have been reviewed in detail previously [8–10], some contrasting features of the HCMV-induced IE and early biochemical and physiologic responses are noteworthy. As noted above, the IE responses identified to date are plasma-membrane-related events, occur very rapidly (minutes) after exposure of cells to HCMV, and do not require infectious virus or de novo synthesis of RNA or protein. In contrast to the IE cellular responses, early biochemical and physiologic cellular responses are observed at later times (several hours or more) and appear to require infectious virus and the synthesis of RNA and protein. Thus, it is possible that the expression of IE and/or early HCMV genes may contribute to the early cellular biochemical and physiologic response.

Cell Membrane Phospholipid Turnover Associated with the Early Phase of HCMV Infection

As described above, a sharp increase in the formation of secondary messengers was observed in HCMV-infected cells between 10 and 60 min PI, followed by a return to mock-infection levels by 120 min PI. Significant increases in intracellular levels of IP_3 and DG [81] and in the release of AA (AbuBakar et al., unpublished data) have been noted also by about 4 hr PI (Table 1). The increases in these secondary messengers are maximal by several hours later and, by 10–11 h PI, detection of these metabolic products of PLC and PLA_2 activity is similar for CMV- and mock-infected cell cultures. Although these increases are temporally associated with early increases in cAMP and $[Ca^{2+}]_i$, there is not sufficient information available at this time to determine if they are interrelated. Contrary to the findings for IE phase responses, UV irradiation, serum neutralization, or heat inactivation of HCMV stocks significantly reduces or eliminates changes in levels of IP_3, DG, and AA during the early phase. These results suggest that the early cellular responses are associated with expression of viral gene(s).

The generation of these short-lived, bioactive intermediates involves two biochemical pathways regulated by PLC and PLA_2 [61, 66, 69]. In the first, PIP_2 is hydrolyzed by PLC to yield IP_3 and DG. DG can bind to cytosolic PKC along with Ca^{2+}, resulting in a membrane-associated complex that actively phosphorylates various proteins involved in cell activation and regulation. IP_3 binds to specific receptors on the endoplasmic reticulum or calciosomes and initiates the release of Ca^{2+} and an increase in cytosolic Ca^{2+} activity. In the second metabolic pathway, PLA_2s release arachidonate and other unsaturated fatty acids from phospholipids. One of the most important of these phospholipids is AA, since it can be metabolized further to prostaglandins (PGs), thromboxanes (TXs), leukotrienes (LTs), hydroxyeicosatetraenoates (HETEs), and lipoxenes (LXs). These shortlived products can be metabolized to longer-lived compounds such as PGE_2, PGD_2, and TXA_2, which may influence cellular functions. For example, PGE_2 can be involved in cAMP generation through activation of protein kinase A (PKA). The HCMV functions involved in the early increases in IP_3, DG, and AA release are not known at this time. Although the IE cellular responses can be explained possibly by the interaction of HCMV with cell membrane (receptor?), the generation of these secondary messengers during early times may be related to protein(s) encoded by HCMV IE or early genes. Furthermore the generation of these secondary messengers during the early phase of cellular responses may be related to the protracted nature of other HCMV-induced cellular physiologic responses.

Early Ca^{2+} Responses to HCMV Infection

Changes in Ca^{2+} homeostasis are observed in all three phases of the cellular responses to HCMV infection. Ca^{2+} influx, which is maximal by 2 h PI and may be an IE phase response, is of relatively short duration, as is the initial change in total cellular Ca^{2+} during the early phase (9–13 h PI; Fig. 2). An increase in $[Ca^{2+}]_i$ is first observed at 6 h PI and $[Ca^{2+}]_i$ doubles by 13 h [58]. Since total cellular Ca^{2+} increases substantially as $[Ca^{2+}]_i$ increases, these findings imply that during the early phase of HCMV infection most of the Ca^{2+} that enters the cell is captured into stores. At later times (13–25 h PI) after the initial influx of Ca^{2+}, both the influx rate and total cellular Ca^{2+} decrease, while $[Ca^{2+}]_i$ increases significantly. This implies that a major source of the cytosolic Ca^{2+} at this stage is likely to be Ca^{2+} released from intracellular stores.

The Ca^{2+} responses associated with productive HCMV infection are rather intriguing in that they illustrate an aspect of the activation process – protracted responses – that seems to be worthy of some emphasis. The elevation of $[Ca^{2+}]_i$ is prolonged through at least 49 h PI, well into the late phase of HCMV replication. The time course for the increase in $[Ca^{2+}]_i$ in productively infected cells (Fig. 2), thus, differs markedly from that observed in activation of cells by serum or growth factors [48, 63, 69]. The protracted increase in $[Ca^{2+}]_i$ requires infectious virus and is reduced substantially in the presence of inhibitors of either transcription or translation. Accordingly, HCMV-directed synthetic events may be required for the sustained increase in $[Ca^{2+}]_i$. Protracted physiologic cellular responses are most apparent during the late phase of productive HCMV replication.

Early Changes in the Cellular Levels of Cyclic Nucleotides in Response to HCMV Infection

As noted in Fig. 1, activation of cells by serum or growth factors may be accompanied by increases in cyclic nucleotide secondary messengers. Thus, we have monitored the effects of HCMV infection on the cellular levels of cAMP and cGMP [8, 49]. Infection of permissive cells with HCMV results in sequentially ordered increases in cAMP and cGMP (Fig. 2). Increases in the cellular levels of cAMP are observed first at 3 h PI and reach their maximum level by 7 h. By 13 h PI the cAMP levels return to the level observed for mock-infected cells and remain at about this level through 49 h. The cellular level of cGMP is increased from 7 to 25 h PI, with the maximum increase observed at 13 h. Thereafter, the cellular levels of cGMP return to the basal level and remain so through 97 h PI.

The mechanisms responsible for the increased cellular levels of cyclic nucleotides are unknown at this time, but it is possible that they are related to the changes in $[Ca^{2+}]_i$ (e.g., through activation of the Ca^{2+}-dependent adenylate cyclase [17, 62]). Other factors may also contribute to the cAMP increase, for example, the increases in AA metabolism may be related to an increase in prostaglandins that, as in other tissues, may increase the activity of adenylate cyclase [70]. The mechanisms of induction of the early increase in the cellular levels of cAMP must be somewhat more complex, however, since this increase appears to require infectious virus and the IE increase in AA metabolism does not. We have noted previously the possible relationship of the changes in secondary messenger levels to the rounding and contraction of HCMV-infected cells [8].

Early Na^+ Responses to HCMV Infection

During the early phase, the activity of the Na^+/K^+ ATPase is decreased substantially at 13 and 25 h PI and may reflect changes in intracellular pH.

Late Physiologic and Biochemical Cellular Responses to HCMV Infection: Perturbation of Cell Activation Responses and the Development of Cytomegaly

The physiologic changes associated with the development of cytomegaly are among the most intriguing and often overlooked aspects of HCMV research. Our findings suggest that cytomegaly is a manifestation of protracted molecular alterations in cell physiology that may be closely related to efficient HCMV replication. Support for this view can be found in the observations that virus progeny are not detected until cell enlargement begins [27], even though HCMV DNA synthesis is initiated at a much earlier time (Fig. 6), and that substantial increases in the rate of HCMV DNA synthesis and in yields of infectious virus coincide with cell enlargement (Fig. 6).

We have previously reviewed the evidence that the hallmark of HCMV infection, the cytomegalic cell, does not result from an increased burden of virus products on the cell, but rather from Na^+ entry, which in turn appears to be related to the protracted cell activation signals [8].

Changes in $[Ca^{2+}]_i$ and the Cellular Levels of Cyclic Nucleotides During the Late Phase of HCMV Infection

During the initial stage of the late phase of HCMV replication $[Ca^{2+}]_i$ is substantially elevated (i.e., through at least 49 h PI) and total cellular Ca^{2+} is increased from 49 to 97 h (Fig. 2). Cellular levels of cAMP are increased substantially at 73 and 97 h (Fig. 2), while cellular levels of cGMP remain at or near the levels for mock-infected cells. Although it is likely that these late

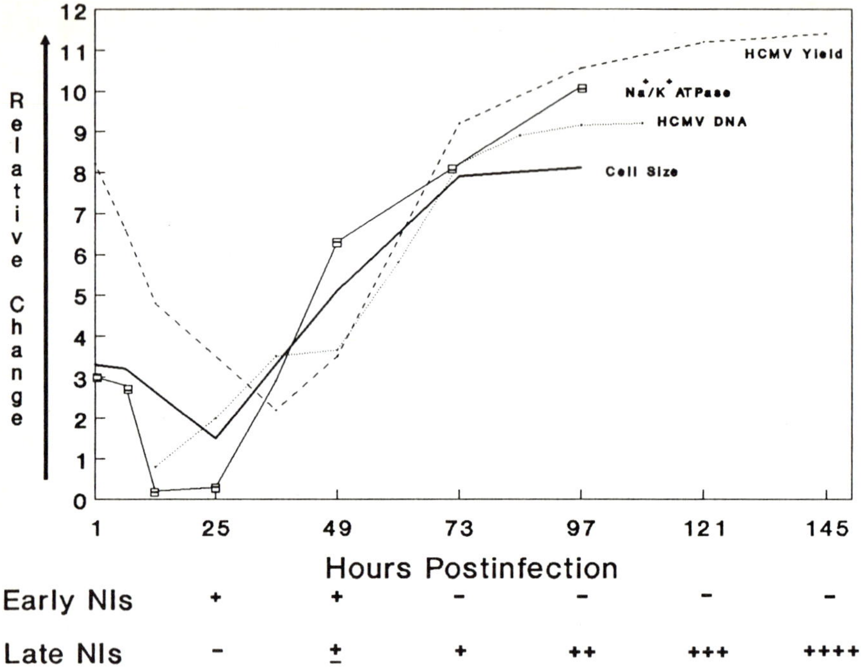

Fig. 6. The relationship between cell size, activity of the Na^+/K^+ *ATPase*, and other crossed through material *HCMV* DNA synthesis, and yields of infectious HCMV. The development and progression of HCMV-induced nuclear inclusions (NIs) is indicated as follows: −, no NI; +, early NI present in most cells without detectable progeny virus; + +, developing late NI demonstrating incomplete cellulae [5, 27] and progeny virus; + + +, mature NI demonstrating numerous well-developed cellulae and abundant progeny virus; + + + +, end stage NI, cellulae beginning to deteriorate

changes in the cellular levels of secondary messengers are related to specific movements of Na^+ (Albrecht et al., unpublished observations), the precise relationship of these secondary messenger responses to Na^+ regulation and the development of cytomegaly remain to be investigated.

Na^+ Responses and Development of Cytomegaly

Entry of Na^+ appears to be closely associated with activation of cells, including progression through the cell cycle and stimulation of cellular DNA synthesis by growth factors and tumor promoters [39]. The gradient between high extracellular [Na^+] and low intracellular [Na^+] is maintained by extrusion of Na^+ through the ouabain-sensitive Na^+/K^+ ATPase [71]. Accordingly, it is not surprising that a transient increase in Na^+/K^+ pump activity is noted in fibroblasts after stimulation with serum, growth factors, or tumor promoters [39].

For HCMV-infected cells the entry of Na^+ appears to be substantially protracted and related to both the development of cytomegaly and to the replication of HCMV. Our findings for the relationship between Na^+ entry and the development of cytomegaly have been reviewed in detail previously [8]. As illustrated in Fig. 6, the time course for the HCMV-induced changes in Na^+/K^+ ATPase activity parallels the increase in cell size from 25 h to 73 h PI. Both the increase in cell size and Na^+/K^+ ATPase activity are blocked by either physiologic inhibition of Na^+ entry by substitution of *N*-methyl-D-glutamine (NMDG) for Na^+ in the cultural fluids or pharmacological inhibition of Na^+ entry by amiloride and amiloride analogues that interfere with Na^+ entry through Na^+ channels or Na^+/H^+ exchange [34, 59]. The protracted increase in Na^+/K^+ ATPase activity and presumably Na^+ entry observed in HCMV-infected cells contrast sharply to the transient increase observed in serum-stimulated cells. Why Na^+ responses to HCMV infection are prolonged is not known. The initial increases in Na^+ entry could result from DG stimulation of PKC [16], however, that would not explain the protracted time course for the increase in Na^+/K^+ ATPase activity or the development of cytomegaly. Protracted Na^+ entry may be associated with protracted cell activation signals (e.g., $[Ca^{2+}]_i$), intracellular acidification related to the HCMV-induced increases in metabolic activity, with the insertion of new molecules into cell membrane [28, 59], or with a combination of these effects.

Correlation of Protracted Cellular Responses with HCMV Replication

Regardless of how HCMV infection protracts cellular Na^+ responses, cellular changes associated with these responses appear to be related to HCMV replication. As illustrated in Fig. 6 and reviewed in detail elsewhere [8], the increase in Na^+/K^+ ATPase activity and cell size parallel the development of the late phase of the HCMV replication cycle including: increases in the rate of HCMV DNA synthesis (the second phase [5, 6, 8, 27]) and protein synthesis [8], the development of late nuclear inclusions [5, 27], the formation of progeny virus [27], and an increase in infectious yields [5, 27]. Inhibition of Na^+ entry by either physiologic (substitution of NMDG for Na^+) or pharmacological (treatment with amiloride) approaches, as previously observed for the increases in Na^+/K^+ ATPase activity and cell size, substantially inhibits HCMV DNA synthesis, the formation of late nuclear inclusions, and the increase in infectious yields (Table 3) [34].

The biochemical and physiologic responses observed in HCMV-infected cells, including those for Na^+, appear to be associated with a cascade of interrelated signals [8], as has been reported for cells activated by serum or growth factors [39, 48, 61, 63]. Thus, inhibition of other physiologic or biochemical responses to HCMV infection also quantitatively affects infectious HCMV yields. For example, the Na^+ responses appear to be related to Ca^{2+}

Table 3. Effects of inhibitors of the HCMV-induced cellular physiologic responses on HCMV yields

Drug	Log_{10}-fold reduction in infectious yields
Cyclic nucleotide modulators	
Papaverine (100 μ*M*)	5+
Nitroprusside (100 μ*M*)	3+
Forskolin (30 μ*M*)	–
IBMX (100 μ*M*)	–
Na^+ entry blockers	
Amiloride (150 μ*M*)	4+
Bumetanide (30 μ*M*)	–
SITS (300 μ*M*)	–
Ca^{2+} modulating drugs	
Ryanodine (1000 μ*M*)	3+
Verapamil (100 μ*M*)	1+
Nifedipine (100 μ*M*)	1+
TFP (10 μ*M*)	1+
Diltiazem (100 μ*M*)	–
TMB-8 (10 μ*M*)	–
Quin2 (10 μ*M*)	–

–, no adverse effect on infectious yields; IBMX, isobutylmethylxanthine; SITS, 4-acetamido-4′-isothiocyanatostilbene-2,2′-disulfonic acid; TFP, trifluoperazine; TMB-8, 8-(*N*,*N*-diethylamino)octyl-3,4,5-trimethoxybenzoate-hydrochloride; Quin2, (2[(2-bis-[carboxymethyl]amino-s-methylphenoxy)-methyl]-6-methoxy-8-bis-[carboxymethyl]aminoquinoline

responses. When Ca^{2+} influx is reduced with Ca^{2+} influx blockers (verapamil, nifedipine), the increase in Na^+/K^+ ATPase is reduced (Albrecht et al., unpublished observations) along with the increase in infectious HCMV yields [7]. Drugs that increase the cellular levels of cGMP (e.g., sodium nitroprusside, papaverine), but not cAMP (e.g., forskolin), significantly reduce HCMV infectious yields [7]. Tanaka et al. [77] have observed that indomethacin, an inhibitor of prostaglandin synthesis, reduces HCMV yields.

Although each of these drugs that are noted for inhibition of biochemical or physiologic responses in a wide range of experimental systems reduces HCMV infectious yields by 1–3 $\log_{10}$, none (except papaverine) quantitatively eliminate infectious yields (Table 3). Ignoring the data for papaverine, it could be argued that the HCMV-induced cellular responses only marginally influence infectious HCMV yields. The reductions of 10- to 1000-fold, however, are significant. Furthermore, when it is considered that, except for papaverine, each of these drugs is recognized for a rather specific effect that results in inhibition of a single step in a branched cascade, it is not surprising that a single drug does not completely eliminate HCMV infectious yields. On the other hand, papaverine, which inhibits the hydrolysis of PIP_2, reduces the increases in $[Ca^{2+}]_i$ and Na^+/K^+ ATPase activity, and substantially increase the cellular level of cGMP during the late phase, at concentrations between 80 and 100 μM often eliminates infectious yields.

Thus, it is likely that cellular responses may be related not only to the initiation of HCMV replication, but also, through protraction of some responses, to changes in the intracellular environment that favor selected HCMV-specific macromolecular synthesis (e.g., HCMV DNA synthesis) over some potentially competing cellular macromolecular synthetic events (e.g., cellular DNA synthesis). A detailed discussion of this point has been presented previously [8].

The Potential for Novel Therapeutic Approaches to Control HCMV Infections Through Interference with Cell Activation Responses

The forgoing observations for the inhibition of HCMV replication by drugs recognized for their inhibition of cell activation phenomena (e.g., work, proliferation) not only suggest that the HCMV-induced cell activation responses are directly or indirectly involved in the synthesis of high yields of HCMV, but that these drugs may offer opportunities for the development of novel therapeutic approaches for HCMV infections. For example, papaverine, a smooth muscle relaxing agent, is an extraordinarily potent inhibitor of HCMV replication [7]. Papaverine is reported to be a specific inhibitor of phosphodiesterases that break down cAMP and cGMP [79]; but in our hands, it appears to be less specific since papaverine also blocks the phosphodiesterase (PLC) mediated hydrolysis of PIP_2. The 50% effective dose (ED_{50}) for reduction of infectious yields by papaverine (about 0.6 μM) is similar to the ED_{50} for DHPG, suggesting that papaverine is among the most potent anti-HCMV drugs in vitro [7].

For drugs that block normal physiologic and/or biochemical responses there is always concern about possibly doing more harm that good. Yet, many of the drugs described in this review are presently in use in humans (e.g., papaverine, nitroprusside, amiloride) because of their efficacy in blocking pathologic responses (e.g., hypertension). It seems possible that it is the protracted biochemical and physiologic cellular responses resulting from perturbation of the cell activation process by HCMV infection that are most sensitive to these inhibitors. An illustration supporting this possibility is found in the observations that papaverine and amiloride appear to block the second, but not the first phase of HCMV DNA synthesis. Therefore, they block the formation of the late nuclear inclusion, and in papaverine-treated cells, early nuclear inclusions are observed almost exclusively. In amiloride-treated cells, poorly developed late nuclear inclusions of a small size are observed [34]. These findings suggest that there may be sufficient differences between critical HCMV-induced cellular responses and those of uninfected cells to develop successful treatment strategies that cause minimal harm to the patient while arresting HCMV infections.

In developing these treatment strategies, it should be borne in mind that the biochemical and physiologic responses to HCMV infection are complex and that inhibition of one arm of the activation cascade may not adequately reduce HCMV infectious yields. Thus, drugs that have multiple effects, or combinations of drugs affecting different HCMV-induced events may prove useful in developing new strategies for treating these infections.

The Possible Involvement of HCMV-Induced Cell Activation Responses in the Pathogenesis of HCMV-Related Disease

The cellular changes induced by HCMV infection in the absence of expression of HCMV genes (e.g., the IE cellular responses) or with limited expression of HCMV genes suggest that HCMV infection is capable of causing important cellular pathologic effects without completing its replication cycle. HCMV-induced unscheduled gene activation may perturb the cell cycle leading to, for example, premature chromosome condensation or C-mitosis [1]. HCMV infection also induces a number of other types of chromosome abnormalities including chromosome breaks [1]. The specific damage induced by the virus is dependent on the cell cycle stage at the time of infection, the permissivity of the cells, and the extent of HCMV expression. The effects of HCMV infection on gene activity, chromosome aberrations, and progression through the cell cycle may explain some of the pathology associated with HCMV disease. Furthermore, HCMV infection enhances the extent of chromosome damage induced by genotoxic chemicals and drugs [33].

A number of chronic diseases have been associated with HCMV infection (e.g., cancer, atherosclerosis), though establishing a causative relationship to these diseases has proven to be difficult. For example, HCMV infection has been associated with several human cancers, including Kaposi's sarcoma [19, 42, 43], colon carcinoma [65], prostate adenocarcinoma [20], and cervical carcinoma [41, 74], as well as neuroblastoma and Wilms' tumor [82]. Definitively establishing a causative role for HCMV in the development of these neoplasias, however, has been elusive, since HCMV-specific components (RNA, DNA) are not detected after long-term subculturing of tumor tissues [19, 21].

Several series of in vitro experiments have supported the view that HCMV has oncogenic potential. HCMV has been demonstrated to induce a mitogenic signal [11, 13, 18, 51, 76] that may be related to IE and early cell activation responses. Malignant transformation of hamster and human cells has been observed after in vitro infection with HCMV or its DNA [4, 18, 22, 35, 72]. While these findings are consistent with an oncogenic potential, they do not definitively establish such a role in vivo. Particularly problematic in establishing a causative relationship has been the accumulating evidence that HCMV gene expression is not necessary for maintenance of a malignant phenotype [21, 41]. Accordingly, it is reasonable to propose that HCMV may be involved in neoplastic processes through "hit and run" mechanisms such as activation of cellular genes, induction of genetic abnormalities, or inappropriate stimulation of cell proliferation, consistent with the comments of Macnab [51].

Conclusion

When considered together, the available data suggest that the interaction of the HCMV particle with the plasmalemma can activate the cell through cellular pathways, resulting in the generation of a mitogenic signal. It is likely that the activating effect of the HCMV particle on the cell is involved in the initiation of HCMV infection through regulation of HCMV IE gene expression. Perturbation of the activation process leading to protracted cellular signals appears to contribute to the efficiency of HCMV infections and may, along with other features of the activation process, be related to the regulation of HCMV infections. The ability of HCMV to influence expression of cell-cycle-associated genes and cellular proliferation may be related to the pathophysiology of HCMV disease.

Significant aspects of this view are that it proposes that there are steps in HCMV replication that have not been fully appreciated and that may result in the induction of cell damage. If this view is correct, then it may present opportunities for new approaches in the development of therapies for HCMV and other viral infections.

Acknowledgements. These studies were supported by USEPA research grants R81 5048 and R81-9394. M.P. Fons is the recipient of a J. W. McLaughlin Fellowship.

References

1. AbuBakar S, Au WW, Legator MS, Albrecht T (1988) Induction of chromosome aberrations and mitotic arrest by cytomegalovirus in human cells. Environ Mol Mutagen 12:409–420
2. AbuBakar S, Boldogh I, Albrecht T (1990) Human cytomegalovirus: Stimulation of [^{3}H] release from [^{3}H]-arachidonic acid prelabelled cells. Arch Virol 113:255–266
3. AbuBakar S, Boldogh I, Albrecht T (1990) Human cytomegalovirus stimulates arachidonic acid metabolism through pathways that are affected by inhibitors of phospholipase A2 and protein kinase C. Biochem Biophys Res Commun 166:953–959
4. Albrecht T, Rapp F (1973) Malignant transformation of hamster embryo fibroblasts following exposure to ultraviolet-irradiated human cytomegalovirus. Virology 55:53–61
5. Albrecht T, Cavallo T, Cole NL, Graves K (1980) Cytomegalovirus: development and progression of cytopathic effects in human cell culture. Lab Invest 42:1–7
6. Albrecht T, Li J-L, Speelman D, Ball R, Nokta M, Fons M, Lee CH, Steinsland O, Thompson WC, Carney DH (1984) Cellular responses to human cytomegalovirus infection. Birth Defects 20:21–34

7. Albrecht T, Lee CH, Speelman DJ, Steinsland OS (1987) Inhibition of cytomegalovirus replication by smooth-muscle relaxing agents. Proc Soc Exp Biol Med 186:41–46
8. Albrecht T, Boldogh I, Fons M, Lee CH, AbuBakar S, Russell JM, Au WW (1989) Cell activation responses to cytomegalovirus infection: relationship to the phasing of CMV replication and to the induction of cellular damage. Subcell Biochem 15:157–202
9. Albrecht T, Boldogh I, Fons M, AbuBakar S, Deng CZ (1990) Cell activation signals and the pathogenesis of human cytomegalovirus. Intervirology 31:68–75
10. Albrecht T, Fons MP, Boldogh I, AbuBakar S, Deng CZ, Millinoff D (1991) Metabolic and cellular effects of human cytomegalovirus infection. Transplant Proc 23:48–55
11. Albrecht T, Nachtigal M, St Jeor SC, Rapp F (1976) Induction of cellular DNA synthesis and increased mitotic activity in Syrian hamster embryo cells abortively infected with human cytomegalovirus. J Gen Virol 30:167–177
12. Alkon DL, Rasmussen H (1988) A spatial-temporal model of cell activation. Science 239:998–1005
13. Ball RL, Carney DH, Albrecht T (1990) Taxol inhibits stimulation of cell DNA synthesis by human cytomegalovirus. Exp Cell Res 191:37–44
14. Barry PA, Pratt-Lowe E, Peterlin BM, Luciw PA (1990) Cytomegalovirus activates transcription directed by the long terminal repeat of human immunodeficiency virus type 1. J Virol 64:2932–2940
15. Berridge MJ (1987) Inositol triphosphate and diacylglycerol: two interacting second messengers. Annu Rev Biochem 56:159–193
16. Berridge MJ, Irvine RF (1984) Inositol triphosphate, a novel second messenger in cellular signal transduction. Nature 312:315–321
17. Blumenthal DK, Stull JT (1980) Activation of skeletal muscle myosin light chain kinase by Ca^{2+} and calmodulin. Biochemistry 19:5608–5614
18. Boldogh I, Gonczol E, Vaczi L (1978) Transformation of hamster embryo fibroblast cells by UV-irradiated human cytomegalovirus. Acta Microbiol Acad Sci Hung 25:269–275
19. Boldogh I, Beth E, Huang E-S, Kyalwazi SK, Giraldo G (1981) Kaposi's sarcoma. IV. Detection of CMV DNA, CMV RNA, and CMNA in tumor biopsies. Int J Cancer 28:469–474
20. Boldogh I, Baskar JF, Mar E-C, Huang E-S (1983) Human cytomegalovirus and herpes simplex type 2 in normal and adenocarcinomatous prostate glands. JNCI 70:192–211
21. Boldogh I, Brichacek B, Gonczol E, Hirsch I, Vaczi L (1985) Viral DNA sequences in human cytomegalovirus transformed hamster cell lines at low passage levels. Acta Microbiol Hung 32:160–166
22. Boldogh I, Huang E-S, Baskar JF, Vaczi L (1985) HCMV-specific expression in HEL cells transformed by Xba I endonuclease-fragmented HCMV DNA. Acta Microbiol Hung 32:167–173
23. Boldogh I, AbuBakar S, Albrecht T (1990) Activation of proto-oncogenes: an immediate early event in human cytomegalovirus infection. Science 247:561–564
24. Boldogh I, AbuBakar S, Deng CZ, Albrecht T (1991) Transcriptional activation of cellular oncogenes, *fos*, *jun* and *myc* by human cytomegalovirus. J Virol 65:1568–1571
25. Boldogh I, AbuBakar S, Millinoff D, Deng CZ, Albrecht T (1991) Cellular oncogene activation by human cytomegalovirus. Lack of correlation with virus infectivity and immediate early gene expression. Arch Virol 118:163–177
26. Boldogh I, AbuBakar S, Fons MP, Deng CZ, Albrecht T (1991) Activation of cellular oncogenes by clinical isolates and laboratory strains of human cytomegalovirus. J Med Virol 34:241–247
27. Cavallo T, Graves K, Cole NL, Albrecht T (1981) Cytomegalovirus: an ultrastructural study of the morphogenesis of nuclear inclusions in human cell culture. J Gen Virol 56:97–104
28. Chee MS, Satchwell SC, Preddie E, Weston KM, Barrell BG (1990) Human cytomegalovirus encodes three G protein-coupled receptor homologues. Nature 344:774–777
29. Cooper JA (1990) Oncogenes and anti-oncogenes. Curr Opin Cell Biol 2:285–295

30. Davis MG, Kenney SC, Kamine J, Pagano JS, Huang E-S (1987) Immediate-early gene region of human cytomegalovirus trans-activates the promoter of human immunodeficiency virus. Proc Natl Acad Sci USA 84:8642–8646
31. DeMarchi JM (1983) Correlation between stimulation of host cell DNA synthesis by human cytomegalovirus and lack of expression of a subset of early virus genes. Virology 129:274–286
32. DeMarchi JM, Kaplan AS (1977) The role of defective cytomegalovirus particles in the induction of host cell DNA synthesis. Virology 82:93–99
33. Deng CZ, AbuBakar S, Fons MP, Boldogh I, Hokanson J, Au WW, Albrecht T (1991) Human cytomegalovirus-enhanced induction of chromosome aberrations in human peripheral blood lymphocytes treated with potent genotoxic agents. Environ Mol Mutagen 19:304–310
34. Fons M, Nokta M, Cerruti-Sola S, Albrecht T (1991) Amiloride inhibition of human cytomegalovirus replication. Proc Soc Exp Biol Med 196:89–96
35. Geder L, Lausch R, O'Neill F, Rapp F (1976) Oncogenic transformation of human embryo lung cells by human cytomegalovirus. Science 192:1134–1137
36. Gibson W (1981) Immediate-early proteins of human cytomegalovirus strains AD169, Davis, and Towne differ in electrophoretic mobility. Virology 112:350–354
37. Greenberg ME, Ziff EB (1984) Stimulation of 3T3 cells induces transcription of the c-*fos* proto-oncogene. Nature 311:433–438
38. Greenberg ME, Hermanowski AL, Ziff EB (1986) Effect of protein synthesis inhibitors on growth factor activation of c-*fos*, c-*myc* and actin gene transcription. Mol Cell Biol 6:1050–1057
39. Grinstein S, Rotin D, Mason MJ (1989) Na^+/H^+ exchange and growth factor-induced cytosolic pH changes: Role in cellular proliferation. Biochim Biophys Acta 988:73–97
40. Hagemeier C, Sissons JGP, Sinclair JH (1990) The binding of nuclear factors to the cAMP responsive element is associated with major immediate-early gene mediated transactivation of c-*fos* upon infection with human cytomegalovirus (Abstr). 15th International Herpesvirus Workshop, Aug 2–Aug 8, Washington
41. Huang E-S, Boldogh I, Mar E-C (1983) Human cytomegaloviruses: evidence for possible association with human cancer. In: Philips LA (ed) Viruses associated with human cancer. Dekker, New York, pp 161–194
42. Huang E-S, Boldogh I, Baskar JF, Mar E-C (1984) The molecular biology of human cytomegalovirus and its relationship to various human cancers. In: Giraldo G, Beth E (eds) The role of viruses in human cancer, vol 2. Elsevier, New York, pp 169–198
43. Huang ES, Mar EC, Boldogh I, Baskar J (1984) The oncogenicity of human cytomegalovirus. Birth Defects 20:193–211
44. Kamm KE, Stull JT (1989) Regulation of smooth muscle contractile elements by second messengers. Annu Rev Physiol 51:299–313
45. Lafemina RL, Pizzorno MC, Mosca JD, Hayward GS (1989) Expression of the acidic nuclear immediate early protein (IE1) of human cytomegalovirus in stable cell lines and its preferential association with metaphase chromosomes. Virology 172:584–600
46. Landschulz WH, Johnson PF, McKnight SL (1988) The leucine zipper: a hypothetical structure common to a new class of DNA binding proteins. Science 240:1759–1764
47. Lau LF (1990) Growth factors and growth control. Curr Opin Cell Biol 2:280–284
48. Laychock SG (1989) Coordinate interactions of cyclic nucleotide and phospholipid metabolizing pathways in calcium-dependent cellular processes. Curr Top Cell Regul 30:203–242
49. Lee CH, Albrecht T (1987) Cyclic nucleotide responses to cytomegalovirus (CMV) infection: partial correlation with inhibition of CMV yields by papaverine (Abstr). 12th International Herpesvirus Workshop, July 30–Aug 4, Philadelphia
50. Macara IG (1989) Oncogenes and cellular signal transduction. Physiol Rev 69:797–820
51. Macnab JCM (1987) Herpes simplex virus and human cytomegalovirus: their role in morphological transformation and genital cancers. J Gen Virol 68:2525–2550
52. Mar EC, Patel PC, Huang ES (1981) Human cytomegalovirus associated DNA polymerase and protein kinase activities. J Gen Virol 57:149–156

53. Martelly I, Castagna M (1989) Protein kinase C and tumor promoters. Curr Opin Cell Biol 1:206–210
54. McNabb DS, Courtney RJ (1990) Characterization of the large tegument protein (ICP1/2) of herpes simplex virus type 1 (Abstr). 15th International Herpesvirus Workshop, Aug 2–8, Washington
55. Michelson-Fiske S, Horodniceanu F, Guillon JC (1977) Immediate early antigens in human cytomegalovirus infected cells. Nature 270:615–617
56. Mocarski ES Jr, Abenes GB, Manning WC, Sambucetti LC, Cherrington JM (1990) Molecular genetic analysis of cytomegalovirus gene regulation in growth, persistence and latency. Curr Top Microbiol Immunol 154:47–74
57. Nelson JA, Gnann JW Jr, Ghazal P (1990) Regulation and tissue-specific expression of human cytomegalovirus. Curr Top Microbiol Immunol 154:75–100
58. Nokta M, Eaton D, Steinsland OS, Albrecht T (1987) Ca^{2+} responses in cytomegalovirus-infected fibroblasts of human origin. Virology 157:259–267
59. Nokta M, Fons MP, Eaton DC, Albrecht T (1988) Cytomegalovirus: sodium entry and development of cytomegaly in human fibroblasts. Virology 164:411–419
60. Prywes R, Roeder RG (1986) Inducible binding of a factor to the c-*fos* enhancer. Cell 47:777–784
61. Rana RS, Hokin LE (1990) Role of phosphoinositides in transmembrane signaling. Physiol Rev 70:115–164
62. Rasmussen H, Barrett PQ (1984) Calcium messenger system: An integrated view. Physiol Rev 64:938–984
63. Rasmussen H, Rasmussen JE (1990) Calcium as intracellular messenger: from simplicity to complexity. Curr Top Cell Regul 31:1–109
64. Roby C, Gibson W (1986) Characterization of phosphoproteins and protein kinase activity of virions, noninfectious enveloped particles, and dense bodies of human cytomegalovirus. J Virol 59:714–727
65. Roche JK, Cheung KS, Boldogh I, Huang E-S, Lang DJ (1981) Cytomegalovirus: detection in human colon and circulating mononuclear cells and presence in gastrointestinal diseases. Int J Cancer 27:659–667
66. Rodriguez-Pena A, Rozengurt E (1984) Disappearance of Ca^{2+}-sensitive, phospholipid-dependent protein kinase activity in phorbol ester-treated 3T3 cells. Biochem Biophys Res Commun 120:1053–1059
67. Rozengurt E (1986) Early signals in the mitogenic response. Science 234:161–166
68. Santomenna LD, Colberg-Poley AM (1990) Stimulation of cellular HSP70 expression by human cytomegalovirus immediate early gene products (Abstr). 15th International Herpesvirus Workshop, Aug 2–8, Washington
69. Siess W (1989) Molecular mechanisms of platelet activation. Physiol Rev 69:58–178
70. Sha'afi RI, Naccache PH (1985) Relationship between calcium, arachidonic acid metabolites and neutrophil activation. In: Rubin RP, Weiss GB, Putney JW (eds) Calcium in biological systems. Plenum, New York, pp 137–146
71. Skou JC (1965) Enzymatic basis for active transport of Na^+ and K^+ across cell membrane. Physiol Rev 45:596–617
72. Smiley ML, Mar E-C, Huang ES (1988) Cytomegalovirus infection and viral-induced transformation of human endothelial cells. J Med Virol 25:213–226
73. Sporn MB, Roberts AB (1988) Peptide growth factors are multifunctional. Nature 332:217–219
74. Stevenson K, Macnab JCM (1989) Cervical carcinoma and human cytomegalovirus. Biomed Pharmacother 43:173–176
75. Stamminger T, Fleckenstein B (1990) Immediate-early transcription regulation of human cytomegalovirus. Curr Top Microbiol Immunol 154:3–19
76. St Jeor SC, Albrecht TB, Funk FD, Rapp F (1974) Stimulation of cellular DNA synthesis by human cytomegalovirus. J Virol 13:353–362

77. Tanaka J, Ogura T, Iida H, Sato H, Hatano M (1988) Inhibitors of prostaglandin synthesis inhibit growth of human cytomegalovirus and reactivation of latent virus in a productively and latently infected human cell line. Virology 163:205–208
78. Treisman R (1986) Identification of a protein-binding site that mediates transcriptional response of the c-*fos* gene to serum factors. Cell 46:567–574
79. Triner L, Vulliemoz Y, Schwartz I, Nahas GG (1970) Cyclic phosphodiesterase activity and the action of papaverine. Biochem Biophys Res Commun 40:64–69
80. Valyi-Nagy T, Bandi Z, Boldogh I, Albrecht T (1988) Hydrolisis of inositol lipids: an early signal of human cytomegalovirus infection. Arch Virol 101:199–207
81. Valyi-Nagy T, Bandi Z, Boldogh I, Horvath A, Albrecht T (1989) Changes in levels of inositol triphosphate and diacylglycerol in fibroblasts infected by cytomegalovirus. Kiserletes Orvostud 41:152–156
82. Wertheim PME, Voute PA (1976) Neuroblastoma, Wilms' tumor and cytomegalovirus. JNCI 57:701–703
83. Yao F, Courtney RJ (1989) A major transcriptional regulatory protein (ICP4) of herpes simplex type 1 is associated with purified virions. J Virol 63:3338–3344

Chapter 20 Potential Oncogenicity of Human Cytomegalovirus

Leonard J. Rosenthal and Sukhendra Choudhury

Summary

Human cytomegalovirus (HCMV) infection has been implicated in the etiology of several human malignancies because of seroepidemiologic evidence as well as the detection of viral DNA in tumor tissues. However, no consistent findings have directly linked HCMV with human cancer. On the other hand, the oncogenic potential of HCMV has been well established by in vitro studies demonstrating the ability of UV-irradiated or infectious HCMV to transform a variety of mammalian cells. This has led to the identification of specific transforming regions within the HCMV genome. Specifically, three HCMV morphological transforming regions (mtrI, II, III) have been found. Of these, only mtrII is retained in focal and tumor-derived lines. Sequence analysis of mtrII showed the presence of open reading frames (ORF) of 79, 83, and 34 amino acids (aa). Analysis of colinear regions within three HCMV strains implicated the 79-aa ORF as the transforming gene. The transformation of NIH 3T3 cells by the 79-aa ORF cloned into a mammalian expression vector provided direct evidence for its role in carcinogenesis.

Introduction

Members of the herpesvirus family have been implicated in the etiology of several human cancers. These include the Epstein-Barr virus, a candidate etiological agent in nasopharyngeal carcinoma and African Burkitt's lymphoma [84]; herpes simplex virus type 2 (HSV-2), linked by serologic and molecular studies with cervical carcinoma [53, 54, 64]; human cytomegalovirus (HCMV) associated with cervical carcinoma [39, 59, 79], adenocarcinomas of the prostate [6, 71] and colon [35, 38] and Kaposi's sarcoma (KS) [5, 29, 30]; and human herpesvirus type 6 (HHV-6) associated with lymphoproliferative disorders [1, 69]. The postulated involvement of herpesviruses in the etiology of human cancer has led to the development of experimental systems in which

---

Department of Microbiology, Georgetown University Medical Center, 3900 Reservoir Rd. N.W., Washington, DC 20007, USA the transforming ability of these viruses is being investigated. This has led to the identification of specific DNA fragments containing transcriptional regulatory elements or coding sequences that are responsible for transformation.

This review is an update of our current knowledge on the transforming sequences of HCMV. It is divided into three main sections, each of which deals with a different aspect of HCMV transformation. The following section describes the background for the association of HCMV with malignant diseases in humans; the second major section focuses on the in vitro transformation of mammalian cells with either infectious or ultraviolet- (UV)-irradiated HCMV; and the third main section describes experimental data on the identification and localization of the morphological transforming regions (mtr) in HCMV DNA, including recent observations from our laboratory.

Association of HCMV Infection with Human Malignancies

Cytomegalovirus is a ubiquitous human pathogen that has the ability to remain latent in the host and to produce reactivated infections following blood transfusions, pregnancy, organ/bone marrow transplantation, immunosuppressive therapy, and other viral infections [62, 76]. HCMV infects leukocytes, endothelial cells, connective tissue cells, and epithelial cells [36, 56, 62]. The virus sheds through milk, semen, urine, saliva, and cervical secretions [12, 14, 15, 49, 50, 61]. Acquisition of HCMV infection may occur via transplacental, perinatal and sexual routes, and through blood transfusion and organ/bone marrow transplantation. Because of the ubiquitous distribution of HCMV and high seroconversion rates [37], an etiological association between HCMV infection and human cancer has been difficult to establish. However, the available virologic, epidemiologic, and molecular studies implicating HCMV with specific human cancers are reviewed in Table 1.

Carcinoma of the Cervix

HCMV has been isolated from cervical cancer biopsies and their derived cell cultures [40, 41, 55]. However, seroepidemiologic studies linking HCMV infection with cervical cancer have yielded conflicting results. Some investigators have found significantly higher levels of antibodies to HCMV in patients with cervical carcinoma than in controls [59, 79, 82] while other groups have found no correlation [23, 34, 48, 75].

Both Huang et al. [39] and Fletcher et al. [20] have detected HCMV sequences in cervical cancer specimens. As shown by Southern blot analysis, two biopsies examined by Fletcher et al. [20] contained sequences that hybridized to the *Hin*dIII-E fragment of HCMV strain AD169. In one of the biopsies, the HCMV sequences were present at 20 copies per cell and were found integrated into cellular DNA [19]. The HCMV insert DNA showed homology to the HCMV major immediate early (IE) gene.

Table 1. Association of HCMV infection with human malignancies

Tumor	HCMV Markers	Detection techniques	Comments	References
Carcinoma of the cervix	Antibody	Complement fixation	Antibody levels higher in carcinoma patients than controls	Pacsa et al. [59] Stoian et al. [79] Vestergaard et al. [82]
	Antibody, immune lymphocytes	Complement fixation Indirect hemagglutination Lymphocyte stimulation	No difference in humoral and cellular immunity between cancer patients and controls	Kumar et al. [48]
	Antibody	ELISA Immunofluorescence Neutralization	No association between HCMV infection and cervical dysplasia	Hart et al. [34]
	Virus	Cell culture	HCMV isolated from tumor-derived cultures	Melnick et al. [55]
	Viral genome	DNA–DNA reassociation	HCMV DNA in tumor tissues	Huang et al. [39]
	*Hin*dIII-E (AD169)	Southern blot	Two CIN biopsies positive HCMV sequences integrated	Fletcher et al. [20] Fletcher and Macnab [19]
Adenocarcinoma of the prostate	Virus	Cell culture	Mj strain isolated from normal prostate Mj strain transforms HEL	Rapp et al. [63] Geder et al. [26]
	Membrane antigens	Cytotoxicity assay	Lymphocytes cytotoxic to infected and transformed cells	Sanford et al. [71]
	DNA RNA Antigens	DNA–DNA reassociation In situ hybridization Immunofluorescence	HCMV DNA, RNA, and antigens in tumor tissues	Boldogh et al. [6]
Adenocarcinoma of the colon	Virus	Cell culture	HCMV isolated from tumor-derived cultures	Hashiro et al. [35]
	Viral DNA	DNA–DNA hybridization	Detected in normal and tumor tissues	Huang and Roche [38]
	Viral DNA	DNA–DNA reassociation	Not detected in tumor biopsies	Brichacek et al. [7]
	Viral RNA Antigens Virus	In situ hybridization Immunofluorescence Cell culture	Not detected in tumor tissues	Hart et al. [33]

ELISA, enzyme-linked immunosorbent assay; CIN, cervical intraepithelial neoplasia; HEL, human embryo lung cells

In human cervical carcinoma, several viruses, including HSV-2, HCMV, and human papilloma virus (HPV) sequences, have been detected in the same tumors, indicating multiple infections [54]. The synergistic interaction among these viruses in the infected cell may occur in the process leading to cervical cancer.

Adenocarcinoma of the Prostate

The demonstration that prostatic carcinoma cells contained herpesvirus nuclear antigens and DNA suggested a viral association [10]. Furthermore, HCMV strain Mj was isolated from a primary culture of human prostatic tissue [63].

Serologic investigation of prostatic cancer patients showed that a large percentage had high antibody titers against HCMV [71]. Lymphocytes from these patients were cytotoxic to both HCMV-infected and transformed cells, indicating the presence of HCMV-specific membrane antigen [70]. This cytotoxicity was blocked by sera from prostatic carcinoma patients. In later investigations, Boldogh et al. [6] detected both HCMV and HSV-2 DNA, RNA, and antigens in both normal and prostatic cancer tissues. Their presence may indicate that both viruses may play some cofactor role in the development of this cancer or may merely represent reactivated viral infections in these tissues.

Adenocarcinoma of the Colon

HCMV persistently infects [6] and has been isolated from the gastrointestinal tract of patients with regional enteritis and ulcerative colitis [17, 60]. HCMV has also been isolated from cell cultures derived from adenocarcinomas of the colon [35]. In contrast, Hart et al. [33] have failed to isolate HCMV from similar cell cultures.

Employing DNA hybridization, Huang and Roche [38] have demonstrated HCMV DNA in adenocarcinomas of the colon. However, in other studies [7, 33] no HCMV DNA sequences were detected in tumor biopsies from adenocarcinomas of the colon and rectum. In light of these conflicting findings, no clean-cut association has been demonstrated.

Kaposi's Sarcoma

Since a comprehensive review of KS is being presented elsewhere in this volume, the association of HCMV with KS will only be briefly discussed.

Until recently, KS was a rare tumor affecting the elderly white men of Mediterranean or Jewish descent, the black population of equatorial Africa, and organ transplant recipients. However, since 1979, the occurrence of a more aggressive form of KS in young male homosexuals with acquired immunodeficiency syndrome (AIDS) has been reported [21, 22]. HCMV infection has been linked to KS by high levels of HCMV antibodies in patients with KS [29], detection of HCMV-related nuclear antigens in KS biopsies and KS-derived lines [5, 30] and the demonstration of HCMV-specific DNA and RNA [5, 18, 30, 44] in KS biopsies. In addition, HCMV strain K9V, isolated from a KS-derived line [28] was shown to transform human endothelial cells [74]. In contrast to the above associations linking HCMV with KS, other investigators have not found evidence linking HCMV infection with KS [3, 32, 68, 81]. Moreover, in addition to HCMV, hepatitis B virus DNA has been detected in several KS biopsies [44, 73].

Transformation of Mammalian Cells In Vitro

The oncogenic potential of HCMV was originally demonstrated by the ability of both infectious and UV-inactivated virus to transform a variety of rodent and human cells in vitro (Table 2). Albrecht and Rapp [2] first showed that UV-inactivated HCMV transformed hamster embryo fibroblasts. The transformed cells induced poorly differentiated malignant fibrosarcomas after subcutaneous injection into newborn and weanling golden Syrian hamsters. HCMV-specific antigens were demonstrated in the transformed and tumor-derived lines; however, no HCMV DNA sequences were detected. Similarly, Boldogh et al. [4] have transformed hamster embryo fibroblasts with UV-irradiated HCMV and both the transformed and tumor-dervied lines retained HCMV specific antigens.

Geder et al. [26] transformed human embryo lung cultures following infection with HCMV strain Mj. Expression of HCMV-specific antigens decreased in the transformed and tumor-derived lines with increasing passage level. Despite this, the cell lines demonstrated enhanced tumorigenicity in the nude mice [27]. At early passage, HCMV DNA was detected in the transformed cells at 0.3 genome equivalents per cell, but was undetectable after prolonged passage [39]. Similarly, Huang et al. [41] transformed human embryo lung cells by infecting with HCMV strains BT1757 or Towne at low multiplicity of infection. HCMV-specific antigens and messenger RNA (mRNA) were detected in the transformed cells by anticomplement immunofluorescent assay and by in situ DNA–RNA hybridization, respectively. The HCMV-transformed cells were tumorigenic in nude mice.

Infections by HCMV strains Towne and K9V have each been used to transform human endothelial cells to anchorage-independent growth [74]. Low passage HCMV strain Towne transformed these cells more efficiently than with high passage virus. UV-inactivated Towne was also capable of transforming human endothelial cells, but at a reduced frequency as compared to infectious virus. Pretreatment of cells with a tumor promoter, TPA, followed by viral infection did not enhance transformation frequency.

Guinea pig hepatocyte cells have been transformed following infection with strain AD169 [42]. Morphologically transformed lines were established that

Table 2. In vitro transformation of mammalian cells by HCMV

Virus (strain)	Cell type	Transformation criteria	HCMV-specific markers	Oncogenicity of transformed cells	References
UV-inactivated HCMV (C-87)	Hamster embryo fibroblast	Morphological and immortalization	Intracellular and membrane antigens	Hamsters	Albrecht and Rapp [2]
Infectious HCMV (Mj)	Human embryo lung	Morphological and immortalization	Nuclear and membrane antigens	Nude mice	Geder et al. [26]
			HCMV DNA (0.3 genome equivalent per cell) in transformed cells at early passage		Huang et al. [39]
UV-inactivated HCMV (C-87)	Hamster embryo fibroblast	Morphological	Intracellular and membrane antigens	Hamsters	Boldogh et al. [4]
Infectious HCMV (AD169)	Guinea pig hepatocyte	Morphological and and growth in soft agarose		Nude mice	Isom et al. [42]
Infectious HCMV (BT1757, Towne)	Human embryo lung	Morphological, immortalization, growth in soft agar, and low serum	Viral antigens, messenger RNA	Nude mice	Huang et al. [41]
Infectious HCMV (AD169)	Dog embryo kidney	Immortalization and growth in soft agarose	Viral antigens		Yelle et al. [83]
UV-inactivated HCMV (AD169)	Rat embryo			Rats	Fletcher et al. [20]
Infectious HCMV (Towne, K9V) UV-inactivated HCMV (Towne)	Human endothelial	Growth in soft agarose	Immediate early and late nuclear antigens		Smiley et al. [74]

produced spindle cell fibrosarcomas upon subcutaneous inoculation into nude mice. In other studies, primary rat embryo cells have been transformed by UV-irradiated AD169, and the transformed cells were tumorigenic in syngeneic animals [20].

Canine cells have also been employed in transformation studies. Yelle et al. [83] transformed primary dog embryo kidney cells following infection with HCMV strain AD169. The transformed cells showed intracellular viral antigens, formed colonies in soft agarose, and were weakly tumorigenic in mice.

In summary, both infectious and UV-inactivated HCMV have been used to transform a variety of mammalian cells in vitro. Loss of HCMV antigens and DNA together with the increased tumorigenicity of the cells resulted from long-term passaging. Thus, the transformed cell phenotype was maintained in the absence of viral sequences. As a result of not being able to correlate HCMV infection with defined events in the transformation process, transfection of rodent cells with HCMV DNA restriction fragments has been employed to elucidate the specific HCMV transforming genes and mechanisms of viral transformation.

Multiple Transforming Regions in HCMV DNA

mtrI in AD169

Transfection of rodent cells with either *Hin*dIII or *Xba*I-digested DNA of HCMV strain AD169 left the transforming activity of the DNA intact [57]. By employing a series of overlapping *Hin*dIII fragments cloned into cosmids, the transforming region was first localized to the *Hin*dIII-E fragment and then to a 2.9-kb *Xba*I–*Hin*dIII-NE fragment (Fig. 1). Deletion analysis finally localized the minimal mtr to a 558-bp fragment (pCM4127), designated mtrI [24, 58]. Upon digestion of mtrI with *Eco*RI, transformation potential was inactivated, indicating an important site required for transforming activity. Sequence analysis located the *Eco*RI site 21 bp from the *Hin*dIII right-hand

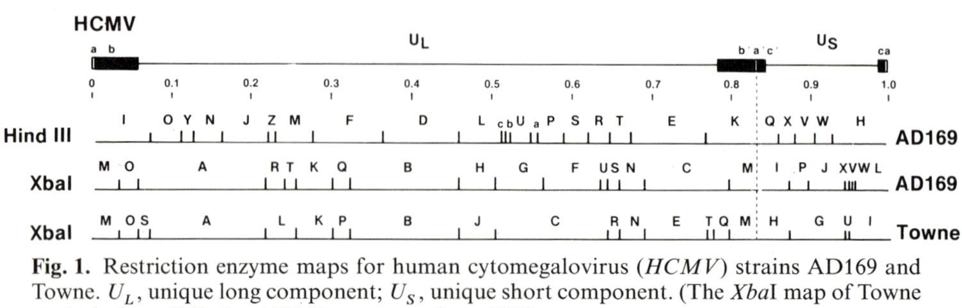

Fig. 1. Restriction enzyme maps for human cytomegalovirus (*HCMV*) strains AD169 and Towne. U_L, unique long component; U_S, unique short component. (The *Xba*I map of Towne strain is from [80]; the AD169 maps are from [46])

border and also identified a 41-amino-acid (aa) open reading frame (ORF) within mtrI. However, based upon the multiple stop codons in all reading frames, Nelson et al. [58] concluded that the 41-aa ORF was not involved in transformation.

Though AD169 mtrI-induced lines were tumorigenic in nude mice, the retention of viral sequences was generally not observed [57]. In the one case where mtrI sequences were retained, experiments were carried out by cotransfecting cells with mtrI and pSV2neo. The analysis of the integration site showed that a complicated recombination had occurred between mtrI and pSV2neo sequences. In fact, pSV2neo sequences, not mtrI, were found flanked on either side by cellular sequences [8].

Since mtrI of HCMV strain AD169 and the *Bgl*II-N minimal transforming region of HSV-2 resided in noncoding 558-bp and 737-bp fragments, respectively, Galloway et al. [24] proposed that these stem-loop structures, resembling insertion-like elements, caused "hit and run" transformation of cells by functioning as either transcriptional enhancers of cellular oncogenes or as insertional mutagens. Indeed, HCMV mtrI has been shown to increase cellular transcription and function as an enhancer [25]. The involvement of an insertion- (IS)-like sequence in the activation of a cellular oncogene has been described in which the 5′ end of c-*mos* in a mouse myeloma cell line has been replaced by a sequence which conforms to a stem-loop structure and is flanked by direct repeats [66]. Transformation by HCMV mtrI and HSV-2 DNA fragments has been extensively reviewed by MacNab [52].

mtrII and mtrIII Identified Within Towne *Xba*I-E

The *Xba*I-E fragment of HCMV strain Towne DNA was identified by nonstringent hybridization conditions to the *Bgl*II-C and *Bgl*II-N transforming regions of HSV-2 [13]. Towne *Xba*I-E was shown to immortalize primary diploid Syrian hamster embryo (SHE) cells and to transform established NIH3T3 cells. Furthermore, Towne *Xba*I-E lacked homology to the transforming *Xba*I-N fragment of AD169 and exhibited homology exclusively to AD169 *Xba*I-C fragment (Fig. 1).

Since *Bam*HI digestion did not affect the transforming activity of Towne *Xba*I-E [16], *Bam*HI and *Xba*I–*Bam*HI subclones of Towne *Xba*I-E were constructed (Fig. 2) and used to localize the transforming region. Subclones containing *Xba*I–*Bam*HI fragments EM, designated mtrII, and EJ, designated mtrIII, were each found to transform NIH3T3 and Rat-2 cells. All Rat-2 lines induced by *Xba*I–*Bam*HI EM and EJ were tumorigenic in immunocompetent 5-week-old Fisher rats [16].

The minimal size, sequence, and structural elements associated with mtrIII are presently unknown. While mtrIII encodes the major IE protein, it is not known if the minimal transforming domain falls within the IE gene region. Since mtrIII-transformed and tumor-derived lines did not retain mtrIII sequences, it is, in this respect, similar to mtrI-transformed cells.

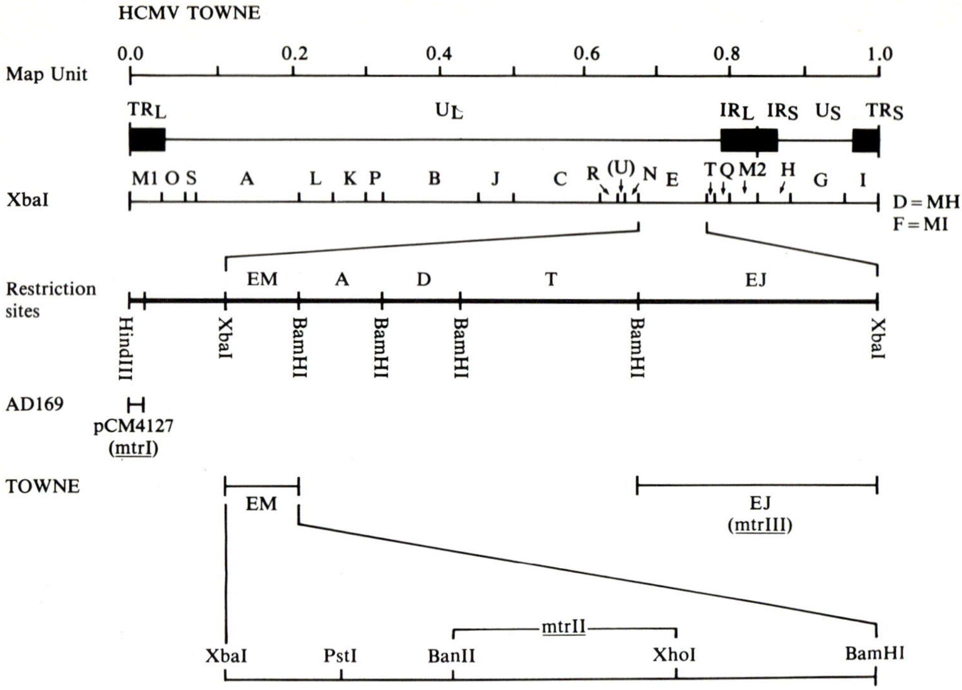

Fig. 2. Restriction map of human cytomegalovirus (*HCMV*) DNA and the locations of the Towne *Xba*I-E fragment and the *Xba*I-*Bam*HI subfragments. The location of the three morphological transforming regions (*mtr*) are identified together with important restriction sites within Towne *Xba*I-*Bam*HI-EM. *D*, MH in one orientation; *F*, MI in the opposite orientation; IR_L, internal repeat of long component; IR_S, internal repeat of short component; TR_L, terminal repeat of long component; TR_S, terminal repeat of short component; U_L, unique long component; U_S, unique short component

Some insight into possible mechanisms of transformation was recently observed when Rat-2 cells transfected with mtrII plus mtrIII showed a sevenfold increase in transformation activity than cells transfected with either mtrII or mtrIII [45]. The lines transformed by mtrII plus mtrIII produced tumors in syngeneic rats at a much faster rate (5–7 days) than those transformed by either alone (25–35 days). Southern blot hybridization showed multiple and amplified mtrII sequences in mtrII-plus-mtrIII lines as compared to mtrII-induced lines. Consistent with previous results [16], mtrIII sequences were not detected in either the single or double transformants. Further analysis of the transformed lines revealed that the levels of p29, a 29-kd transformation-sensitive marker in Rat-2 cells, were decreased 10- to 100-fold in cell lines transformed by mtrII or mtrIII alone. However, no p29 at all was detected in mtrII-plus mtrIII transformants.

Since mtrIII encodes the major IE protein involved in transactivation and viral autoregulation [77, 78], several mechanisms for the enhanced tumorigenic involvement of mtrIII can be proposed [45]. First, mtrIII may regulate the mtrII-encoded ORFs; second, mtrIII may promote insertion or amplification of mtrII; and third, mtrII and mtrIII each may exert independent effects on cellular functions in established cells. The first mechanism would involve the transactivation by mtrIII sequences. However, since mtrIII is not maintained in the transformed and tumor-derived lines, its interaction with mtrII must be transient. In the second mechanism, mtrIII may induce chromosomal aberrations, promoting integration of mtrII into host cell DNA. In support of this, HCMV infection has been shown to damage metaphase chromosomes [51]. Thirdly, mtrII and mtrIII may cooperate to enhance tumorigenesis. Evidence for this possibility is the downregulation of p29 in the double transformants. What role they each play and whether or not mtrII and mtrIII interact with cellular proto-oncogenes remains to be determined.

EM-(mtrII)-Transformed and Tumor-Derived Lines Retain Viral DNA

In contrast to mtrI and mtrIII, the retention of the Towne *Xba*I–*Bam*HI-EM fragment has been demonstrated in both transformed and tumor-derived lines [16]. Using a 1.5-kb *Pst*I–*Xho*I subfragment of EM (Fig. 2), genomic DNA from an EM-induced rat tumor-derived line (RBM 2T1), was shown to have retained a multicopy 3-kb band (Fig. 3; *Xba*I–*Bam*HI, 2-cut digest). In the genomic *Xba*I–*Bam*HI–*Pst*I–*Xho*I (4-cut) digest, a multicopy band comigrating with the 1.5-kb *Pst*I–*Xho*I subfragment of EM was detected. Another independently derived EM-transformed line (RBM 3T1) also retained the 3- and 1.5-kb bands in the 2-enzyme and 4-enzyme digests, respectively (Fig. 3 B). The consistent retention of single or multicopy virus-specific bands may indicate a maintenance role for the retained viral DNA sequences. The nature and state of the viral EM sequences in the transformed cells is unknown. However, bands hybridizing (in Fig. 3 A) higher than 3 kb in size are suggestive of integration.

Determination and Sequence Analysis of the mtrII Minimal Transforming Domain

To define the minimal transforming region of the Towne EM fragment, the three subfragments of *Pst*I–*Xho*I-digested EM (Fig. 2) were subcloned in pUC18 and assayed for transforming activity [65]. As shown in Table 3, the 1.5-kb *Pst*I–*Xho*I subfragment of EM showed transforming activity. To delineate the transforming region within the *Pst*I–*Xho*I subfragment, a 980-bp subclone extending from the *Ban*II site (located 610 bp to the right of the *Pst*I site) to the *Xho*I site was constructed. The *Ban*II–*Xho*I clone showed overall transforming activity similar to that of intact EM. The relative proportion of large foci previously shown to be an in vitro correlate of tumorigenicity [16], was higher in *Ban*II–*Xho*I-transfected than in EM-transfected cultures. Upon

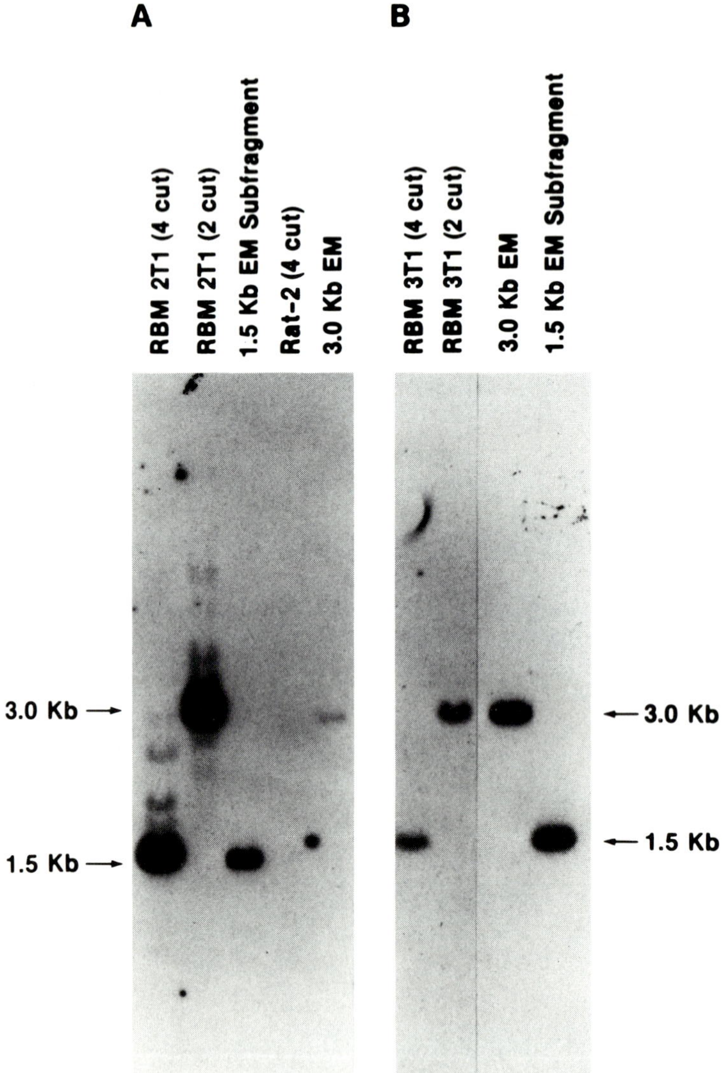

Fig. 3 A, B. Southern hybridization of *Xba*I-*Bam*HI-EM transformed rat tumor-derived cellular DNAs to ^{32}P-labeled *Pst*I-*Xho*I 1.5-kb EM subfragment. **A** Normal Rat-2 and rat tumor (RBM 2T1) DNAs (10 μg each) were digested with *Xba*I-*Bam*HI (*2 cut*) or with four enzymes (*Xba*I, *Bam*HI, *Pst*I, and *Xho*I) (*4 cut*) and hybridized with ^{32}P-labeled 1.5-kb EM subfragment as probe. Markers used were 3-kb EM and 1.5-kb EM subfragment. **B** DNA (10 μg) from another independent rat tumor-derived line (RBM 3T1) was digested with two (*2 cut*) or four enzymes (*4 cut*) as above and hybridized with ^{32}P-labeled *Pst*I-*Xho*I 1.5 kb EM subfragment as probe. The 1.5-kb subfragment and one genome equivalent of 3.0-kb EM were used as markers. kb, kilobase pairs. (Reprinted with permission from [16])

Table 3. Transforming activities of the HCMV EM subclones (after [65])

DNA	Foci per dish	
	NIH 3T3	Rat-2
Xba I EM *Bam*HI	8L, 12M, 14S	2M, 22S
Xba I *Pst* I	0	1M, 5S
Pst I *Xho* I	11L, 23M, S	5M, 45S
Ban II *Xho* I	21L, 9M, 4S	17L
Bgl II *Bam*HI	4L, 9M, S	2M, 6S
Xho I *Bam*HI	0	1M, 2S
Vector pUC18	1	3S
Vector pBR327	1	ND
Salmon testes	0	ND

Focus-formation data are averages of two experiments (focus sizes: L, large; M, medium, S, small)

testing a *Bgl*II–*Bam*HI fragment, a 62%–66% reduction in transforming activity was detected and the focal lines tested were nontumorigenic. Therefore, *Bgl*II cleaved within the transforming domain of the *Ban*II–*Xho*I fragment, approximately 1-kb to the left of the *Bam*HI site. This 980-bp fragment was designated mtrII [65].

The nucleotide sequence of the mtrII (Fig. 4) revealed three putative ORFs of 79, 83, and 34 aa located between map positions 294 and 530, 612 and 860, and 622 and 723, respectively. The sequences at the 5′ terminus of the ORFs contained regulatory elements that included CAAT boxes, SpI binding sites, and TACAAA and ATA transcriptional initiation signals. In addition, six copies of the heptanucleotide sequence GGTGA/GTC which has similarity to the simian virus (SV40) enhancer core consensus sequence were observed. All of these were found in the first 300 nucleotides upstream of the ORFs. The 79- and 34-aa ORFs also contained motifs which have 55%–78% homology to the Kozak consensus translational initiation sequence of CCA/GCCATGG, suggesting that these ORFs may be expressed.

Expression of Towne mtrII in HCMV-Infected Cells

To determine if mtrII transcripts were expressed, human fibroblasts were infected with HCMV strain Towne. IE RNA was isolated at 14 h postinfection and early RNA at 24 h. Two single-stranded 5′-end-labeled DNA probes for S1 nuclease analysis were generated (Fig. 5) from a clone containing the 980-bp *Ban*II–*Xho*I (mtrII) fragment inserted into M13 map position (mp) 10. One probe was a 980-base *Ban*II–*Xho*I probe that covered the entire mtrII sequence

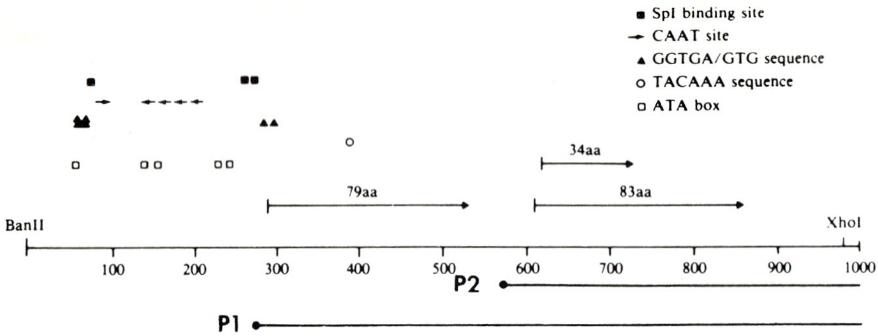


```
AGCCCACCAC CTTTTTTTTA AGAGAGGAGG AATTTCGTCT TGATCTCCAG CCGGAGATAA ( 60)
CGGCGGTGGT GGTGGTGGCG GGAGAGACTT CAAGGCAATG AAAAAAAAAA ATTTCGTTTT ( 120)
GCCATCAAGT GGTGACGATA ACCCGTCAGA TTGATAATTG GTTCCTACAG AAACTATTCT ( 180)
AACCGCGGAA GAAAGAAATT GAAAAAAAAA AATTGACAAA AAACATCATA ACATAAAGGA ( 240)
CCACCTACCT GGGACGCGCA GTTGGGCGGC GGACTGGGCG GCATGCTGCG GTGATGCTGT ( 300)
                                                        Start-79aa
CGGTGATGGT CTCTTCCTCT CTGGTCCTGA TCGTCTTTTT TCTAGGCGCT TCCGAGGAGG ( 360)
CGAAGCCGGC GACGACGACG ACGATAAAGA ATACAAAGCC GCAGTGTCGT CCAGAGGATT ( 420)
ACGCGACCAG ATTGCAAGAT CTCCGCGTCA CCTTTCATCG AGTAAAACCT ACGTTGGTAG ( 480)
GTCACGTAGG TACGGTTTAT TGTGACGGTC TTTCTTTTCC GCGTGTCGGG TGACGTAGTT ( 540)
                                                   End 79aa
TTCCTCTTGT AGCAACGTGA GGACGACTAC TCCGTGTGGC TCGACGGTAC GGTGGTCAAA ( 600)
GGCTGTTGGG GATGCAGCGT CATGGACTGG TTGTTGAGGC GGTATCTGGA GATCGTGTTC ( 660)
   Start 83aa               Start 34aa
CCCGCAGGCG ACCACGTCTT AATCCCGGAC TCAAGACGGA ATTGCATAGT ATGCGCTCGA ( 720)
CGCTAGAATC CATCTACAAA GACATGCGGC AATGCGTAAG TTGGTTCCTC TGTGGCGGCG ( 780)
    End 34aa
CTGTCCCGAG AGGTAACAAC GTGTTCATAG CACGCTGTTT TACTTTTGTC GGGCTCCCAG ( 840)
CCTCTGTTAG GTTGCGGAGA TAAGTCCGTG ATTAGTCGGC TGTCTCAGGA GGCGGAAAGG ( 900)
             End 83aa
AAATCGGATA ACGGCACGCG GAAAGGTCTC AGCGAGTTGG ACACGTTGTT TAGCCGTCTC ( 960)
GAAGAGTATC TGCACTCGAG                                             (1020)
```

Fig. 4. Map positions of the 79-, 34-, and 83-aa ORFs and the upstream regulatory sequences are shown, together with the complete nucleotide sequence of mtrII. *P1* and *P2* indicate the RNA transcripts detected in infected cells by S1 nuclease protection assay. The *Bql*II site is located at nucleotide 436. (Reprinted from [65])

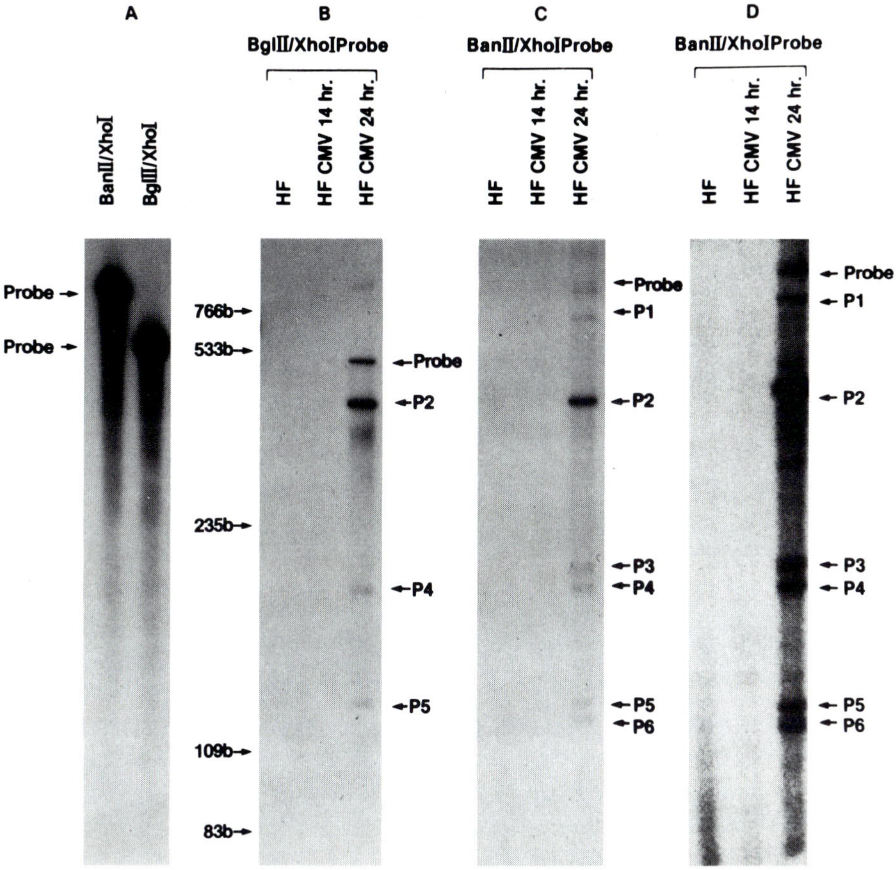

Fig. 5 A–D. S1 nuclease analysis of mtrII RNA in human cytomegalovirus- (HCMV-)infected cells. **A** Analysis of 980-base -*Ban*II-*Xho*I and 540-base *Bgl*II-*Xho*I probes. **B** S1 nuclease analysis of RNAs in uninfected human fibroblasts (*HF*) or human fibroblasts infected with HCMV for 14 or 24 h (*HF CMV 14 h* and *HF CMV 24 h*), using the *Bgl*II-*Xho*I probe. *b*, bases. **C** S1 nuclease analysis of RNAs as in **B**, using the *Ban*II-*Xho*I probe. **D** Longer exposure of **C**. Molecular weight markers: *Hin*fI restriction digest of simian virus 40 DNA. (From [65])

and the other a *Bgl*II–*Xho*I probe that encompassed the 3′ 540 bases. When the full-length *Ban*II–*Xho*I probe was used (Fig. 5 C), several distinct early RNA species, designated P1 through P6, were detected in the 24-h infected cultures, but not in the 14-h cultures. The transcripts P1 and P2 were of particular interest because the length of the protected DNA fragments positioned the 5′ end of the RNAs upstream of the putative ORFs (Fig. 4). The P1 transcript was found to be approximately 720 bases in length and, depending upon the exact position of the 5′ end, contained the coding sequences for the 79-, 83-, and 34-aa proteins. The P1 transcript was also detected in Fig. 5 B as an mRNA that hybridized to the full length of the *Bgl*II–*Xho*I probe, resulting in a protected 540-base DNA fragment. The major RNA transcript, P2, was 410 bases in length, which positioned the 5′ end of the RNA at approximately nucleotide 570 ± 10, 30–40 bases upstream of the AUG initiation codons for the 83- and 34-aa proteins. An identical size, protected DNA fragment was detected with both the *Ban*II–*Xho*I and *Bgl*II–*Xho*I probes (Fig. 5 A), demonstrating the validity of the S1 mapping technique used. It is believed that the RNA species represented authentic 5′ ends, since no homologies to the consensus splice donor, AG↓GTAAGT, and splice acceptor, Py_{10}CAG↓, sequences were detected.

Stem-Loop Structures Within mtrII

Sequence analysis of mtrII also revealed numerous repetitive elements that may form stem-loop structures (Fig. 6). These were identified on the basis of the thermodynamic stability of the stem, size of the loop, and the presence of repetitive sequences in the flanking region of the stem structure. The first three (a–c) were located in the presumed promoter region. Stem-loop structures d and e contained small loops and stable stems and were located within the 79- and 83-aa ORFs, respectively. The stem-loop in f was from the AD169 mtrI and is the structure that Galloway et al. [24] associated with transformation.

Transforming Activity of mtrII Colinear Regions

The colinear mtrII of HCMV strain Tanaka as well as the colinear 2.2-kb fragment of strain AD169 were isolated and tested for transforming activity (Table 4) [43]. Compared with Towne mtrII, the AD169 2.2-kb colinear region showed the similar transforming activity. In contrast, Tanaka mtrII showed a 75% reduction in transforming activity compared with Towne mtrII and only 4.3%–5.5% of the activity for large-focus formation. All lines induced by either Towne mtrII or by the AD169 colinear 2.2-kb fragment exhibited cloning efficiencies ranging from 0.48% to 3.5%, and the colonies which grew were macro (> 0.5 mm) in size. Production of macro colonies have been correlated previously with tumorigenicity [16]. Focal lines induced by Tanaka mtrII exhibited a negligible cloning efficiency similar to that of the controls. Moreover, Tanaka-induced colonies that grew were predominantly micro in size (0.1–2.5 mm). The results indicated that Tanaka mtrII was transformation defective.

The Tanaka mtrII sequence was next compared with the sequences of Towne mtrII and the colinear region in strain AD169. The resulting differences in the mtrII ORFs are schematically presented in Fig. 7. The 79-aa ORF of Towne mtrII was found in strain AD169 but not in Tanaka mtrII. The 83-aa ORF of Towne was truncated in AD169, and the N-terminal end of the 34-aa ORF was fused by a frameshift mutation to the C-terminal end of the 83-aa ORF, creating a somewhat larger ORF. In Tanaka, the 83- and 34-aa ORFs

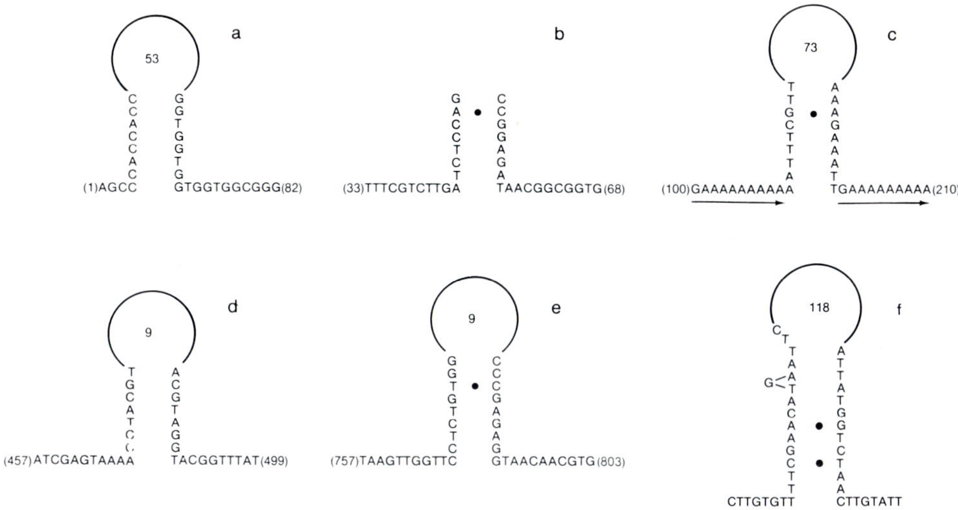

Fig. 6 a–f. Stem-loop structures within Towne mtrII (**a–e**) and the stem-loop structure from AD169 mtrI (**f**). A *small circle* indicates a base mismatch in the stem. Nucleotide positions are indicated in *parentheses*. *Arrows* indicate direct repeats in flanking 10 nucleotides of the stem-loop structure. The size of the loop in nucleotides is indicated by the *number in the loop*. (Stem-loop **a–e** are from [65] and stem-loop structure in **f** from [24])

Table 4. Transforming potential of HCMV colinear mtrII regions in established NIH 3T3 cells (from [43])

Transfected DNA	Focus formation [a]	Cloning in agarose [b]	
		Colony efficiency	Colony size
Towne mtrII (980 bp)	43 (23L, 11M, 9S)	1.4–3.5	Macro
Tanaka mtrII (980 bp)	11 (1L, 6M, 4S)	0.005–0.01	Micro
Towne mtrII (*Bgl*II digested)	19 (10L, 5M, 5S)	NT	
AD169 colinear 2.2-kb region	43 (18L, 14M, 11S)	0.48–1.09	Macro
Salmon testes	2 (1M, 1S)	0.003	Micro
Control	2 (1M, 1S)	0.003	Micro

NT, not tested

[a] Average number of foci per 100-mm-diameter dish from two experiments. NIH 3T3 cells were transfected with 15 μg of each HCMV DNA together with 5 μg of salmon testes DNA use as a carrier. After 48 h, cells were trypsinized and divided at a 1:3 ratio, and morphologically transformed foci were scored 5–6 weeks later. Focus diameter: L, >2.5 mm; M, 1.5–2.5 mm; S, >1.0 mm

[b] Cells were seeded in 0.3% agarose at 10^5 cells per 60-mm-diameter dish, and 3–4 weeks later, colonies were scored. Colony efficiency is defined as (number of colonies × 100)/(number of seeded cells). Data shown are the range for colony efficiency for all focal lines tested. Colony diameter size: micro, 0.1–0.25 mm; macro, >0.5 mm

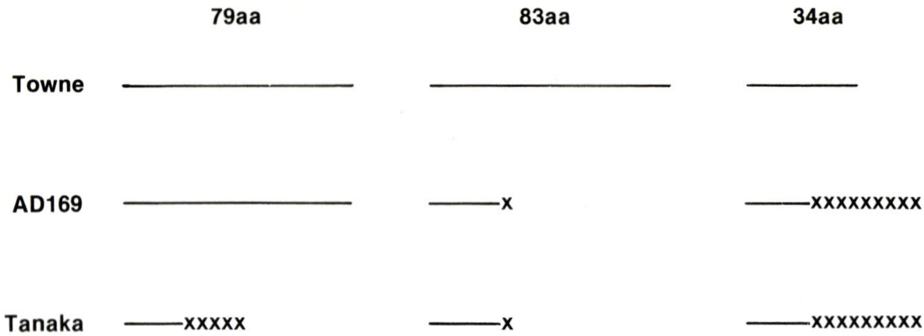

Fig. 7. Comparison of the translated mtrII open reading frames (ORFs) from human cytomegalovirus strains Towne, AD169, and Tanaka. Data taken from sequence analyses on Towne and Tanaka mtrII [43] and compared with the sequence of AD169 [47]. *Solid line*, homology; *X*, changes in amino acid (*aa*) sequence. (From [43])

were similar to those in AD169. Since the colinear fragment in strain AD169 containing the 79-aa ORF was transforming while the colinear fragment in strain Tanaka lacking the 79-aa ORF was transformation defective, the data implicated a role for the 79-aa ORF in transformation. This conclusion is further substantiated by the reduced transforming activity (Table 3) seen with a *Bgl*II–*Bam*HI subclone of EM because the *Bgl*II site is within the 79-aa ORF. Further importance of the putative 79-aa ORF within mtrII was found when cells transfected with *Bgl*II-digested Towne mtrII showed a 56% reduction in transforming activity as compared with intact Towne mtrII.

Comparison of the colinear regions for stem-loop structures in mtrII suggested no role in transformation as was reported for mtrI [24, 25]. Stem-loops in Fig. 6a–c were virtually unaltered in their sequence in the Tanaka mtrII, the transforming AD169 2.2-kb, and the Towne mtrII. Similarly, the stem-loop structure (Fig. 6d) located within the Towne mtrII 79-aa ORF was unchanged in the others. Thus, the reduction in transforming activity of Tanaka mtrII was consistent with the truncation of the 79-aa ORF. The residual transforming activity associated with Tanaka mtrII may be due to some partial activity of the truncated 79-aa ORF. Finally, the stem-loop structure in Fig. 6e was dramatically altered in both AD169 and Tanaka colinear regions.

Promoter Activity of mtrII

The identification of the 5′ ends of early RNA transcripts that mapped within Towne mtrII as well as its sequence analysis suggested the presence of promoter elements. Along these lines, promoter activity has been reported for Towne mtrII using the in vitro chloramphenicol acetyltransferase (CAT) expression system (Fig. 8) [67]. MtrII (980S) cloned in front of the CAT gene in the sense (S) orientation with reference to the ORFs exhibited promoter activity that was almost 40-fold higher than the promoterless CAT plasmid,

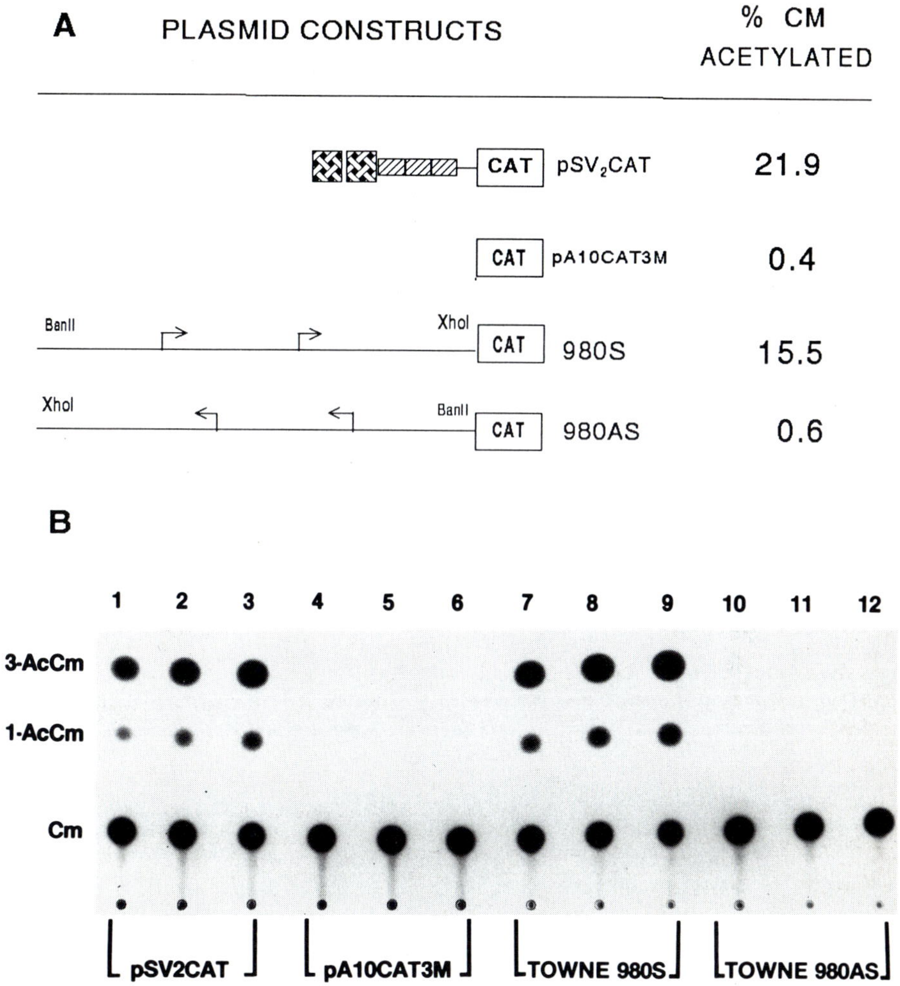

Fig. 8 A, B. Promoter activity of mtrII. **A** the *Ban*II-*Xho*I sites of mtrII were converted to *Xba*I sites and ligated into the promoterless plasmid, pA10CAT3M. Clones representing the positive and negative orientations of 980 bp to the chloramphenicol acetyltransferase (CAT) gene were selected with *Bgl*II. CV-1 cells were transfected with each plasmid DNA (10 μg) together with carrier DNA (15 μg) according to Chen and Okayama [11]. At 48 h, cell extracts were assayed for CAT activity [31]. The data presented are for 1 μl of pSV2CAT cell extract and 10 μl for all other cell extracts. **B** CAT activity is presented as percentage conversion of [^{14}C]chloramphenicol (*Cm*) to 1′-acetyl-Cm and 3′-acetyl-Cm forms. *Lanes 1–3* represent 0.5, 1.0, and 1.5 μl of pSV2CAT respectively; *lanes 4–6:* 20, 30, and 40 μl of pA10CAT3M; *lanes 7–9:* 20, 30, and 40 μl of Towne 980S (sense orientation); *lanes 10–12:* 20, 30, and 40 μl of Towne 980AS (antisense orientation). (Modified from [67])

pA10CAT3M. The data supported the sequence analysis of mtrII that indicated transcriptional control elements in the sense but not antisense orientation. Furthermore, the demonstration of mtrII promoter activity was consistent with and strengthened the S1 nuclease data that mapped early RNAs within mtrII, suggesting two separate promoters [65]. Making use of the unique *Bgl*II restriction site within mtrII, constructs were generated which separated the two putative promoter regions. When tested in the CAT assay system both the Towne mtrII 440-bp and 540-bp subfragments demonstrated promoter activity in the sense orientation only (Inamdar et al., in preparation). Furthermore, both intact Tanaka mtrII and its 440-bp subfragment (containing the promoter for the 79-aa ORF) also exhibited promoter activity. These results demonstrate that the lack of transforming ability of Tanaka mtrII was not due to the absence of promoter activity.

mtrII is a 79-aa ORF

Direct evidence for the role of the 79-aa ORF was recently obtained by cloning the 79-aa ORF into a mammalian expression vector, pCHC6, followed by transfection of NIH3T3 cells (Thompson et al., in preparation). Transformation of NIH3T3 cells was demonstrated with the expression construct containing the intact 79-aa ORF. Constructs containing either the 440-bp or 540-bp subfragments, each with its respective promoter, were nontransforming. Since the 79-aa ORF is interrupted in the 440-bp construct, the data further support the concept that an intact 79-aa ORF is required for transforming activity.

Other small viral polypeptides have been associated with transformation. The E5 transforming domain of bovine papilloma virus is a 44-aa polypeptide with a molecular weight of 7 kDa [9, 72]. Additionally, transformation by Marek's disease virus is thought to involve a small ORF (Bradley, personal communication).

Summary and Conclusions

Human cytomegalovirus infection has been associated with cervical cancer, adenocarcinomas of the colon and rectum, and the classic and aggressive forms of KS. However, in no case has HCMV been consistently detected in these malignant tissues. Therefore, direct evidence linking HCMV infection with these malignancies is lacking.

On the other hand, data exist on the transformation of both human and nonhuman cells following infection with either infectious or UV-irradiated virus. These results provide the framework for studying the oncogenic potential of the virus.

A summary of transfection experiments employing HCMV restriction enzyme DNA fragments is shown in Table 5. These studies have identified three

Table 5. Morphological transforming regions of HCMV

Virus strain	DNA fragment (size)	Cells trans-formed	mtr	Minimal size (bp)	Sequence		Proposed function	Tumors in animals	Fragment retained	References
					Structure	ORF				
AD169	*Xba*I/*Hin*dIII-NE (2.9 kb)	NIH 3T3						Yes	No	Nelson et al. [57]
AD169	pCM4115 * pCM4127 *	NIH 3T3	mtrI **	490 * 558 **	Stem-loop	41 aa	Transcriptional enhancer ***	Yes	No	Nelson et al. [58] * Galloway et al. [24] ** Galloway et al. [25] ***
Towne	*Xba*I-E (20 kb)	Primary SHE NIH 3T3						Yes	Yes *	Clanton et al. [13] El-Beik et al. [16]
Towne	*Xba*I/*Bam*HI-EM (3 kb)	NIH 3T3 Rat-2						Yes	Yes	El-Beik et al. [16]
Towne	*Ban*II-*Xho*I subfragment of EM (980 bp)	NIH 3T3 Rat-2	mtrII	980	Stem-loops	79, 83, 34 aa	Putative transforming polypeptides	Yes	Yes	Razzaque et al. [65]
Tanaka	Colinear *Ban*II-*Xho*I subfragment of EM (980 bp)	NIH 3T3	mtrII	980	Stem-loops	79 aa absent	Defective in transformation			Jahan et al. [43]
Towne	*Xba*I/*Bam*HI-EJ (7.6 kb)	NIH 3T3 Rat-2	mtrIII	Unknown		IE region I	Autoregulation, transactivation	Yes	No	El-Beik et al. [16] Razzaque et al. [65]

HCMV mtr, each of which is likely to transform cells by a different mechanism. For mtrI of AD169 and mtrIII of Towne, the absence of viral sequences in transformed and tumor-derived lines mimics studies employing infectious and UV-irradiated virus. In the latter case, viral sequences were also not maintained in the transformed cells. This is in constrast to other DNA virus transformation studies (e.g., SV40, polyomavirus, and adenovirus) where viral sequences are required for maintenance. For Towne mtrII, viral sequences have been routinely detected in the transformed and tumor-derived lines. Moreover, Towne mtrII was shown to contain two promoters, each of which was insufficient to transform NIH3T3 cells (Inamdar et al., in preparation). Since the 79-aa ORF was found truncated in the colinear mtrII of transformation-defective strain Tanaka it was implicated in viral transformation. The direct demonstration of the transforming ability of the 79-aa ORF was recently obtained (Thompson et al., in preparation), employing an expression vector containing the intact 79-aa ORF.

The enhanced transformation employing mtrII plus mtrIII indicated their possible interaction. Based upon the multistep process of human cancer, the initiating and transforming steps for mtrII and mtrIII need to be delineated. This will require further dissection of the transforming events in primary rodent as well as in human cells. The use of relevant human target cell systems will be most important to validate the oncogenic potential of HCMV.

Acknowledgements. The authors wish to express their gratitude to R. Jariwalla and J. Brady for their participation throughout the studies reviewed in this chapter. We would also like to thank E.-S. Huang and J. Macnab for preprints of unpublished work. We are grateful to J. Doniger for critical review of the chapter. This work was supported in part by a National Institute of Health grant (CA 37259) and by a contract from the National Foundation for Cancer Research.

References

1. Ablashi DV, Josephs SF, Buchbinder A, Hellman K, Nakamura S, Llana T, Lusso P, Kaplan M, Dahlberg J, Memon S, Imam F, Ablashi KL, Markham PD, Krmarsky B, Krueger GRF, Biberfeld P, Wong-Staal F, Salahuddin SZ, Gallo RC (1988) Human B-lymphotropic virus (human herpesvirus-6). J Virol Methods 21:29–48
2. Albrecht T, Rapp F (1973) Maligant transformation of hamster embryo fibroblasts following exposure to ultraviolet-irradiated human cytomegalovirus. Virology 55:53–61
3. Ambinder RF, Newman C, Hayward GS, Biggar R, Melbye M, Kestens L, van Marck E, Piot P, Gigase P, Wright PB, Quinn TC (1987) Lack of association of cytomegalovirus with endemic African Kaposi's sarcoma. J Infect Dis 156:193–197
4. Boldogh I, Gonczol E, Vaczi L (1978) Transformation of hamster embryonic fibroblast cell by UV-irradiated human cytomegalovirus. Acta Microbiol Hung 25:269–275
5. Boldogh I, Beth E, Huang E-S, Kyalwazi SK, Giraldo G (1981) Kaposi's sarcoma. IV. Detection of CMV DNA, CMV RNA and CMNA in tumor biopsies. Int J Cancer 28:469–474

6. Boldogh I, Baskar JF, Mar EC, Huang E-S (1983) Human cytomegalovirus and herpes simplex type 2 virus in normal and adenocarcinomatous prostate glands. JNCI 70:819–825
7. Brichacek B, Hirsch I, Zavadova H, Prochazka M, Faltyn J, Vonka V (1980) Absence of cytomegalovirus DNA from adenocarcinoma of the colon. Intervirology 14:223–227
8. Buonaguro FM, McDougall JK, Galloway DA (1987) Characterization of the integration site of the CMV mtr in a tumor cell line. Virology 156:74–83
9. Burkhardt A, DiMaio D, Schlegel R (1987) Genetic and biochemical definition of the bovine papilloma virus E5 transforming protein. EMBO J 6:2381–2385
10. Centifanto YM, Kaufman HE, Zam ZS, Drylie DM, Deardourff SL (1973) Herpesvirus particles in prostatic carcinoma cells. J Virol 12:1608–1611
11. Chen C, Okayama H (1987) High-efficiency transformation of mammalian cells by plasmid DNA. Mol Cell Biol 7:2745–2752
12. Chretien JH, McGinnis CG, Muller A (1977) Venereal causes of cytomegalovirus mononucleosis. JAMA 238:1644–1645
13. Clanton DJ, Jariwalla RJ, Kress C, Rosenthal LJ (1983) Neoplastic transformation by a cloned human cytomegalovirus DNA fragment-uniquely homologous to one of the transforming regions of herpes simplex virus type 2. Proc Natl Acad Sci USA 80:3826–3830
14. Drew WL, Mintz L, Miner RC, Sands M, Ketterer B (1981) Prevalence of cytomegalovirus infection in homosexual men. J Infect Dis 143:188–192
15. Drew WL, Conant MA, Miner RC, Huang ES, Ziegler JL, Groundwater JR, Gullett JH, Abrams DI, Volberding P, Mintz L (1982) Cytomegalovirus and Kaposi's sarcoma in young homosexual men. Lancet 2:125–127
16. El-Beik T, Razzaque A, Jariwalla R, Cihlar RL, Rosenthal LJ (1986) Multiple transforming regions of human cytomegalovirus DNA. J Virol 60:645–652
17. Farmer GW, Vincent MM, Fuccillo DA (1973) Viral investigations in ulcerative colitis and regional enteritis. Gastroenterology 65:8–18
18. Fenoglio CM, Oster MW, Gerfo PL, Reynolds T, Edelson R, Patterson JAK, Madeiros E, McDougall JK (1982) Kaposi's sarcoma following chemotherapy for testicular cancer in a homosexual man: demonstration of cytomegalovirus RNA in sarcoma cells. Hum Pathol 13:955–959
19. Fletcher K, Macnab JCM (1989) Molecular cloning of DNA sequences from cervical intraepithelial neoplasia that hybridize to human cytomegalovirus DNA. Virus Genes 2:323–333
20. Fletcher K, Cordiner JW, Macnab JCM (1986) Detection of sequences that hybridize to human cytomegalovirus DNA in cervical neoplastic tissue. Dis Markers 4:219–229
21. Friedman-Kien AE (1981) Disseminated Kaposi's sarcoma syndrome in young homosexual men. J Am Acad Dermatol 5:468–471
22. Friedman-Kien AE, Ostreicher R (1984) Overview of classical and epidemic Kaposi's sarcoma. In: Friedman-Kien AE, Laubenstein LJ (eds) AIDS: the epidemic of Kaposi's sarcoma and opportunistic infections. Masson, New York, pp 23–34
23. Fucillo DA, Sever JL, Moder FL, Chen TC, Catalano LW, Johnson LD (1971) Cytomegalovirus antibody in patients with carcinoma of the uterine cervix. Obstet Gynecol 38:599–601
24. Galloway DA, Nelson JA, McDougall JK (1984) Small fragments of herpesvirus DNA with transforming activity contain insertion sequence-like structures. Proc Natl Acad Sci USA 81:4736–4740
25. Galloway DA, Buonaguro FM, Brandt CR, McDougall JK (1986) Herpes simplex virus and cytomegalovirus: unconventional DNA tumor viruses. In: Botcham M, Grodzicker T, Sharp PA (eds) DNA tumor viruses. Cancer Cells 4:355–361
26. Geder L, Lausch R, O'Neill F, Rapp F (1976) Oncogenic transformation of human embryo lung cells by human cytomegalovirus. Science 192:1134–1137
27. Geder L, Laychock AM, Gorodecki J, Rapp F (1978) Alterations in biological properties of different lines of cytomegalovirus-transformed human embryo lung cells following in vitro cultivation. IARC Sci Publ 24:591–601

28. Giraldo G, Beth E, Haguenau F (1972) Herpes-type virus particles in tissue culture of Kaposi's sarcoma from different geographic regions. JNCI 49:1509–1526
29. Giraldo G, Beth E, Henle W, Henle G, Mike V, Safai B, Huraux JM, McHardy J, De-The G (1978) Antibody patterns to herpesviruses in Kaposi's sarcoma. II. Serological association of American Kaposi's sarcoma with cytomegalovirus. Int J Cancer 22:126–131
30. Giraldo G, Beth E, Huang E-S (1980) Kaposi's sarcoma and its relationship to cytomegalovirus (CMV). III. CMV DNA and CMV early antigens in Kaposi's sarcoma. Int J Cancer 26:23–29
31. Gorman CM, Moffat LF, Howard BH (1982) Recombinant genomes which express chloramphenicol acetyltransferase in mammalian cells. Mol Cell Biol 2:1044–1051
32. Grody WW, Lewin KJ, Naeim F (1988) Detection of cytomegalovirus DNA in classic and epidemic Kaposi's sarcoma by in situ hybridization. Hum Pathol 19:524–528
33. Hart H, Neill WA, Norval M (1982) Lack of association of cytomegalovirus with adenocarcinoma of the colon. Gut 23:21–30
34. Hart H, Springbett A, Norval M (1982) Lack of association of cytomegalovirus antibody level with carcinoma of the uterine cervix. Gynecol Obstet Invest 14:300–308
35. Hashiro GM, Horikami S, Loh PC (1979) Cytomegalovirus isolation from cell cultures of human adenocarcinoma of the colon. Intervirology 12:84–88
36. Hirsch MS (1984) Cytomegalovirus–Leukocyte interactions. Birth Defects 20:161–173
37. Ho M (1982) Cytomegalovirus biology and infection. In: Greenough WB, Merigan TC (eds) Current topics in infectious disease. Plenum, New York, pp 79–104
38. Huang E-S, Roche JK (1978) Cytomegalovirus DNA and adenocarcinoma of the colon: evidence for latent viral infection. Lancet 1:957–960
39. Huang E-S, Boldogh I, Mar E-C (1983) Human cytomegaloviruses: evidence for possible association with human cancer. In: Philips LA (ed) Viruses associated with human cancer. Dekker, New York, pp 161–193
40. Huang E-S, Boldogh I, Baskar JF, Mar E-C (1984) The molecular biology of human cytomegalovirus and its relationship to various human cancers. In: Giraldo G, Beth E (eds) The role of viruses in human cancers, vol 2. Elsevier, New York, pp 169–194
41. Huang E-S, Davis MG, Baskar JF, Huong S-M (1986) Molecular epidemiology and oncogenicity of human cytomegalovirus. In: Harris CC (ed) Biochemical and molecular epidemiology of cancer. Liss, New York, pp 323–344
42. Isom HC, Mummaw J, Kreider JW (1983) Malignant transformation of guinea pig cells after exposure to ultraviolet-irradiated guinea pig cytomegalovirus. Virology 126:693–700
43. Jahan N, Razzaque A, Brady J, Rosenthal LJ (1989) The human cytomegalovirus mtrII colinear region in strain Tanaka is transformation defective. J Virol 63:2866–2869
44. Jahan N, Razzaque A, Greenspan J, Conant MA, Josephs SF, Nakamura S, Rosenthal LJ (1989) Analysis of human KS biopsies and cloned cell lines for cytomegalovirus, HIV-1 and other selected DNA virus sequences. AIDS Res Hum Retroviruses 5:225–231
45. Jariwalla RJ, Razzaque A, Lawson S, Rosenthal LJ (1989) Tumor progression mediated by two cooperating DNA segments of human cytomegalovirus. J Virol 63:425–428
46. Kemble GW, McCormick AL, Pereira L, Mocarski E (1987) A cytomegalovirus protein with properties of herpes simplex virus ICP8: partial purification of the polypeptide and map position of the gene. J Virol 61:3143–3151
47. Kouzarides T, Bankier AT, Barrell BG (1983) Nucleotide sequences of the transforming region of human cytomegalovirus. Mol Biol Med 1:47–58
48. Kumar A, Selim MS, Madden DL, Wallen WC, Vasquez HH, Nankervis GA (1980) Humoral and cell-mediated immune responses to herpesvirus antigens in patients with cervical carcinoma. Gynecol Oncol 10:18–25
49. Lang DJ, Kummer JF (1972) Demonstration of cytomegalovirus in semen. N Engl J Med 287:756–758
50. Lang DJ, Kummer JF (1975) Cytomegalovirus in semen: observations in selected population. J Infect Dis 132:472–473

51. Lüleci G, Sakizli M, Günalp A (1980) Selective chromosomal damage caused by human cytomegalovirus. Acta Virol (Praha) 24:341–345
52. Macnab JCM (1987) Herpes simplex virus and human cytomegalovirus: their role in morphological transformation and genital cancers. J Gen Virol 68:2525–2550
53. McDougall JK, Galloway DA, Fenoglio CM (1980) Cervical carcinoma: detection of herpes simplex virus RNA in cells undergoing neoplastic change. Int J Cancer 25:1–8
54. McDougall JK, Nelson JA, Myerson D, Beckmann AM, Galloway DA (1984) HSV, CMV, and HPV in human neoplasia. J Invest Dermatol 83:72–76
55. Melnick JL, Lewis R, Wimberly I, Kaufman RH, Adam E (1978) Association of cytomegalovirus (CMV) infection with cervical cancer: isolation of CMV from cell cultures derived from cervical biopsy. Intervirology 10:115–119
56. Myerson D, Hackman RC, Nelson JA, Ward DC, McDougall JK (1984) Widespread presence of histologically occult cytomegalovirus. Hum Pathol 15:430–439
57. Nelson JA, Fleckenstein B, Galloway DA, McDougall JK (1982) Transformation of NIH3T3 cells with cloned fragments of human cytomegalovirus strain AD169. J Virol 43:83–91
58. Nelson JA, Fleckenstein B, Jahn G, Galloway DA, McDougall JK (1984) Structure of the transforming region of human cytomegalovirus AD169. J Virol 49:109–115
59. Pacsa AS, Kummerländer L, Pejtsik B, Pali K (1975) Herpesvirus antibodies and antigens in patients with cervical anaplasia and in controls. JNCI 55:775–781
60. Powell RD, Warner NE, Levine RS, Kirsner JB (1961) Cytomegalic inclusion disease and ulcerative colitis. Am J Med 30:334–340
61. Quinnan GV Jr, Mazur H, Rook AH, Armstrong G, Frederick WR, Epstein J, Manischewitz JF, Macher AM, Jackson L, Ames J, Smith HA, Parker M, Pearson GR, Parrillo J, Mitchell C, Straus SE (1984) Herpes infections in the acquired immune deficiency syndrome. JAMA 252:72–77
62. Rapp F (1984) Cytomegalovirus and carcinogenesis. JNCI 72:783–787
63. Rapp F, Geder L, Murasko D, Lausch R, Ladda R, Huang E-S, Webber MM (1975) Long-term persistence of cytomegalovirus genome in cultured human cells of prostatic origin. J Virol 16:982–990
64. Rawls WE, Bacchetti S, Graham FL (1977) Relation of herpes simplex viruses to human malignancies. Curr Top Microbiol Immunol 77:71–95
65. Razzaque A, Jahan N, McWeeney D, Jariwalla RJ, Jones C, Brady J, Rosenthal LJ (1988) Localization and DNA sequence analysis of the transforming domain (mtrII) of human cytomegalovirus. Proc Natl Acad Sci USA 85:5709–5713
66. Rechavi G, Givol D, Canaani E (1982) Activation of a cellular oncogene by DNA rearrangement: possible involvement of an IS-like element. Nature 300:607–611
67. Rosenthal LJ, Shi-Zhang S, Inamdar A (1991) Identification of the morphological transforming regions of human cytomegalovirus. Virolog Sin (in press)
68. Rüger R, Colimon R, Fleckenstein B (1983) Search for DNA sequences of human cytomegalovirus in Kaposi's sarcoma tissues with cloned probes. Preliminary report. Antibiot Chemother 32:43–47
69. Salahuddin SZ, Ablashi DV, Markham PD, Josephs SF, Sturzenegger S, Kaplan M, Halligan G, Biberfeld P, Wong-Staal F, Kramarsky B, Gallo RC (1986) Isolation of a new virus. HBLV in patients with proliferative disorders. Science 234:596–601
70. Sanford EJ, Dagen JE, Geder L, Rohner TJ Jr, Rapp F (1977) Lymphocyte reactivity against virally transformed cells in patients with urologic cancer. J Urol 118:809–810
71. Sanford EJ, Geder L, Laychock A, Rohner TJ Jr, Rapp F (1977) Evidence for the association of cytomegalovirus with carcinoma of the prostate. J Urol 118:789–792
72. Schlegel R, Wade-Glass M, Rabson M, Yang YC (1986) The E5 transforming gene of bovine papillomavirus encodes a small, hydrophobic polypeptide. Science 233:464–467
73. Siddiqui A (1983) Hepatitis B virus DNA in Kaposi's sarcoma. Proc Natl Acad Sci USA 80:4861–4864
74. Smiley ML, Mar E-C, Huang E-S (1988) Cytomegalovirus infection and viral-induced transformation of human endothelial cells. J Med Virol 25:213–226

75. Sprecher-Goldberger S, Thiry L, Lefebvre N, Dekegel D, DeHalleux F (1971) Complement-fixation antibodies to adenovirus-associated viruses, adenoviruses, cytomegaloviruses, and herpes simplex viruses in patients with tumours and in control individuals. Am J Epidemiol 94:351–358
76. Stagno S, Reynolds DW, Pass RF, Alford CA Jr (1980) Breast milk and the risk of cytomegalovirus infection. N Engl J Med 302:1073–1074
77. Stenberg RM, Stinski MF (1985) Autoregulation of the human cytomegalovirus major immediate-early gene. J Virol 56:676–682
78. Stenberg RM, Thomsen DR, Stinski MF (1984) Structural analysis of the major immediate-early gene of human cytomegalovirus. J Virol 49:190–199
79. Stoian M, Hozoc M, Iasipenco M, Bolocan J, Nastac E (1982) Presence of antibodies to human cytomegalovirus in patients with different forms of cancer and in other categories of subjects. Rev Roum Med Virol 33:153–161
80. Thomsen DR, Stinski MF (1981) Cloning of the human cytomegalovirus genome as endonuclease XbaI fragments. Gene 16:207–216
81. Vandenberg F, Schipper M, Jiwa M, Rook R, van de Rijke F, Tigges B (1989) Implausibility of an aetiological association between cytomegalovirus and Kaposi's sarcoma shown by four techniques. J Clin Pathol 42:128–131
82. Vestergaard BF, Hurnsleth A, Pedersen SN (1972) Occurrence of herpes and adenovirus antibodies in patients with carcinoma of the cervix uteri. Cancer 30:68–74
83. Yelle J, Dion M, Hamelin C (1986) Distinct regions of the human cytomegalovirus genome are responsible for the immortalization and tumorigenicity of animal cells. Cancer Lett 32:101–106
84. Zur Hausen H, Schulte-Holthausen H, Klein G, Henle W, Henle G, Clifford P, Sanesson L (1970) EBV DNA in biopsies of Burkitt tumors and aplastic carcinomas of the nasopharynx. Nature 228:1056–1058

Chapter 21 Proteins of Human Cytomegalovirus that Elicit Humoral Immunity

Lenore Pereira [1], David Navarro [2], and Gerhard Jahn [3]

Summary

Several of the cytomegalovirus (CMV) genes encoding glycoproteins, structural proteins, and infected-cell proteins that elicit an immune response in human infection have been mapped. Human sera and monoclonal antibodies react with these viral polypeptides made as native molecules in CMV-infected cells, as genetically engineered proteins, as truncated derivatives expressed in eukaryotic cells, and as bacterial fusion proteins from portions of the reading frames cloned into prokaryotic expression vectors. Synthetic oligopeptides from immunodominant regions of these molecules have also been used as antibody targets. Studies on proteins encoded by reading frames UL55, UL32, and UL44, on glycoprotein B, and on phosphoproteins pp150 and pp65 have been particularly fruitful. Recent developments employing these and other immunogenic CMV proteins as antigens for serodiagnosis of primary, recurrent, and past CMV infections are discussed.

Introduction

Human cytomegalovirus (CMV) is a complex virus with a large genome that contains over 200 reading frames [15, 63, 112]. CMV has been more difficult to study than herpes simplex virus 1 (HSV-1), for several reasons: (1) it has a restricted host range, growing mainly in human diploid cells; (2) it fails to turn off host-cell protein synthesis; (3) several of the infected-cell proteins have similar electrophoretic properties and comigrate on polyacrylamide gels; (4) some proteins are viral gene products that undergo posttranslational modifications, including glycosylation, phosphorylation, and cleavage; and (5) in addition, several viral transcripts undergo complex splicing patterns.

[1] University of California San Francisco, Department of Stomatology, Division of Oral Biology, HSW-604, San Francisco, CA 94143, USA

[2] University of Valencia, School of Medicine, Valencia, Spain

[3] Institute for Clinical and Molecular Virology, University of Erlangen-Nürnberg, W-8520 Erlangen, Germany

To date, fewer than 20 proteins have been mapped on the viral genome, and many of these were identified with the aid of CMV-immune serum and monoclonal antibodies. A comparison of the predicted amino acid sequence of CMV genes with genes of HSV-1 showed that many reading frames in the unique long (UL) component of the viral genome are conserved between these viruses and other herpesviruses, but not those in the unique short (US) component [15]. Four comprehensive reviews discuss the properties of most of the known CMV proteins [34, 42, 63, 85].

In studies on CMV proteins, immune precipitation reactions with sera from infected patients showed a specific immune response to viral proteins that were identified by their electrophoretic properties in polyacrylamide gels. Among these were the immediate-early (IE) proteins [5], virion structural proteins [10, 24, 68, 93, 101, 103] and virus-specific proteins synthesized in infected cells [76, 77, 114]. The immune response to CMV proteins was also determined by immunoblot analyses of denatured, electrophoretically separated virion proteins reacted with patient sera [20, 28, 43, 44, 74, 80a].

Monoclonal antibodies and antisera to purified virions have facilitated the mapping of genes encoding immunogenetic CMV proteins. A particularly advantageous technique for mapping the loci of CMV proteins has been the use of λgt11 CMV DNA expression libraries [64]. In this strategy, fragments of viral genomic DNA (400–500 bp in length) or complementary DNAs (cDNAs) are cloned into *Escherichia coli* prokaryotic expression vectors. Portions of reading frames expressed by these DNA sequences are then reacted with the CMV-specific serological reagents. An important requirement is that the antisera recognize a segment of linear or continuous amino acids on the gene product, since only a small portion of the protein is expressed. To map the gene encoding the protein segment, DNA from the positive λgt11 clone is amplified, radiolabeled, and hybridized to restriction fragments of genomic DNA. Examples of CMV proteins that have been mapped with this approach are the DNA-binding proteins [1, 39, 64], phosphoproteins [35, 36, 113], glycoproteins [54], other virion structural proteins [51, 59, 71], and infected-cell proteins [65].

Several strategies have been used successfully to map CMV glycoproteins that are highly dependent on conformation by expressing them in eukaryotic cells. Cloned reading frames have been expressed transiently from eukaryotic expression vectors in COS-1 cells [2] and stably in CHO cell lines [69, 97]. CMV glycoproteins have also been expressed in cells infected with viral vectors, in particular vaccinia virus [12, 18, 19] and adenovirus [55]. Baculovirus vectors have been particularly suited to producing larger quantities of CMV glycoproteins in insect cells [111].

Immunodominant regions of CMV proteins have been identified by expressing different regions as *E. coli* β-galactosidase fusion proteins from DNA sequences derived from a single reading frame. Systematic analysis of CMV-immune patient sera in reactions with the fusion proteins has led to the development of an immune response profile in infected individuals [46–48, 80, 92, 108, 109]. In this chapter, we summarize recent studies on the properties of

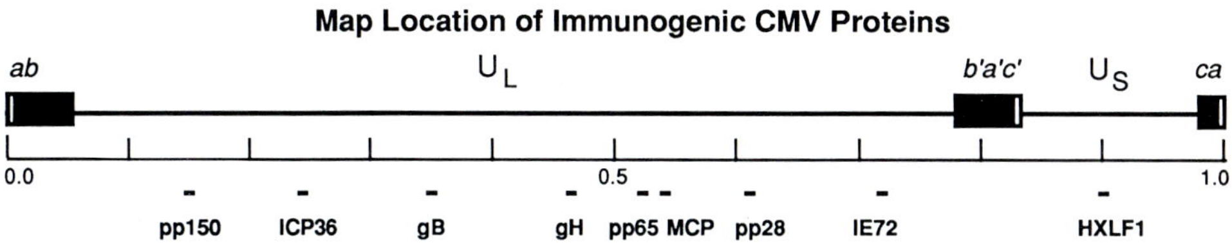

Fig. 1. Schematic drawing of open reading frames in the cytomegalovirus genome encoding the proteins that are immunogenic in human infection. U_L, unique long component; U_S, unique short component

Table 1. Properties of CMV proteins that elicit antibodies in human infection

Protein	Other names	Reading frame [15]	Map location in AD169 genome	Molecular mass (kDa)	Posttranslational modification
gB	gA family p150/p55 gp58, gcI gp58/gp116	UL55	*Xma*I fragment of *Hin*dIII F	145, 116, 58	Glycosylation Proteolytic cleavage Virion envelope
gH	gp86 gcIII	UL75	*Hin*dIII L	86	Glycosylation Virion envelope
HXLF1	gcII	US6	*Hin*dIII X	47–52	Glycosylation Virion envelope
ICP36	p52	UL44	*Hin*dIII M	50, 48	Phosphorylation DNA binding
pp150	BPP[a]	UL32	*Hin*dIII J and N	150	Phosphorylation Addition of O-linked *N*-acetylglucosamine Virion component
pp65	Lower matrix Tegument gp64 ICP27 Major structural	UL83	*Hin*dIII L, b, c	65	Phosphorylation
pp28	25-, 32-kDa proteins	UL99	*Hin*dIII R	25–32	Phosphorylation
MCP	Capsid protein	UL86	*Hin*dIII U, b, a	150	Virion component
IE72	IE1 IE2 α proteins	UL122 UL123	*Hin*dIII E	68–72 86	Phosphorylation

[a] BPP, basic phosphoprotein

CMV proteins known to elicit humoral immunity in natural infection and to have potential use in serodiagnostic tests. The approximate locations of the genes encoding these proteins in the CMV genome are shown in Fig. 1, and the properties of the proteins are summarized in Table 1.

2. Glycoproteins that Elicit Humoral Antibodies

CMV Glycoprotein B Homologue, Encoded by UL55

Cytomegalovirus encodes a major glycoprotein in a family of related proteins that were identified by reactions with CMV-immune patient sera [75, 77] and with monoclonal antibodies to CMV [76]. We first named this family of glycoproteins with different electrophoretic properties as gA [76, 78]; others designated it as p150/p55 [87], gp 58 [9], gcI [32, 37], and gp58/gp116 [60]. Later, the gene encoding this glycoprotein was mapped on the genome of strain AD169 [18, 54] and Towne [97], and its product, characterized with monoclonal antibodies, was shown to correspond to gA [2]. Nucleotide sequence analysis of the AD169 genome showed that this glycoprotein is the homologue of HSV-1 gB [18] (reviewed by [15]). CMV gB in the AD169 genome maps within an *Xma*I subfragment of *Hin*dIII fragment F [18] and in the corresponding region of the Towne genome in *Hin*dIII fragment D [2, 97]. Northern blot analysis showed that three transcripts arise from this region of the genome; the 3.9-kb RNA (mRNA) encodes the gB gene [97]. The RNA was abundantly made and was detected as early as 4 h postinfection, preceding the synthesis of the gene product [78, 88].

Synthesis and Processing of gB

Studies on the synthesis and processing of gB in CMV-infected cells revealed that a subset of the related family members differed significantly in their electrophoretic properties [74, 78]. Six electrophoretically distinct, antigenically related forms were immunoprecipitated with a panel of monoclonal antibodies to CMV gB. Precursors were identified by treating CMV-infected cells with inhibitors of glycosylation [78, 89]. gB is a disulfide-linked glycoprotein that is contained in virions [7, 23]. Pulse-chase experiments revealed that the fastest-migrating form, 55–58.5 kDa, was derived from the larger molecule at about 1 h after synthesis [9, 78]. The smaller fragment was later shown to be a proteolytic cleavage product [97]. The cleavage site on gB, which maps between residues 460 and 461, is composed of hydrophilic residues between two *N*-glycosylation sites at residues 456–458 and 466–468. The sequence of amino acids at or proximal to the cleavage site was critical for cleavage by a cellular protease [98]. Substitution of threonine for arginine at either residue 457 or 460, substitution of glutamine for lysine at residue 459, or all three substitutions, blocked cleavage of the full-length gB molecule. In CMV-infected cells, inhibition of gB cleavage by palmitoyl-peptidyl-chloromethyl ketone had no effect on gB transport to the cell surface or production of infectious progeny, but interfered with virion release from cells [13]. Glycosylation and transport through the exocytic pathway were shown to be required for the subsequent cleavage of gB [84]. In eukaryotic cells stably transformed with a truncated derivative of the gB gene, cleavage of the molecule was inhibited by a calcium-specific ionophore [98].

Humoral Immune Response to gB in Infection

Several studies have demonstrated that CMV gB is immunogenic and elicits neutralizing antibodies in natural infection and in animals immunized with the glycoprotein. Detection of antibodies to gB in CMV-infected patients is a serological marker for seroconversion to CMV [10, 20, 90] (Pereira et al., in preparation). A major fraction of neutralizing antibodies in sera from CMV-infected patients is directed to gB [11, 12, 41, 85, 90].

Antibodies to gB were detected in patient sera by immunoprecipitation reactions with extracts of CMV-infected cells or purified virions. Analysis of sera from CMV-infected babies with congenital and perinatal infections showed that gB is a target of antibodies, particularly in babies with symptomatic infections [10, 77] (Fig. 2, compare panels A–C with panel CH51). We found that the seropositive response to gB in babies with symptomatic CMV infections continues for years after birth. A weaker but detectable reaction to gB was also found in sera from asymptomatic, perinatally infected babies [77]. In a subsequent report [20], specific proteins isolated from extracts of CMV-infected cells by means of monoclonal antibodies were evaluated in im-

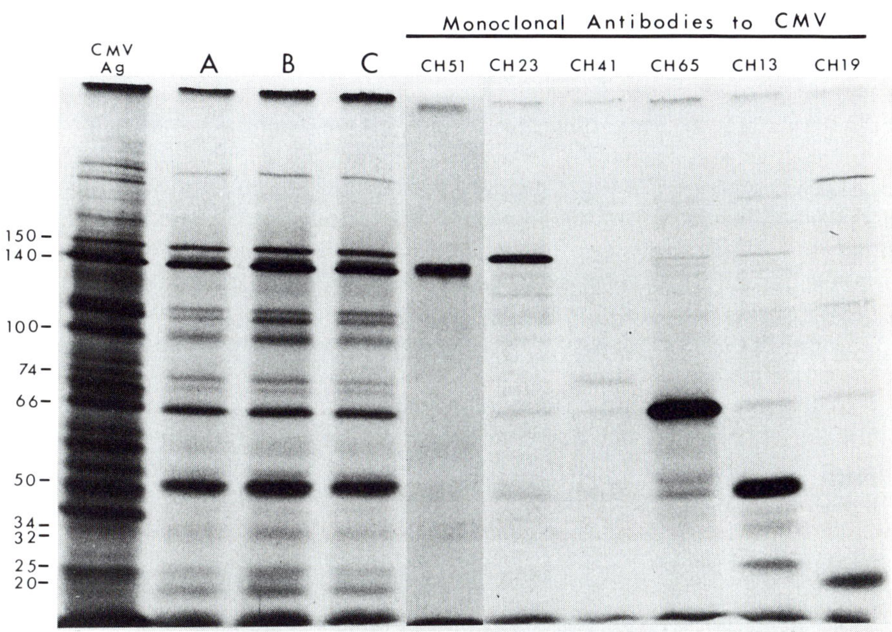

Fig. 2. Immunoprecipitates of [^{35}S]methionine-labeled cytomegalovirus- (*CMV*-)infected cells, formed by sera from babies with congenital, symptomatic CMV infections (*lanes A–C*). Sera were obtained between 7 and 18 months after birth. The patient profiles are compared with immunoprecipitates obtained from infected cells with monoclonal antibodies to CMV (*right panel*). The profile of immunogenic proteins shown in the *right panel* is as follows: gB (*CH51*), major capsid protein (*CH23*), matrix protein (*CH65*), ICP36 (*CH13*), and pp28 (*CH19*). (From [7])

munoassays for use in diagnosing primary or recurrent infections. Sera from transplant recipients undergoing primary or recurrent CMV infections reacted with CMV gB and other proteins. A comparison of the immune responses to these proteins showed that antibody to gB appeared earlier in primary infection, increased quickly in concentration, and persisted at a higher concentration than did antibody to the other CMV proteins tested. Subsequently, we showed that antibodies to gB were detected in immunoblot reactions with immunoaffinity-purified gB in both acute- and convalescent-phase sera from patients undergoing recurrent CMV infections [74]. Results of these studies showed that patients with recurrent infections have antibodies to conformational epitopes on gB, detected by immunoprecipitation of the native molecule, and also to continuous epitopes, detected in immunoblot reactions.

The presence of serum antibodies to CMV has also been assessed against genetically engineered forms of gB. Analysis of the human neutralizing antibody response to CMV gB cloned into the vaccinia virus genome and made in cells infected with the vaccinia virus-gB recombinant showed that 40%–70% of the total serum virus-neutralizing activity of individuals with past CMV infections was directed against gB [12]. Moreover, sera from a small number of women with primary CMV infections reacted predominantly with gB. It was shown recently that sera from CMV-immune patients recognized recombinant gB made in CHO cell lines genetically engineered to produce a truncated form of the molecule that lacked the transmembrane region and carboxy terminus [90, 97]. Approximately 60% of the sera from immunocompetent individuals reacted with the recombinant gB molecule in immunoblot and immunoprecipitation assays. Analysis of the immune response to a genetically engineered form of CMV gH included in the study by the same investigators is discussed below. From their findings, the authors concluded that the level of antibody to each glycoprotein was influenced by the antigenic stimulus, or amount of replicating virus from reactivated infections, or repeated exposures to CMV. This observation was consistent with the potent immune response to gB found in studies on sera from infected babies and transplant recipients, described above.

To fine-map the immunodominant regions on CMV gB recognized by immune sera, particularly domains dependent on conformation, we assessed the presence of antibodies to truncated forms of the molecule made transiently in eukaryotic cells (Pereira et al., in preparation). These findings will be discussed below (see "Human Immune Response to Regions of gB").

CMV gB Elicits Neutralizing Antibodies in Immunized Animals

The results of studies with patient sera suggest CMV gB as a potential vaccine candidate, and several strategies have been employed to produce and purify large amounts of the glycoprotein. Immunoaffinity-purified forms of gB isolated from extracts of CMV-infected cells elicit neutralizing antibodies in immunized laboratory animals [29, 30, 87]. Engineered forms of the molecule have also been expressed from the adenovirus genome [55] and in vaccinia virus vectors [12, 18]. These forms of recombinant gB elicit neutralizing antibodies in immunized mice. Truncated forms of gB lacking the transmembrane region and carboxy terminus that are produced in CHO cell lines retain many of the conformational epitopes of the native molecule and are likely candidates for human vaccination [2, 97]. Large quantities of gB can be generated in insect cells by using a baculovirus expression system; however, this form contained predominantly high-mannose sugars and was less efficiently cleaved in these cells [111]. CMV-immune patient sera immunoprecipitated gB from extracts of baculovirus-infected cells, as did a monoclonal antibody to a linear epitope. Mice immunized with the baculovirus-derived gB developed neutralizing antibodies to CMV. A nonglycosylated form of gB produced in a prokaryotic expression system appears to be less immunogenic than the glycosylated protein made in eukaryotic cells [11]. The absence of carbohydrates on gB appears to alter its conformation and immunogenic properties. Many of the antibodies produced against gB made in prokaryotic cells have complement-independent neutralizing activity, whereas those produced against native forms of the molecule made in eukaryotic cells are primarily complement dependent.

Mapping Continuous Antigenic Regions Within the Domain of gB

Certain regions of CMV gB are immunodominant, as indicated by the reactivity of monoclonal antibodies and convalescent-phase sera with this glycoprotein. The antigenic domains on gB identified with our panel of monoclonal antibodies and published in several reports are summarized in Table 2. Figure 3 illustrates the domains on gB mapped by our group and the antigenic sites identified by others, using murine and human monoclonal antibodies with different properties.

In a recent study [3, 79], it was shown that monoclonal antibodies to continuous epitopes react with deletion mutants lacking the amino or the carboxy terminus of gB from strains Towne and AD169. Three domains, $DC1_v$, DC2, and DC3, composed of continuous amino acids were recognized by these antibodies (Table 2). Domain $DC1_v$ maps in the very amino terminus of the molecule and contains epitopes that vary among CMV strains. Comparison of the nucleotide sequence of gB encoded by strains AD169 and Towne indicates that differences in the amino acid sequences of these molecules cluster between residues 28 and 67 of their coding sequences [97]. From our work and that of others, it appears that these differences in amino acid sequence affect the antigenic properties of the amino terminus [3, 58, 79]. It was recently reported that a linear epitope of a human monoclonal antibody with complement-independent neutralizing activity maps in the very amino terminus between residues 27 and 84 [60]. It was later shown that this epitope was conserved among CMV strains and mapped to amino acids 68–77, close to an antigenic site between amino acids 50 and 54 that varies among strains [58]. Both the

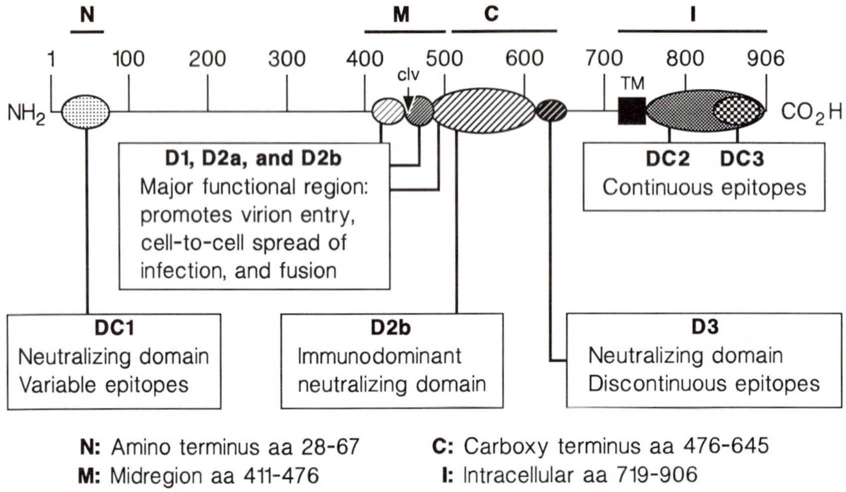

Fig. 3. Schematic representation of the antigenic and functional domains on cytomegalovirus (CMV) gB. Domains containing epitopes of neutralizing antibodies and other antigenic regions are indicated by *ellipses*. Types of epitopes are described in *boxes*. Amino acids are indicated by *numbers* inclusive of the signal sequence. The cleavage site between amino acids 460 and 461 [97] is marked by a *downward arrow*. The transmembrane anchor domain (*box*) and the amino (NH_2) and carboxy (CO_2H) termini are indicated [18]. A panel of monoclonal antibodies to CMV gB produced by Pereira and Hoffman [74–76, 78] was used to obtain the mapping results published in several reports [2, 3, 66, 79, 83]. Epitopes mapped with antibodies from other laboratories are included in the domains shown [41, 60, 97, 109]

conserved and the variable sites are contained within domain $DC1_v$. It is notable that antibody CH408-1, which maps in domain $DC1_v$, has complement-dependent neutralizing activity for strain AD169 [74].

Continuous (or sequential) epitopes have been mapped in other regions of gB. Several laboratories have shown that neutralizing antibodies to continuous epitopes react with the carboxy-terminal half of gB [11, 41, 109]. Two epitopes are located in the extracellular domain, between amino acids 589–645 [41] and 608–625 [109] (Fig. 3). The very carboxy terminus of gB contains a domain of continuous epitopes, DC2, which are expressed by all of the CMV strains tested thus far (Table 2). After antibodies to these continuous epitopes were reacted with a set of overlapping synthetic peptides, the epitopes were subdivided, with the linear ones grouped into domain DC3 [3, 79]. Kniess et al. [41] also identified an immunogenic region of continuous residues at the carboxy terminus; mapping between residues 703 and 906, it overlaps domains DC2 and DC3. Complement-independent neutralizing antibodies to continuous epitopes on CMV gB have also been generated, but their binding sites have not been mapped [38]. Three other continuous epitopes are contained in this region of gB [53], but their location relative to the neutralizing epitopes has not been established.

Table 2. Neutralizing epitopes in immunodominant domains on CMV (AD169) gB mapped with amino-terminal deletion mutants

Antigenic domain	Monoclonal antibody	Complement dependent	gB mutants (1-258)	(1-411)	(1-447)	(1-618)	(1-645)	(1-832)
Continuous epitopes								
$DC1_v$ [a]			+	+	+	+	+	+
	CH408-1	+						
DC2			–	–	–	–	–	–
DC3 [b]			–	–	–	–	–	–
Discontinuous epitopes								
D1 [c]			–	–	+	+	+	+
	CH177-3	–						
	CH358-5	–						
	CH382-2	–						
	CH388-4	–						
	CH395-1	+						
	CH87-1 [e]	+						
	CH92-1 [e]	+						
	CH105-7 [e]	+						
	CH112-1 [e]	+						
	CH244-4 [e]	+						
	CH253-1 [e]	–						
D2 [d]			–	–	–	+	+	+
	CH130-9	+						
	CH143-13	+						
	CH424-1	+						
	CH432-1	–						
	CH442-1	–						
	CH446-2	–						
D3 [d]			–	–	–	–	+	+
	CH51-4	+						
	CH114-5	+						
	CH436-1	–						

[a] Fine-mapped using β-galactosidase fusion proteins of CMV (AD169) gB spanning amino acids 28–67 [58]

[b] Fine-mapped with overlapping synthetic oligopeptides containing amino acids 833–853 and 878–898 [3, 79]

[c] Conformation-dependent domain containing discontinuous epitopes mapped by Qadri et al. [83]

[d] Conformation-dependent domain containing discontinuous epitopes mapped by Banks et al. [2]

[e] Weakly reactive by immunofluorescence with CMV gB-(1-447)

Mapping Conformational Epitopes of Neutralizing Antibodies with Complement-Dependent and -Independent Activity

Discontinuous, or conformation-dependent, epitopes on CMV gB have been mapped by expressing amino-terminal derivatives that lack portions of the carboxy terminus in eukaryotic cells. In this system conformational epitopes are maintained, provided that the residues required for their assembly are present and accessible. Derivatives of gB were expressed transiently in transfected COS-1 cells [2, 82, 83] or in CHO cell lines stably transformed with a derivative of the gB gene [97], and the epitopes were mapped by reactions with monoclonal antibodies (Table 2). Antibodies with complement-dependent and -independent neutralizing activity reacted with a 619-residue amino-terminal derivative of gB in transient expression assays [2]. These antibodies and others reacted with a 680-residue amino-terminal derivative expressed by CHO cells. We subsequently found that these antibodies recognize a derivative 645 amino acids in length, but not a shorter one with 447 residues [82, 83]. It was concluded that the complement-dependent neutralizing epitopes map in two separate domains, D2 and D3. Domain D2 maps between amino acids 447 and 618 in the midregion of gB and domain D3 between 618 and 645 in the carboxy-terminal half of the molecule (Fig. 3). It appears that the antigenic region designated as AD-1 by Kniess et al. [41], which contains a linear epitope and maps between residues 589 and 645, partially overlaps domains D2 and D3 (Fig. 3). Nucleotide sequence analysis of the gB gene encoded by several clinical isolates showed that the sequences that surround the cleavage site vary among strains [16]. Although this region overlaps D2, preliminary analysis of CMV strains indicates that the epitopes mapping in this region of the molecule are conserved in other CMV isolates [79] (Pereira, et al., in preparation). Human monoclonal antibodies to CMV gB with complement-dependent and -independent neutralizing activity have also been identified, but their epitopes have not been characterized [107].

Epitopes of complement-independent neutralizing antibodies have also been mapped in a novel neutralizing region consisting of domains D1 and D2a [82, 83]. These domains, mapped by the reactions of potent neutralizing antibodies, were assembled between residues 411 and 476 in the amino-terminal half and midregion of gB (Fig. 3). They were not dependent for conformation on the carboxy-terminal portion of the molecule. Detailed analysis of the neutralizing activities of these antibodies revealed that they prevent virion penetration into cells, transmission of infection from cell to cell, and cell fusion [66]. Since gB plays an important role in CMV infection by promoting infection and the spread of virus, it appears that antibodies directed toward this functional domain may also be important in limiting infection in the host. We recently found that antibodies in convalescent-phase CMV-immune sera compete with murine monoclonal antibodies for a subset of the neutralizing epitopes on gB (Pereira et al., manuscript in preparation).

Human Immune Response to Regions of gB

Based on work from several laboratories using different strategies, we have begun to identify the regions on gB that are targets of antibody in immunocompetent CMV-infected individuals. Studies discussed above using murine antibodies identified four immunodominant domains on the extracellular portion of gB: two in the amino-terminal half, one continuous ($DC1_v$) and one discontinuous (D1); and two in the carboxy-terminal half, both discontinuous (D2 and D3) (Fig. 3). The latter region also contains continuous neutralizing and nonneutralizing epitopes mapped by others [109]. It was recently shown that antibodies in CMV-immune human sera bind to a gB β-galactosidase fusion protein containing amino acids 589–645, which overlap domains D2 and D3 on the native molecule [41]. When competition assays were carried out using baculovirus-derived gB made in insect cells [111], monoclonal antibodies to this region significantly reduced the binding of human sera to the recombinant molecule [41]. This finding indicated that a limited region of the carboxy-terminal half of gB, first mapped with murine antibodies, is also immunodominant in human infection. In a study to determine the levels of neutralizing antibodies to gB in CMV-immune sera, the sera were adsorbed with intact cells expressing gB after being infected with a vaccinia virus recombinant [12]. After adsorption, the sera lost most of the CMV-neutralizing activity, indicating that the extracellular domain of gB presented on eukaryotic cells is the target of neutralizing antibodies; the specific region targeted, however, was not mapped.

The intracellular domain of the carboxy terminus of gB is also recognized in CMV infection. Kniess et al. [41] expressed a β-galactosidase fusion protein containing residues 783–906 of gB and found that this region was strongly reactive by immunoblot analysis with convalescent-phase sera. In a recent study to map continuous epitopes of monoclonal antibodies, we expressed a carboxy-terminal fragment of gB composed of residues 716–906, which contains domains DC2 and DC3 (Fig. 2) [3, 79]. When this region was expressed in eukaryotic cells and reacted by immunofluorescence with high-titered sera from CMV-infected patients, a smaller number of sera reacted than react with the intact molecule (Pereira et al., in preparation). This finding indicates that although the intracellular region of gB is immunogenic, it is less so than the extracellular portion of the carboxy terminus.

Recently published work indicates that the amino-terminal half of CMV gB also is a target of neutralizing antibodies in infected patients. To determine whether this region of the molecule binds neutralizing antibodies, Liu et al. [52] expressed a derivative of gB, containing the entire amino-terminal half of the molecule (513 residues), in cells infected with a vaccinia virus recombinant. Sera from seropositive donors were then adsorbed with fixed cells expressing the amino-terminal derivative and with vaccinia virus-infected cells expressing intact gB. It was found that the amino-terminal half of gB adsorbed 25%–30% of the neutralizing activity in seropositive individuals, whereas intact gB adsorbed 50% of the activity. This was the first demonstration that the amino terminus is a target of neutralizing antibodies in human infection.

In a recent study, we analyzed sera from patients with CMV infection to determine whether conformational domains identified with murine antibodies are recognized in cases of primary or reactivated infections (Pereira et al., in preparation). Amino-terminal gB derivatives of different lengths and the intact gB molecule were expressed in eukaryotic cells and reacted by immunofluorescence with sera from patients with recurrent infections and IgM-positive paired sera from patients with primary infections who had seroconverted. In recurrent CMV infections with high-titered sera, all of the sera reacted with intact gB, with a derivative containing 687 residues, and with the amino-terminal 447-residue derivative. In contrast, fewer than half of these sera recognized the very amino-terminal derivative containing 258 residues of gB. Analysis of sera from patients with primary infections showed that most of them reacted with intact gB and with the 687-residue derivative. Approximately half recognized the 447-residue derivative, and very few reacted with the 258-residue derivative. Our results showed that the amino-terminal half of gB, including the conformation-dependent domain between residues 411 and 447, is an antibody target in recurrent infection and in some patients with primary infection. Compared with the titers of antibody developed against intact gB, particularly to residues in the midregion and carboxy-terminal half of the molecule, antibody titers to the amino-terminal half may rise more slowly. The failure of many sera to react with the 258-residue construct containing the very amino terminus of gB is consistent with the observation that epitopes in this region vary among CMV strains [79]. Since the amino-terminal derivatives in this study were constructed from the AD169 gB gene, only those patients infected with a strain having gB that is AD169-like will recognize this region of the molecule. It is notable that sera from patients with recurrent CMV infections, all of which reacted with the 447-residue derivative, had neutralizing antibody titers (50% plaque reduction) ranging from 1:100 to 1:800. From these data one might speculate that a high titer of neutralizing antibody to the amino-terminal domain, which functions in virion penetration and the spread of infection from cell to cell, would limit the spread of disease in the host. Assuming that neutralizing antibodies with complement-dependent activity, which bind primarily to the mid-region and carboxy-terminal half of gB, facilitate lysis of infected cells displaying gB on their surfaces, then a repertoire of antibodies to both regions could potentially eliminate the virus-infected cells and free virions from circulation.

CMV Glycoprotein H (gH) Homologue, Encoded by UL75

A CMV glycoprotein 86 kDa in apparent molecular weight was identified by immunoprecipitation from extracts of infected cells, using a monoclonal antibody with complement-independent neutralizing activity [86, 87]. A glycoprotein with similar electrophoretic properties was shown to be a component of the protein complex gcIII isolated from CMV-infected cells [32]. Analysis of the nucleotide sequence showed that the CMV genome encodes a homologue of HSV-1 gH [19], varicella-zoster virus gpIII, and Epstein-Barr virus BXLF2. Figure 1 shows the location of this gene on the AD169 genome. This gene maps in the *Hin*dIII L fragment of the AD169 genome and is approximately colinear in the Towne genome [69]. Transcriptional analysis of the gH gene showed that a 2.9-kb transcript was detected at late times postinfection, indicating that this glycoprotein belongs to the late kinetic class of proteins. Analysis of the antigenic properties of truncated forms of gH with monoclonal antibodies showed that this glycoprotein was highly conformation dependent.

Immune Response to gH

CMV gH is also a target of the human immune response in immunocompetent individuals. Studies on the immune response to recombinant-derived gH made in a eukaryotic cell line stably transformed with this gene showed that antibodies to gH were detected less frequently than those to gB, i.e., in less than 10% of the sera from patients with symptomatic infections [90]. In comparison to patients with symptomatic infections, those with asymptomatic infections who seroconverted to CMV responded weakly to gH. After seroconversion to gH, antibodies to this glycoprotein rapidly waned over time without repeated exposure to the virus. Immune serum globulin administered prophylactically to transplant recipients was frequently deficient in antibody to the recombinant-derived gH, but not to gB. At a recent meeting [108], it was reported that CMV-immune human sera react with sequential antigenic sites on gH, expressed as β-galactosidase fusion proteins spanning this reading frame. An immunodominant region between amino acids 34 and 111 within the amino terminus of gH was identified by 40% of the sera from CMV-infected individuals. When antibodies specific for this region of gH were isolated from CMV-immune sera, they exhibited complement-independent neutralizing activity. Monoclonal antibodies produced against the amino-terminal gH fusion protein recognized a linear epitope mapping between residues 35 and 46 and neutralized CMV without complement. Like the epitopes that mapped at the amino terminus of gB, a subset of those located in this region of gH were found to be strain-specific.

Glycoprotein Family Encoded by Reading Frame HXLF1, US6 Family

HXLF1 reading frame in *Hin*dIII fragment X of the unique short component of the genome was predicted to encode a protein of 25 265 Da and has both a signal and an anchor sequence and one *N*-glycosylation site [112]. Figure 1 shows the location of this gene on the AD169 genome. Expression of these genes in an SP6 expression vector showed that this reading frame encodes a 47–52 kDa glycoprotein in CMV-infected cells [31, 37]. This family of proteins is a component of the virion envelope and elicits complement-independent neutralizing antibodies in infection. Little is known about the immune response to this protein in CMV infection.

Phosphoproteins as Targets of Humoral Immunity

The Major Family of DNA-Binding Proteins, ICP36 (p52), Encoded by UL44

In studies with CMV-immune patient sera, a family of related proteins of approximately 48–50 kDa was immunoprecipitated from extracts of CMV-infected cells [75, 77]. Immunoprecipitation and immunoblot reactions with monoclonal antibodies showed that this set of proteins was antigenically related [74, 76]. These bands were present in the immune response profile of sera from congenitally infected babies and were specifically precipitated by monoclonal antibody CH13 (Fig. 2) [77]. Early studies showed that this protein had DNA-binding properties [26, 27]. The coding sequence of the gene for this protein family, also called infected-cell protein (ICP)36, was localized to a 2800-bp *Eco*RI fragment on the Towne and AD169 genomes [81 a] by using DNA from an immunoreactive λgt11 clone as a probe [64]. Figure 1 shows the location of this gene on the AD169 genome. A 5000-nucleotide transcript from this region was detected during the early and late phases of the CMV growth cycle. When hybrid-selected and translated in vitro, this transcript directed the synthesis of the predominant member of the ICP36 family; immunoprecipitation of the translation product confirmed the map position. The ICP36 a and b gene products were phosphorylated in CMV-infected cells and were shown to have DNA-binding properties. The transcription of the ICP36 gene was analyzed, revealing a complex early- and late-transcriptional regulation [50]. The transcription initiates at three different sites. At early times two of the start sites were active, whereas at late times the third start site was active. Characteristic TATA-like elements were found upstream of all three start sites, and in transient assays the two early start sites functioned as independently regulated promoters.

Immune Response to ICP36

In recent studies, β-galactosidase fusion proteins containing regions of the ICP36 protein were expressed as antigens to screen sera from CMV-infected patients. Ripalti et al. [92] screened a λgt11 DNA library with CMV-positive human sera and identified a clone that encoded a 52-kDa protein. The identity of this protein was confirmed by hybridization with cloned DNA fragments of the CMV genome. The protein reacted with monoclonal antibodies to ICP36 and also reacted strongly in immunoblot tests with patient sera (Fig. 4). Sera from patients with acute CMV infections preferentially reacted with the ICP36 β-galactosidase fusion protein (Fig. 4 A), whereas sera from healthy CMV-seropositive individuals did not (Fig. 4 B). The DNA insert of the λgt11 clone has been determined, and the immunogenic region was found to map in the amino-terminal 150 residues of this protein. Another fusion protein containing this region of ICP36 was recently expressed in a high-level expression vector and was strongly reactive with CMV-IgM-positive sera [81 a]. Although it is

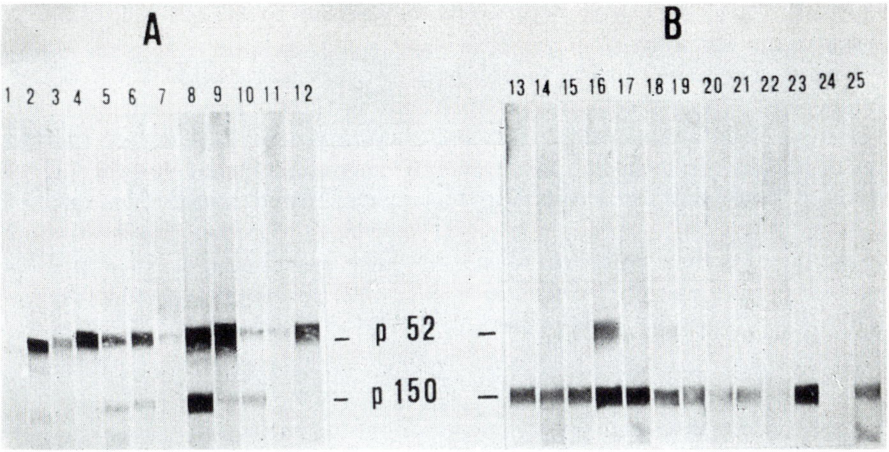

Fig. 4 A, B. Immunoblot reactions showing differential detection of β-galactosidase CMV fusion proteins of ICP36 (p52) and pp150 by sera from patients with acute CMV infections (**A**) or from individuals with past infections (**B**). Fusion proteins p52 and pp150 are indicated. (From [92])

not clear whether there are other immunogenic regions of ICP36, it appears that one region of this protein is a suitable antigen for detection of an early humoral immune response in primary and reactivated CMV infection.

The Large Phosphorylated Structural Protein, pp150, Encoded by UL32

In two studies, Landini et al. [43, 44] analyzed the immune response to CMV proteins in immunoblot tests in which electrophoretically separated polypeptides from purified CMV virions were used as antigens. Sera from a large number of CMV-infected patients having different titers of IgG and IgM were tested. At least 15 electrophoretically distinct structural polypeptides were detected. Among the reactive bands, a protein 155 kDa in apparent molecular size was consistently found to react with all CMV-antibody-positive sera regardless of the state of the infection. Two earlier reports showed that two comigrating 150-kDa proteins in this region could be separated under different conditions [93, 110]. One was a phosphorylated tegument protein named the basic phosphoprotein (BPP). The other protein was found to crossreact with antisera prepared against the capsid protein of simian CMV and was designated as the major capsid protein (MCP) of CMV (discussed below). By electrophoretic separation and immunoblot analysis, all sera were found to react with the BPP protein [36]. It was concluded that the most immunogenic of these bands was the phosphoprotein, which was named originally pp150 [68]. pp150 is a major constituent of CMV virions and constitutes about 20% of the virion protein content [33]. It was shown that pp150 not only undergoes phosphorylation but is also modified by the addition of an O-linked residue of *N*-acetylglucosamine [4].

The gene encoding pp150 was mapped by screening a λgt11 CMV cDNA library with a monospecific rabbit antiserum produced against sodium dodecyl sulfate-denatured proteins from polyacrylamide gels [35]. Figure 1 shows the location of this gene mapping in *Hin*dIII fragments J and N, on the AD169 genome. Analysis of transcripts from this region showed that pp150 is encoded by a late mRNA of approximately 6 kb and that the transcription initiation site is preceded by a TATA consensus sequence. Pande et al. [72] mapped the gene for pp150 in strain Towne and showed that the encoding sequence maps to a corresponding location of the strain AD169 [35] genome.

Immune Response to pp150

Several studies have shown that pp150 is a serological marker for CMV infection. It was reported that CMV-immune sera recognize different portions of pp150, particularly an internal region of the pp150 reading frame, which proved to be highly immunogenic [96]. Immunoblot reactions of CMV-immune human sera with a β-galactosidase fusion protein containing amino acids 555–705 of pp150 are shown in Fig. 5 (lanes 4 and 6). In a study to identify serological markers of CMV infection, Ripalti et al. [92] screened a λgt11 DNA library with human sera and found a strongly reactive clone that hybridized with DNA fragments containing the pp150 gene. Monospecific antiserum confirmed the identity of this protein as pp150. They subsequently determined the sequence of the DNA insert and mapped it to the carboxy-terminal 25 amino acids of this protein, which are highly charged. Analysis of human sera showed that antibodies to this region of pp150 were slow to develop but were long-lasting markers of CMV infection. Figure 4 shows sera from patients with acute CMV infections (Fig. 4A) and sera from healthy seropositive individuals with past infections (Fig. 4B) in immunoblot reactions with β-galactosidase fusion proteins of pp150 and of ICP36 [92]. These results showed that the presence of antibody to pp150 is a serological marker for past infection, whereas antibody to ICP36 is more a marker for acute CMV disease (discussed above).

Immunodominant regions of pp150 recognized by patient sera early in CMV infection have been located on the protein. In a recent study, portions of the pp150 reading frame were expressed as β-galactosidase fusion proteins [81b]. Immunoblot analysis with patient sera showed that recombinant proteins of pp150 are recognized reproducibly by a broad spectrum of CMV-positive sera and reacted strongly with three regions of pp150. Antibodies to these regions were detected early in infection and were long-lasting serological markers of past infection. Immunodominant regions were were fine-mapped [48, 81b], using oligopeptides deduced from various regions of pp150. Synthetic peptides from several regions of pp150 were reacted with sera containing CMV-specific IgG from healthy individuals with past infections, and sera

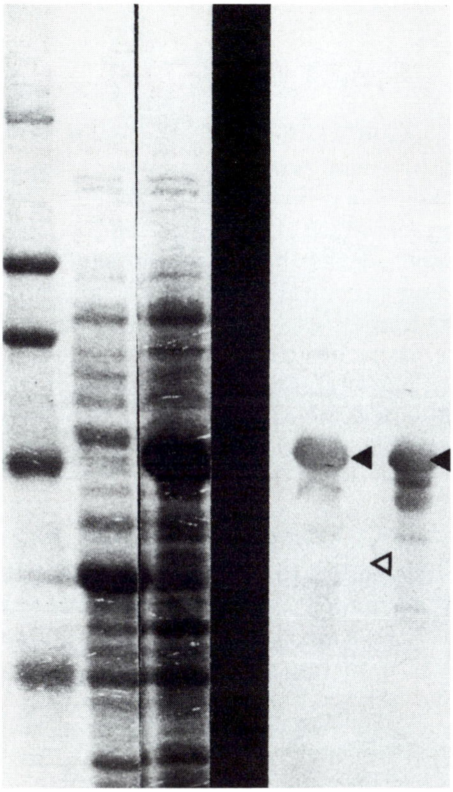

Fig. 5. Immunoblot reactions of cytomegalovirus- (CMV-)immune human sera with a β-galactosidase-CMV pp150 fusion protein. *Lane 1,* molecular weight markers. *Lane 2,* total protein extracts of *Escherichia coli* with prokaryotic vector expressing a portion of β-galactosidase alone or, *lane 3,* β-galactosidase-pp150 fusion protein containing amino acids 555–705 of pp150. *Lanes 4 and 6,* immunoblot reactions with human sera against extracts containing β-galactosidase-pp150 fusion protein. *Lane 5,* immunoblot reaction with *E. coli* extracts. *Solid traingle* shows β-galactosidase = pp150 band recognized by human sera. *Open triangle,* β-galactosidase alone. (From [96])

containing CMV-specific IgM from renal transplant patients who had active infections and were shedding virus. The peptides were predicted to be immunogenic, based either on analysis of immune reactions with a fusion protein [46, 81 b, 92, 96] or on their high content of hydrophilic amino acids deduced from the nucleotide sequence of the gene [15]. A series of overlapping peptides were synthesized to contain amino acids 990–1048, 961–1022, 692–724, 501–537, and 407–440. An important IgM-binding epitope mapped in the last 38 amino acids at the carboxy terminus of the molecule. This region reacted with CMV-specific IgM present in most of the IgM-positive human sera. Adsorption experiments showed that IgM titers to the entire pp150 decrease 25% – 50% in most sera after adsorption with peptides from this region.

The Lower Phosphorylated Matrix Protein, pp65, Encoded by UL83

Immunoprecipitation reactions of extracts of CMV-infected cells with CMV-immune patient sera suggested that a 65-kDa viral protein was a potent inducer of humoral immunity in infection [75, 77]. Monoclonal antibodies also recognized this protein in immune reactions with CMV-infected cells [74, 76]. This phosphorylated matrix protein, pp65, which has also been called the tegument protein and is the most abundant structural constituent of laboratory strains of CMV, is encoded by reading frame UL63 [15]. Other designations for this polypeptide include the lower matrix protein [33], major structural phosphoprotein pp65 [67], glycoprotein gp64 [17, 70], and ICP27 [73]. The DNA coding sequence was independently determined for strains AD169 and Towne, and the predicted sequences were shown to be identical. The pp65 reading frame in the AD169 genome maps within *Hin*dIII fragments L, b, and c [95], and the corresponding gene of Towne maps within *Hin*dIII fragments H and N [17]. Figure 1 shows the location of this gene on the AD169 genome. An abundant 4-kb mRNA corresponding to the pp65 reading frame was detected at early and late times, but no characteristic TATA sequence was found proximal to the RNA unit [40, 95]. This mRNA was produced during the early and late phases of viral replication but appeared to be translated to high levels at late times [25]. Recent studies showed that the level of the mRNA correlates with the amount of pp65 synthesized, indicating that the expression of the gene is transcriptionally regulated [22, 40]. Another phosphorylated viral polypeptide of 67 kDa was also mapped on the Towne genome to the *Eco*RI G fragment [21]. Nucleotide sequence comparison showed that this protein is not related to pp65 [15].

Immune Response to pp65

When CMV-immune sera were reacted by immunoprecipitation with CMV-infected-cell proteins [75, 77] and by immunoblot with purified CMV virions [44], a protein of 65 kDa was one of the most highly immunogenic proteins recognized. Figure 2 compares the immune response profiles of sera from babies with congenital symptomatic CMV infections with the profile of monoclonal antibody CH65, which precipitates pp65 [77]. In this study, sera from babies with either symptomatic or asymptomatic CMV infections immunoprecipitated pp65 from extracts of infected cells. Others subsequently found that unlike the broad reactivity of sera to pp150, pp65 was reactive with some, but not all, CMV-immune sera [36] and was preferentially reactive with IgM-positive sera. Several problems have been encountered with analysis of the immune response to pp65. First, in comparison to clinical isolates, laboratory strains overproduce pp65 [36, 40]. Thus, when sera are tested against the protein derived from cell culture, a problem arises in assessing the immune response to pp65 relative to other viral proteins. Second, some human sera, monospecific immune sera, and monoclonal antibodies react nonspecifically with pp65 [8, 80].

In a recent study, three different regions of pp65, representing portions of 26, 70, and 196 amino acids, were expressed as β-galactosidase fusion proteins and tested with CMV-positive sera [80]. The three pp65 recombinant peptides represented about 50% of the reading frame. Using these defined fusion proteins in immunoblot analysis allowed the reactivity against specific regions of pp65 to be analyzed without interference from other proteins of similar size. Also, by using controlled amounts of the recombinant pp65 proteins, the relative immune response to this protein could be compared with that of fusion proteins constructed from other CMV genes. Approximately one third of the CMV-positive sera reacted with the pp65 fusion proteins. These results indicate that it would be advantageous to use portions of pp65 together with other recombinant antigens to optimize large-scale screening of human sera for CMV-specific antibodies. Insofar as reactivity did not correlate with acute CMV infection, antibody to pp65 seem not to be a reliable serological marker for primary infections.

In another report recombinant proteins of pp65 have been shown to be suitable antigens for large-scale screening of human sera. Landini et al. [47] screened a large panel of human sera against ten recombinant CMV antigens by immunoblot analysis. Among these antigens were defined regions of the structural proteins, 150, 71, 65, 38 and 28 kDa, and the nonstructural protein, ICP36. It was concluded that recombinant proteins containing immunoreactive regions can replace cell-culture-derived viral antigens for serological evaluation of CMV-specific antibodies. Comparison of the pp65 fusion protein containing 70 residues spanning positions 401–470 with that spanning residues 297–458 showed that sera were more reactive with the latter fusion protein. In a recent report describing the properties of human monoclonal antibodies to CMV, antibody HMZ01, which recognizes the lower matrix protein, reacted with a fusion protein from this open reading frame expressing amino acids 106–253 [6]. This finding locates yet another antigenic site on this phosphoprotein.

The 28-kDa Phosphoprotein, pp28, Encoded by UL 99

CMV virions contain a phosphorylated structural protein 28 kDa in apparent molecular mass, which was identified by immunoelectron microscopy and located on the surface of cytoplasmic nucleocapsids [45]. The gene encoding pp28 was mapped to the *Hin*dIII fragment R of strain AD169 by use of a pp28-specific monoclonal antibody to screen a λgt11 cDNA library [59] (see Fig. 1). The transcript for this gene is a late 1.3-kb mRNA. St. Jeor and coworkers mapped a 25-kDa protein to the same locus in the AD169 genome and detected a 1.6-kb mRNA that encodes this protein [56, 57]. The corresponding polypeptide of Towne strain migrates as a 32-kDa protein and was shown to be encoded by a 1.4-kb mRNA that mapped to this region of the genome [71].

Several studies have shown that pp28 is highly immunogenic in human infection. Figure 2 compares the reactivities of sera from congenitally infected babies having symptomatic CMV infections with the reactivity of monoclonal antibody CH19 to pp28 [77] (Gimeno and Pereira, unpublished data). All of these sera precipitated pp28 from extracts of CMV-infected cells. The pp28 polypeptide is also reactive in immunoblot assays with most of the CMV-positive sera tested [43] and with a monoclonal antibody to CMV [91]. In recent studies, β-galactosidase fusion proteins containing amino acids 7–99 of pp28, representing 87% of the polypeptide, were reactive when tested by immunoblot analysis with CMV-positive human sera [47, 59]. IgG, but not IgM, titers to the authentic viral protein and the recombinant protein rose on recurrent infection, indicating that antibody to pp28 is a reliable serological marker for reactivated, but not primary, infections.

Other Immunogenic CMV Proteins

The Major Capsid Protein (MCP) Encoded by UL86

Purified CMV particles contain at least two prominent large proteins with an apparent molecular mass of approximately 150 kDa. One of these, a phosphorylated protein called pp150, was discussed above. The other does not undergo posttranslational modification and was designated the MCP [26]. The gene encoding CMV MCP was identified by sequence comparisons with the MCP sequences of other human herpesviruses and was confirmed immunologically [14]. The MCP of CMV has an amino acid identity of 25% with VP5, the capsid protein of HSV-1, 29% with MCP of Epstein-Barr virus, and 23% with MCP of varicella-zoster virus (VZV). The sequence of the MCP of human herpesvirus 6 shows an amino acid identity of 43% with CMV MCP, which underscores their close evolutionary relatedness [49]. CMV MCP is encoded by a reading frame, UL86, which spans *Hin*dIII fragments U, b, and a of AD169 (Fig. 1). A late 8-kb mRNA coding for the MCP was mapped to this region of the genome [94]. The mRNA is synthesized late in infection and was not detected prior to viral DNA replication. The 3′ end of the gene mapped within the *Hin*dIII fragment b [94a].

Human Immune Response to the MCP

Figure 2 compares immunoprecipitation reactions of sera from babies with congenital CMV infections with the reactivity of monoclonal antibody CH23, which precipitates the MCP of CMV [77]. In this study, we showed that sera from patients with active CMV infections reacted with the MCP. We and others have found that about one third of CMV-immune sera react with the MCP in immunoblots, suggesting that in contrast to the other herpesviruses, the MCP of CMV is of limited antigenicity [20, 36, 94]. For a detailed analysis of the immunoreactive and immunogenic properties of the MCP, three portions of this protein were expressed as β-galactosidase fusion proteins [94]. MCP recombinants that covered about 75% of the reading frame were tested in immunoblot reactions for their reactivity with CMV-immune sera. One fusion protein from the midregion of the gene was found to represent the immunodominant portion of the protein. The MCP recombinant proteins were also used to study cross-reactivity with VP5, the HSV-1 capsid protein. In immunoblot analyses and immunofluorescence assays, both a monospecific rabbit antiserum raised against the recombinant peptide close to the amino terminus and a monoclonal antibody to the authentic viral MCP of CMV cross-reacted with the HSV-1 capsid protein. To identify antibodies to common epitopes in human sera reactive with the HSV-1 and CMV capsid proteins, the recombinant proteins were conjugated to CNBr-activated sepharose and used to select antibodies from CMV- and HSV-1-positive sera [94]. This approach detected antibodies that cross-reacted with CMV and HSV-1 but failed to identify antibodies to nonlinear epitopes or to discriminate between unidirectional and bidirectional cross-reactivity of these herpesviruses. Proteins eliciting antibodies that cross-react with other herpesviruses would not be suitable antigens for use in serodiagnostic tests.

The Immediate-Early (IE) Proteins Encoded by UL122 and UL123

At least three distinct regions of the CMV genome are transcribed at IE times after infection [104–106]. Most of these transcripts originate from the *Hin*dIII fragment E of strain AD169 and the corresponding region of the Towne strain genome. This major transcription unit is directed by a single strong promoter/enhancer region. The mRNA species contain multiple exons that are differentially spliced to produce distinct transcripts that result in the synthesis of multiple related and unrelated polypeptides [99, 100]. The predominant IE proteins originating from regions 1 and 2 have a predicted size of about 68–72 kDa and 86 kDa, respectively [5, 61, 62, 102]. The 72-kDa gene product is phosphorylated.

CMV IE proteins might be targets of humoral antibodies. In an early study to show the virus-specific nature of proteins in CMV-infected cells, CMV-immune sera immunoprecipitated these gene products [5]. Detailed analysis of the immunogenic properties of the IE proteins has been slow. In a recent study, it was reported that β-galactosidase fusion proteins containing coding regions of the IE1 and IE2 reading frames are recognized by monoclonal antibodies to CMV and by CMV-immune sera [81, 81c]. The fusion proteins expressed the amino-terminal portions of the IE1 and IE2 gene products. Immunoblot analysis showed that the epitopes of most monoclonal antibodies mapped within exons 2 and 4 of IE region 1. Analysis of CMV-immune sera from patients with primary infections indicated that they reacted with IE exon 4 coding sequences early in infection. It was concluded that reactivity of antibodies to the IE proteins might be useful serological markers for the early phase of primary infection.

Conclusions

Research on CMV proteins that elicit an immune response in human infection has made significant progress over the last 10 years. Many of these gene products have already been identified, their nucleotide sequence characterized, and the regions that serve as antibody targets determined. The next phase of study, which involves fine-mapping the immunodominant sites and determining whether antibodies to them are present in sera from individuals with primary, recurrent, or past CMV infections, is underway. Although multiple serological markers for the convalescent phase and for recurrent CMV infections have already been elucidated, those for acute infection that are recognized by IgM are not well defined. From the studies on the immune response profile in different CMV infections, it seems that a mixture of viral proteins would be optimal for use as antigens in serodiagnostic tests. Serological markers for the convalescent phase, in patients with primary infections and reactivated infections, include antibodies to glycoproteins gB and gH, and also to proteins pp150, pp65 and pp28. Both IgG and IgM antibodies to ICP36 (p52) are markers for acute and primary infections. Recent studies indicate that IgM antibodies to pp150 and IE72 are also markers for primary infections. Antibodies to pp150 are long lasting and serve as reliable indicators of past CMV infections in immunocompetent individuals. Much work still remains to broaden the spectrum of serological markers for different stages of infection and to produce these protein products on a large scale for screening of sera from blood donors and pregnant women. Perhaps the near future will see the evolution of specifically defined mixtures of CMV proteins with which to identify patients in various stages of infection, to assist in the course of treatment with antiviral drugs, and to better determine the prognosis for recovery from CMV disease.

References

1. Anders DG, Gibson W (1988) Location, transcript analysis, and partial nucleotide sequence of the cytomegalovirus gene encoding an early DNA-binding protein with similarities to ICP8 of herpes simplex virus type 1. J Virol 62:1364–1372
2. Banks T, Huo B, Kousoulas K, Spaete R, Pachl C, Pereira L (1989) A major neutralizing domain maps within the carboxyl terminal half of the cleaved cytomegalovirus B glycoprotein. J Gen Virol 70:979–985
3. Basgoz N, Quadri I, Navarro D, Sears A, Lennette E, Youngblom J, Pereira L (1992) Antigenic properties of human cytomegalovirus glycoprotein B: continuous epitopes

that vary among strains map at the amino terminus and conserved epitopes at the carboxy terminus. J Gen Virol 73:983–988

4. Benko D, Haltiwanger R, Hart G, Gibson W (1988) Virion basic phosphoprotein from human cytomegalovirus contains O-linked N-acetylglucosamine. Proc Natl Acad Sci USA 85:2573–2577
5. Blanton RA, Tevethia MJ (1981) Immunoprecipitation of virus-specific immediate-early and early polypeptides from cells lytically infected with human cytomegalovirus strain AD169. Virology 112:262–273
6. Bradshaw PA, Duran MR, Foung SKH (1991) Anti-CMV human monoclonal antibodies: epitope identification and immune response analysis. In: Landini PM (ed) Progress in submegalovirus research. International congress series 978. Excerpta Medica, Amsterdam
7. Britt WJ (1984) Neutralizing antibodies detect a disulfide-linked glycoprotein complex within the envelope of human cytomegalovirus. Virology 135:369–378
8. Britt WJ, Auger D (1985) Identification of a 65,000 dalton virion envelope protein of human cytomegalovirus. Virus Res 4:31–36
9. Britt WJ, Auger D (1986) Synthesis and processing of the envelope gp55-116 complex of human cytomegalovirus. J Virol 58:185–191
10. Britt WJ, Vugler LG (1990) Antiviral antibody responses in mothers and their newborn infants with clinical and subclinical congenital cytomegalovirus infections. J Infect Dis 161:214–219
11. Britt WJ, Vugler L, Stephens EB (1988) Induction of complement-dependent and -independent neutralizing antibodies by recombinant-derived human cytomegalovirus gp55-116 (gB). J Virol 62:3309–3318
12. Britt WJ, Vugler L, Butfiloski EJ, Stevens EJ (1990) Cell surface expression of human cytomegalovirus (HCMV) gp55-116 (gB); use of HCMV-recombinant vaccinia virus-infected cells in analysis of the human neutralizing antibody response. J Virol 64:1079–1085
13. Brucher KH, Garten W, Klenk HD, Shaw E, Radsak K (1990) Inhibition of endoproteolytic cleavage of cytomegalovirus (HCMV) glycoprotein B by palmitoyl-peptidyl-chloromethyl ketone. Virology 178:617–620
14. Chee MS, Rudolph S-A, Plachter B, Barrell B, Jahn G (1989) Identification of the major capsid protein gene of human cytomegalovirus. J Virol 63:1345–1353
15. Chee MS, Bankier AT, Beck S, Bohni R, Brown CM, Cerny R, Horsnell T, Hutchinson CA III, Kouzarides T, Martignetti JA, Preddie E, Satchwell SC, Tomlinson P, Weston KM, Barrell BG (1990) Analysis of the protein-coding content of the sequence of human cytomegalovirus strains AD169. Curr Top Microbiol Immunol 154:125–170
16. Chou SW, Dennison KM (1991) Analysis of interstrain variation in cytomegalovirus glycoprotein B sequences encoding neutralization-related epitopes. J Infect Dis 163:1229–1234
17. Clark BR, Zaia JA, Balce-Directo L, Ting Y-P (1984) Isolation and partial chemical characterization of a 64,000-dalton glycoprotein of human cytomegalovirus. J Virol 49:279–282
18. Cranage MP, Kousarides T, Bankier AT, Satchwell S, Weston K, Tomlinson P, Barrell B, Hart H, Bell SE, Minson AC, Smith GL (1986) Identification of the human cytomegalovirus glycoprotein B gene and induction of neutralizing antibodies via its expression in recombinant vaccinia virus. EMBO J 5:3057–3063
19. Cranage MP, Smith GL, Bell SE, Hart H, Brown C, Bankier AT, Tomlinson P, Barrell BB, Minson TC (1988) Identification and expression of a human cytomegalovirus glycoprotein with homology to the Epstein-Barr virus BXLF2 product, varicella-zoster virus gpIII, and herpes simplex virus type 1 glycoprotein H. J Virol 62:1416–1422
20. Cremer N, Cossen CK, Shell GR, Pereira L (1985) Antibody response to cytomegalovirus polypeptides captured by monoclonal antibodies on the solid phase in enzyme immunoassays. J Clin Microbiol 21:517–521
21. Davis MG, Huang ES (1985) Nucleotide sequence of a human cytomegalovirus gene fragment encoding a 67-kilodalton phosphorylated viral protein. J Virol 56:7–11

22. Depto AS, Stenberg RM (1989) Regulated expression of the human cytomegalovirus pp65 gene: octamer sequence in the promoter is required for activation by viral gene products. J Virol 63:1232–1238
23. Farrar GH, Greenaway PJ (1986) Characterization of glycoprotein complexes present in human cytomegalovirus envelopes. J Gen Virol 67:1469–1473
24. Fiala M, Honess R, Heiner D, Heine J, Murnane J, Wallace R, Guze L (1976) Cytomegalovirus proteins. I. Polypeptides of virions and dense bodies. J Virol 19:243–254
25. Geballe AP, Leach FS, Mocarski ES (1986) Regulation of cytomegalovirus late gene expression: λ genes are controlled by posttranscriptional events. J Virol 57:864–874
26. Gibson W (1983) Protein counterparts of human and simian cytomegaloviruses. Virology 128:391–406
27. Gibson W, Murphey TL, Roby C (1981) Cytomegalovirus-infected cells contain a DNA-binding protein. Virology 111:251–262
28. Gold D, Ashley R, Handsfield HH, Veron M, Leach L, Mills J, Drew L, Corey L (1988) Immunoblot analyses of the humoral immune response in primary cytomegalovirus infection. J Infect Dis 157:319–326
29. Gonczol E, Hudecz F, Ianacone J, Dietzschold B, Starr S, Plotkin SA (1986) Immune responses to isolated human cytomegalovirus envelope proteins. J Virol 58:661–664
30. Gonczol E, Ianacone J, Ho WZ, Starr S, Meignier B, Plotkin S (1990) Isolated gA/gB glycoprotein complex of human cytomegalovirus envelope induces humoral and cellular immune responses in human volunteers. Vaccine 8:130–136
31. Gretch DR, Kari B, Gehrz RC, Stinski MF (1988) A multigene family encodes the human cytomegalovirus glycoprotein complex gcII (gp47-52 complex). J Virol 62:1956–1962
32. Gretch DR, Kari B, Rasmussen L, Gehrz RC, Stinski MF (1988) Identification and characterization of three distinct families of glycoprotein complexes in the envelopes of human cytomegalovirus. J Virol 62:875–881
33. Irmiere A, Gibson W (1983) Isolation and characterization of a noninfectious virion-like particle released from cells infected with human strains of cytomegalovirus. Virology 130:118–133
34. Jahn G, Mach M (1990) Human cytomegalovirus phosphoproteins and glycoproteins and their coding regions. Curr Top Microbiol Immunol 154:171–185
35. Jahn G, Kouzarides T, Mach M, Scholl BC, Plachter B, Traupe B, Preddie E, Satchwell SC, Fleckenstein B, Barrell BG (1987) Map position and nucleotide sequence of the gene for the large structural phosphoprotein of human cytomegalovirus. J Virol 61:1358–1367
36. Jahn G, Scholl B-C, Traupe B, Fleckenstein B (1987) The two major structural phosphoproteins (pp65 and pp150) of human cytomegalovirus and their antigenic properties. J Gen Virol 68:1327–1337
37. Kari B, Lussenhop N, Goertz R, Wabuke-Bunoti M, Radeke R, Gehrz R (1986) Characterization of monoclonal antibodies reactive to several biochemically distinct human cytomegalovirus glycoprotein complexes. J Virol 60:345–352
38. Kari B, Liu Y-NC, Goertz R, Lussenhop N, Stinski MF, Gehrz R (1990) Structure and composition of a family of human cytomegalovirus glycoprotein complexes designated gC-1 (gB). J Gen Virol 71:2673–2680
39. Kemble G, McCormick AL, Pereira L, Mocarski E (1987) A cytomegalovirus protein with properties of herpes simplex virus ICP8: partial purification of the polypeptide and map position of the gene. J Virol 61:3145–3151
40. Klages S, Ruger B, Jahn G (1989) Multiplicity dependent expression of the predominant phosphoprotein pp65 of human cytomegalovirus. Virus Res 12:159–168
41. Kniess N, Mach M, Fay J, Britt WJ (1991) Distribution of linear antigenic sites on glycoprotein gp55 of human cytomegalovirus. J Virol 65:138–146
42. Landini M, Michelson S (1988) Human cytomegalovirus proteins. Prog Med Virol 35:152–185
43. Landini M, Re M, Mirolo G, Baldassarri B, La Placa M (1985) Human immune response to cytomegalovirus structural polypeptides studied by immunoblotting. J Med Virol 17:303–311

44. Landini M, Mirolo G, Coppolecchia P, Re M, La PM (1986) Serum antibodies to individual cytomegalovirus structural polypeptides in renal transplant recipients during viral infection. Microbiol Immunol 30:683–695
45. Landini M, Severi B, Furlini G, Badiali-De GL (1987) Human cytomegalovirus structural components: intracellular and intraviral localization of p28 and p65-69 by immunoelectron microscopy. Virus Res 8:15–23
46. Landini MP, Lazzarotto T, Ripalti A, Guan MX, La Placa M (1989) Antibody response to recombinant lambda gt11 fusion proteins in cytomegalovirus infection. J Clin Microbiol 27:2324–2327
47. Landini MP, Guan MX, Jahn G, Lindenmaier W, Mach M, Ripalti A, Necker A, Lazzarotto T, Plachter B (1990) Large-scale screening of human sera with cytomegalovirus recombinant antigens. J Clin Microbiol 28:1375–1379
48. Landini MP, Ripalti A, Sra K, Pouletty P (1991) Human cytomegalovirus structural proteins: immune reaction against pp150 synthetic peptides. J Clin Microbiol 29:1868–1872
49. Lawrence GL, Chee M, Craxton MA, Gompels UA, Honess RW, Barrell BG (1990) Human herpesvirus 6 is closely related to human cytomegalovirus. J Virol 64:287–299
50. Leach FS, Mocarski ES (1989) Regulation of cytomegalovirus late-gene expression: differential use of three start sites in the transcriptional activation of ICP36 gene expression. J Virol 63:1783–1791
51. Lehner R, Meyer H, Mach M (1989) Identification and characterization of a human cytomegalovirus gene coding for a membrane protein that is conserved among human herpesviruses. J Virol 63:3792–3800
52. Liu Y-NC, Klaus A, Kari B, Stinski MF, Eckhardt K, Gehrz RC (1991) The N-terminal 513 amino acids of the envelope glycoprotein gB of human cytomegalovirus stimulates both B- and T-cell immune responses in humans. J Virol 65:1644–1648
53. Lussenhop NO, Goertz R, Wabuke-Bunoti M, Gehrz R, Kari B (1988) Epitope analysis of human cytomegalovirus glycoprotein complexes using murine monoclonal antibodies. Virology 164:362–372
54. Mach M, Utz U, Fleckenstein B (1986) Mapping of the major glycoprotein gene of human cytomegalovirus. J Gen Virol 67:1461–1467
55. Marshall GS, Ricciardi RP, Rando RF, Puck J, Ge RW, Plotkin SA, Gonczol E (1990) An adenovirus recombinant that expresses the human cytomegalovirus major envelope glycoprotein and induces neutralizing antibodies. J Infect Dis 162:1177–1181
56. Martinez J, St Jeor SC (1986) Molecular cloning and analysis of three cDNA clones homologous to human cytomegalovirus RNAs present during late infection. J Virol 60:531–538
57. Martinez J, Lahijani RS, St Jeor SC (1989) Analysis of a region of the human cytomegalovirus (AD169) genome coding for a 25-kilodalton virion protein. J Virol 63:233–241
58. Meyer H, Mach M (1991) The glycoprotein gp116 of human cytomegalovirus contains two antibody binding sites in close proximity. J Cell Biochem Suppl 15E:101
59. Meyer H, Bankier A, Landini M, Brown C, Barrell B, Ruger B, Mach M (1988) Identification and procaryotic expression of the gene coding for the highly immunogenic 28-kilodalton structural phosphoprotein (pp28) of human cytomegalovirus. J Virol 62:2243–2250
60. Meyer H, Masuho Y, Mach M (1990) The gp116 of the gp58/116 complex of human cytomegalovirus represents the amino-terminal part of the precursor molecule and contains a neutralizing epitope. J Gen Virol 71:2443–2450
61. Michelson S, Horodniceanu F, Kress M, Tardy PM (1977) Immediate early antigens in human cytomegalovirus. Nature 270:615–617
62. Michelson S, Horodniceanu F, Kress M, Tardy PM (1979) Human cytomegalovirus-induced immediate early antigens: analysis in sodium dodecyl sulfate-polyacrylamide gel electrophoresis after immunoprecipitation. J Virol 32:259–267
63. Mocarski ES (1992) Cytomegalovirus biology and replication. In: Roizman B, Whitley R, Lopez C (eds) Human herpesviruses: biology, pathogenesis, and treatment. Raven, New York (in press)

64. Mocarski ES, Pereira L, Michael N (1985) Precise localization of genes on large animal virus genomes: use of λgt11 and monoclonal antibodies to map the gene for a cytomegalovirus protein family. Proc Natl Acad Sci USA 82:1266–1270
65. Mocarski ES, Pereira L, McCormick L (1988) Human cytomegalovirus ICP22, the product of the HWLF1 reading frame, is an early nuclear protein that is released from cells. J Gen Virol 69:2613–2621
66. Navarro D, Paz P, Tugizov S, Topp K, LaVail J, Pereira L (1992) Glycoprotein B of human cytomegalovirus promotes virion penetration into cells, transmission of infection from cell to cell, and fusion of infected cells (submitted)
67. Nowak B, Gmeiner A, Sarnow P, Levine A, Fleckenstein B (1984) Physical mapping of human cytomegalovirus genes: identification of DNA sequences coding for a virion phosphoprotein of 71 kDa and a viral 65-kDa polypeptide. Virology 134:91–102
68. Nowak B, Sullivan C, Sarnow P, Thomas R, Bricout F, Nicolas JC, Fleckenstein B, Levine AJ (1984) Characterization of monoclonal antibodies and polyclonal immune sera directed against human cytomegalovirus virion proteins. Virology 132:325–338
69. Pachl C, Probert WS, Hermsen KM, Masiarz FR, Rasmussen L, Merigan T, Spaete RR (1989) The human cytomegalovirus strain Towne glycoprotein H gene encodes glycoprotein p86. Virology 169:418–426
70. Pande H, Baak SW, Riggs AD, Clark BR, Shively JE, Zaia JA (1984) Cloning and physical mapping of a gene fragment coding for a 64-kilodalton major late antigen of human cytomegalovirus. Proc Natl Acad Sci USA 81:4965–4969
71. Pande H, Campo K, Churchill MA, Clark BR, Zaia JA (1988) Genomic localization of the gene encoding a 32-kDa capsid protein of human cytomegalovirus. Virology 167:306–310
72. Pande H, Campo K, Churchill MA, Zaia JA (1989) Genomic locus for a 140 kDa structural protein (pp150) of human cytomegalovirus in strains Towne and AD169. Virus Res 12:11–18
73. Pereira L (1984) Glycoproteins specified by human cytomegalovirus. In: Roizman B (ed) The herpesviruses. Plenum, New York, pp 383–404
74. Pereira L, Hoffman M (1986) Immunology of human cytomegalovirus glycoproteins. In: Lopez C, Roizman B (eds) Human herpesvirus infections: pathogenesis, diagnosis, and treatment. Raven, New York, pp 69–92
75. Pereira L, Hoffman M, Cremer N (1982) Electrophoretic analysis of polypeptides immune precipitated from extracts of cytomegalovirus infected cells by human sera. Infect Immun 36:933–942
76. Pereira L, Hoffman M, Gallo D, Cremer N (1982) Monoclonal antibodies to human cytomegalovirus. I. Three cell surface proteins with unique immunologic and electrophoretic properties specify cross-reactive determinants. Infect Immun 36:924–932
77. Pereira L, Stagno S, Hoffman M, Volanakis J (1983) Cytomegalovirus infected cell polypeptides immune precipitated by children with congenital and perinatal cytomegalovirus infections. Infect Immun 39:100–108
78. Pereira L, Hoffman M, Tatsuno M, Dondero D (1984) Polymorphism of human cytomegalovirus glycoproteins characterized by monoclonal antibodies. Virology 139:73–86
79. Pereira L, Basgoz N, Youngblom J, Sears A, Navarro D, Qadri I, Lennette E (1991) Mapping conserved antigenic regions and strain-specific epitopes within the glycoprotein B gene of human cytomegalovirus. In: Landini PM (ed) Progress in cytomegalovirus research. International congress series 978. Excerpta Medica, Amsterdam, pp 195–198
80. Plachter B, Klages S, Hagelmann S, Britt W, Landini MP, Jahn G (1990) Prokaryotic expression of phosphorylated tegument protein pp65 of human cytomegalovirus and application of recombinant peptides for immunoblot analyses. J Clin Microbiol 28:1229–1235
80a. Plachter B, Jahn G (1990) Cytomegalovirus diagnostics: Standard procedures and perspectives. Biotest Bulletin 4: 107–118
81. Plachter B, Hagelmann S, Jahn G (1991) Prokarytic expression of peptides from IE-regions 1 and 2 of human cytomegalovirus. In: Landini PM (ed) Progress in cyto-

megalovirus research. International congress series 978. Excerpta Medica, Amsterdam, pp 165–168

81a. Plachter B, Nordin M, Zweygberg Wirgart B, Mach M, Stein H, Grillner L, Jahn G (1992) The DNA-binding protein P52 of human cytomegalovirus reacts with monoclonal antibody CCH2 and associates with the nuclear membrane at late times after infection. Virus Res 24:265–276

81b. Plachter B, Wieczorek L, Scholl B-C, Ziegelmaier R, Jahn G (1992) Detection of cytomegalovirus antibodies by an enzyme-linked immunosorbent assay using recombinant polypeptides of the large phosphorylated tegument protein pp 150. J Clin Microbiol, pp 201–206

82. Qadri I, Navarro D, Paz P, Pereira L (1991) Analysis of the assembly, antigenic properties, and transport of mutants in glycoprotein B of human cytomegalovirus. 16th International Herpesvirus Workshop, p 41

83. Qadri I, Navarro D, Paz P, Pereira L (1992) Assembly of conformation-dependent neutralizing domains on glycoprotein B of human cytomegalovirus. J Gen Virol 73 (in press)

84. Radsak K, Brucher KH, Britt W, Shiou H, Schneider D, Kollert A (1990) Nuclear compartmentation of glycoprotein B of human cytomegalovirus. Virology 177:515–522

85. Rasmussen L (1990) Immune response to human cytomegalovirus infection. Curr Top Microbiol Immunol 154:221–254

86. Rasmussen LE, Nelson RM, Kelsall DC, Merigan TC (1984) Murine monoclonal antibody to a single protein neutralizes the infectivity of human cytomegalovirus. Proc Natl Acad Sci USA 81:876–880

87. Rasmussen L, Mullenax J, Nelson M, Merigan TC (1985) Human cytomegalovirus polypeptides stimulate neutralizing antibody in vivo. Virology 145:186–190

88. Rasmussen L, Mullenax J, Nelson R, Merigan TC (1985) Viral polypeptides detected by a complement-dependent neutralizing murine monoclonal antibody to human cytomegalovirus. J Virol 55:274–280

89. Rasmussen L, Nelson M, Neff M, Merigan TC (1988) Characterization of two different human cytomegalovirus glycoproteins which are targets for virus neutralizing antibody. Virology 163:309–318

90. Rasmussen L, Matkin C, Spaete R, Pachl C, Merigan TC (1991) Antibody response to human cytomegalovirus glycoproteins gB and gH after natural infection in humans. J Infect Dis 164:835–842

91. Re M, Landini M, Coppolecchia P, Furlini G, La Placa M (1985) A 28,000 molecular weight human cytomegalovirus structural polypeptide studied by means of a specific monoclonal antibody. J Gen Virol 66:2507–2511

92. Ripalti A, Landini MP, Mocarski ES, Placa ML (1989) Identification and preliminary use of recombinant lambda gt11 fusion proteins in human cytomegalovirus diagnosis. J Gen Virol 70:1214–1251

93. Roby C, Gibson W (1986) Characterization of phosphoproteins and protein kinase activity of virions, noninfectious enveloped particles, and dense bodies of human cytomegalovirus. J Virol 59:714–727

94. Rudolph S-A, Kuhn JE, Korn K, Braun RW, Jahn G (1990) Prokaryotic expression of the major capsid protein of human cytomegalovirus and antigenic cross-reactions with herpes simplex virus type 1. J Gen Virol 71:2023–2031

94a. Rudolph S-A, Stamminger T, Jahn G (1990) Transcriptional analysis of the eight-kilobase mRNA encoding the major capsid protein of human cytomegalovirus. J Virol, pp 5167–5172

95. Ruger B, Klages S, Walla B, Albrecht J, Fleckenstein B, Tomlinson P, Barrell B (1987) Primary structure and transcription of the genes coding for the two virion phosphoproteins pp65 and pp71 of human cytomegalovirus. J Virol 61:446–453

96. Scholl BC, von Hintzenstern J, Borisch B, Traupe B, Broker M, Jahn G (1988) Prokaryotic expression of immunogenic polypeptides of the large phosphoprotein of human cytomegalovirus. J Gen Virol 69:1195–1204

97. Spaete RR, Thayer RM, Probert WS, Masiarz FR, Chamberlain SH, Rasmussen L, Merigan TC, Pachl C (1988) Human cytomegalovirus strain Towne glycoprotein B is processed by proteolytic cleavage. Virology 167:207–225
98. Spaete RR, Saxena A, Scott PI, Song GJ, Probert WS, Britt WJ, Gibson W, Rasmussen L, Pachl C (1990) Sequence requirements for proteolytic processing of glycoprotein B of human cytomegalovirus strain Towne. J Virol 64:2922–2931
99. Stenberg RM, Witte PR, Stinski MF (1985) Multiple spliced and unspliced transcripts from cytomegalovirus immediate-early region 2 and evidence for a common initiation site within immediate early region 1. J Virol 56:665–675
100. Stenberg RM, Fortney J, Barlow SW, Magrane BP, Nelson JA (1990) Promoter-specific transactivation and repression by human cytomegalovirus immediate-early proteins involves common and unique protein domains. J Virol 64:1556–1565
101. Stinski MF (1976) Human cytomegalovirus: glycoproteins associated with virions and dense bodies. J Virol 19:594–609
102. Stinski MF (1978) Sequence of protein synthesis in cells infected by human cytomegalovirus: early and late virus-induced polypeptides. J Virol 26:686–701
103. Stinski MF, Mocarski ES, Thomsen DR, Urbanowski ML (1979) Membrane glycoproteins and antigens induced by human cytomegalovirus. J Gen Virol 43:119–129
104. Stinski MF, Thomsen DR, Stenberg RM, Goldstein LC (1983) Organization and expression of the immediate early genes of human cytomegalovirus. J Virol 46:1–14
105. Stinski MF, Stenberg RM, Goins WF (1984) Structure and function of the human cytomegalovirus immediate early genes. In: Rapp F (ed) Herpesvirus. Liss, New York, pp 399–421
106. Thomsen DR, Stenberg RM, Goins WF, Stinski MF (1984) Promoter-regulatory region of the major immediate early gene of human cytomegalovirus. Proc Natl Acad Sci USA 81:659–663
107. Tomiyama T, Matsumoto Y, Sugano T, Fujinaga S, Masuho Y (1990) Preparation of human monoclonal antibodies against a cytomegalovirus glycoprotein complex of 130 and 55 kDa. J Immunol Methods 131:249–255
108. Urban M, Britt WJ, Mach M (1991) Characterization of linear antigenic sites on glycoprotein gp86 of human cytomegalovirus. In: Landini PM (ed) Progress in cytomegalovirus research. International congress series 978. Excerpta Medica, Amsterdam, pp 199–202
109. Utz U, Britt W, Vugler L, Mach M (1989) Identification of a neutralizing epitope on glycoprotein gp58 of human cytomegalovirus. J Virol 5:1995–2001
110. Weiner D, Gibson W (1983) Phosphorylation, maturational processing, and relatedness of strain colburn matrix proteins. Virology 129:155–169
111. Wells DE, Vugler LG, Britt WJ (1990) Structural and immunological characterization of human cytomegalovirus gp55-116 (gB) expressed in insect cells. J Gen Virol 71:873–880
112. Weston K, Barrell BG (1986) Sequence of the short unique region, short repeats, and part of the long repeats of human cytomegalovirus. J Mol Biol 192:177–208
113. Wright DA, Staprans SI, Spector DH (1988) Four phosphoproteins with common amino termini are encoded by human cytomegalovirus AD169. J Virol 62:331–340
114. Zaia J, Forman S, Ting Y, Vanderwal-Urbina E, Blume K (1986) Polypeptide-specific antibody response to human cytomegalovirus after infection in bone marrow transplant recipients. J Infect Dis 153:780–787

Chapter 22 Postscript: What Is the Role of Dendritic Cells in the Pathogenesis of Human Cytomegalovirus in Immunocompetent and Immunocompromised Hosts?

Yechiel Becker

Summary

The information concerning the complications that human cytomegalovirus (HCMV) is capable of inflicting in immunosuppressed people (organ transplant patients and acquired immune deficiency, AIDS, patients) is described in detail in numerous chapters of this book. Yet, the responses of immune cells in the protection against HMCV infections and the role of the dendritic cell system in the defense against virus reactivations is not fully known. From the research on the role of dendritic cells in the cellular defense against Herpes simplex virus-1, it is possible to suggest that further studies on the effect of immunosuppressive drugs (cyclosporin A, cyclophosphamide, FK506) and their inhibitory effect on dendritic cells may lead to differentiation between the antiviral dendritic cells and the dendritic cells involved in graft rejection. Drugs which do not prevent the antiviral activity of dendritic cells but preserve the dendritic cells capable of anti-HMCV activity, while inhibiting the dendritic cells involved in graft rejection, might be the immunosuppressive drugs of choice.

Introduction

The present book provides the reader with an almost complete story of human cytomegalovirus (HCMV) pathogenesis in immunocompetent and immunocompromised hosts. The medical observations of the many diseases caused by HCMV are complemented by molecular analyses of the virus genes and proteins. The advancement in surgery and organ transplants with emphasis on the use of new immunosuppressive drugs is presented in this book from the point of view of the failures due to reactivation of HCMV leading to life-threatening infections in organ transplant patients. The advancement in the chemotherapy of the herpesvirus diseases is equaled to the low efficiency of the drugs in the treatment of HCMV reactivations. While reading the chapters of

Department of Molecular Virology, Faculty of Medicine, The Hebrew University of Jerusalem, Jerusalem, Israel this book I realized that the dendritic cell (DC) system is not discussed and only one of the chapters deals with the role of macrophages in HCMV infections.

The aim of the present review is to present information on the DC system and its importance in the defense against Herpes simplex virus and to address the question of whether DC have a role in the defense against HCMV infections.

HCMV-Related Diseases: From Asymptomatic Infections in Immunocompetent Hosts to Clinical Diseases in the Immunocompromised Host

Table 1 summarizes the clinical diseases caused by HCMV. It was noted that while the infections may be asymptomatic, the virus infection might also affect the immune system. This HCMV–host relationship then dramatically changes when the host immune system is affected by another virus (e.g. human immunodeficiency virus, HIV), by treatment with immunosuppressive drugs or in cancer patients (Tables 1, 2).

Interestingly, HCMV can infect the epithelia of the gastrointestinal tract (GIT) from the gingiva in the mouth to the anus, causing ulcerations and bleeding. The skin can be infected as well (Table 3). It seems that if there were any cellular defense in the epithelia mentioned above in the immunocompetent host, such cellular defenses would be operational in the normal individual and not allow HCMV to damage the tissues. In the immunocompromised hosts such cellular defenses are absent.

How the Immune System Controls HCMV

The interaction of HCMV with macrophages is described by S. Haskill et al. (Chap. 6) and is summarized in Table 3. The macrophages are nonpermissive

Table 1. Clinical diseases caused by HCMV[a]

1. Most infections in immunocompetent individuals are asymptomatic
2. Heterophile-negative infectious mononucleosis is caused by HCMV
3. Increased susceptibility to opportunistic pathogens due to virus-induced immunosuppression
4. Distinctive forms of allograft rejection in actively infected organ transplant recipients
5. Association with particular types of malignancies
6. A possible link to atherosclerosis
7. Post-blood-perfusion syndrome
8. Posttransplantation syndrome

[a] Based on the data presented by J. D. Hamilton (Chap. 9, this volume)

Table 2. HCMV and human diseases – a summary

A. HCMV infection of the immunocompetent host [a]

1. Most infections in healthy individuals are asymptomatic and the virus is latent in kidney and lymphocytes
2. Approximately 1% of live born infants and 60%–80% of adult evidence cytomegalovirus (CMV) infection. Incidence increases with age.
3. Majority of CMV infections consist only of serological changes of CMV antibody titer or asymptomatic viral shedding
4. Cytomegalic cells were initially found within the parotid and salivary gland but also discovered in other sites with a tendency to infect endothelial cells

B. HMCV infection in cancer patients [a]

1. CMV infections in patients with neoplasms such as immunosuppressed individuals with leukemia or lymphoma was often described
2. The CMV infections in cancer patients determined after autopsy revealed inclusions in lung, adrenals, kidneys, spleen, gastrointestinal tract (GIT), liver, pancreas, skin, thyroid, testis, and brain
3. Necrotizing pancreatitis was described

C. HCMV in renal transplant patients [a]

1. In renal transplant patients 30%–40% of CMV infections consist of fever, musculoskeletal pain, abnormal liver function test, penkopenia and respiratory symptoms
2. In about 2%–3% of the patients the CMV infection may be fatal
3. CMV infection of the GIT is an important reason for morbidity and mortality in renal transplant patients – colonic ulcerations and fatal lower GIT bleeding
4. The most common organ affected was the lungs in 38%–75% of cases. Diffuse panlobular interstitial pneumonia, focal intestinal pneumonia, and scattered inclusion-bearing cells. Inclusions in *pneumocytes lining alveoli and in macrophage*
5. Of renal transplant patients 45% develop hepatitis. In necropsy CMV inclusions were noted in adrenal glands, lymph nodes, salivary glands, thymus, parathyroid, prostate, and bladder
6. Central nervous system (CNS) infections were noted in renal transplant patients. Microscopically, all patients showed *microglia nodules* scattered throughout all the areas of central neuroaxis: most in the gray matter

D. HCMV in bone marrow transplant patients [a]

1. Average incidence is 50% during the first 8–9 weeks after transplantation due to latent virus in donor's marrow. Complications: fatal interstitial pneumonitis in about one half of the patients
2. Ulcerations in all parts of GIT

E. HCMV in AIDS patients [b]

1. CMV enhances HIV-1 infection of *CD4+ lymphoblasts, monocytes, and astrocytes*
2. CMV is synergistic with HIV as a cause of severe AIDS encephalopathy and peripheral neuropathy
3. AIDS dementia complex by CMV encephalopathy is distinguished from pure AIDS dementia complex by CMV viremia with high fever, seizures, and rapid demise
4. In AIDS patients disseminated CMV infection also involves the lungs, GIT, adrenal glands, and other organs
5. A predominance of polymorphonuclear leukocytes in the CSF has been suggestive of CMV infection

---

[a] Based on the data presented by H. V. Vinters and J. A. Ferreiro (Chap. 2, this volume)
[b] Based on the data presented by M. Fiala et al. (Chap. 8 in this book)

Table 3. HCMV interaction with monocytes [a]

1.	HCMV infection appears to be limited to the synthesis of IE and early viral gene products
2.	Inactivated HCMV can indirectly activate cytokine production by monocytes
3.	Transcriptional enhancement of IL-1β, TNF-α, CSF-1 and IL-8 genes
4.	A low but significant proportion of monocytes persistently express high levels of IL-*1β* mRNA
5.	HCMV-IE gene regions were capable of transactivating inflammatory mediator genes like IL-1β

[a] From the data presented by S. Haskill et al. (Chap. 6, this volume)
HCMV, human cytomegalovirus; IL, interleukin; TNF, tumor necrosis factor; CSF, colony-stimulating factor; IE, immediate early

for HCMV and the expression of its immediate-early genes is possible. The product of these viral genes transactivate the cellular genes interleukin-1β (IL-1β), tumor necrosis factor-α (TNF-α), colony-stimulating factor-1 CSF-1 and IL-8. These gene products are mediators of inflammation. These cytokine genes can be activated in macrophages by an inactivated HCMV or by viral proteins. Macrophages may also serve as antigen-presenting cells to stimulate the humoral immune response. Immunological cross-reactivity was found between HCMV and HLA-DR [4]. However, no mention of the DC system in HCMV-infected individuals is presented in this book. Since the DC system is involved in antigen presentation, disease mechanisms, graft rejection, and in the cellular defense against viruses, information on this cell system is presented.

The DC System

Table 4 presents the DC lineage. It can be seen that the progenitor cell is present in the bone marrow [6], the precursors are in the blood, and all the epithelia of the body contain DC in a distinctive region of the epidermis [15]. As can be seen in Table 4 the DC are involved in regulatory functions as well as immunological functions such as antigen presentation or in T cell development in the thymus. The microglia cells in the central nervous system are also bone marrow-derived and belong to the DC lineage. Table 5 presents the cellular markers used for the identification of DC in lymphoid tissues, skin (Langerhans cells), and other organs. It is of interest that HCMV encodes a glycoprotein homologous to major histocompatibility complex (MHC) class I antigens [3].

DC were found in human and mouse bronchial epithelium [9] and form a contiguous network of antigen-presenting class II MHC (Ia+) positive DC within the respiratory epithelium [5, 9]. The Ia+ DC of the lung were reported to consist of a heterogeneous population in respect to the expression of surface membrane antigens [19]. The lung DC stimulate resting T cells in the mixed

Table 4. The dendritic cell (DC) lineage

Cell type	Location	Function
1. DC	Bone marrow	Progenitor cells
2. DC	Blood	Precursors of epithelium associated DC
3. DC	Lungs	Antigen-presenting cells involved in T-cell development in liver epithelium (3–5)
4. DC	Thymus	
5. DC, Kupffer cells	Liver	
6. DC	Pancreas	
7. DC	Gut	
8. DC	Spleen	
9. DC (LC)	Skin	– Involved in processing of antigens, haptens, and allergens – Involved in graft rejection – Involved in allergic reactions – Regulation of keratinocytes and melanocytes – Protection against virus infections – Protection against primary tumors
10. Veiled cells	Lymph vessels	Antigen processing LC traveling to afferent lymphatics. Present in T-cell areas of secondary lymphatic tissues
11. Lymphoid DC	Lymphoid tissues	
12. Interdigitating DC	Lymph nodes Thymus	Presentation of antigens to T cells; initiation of the humoral immune response, in the medulla, instruction of T-cells
13. Follicular DC	B-cell areas of secondary lymphoid tissues	
14. Nonlymphoid or interstitial DC	Interstitial area Connective tissues	
15. Factor XIIIa positive dendrocytes	Surrounding the blood vessels	
16. Microglia	Brain	Originate as all other DC from bone marrow progenitor cells; function not fully understood

(Based in part on [2].) DC, dendritic cells; LC, Langerhans cells

lymphocyte response (MLR) test [8]. The lung DC interact with chemical irritants in dust or aerosolized bacterial lipopolysaccharide (LPS), and the number of intraepithelial DC increase by 59% in the large airways. Schon-Hegrad et al. [9] suggested that these airway epithelial DC form a dynamic population constituting "the first line of defense," suggesting "a role in allergic and infectious diseases in the respiratory tract" [5].

A number of activators and inhibitors of DC were described (Table 6). The immunosuppressive drugs cyclophosphamide and cyclosporin A were reported to inhibit DC activity (C. Berkowitz and Y. Becker, unpublished).

Table 5. Markers on lymphoid dendritic cells and Langerhans cells (after [1])

Parameter	Lymphoid dendritic cells	Langerhans cells
Membrane ATPase	−	+
Nonspecific esterase	−	+
MHC class I	+	+
MHC class II	+	+
Birbeck granules	−	+
NLDC 145 (mouse)	+	+
CD1a (human)	−	+
S-100	+	+
CD4	+	+
Complement receptors CR3	+	+
Fc-IgG receptor	−	+
ICAM-1	+	+
LFA-1	+	+
LFA-3	+	+

MHC, major histocompatiblity complex; ICAM-1, intercellular adhesion molecule-1; LFA-1, lymphocyte function associated antigen-1

Table 6. Modulators of Langerhans/dendritic cell activity (from [17])

Activators	Inhibitors
Cytokines	UV light
(IL-1, GM-CSF, IFN-γ)	X-irradiation
Retinoic acid	Steroids
OK-432	Trauma to the skin
Splenopentin	Cyclophosphamide
Monobenzyl ether of hydroquinone	Cyclosporin A

IL, interleukin; GM-CSF, granulocyte-macrophage colony-stimulating factor; IFN, interferon

Immunosuppressive Drugs: Inhibition of DC and Reactivation of HCMV?

The inhibitory effect exerted by cyclophosphamide or cyclosporin A on the immune system is shown to parallel the ability of HCMV to reactivate in immunosuppressed patients (Table 7). It is not yet known whether the reactivation of HCMV is due to the suppression of DC or other elements of the cellular defense system. However, in studies on the role of DC in the defense against Herpes simplex virus 1, it was noted that the virus entry into internal organs is enhanced in mice treated with cyclosporin A or cyclophosphamide [16]. If the immunosuppressive drugs inactivate the lung DC, the cellular defenses against HCMV in the lung might be abolished.

Table 7. Immunosuppressive drugs and their effect on dendritic cells and on HCMV reactivation

Immunosuppressive drug	HCMV reactivation	Mode of action on skin LC
1. Cyclophosphamide	Reactivation	Inactivation [a]
2. Cyclosporin A	Reactivation	Partial inactivation [a]
3. FK506	No reactivation	?

[a] C. Berkowitz and Y. Becker (unpublished)
HCMV, human cytomegalovirus; LC, Langerhans cells

The effect of the new immunosuppressive drug FK506 on the reactivation of HCMV in organ transplant patients is discussed by M. Ho in this book (Chap. 10). Ho indicates that treatment with FK506 of organ transplant patients prevented the reactivation of HCMV infections. Information on the effect of FK506 on DC is lacking.

DC in Herpes Simplex Virus Infections

Skin epidermal Langerhans cells (LC) play a critical role in Herpes simplex virus-1 infection of the skin. LC were shown to transfer the viral antigens to the lymph nodes and to trigger the T cell response to the virus [11–14]. Herpes simplex virus-1 interaction with DC induced the transcription of IL-1β and TNF-α gene expression in the DC [17]. It was also reported (Otani and Mori 1987) that ultraviolet irradiation of the skin LC changed the course of Herpes simplex virus-1 infection and induced its reactivation. Recurrent infections of this virus in the skin occur after treatments of the skin which inactivate the skin LC [18].

Conclusion

It seems that the role DC may have in the cellular defense against infection by HCMV requires careful attention. It is possible that DC in the immunocompetent host are involved in the suppression of the virus infection leading to the asymptomatic infections. Stimulation of DC activity as suggested in Table 6 might be useful in reducing natural HCMV infections. The study of the effects of immunosuppressive drugs on DC might shed light on the mechanism of HCMV reactivation. Use of immunosuppressive drugs that do not affect all the types of DC, but do eliminate the DC involved in graft rejection, will contribute towards prevention of HCMV reactivations in immunosuppressed individuals.

References

1. Austyn JM (1987) Lymphoid dendritic cells. Immunology 62:161–170
2. Austyn JM (1989) Antigen presenting cells. IRL Press, New York
3. Beck S, Barrel BG (1988) Human cytomegalovirus encodes a glycoprotein homologous to MHC class-I antigens. Nature 331:269–272
4. Fujinami RS, Nelson JA, Walker L, Oldstone MB (1988) Sequence homology and immunologic cross reactivity of human cytomegalovirus with HLA-DR beta chain: a means of graft rejection and immunosuppression. J Virol 62:100–105
5. Holt PG, Schon-Hegrad MA, Oliver J, Holt BJ, McMenamin PG (1990) A contiguous network of dendritic antigen-presenting cells within the respiratory epithelium. Int Arch Allergy Appl Immunol 91:155–159
6. Katz SI, Tamaki K, Sachs DH (1979) Epidermal Langerhans cells are derived from cells originating in bone marrow. Nature 282:324–326
7. Otani T, Mori K (1987) The effects of ultraviolet irradiation of the skin on HSV infections: alteration in immune function mediated by epidermal cells and in the course of infection. Arch Virol 96:1–15
8. Pollard AM, Lipscomb MF (1990) Characterization of murine lung dendritic cells: similarities to Langerhans cells and thymic dendritic cells. J Exp Med 172:159–167
9. Schon-Hegrad MA, Oliver J, McMenamin PG, Holt PG (1991) Studies on the density, distribution and surface phenotype of intraepithelial class II major histocompatbility. J Exp Med 173:1345–1356
10. Sertl K, Takemura T, Tschachler E, Ferrans VJ, Kaliner MA, Shevach EM (1986) Dendritic cells with antigen-presenting capability reside in airway epithelium, lung parenchyma and visceral pleura. J Exp Med 163:436–451
11. Sprecher E, Becker Y (1986) Skin Langerhans cells play an essential role in the defense against HSV-1 infection. Arch Virol 91:341–349
12. Sprecher E, Becker Y (1987) Herpes simplex virus type 1 pathogenicity in foot pad and ear skin of mice depends on Langerhans cell density, mouse genetics and virus strain. J Virol 61:2515–2522
13. Sprecher E, Becker Y (1988) Role of epidermal Langerhans cells in viral infections. Arch Virol 103:1–14
14. Sprecher E, Becker Y (1989) Langerhans cell number and activity in the skin and lymph nodes determines HSV-1 pathogenicity. Arch Virol 107:191–205
15. Sprecher E, Becker Y (1991) Dendritic cells in the epidermis and the lymph nodes – a review. In: Becker Y (ed) Skin Langerhans (dendritic) cells in virus infections and AIDS. Kluwer, Boston, pp 3–23
16. Sprecher E, Becker Y (1992a) Role of dendritic cells in disease states. In preparation
17. Sprecher E, Becker Y (1992b) Detection of IL-1β, TNFα and IL-6 gene transcription by the polymerase chain reaction in keratinocytes, Langerhans cells and peritoneal exudate cells during infection with Herpes simplex virus-1. Arch Virol (In press)
18. Williams NA, Blyth WA, Hill TJ (1991) Langerhans cells and recurrent infection with Herpes simplex virus. In: Becker Y (ed) Skin Langerhans (dendritic) cells in virus infections and AIDS. Kluwer, Boston, pp 185–201
19. Xia W, Schneeberger EE, McCarthy K, Kradin RL (1991) Accessory cells of the lung. II. Ia+ pulmonary cells display cell surface antigen heterogeneity. Am J Respir Cell Mol Biol 5:276–283

Subject Index